EMBRYOLOGY AND GENETICS

VOLUME 1
MAPPING THE ORIGINS AND MECHANISMS OF LIFE

Dr. Vijaykumar Deshmukh
and Dr. Jaykumar Deshmukh

ALLIED
HEALTH
PRESS

Embryology and Genetics

Volume 1: Mapping the Origins and Mechanisms of Life

Authors: **Dr. Vijaykumar Deshmukh and Dr. Jaykumar Deshmukh**

Allied Health Press
4164 Lakeshore Road
Burlington ON L7L 1A4
Canada
www.alliedhealthpress.com
Email: orders@arclereducation.com

ISBN: 978-1-77956-772-7

ABOUT THE AUTHORS

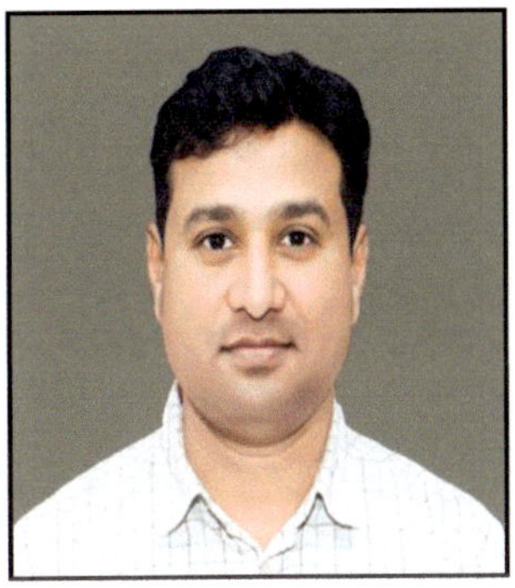

Dr. Vijaykumar D Deshmukh is presently serving as Assistant Professor in Department of Plant Biotechnology, MGM College of Agricultural Biotechnology, Chh. Sambhajinagar (Maharashtra). He obtained his M.Sc. in (Agril. Biotech.) and Ph.D. in (Biotech.). He started his career as an Assistant Professor in 2005. His field of specialisation is Plant Biotechnology and Molecular Biology. He has published Six books and more than 25 research papers in National and international journals. He has participated in International, National and State Level Seminar and Symposiums.

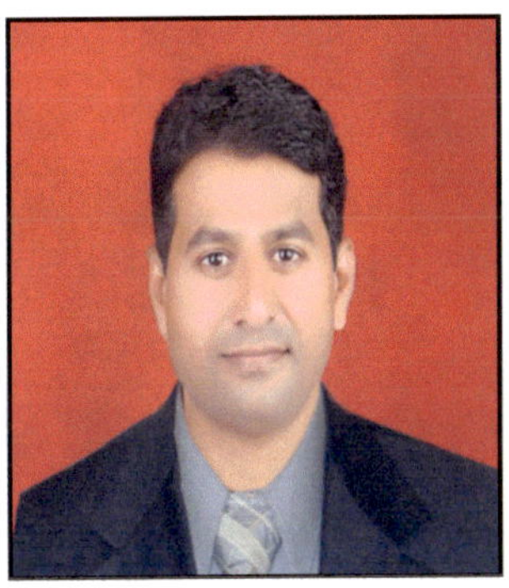

Dr. Jaykumar D. Deshmukh (1981) is presently serving as Assistant Professor in Department of Genetics and Plant Breeding, College of Agriculture Parbhani, Maharashtra, India. He obtained his M.Sc. (GPB) in 2005 and Ph.D. (GPB) in 2013 from Vasantrao Naik Marathwada Krishi Vidyapeeth, Parbhani, Maharashtra. He started his career as an Assistant Professor in 2013. His field of specialisation is Genetics and Plant Breeding. He has published seven books and more than 45 research papers in National and international journals. He has participated in International, National and State Level Seminar and Symposiums.

Brief Table of Contents

Detailed Table of Contents

CHAPTER 3

CHAPTER 4

CHAPTER 5

Gastrulation 131

CHAPTER 6

Neurulation 161

CHAPTER 7

Extraembryonic Membranes and Placenta 193

CHAPTER 8

Genetics 225

CHAPTER 9

Structure and Function of DNA and RNA 261

LIST OF FIGURES

PREFACE

The study of embryology and genetics presents a powerful lens through which the continuity of life can be understood. Beginning with the earliest moments of development, embryology reveals how a single totipotent cell gives rise to the astonishing complexity of a fully formed organism. This field illuminates the sequence of events—from the first cellular divisions to the establishment of body axes—that underpin normal growth and differentiation. At the same time, genetics uncovers the molecular instructions that govern these developmental processes. By studying gene transmission, expression and changes, we can see why life is both similar and different throughout generations. When these areas are combined, one can explore the question of how specific gene products regulate tissue growth. What molecular mechanisms ensure fidelity during cell division? How do changes in genetic information lead to developmental disorders?

In parallel, genetics charts the blueprint that defines an organism's potential. It reveals the dual nature of DNA and RNA as both stable carriers of information and dynamic molecules that can be edited, transcribed, and translated. Genetics also examines how chromosomal architecture and gene regulation work together to produce precise patterns of cellular behavior. Through classical experiments and modern genomic techniques, the field shows how inherited traits emerge, how variation arises within populations, and how mutations can manifest as altered form or function. Both embryology and genetics provide a detailed explanation of regular development as well as the causes of birth defects, many diseases and possible treatments. Exploring these topics together, scholars and clinicians help medicine, biotechnology and our understanding of life's complexity grow.

Embryology and Genetics Volume 1 is organized to link the fields of developmental biology and molecular genetics. The book is designed to guide readers on a logical path, from the formation of embryos to the control of heredity at the molecular level. The book presents history alongside critical new findings, so that the main ideas are set before new approaches are introduced. Emphasis is placed on explaining things clearly and also on how they function. Illustrations and diagrams are included to support the story and explain complex processes. The chapters are connected, so each one adds to the previous one and prepares the reader for more in-depth study in later books.

Chapter 1 provides an overview of embryology by examining its history and defining key terms. It discusses the importance of model organisms, describes the main theories of induction and competence and describes the early stages of embryonic development.

Chapter 2 describes the processes involved in gametogenesis, which produce haploid gametes. It explains the meiotic divisions, maturation of the cytoplasm, and the checkpoints that maintain the correctness of the genome in oocytes and spermatozoa.

Chapter 3 explains fertilization and covers the steps of sperm and egg membrane interactions, the prevention of multiple sperm entering, and how genes in the zygote are activated. It highlights the role of calcium signals and the proteins that alter the structure of the oocyte's cytoskeleton.

Chapter 4 explains how the zygote goes through many mitotic divisions, shifts from being able to develop into any cell to being able to develop into only certain kinds, and begins choosing which cells to become. This chapter explains the different ways cleavage occurs in other species and covers the creation of the blastocoel.

Chapter 5 investigates gastrulation by describing the coordinated cell movements that give rise to the three primary germ layers: ectoderm, mesoderm, and endoderm. It covers the molecular cues that drive invagination, ingression, and epiboly, as well as the role of morphogen gradients.

Chapter 6 examines neurulation, elucidating the shaping of the neural plate, the elevation and fusion of neural folds, and the formation of the neural tube. It also addresses neural crest cell migration and the signaling pathways, such as BMP and Wnt, that pattern the nervous system.

Chapter 7 focuses on extraembryonic membranes and the placenta, detailing the origin and function of the amnion, chorion, yolk sac, and allantois in mammals. It discusses placental architecture, maternal–fetal exchange mechanisms, and the endocrine roles of trophoblast derivatives.

Chapter 8 transitions to genetics with an introduction that explains basic genetic terms, inheritance patterns, and the central dogma of molecular biology. It also touches on genetic mapping and the principles of linkage analysis.

Chapter 9 provides insight into the structure and function of DNA and RNA, detailing nucleotide chemistry, the double-helix architecture, chromatin organization, and the roles of mRNA, tRNA, and rRNA in protein synthesis. It examines replication fidelity mechanisms and RNA processing events.

Chapter 10 addresses chromosomes and cell division by tracing the processes of mitosis and meiosis at both the cellular and molecular levels. The chapter details spindle assembly, checkpoint controls, and the segregation of homologues and sister chromatids.

Chapter 11 presents Mendelian genetics by revisiting Gregor Mendel's experiments and extending the discussion to include non-Mendelian inheritance phenomena such as incomplete dominance, codominance, and gene interactions. It illustrates how genetic crosses are analyzed and interpreted.

Chapter 12 explores genetic mutations and disorders, categorizing mutation types—point mutations, insertions, deletions, chromosomal rearrangements—and explaining how these alterations can disrupt gene function. It also considers the genetic basis of common congenital syndromes and modern approaches to diagnosis and therapy.

This volume is written for a broad audience, including graduate and advanced undergraduate students in developmental biology, genetics, and related biomedical fields. It will also serve as a valuable reference for medical trainees, particularly those in anatomy, obstetrics and gynecology, pediatrics, and pathology. An individual starting in developmental genetics will find the detailed descriptions of the main mechanisms very helpful. Some teachers may choose individual chapters for their courses in embryology or molecular genetics, and the book's wide coverage will be helpful in academic libraries. The purpose of this work is to help readers understand the fundamental processes that influence life from the outset, providing them with the knowledge necessary for research and clinical work.

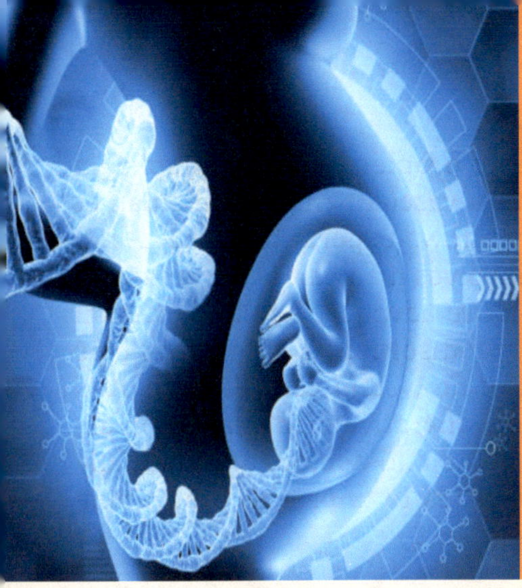

Chapter 1

EMBRYOLOGY

Contents

Introduction

Embryology is at the heart of biology because it describes how a fertilized cell can develop into a fully grown organism. Instead of presenting neatly organized steps, think of it like a journey that begins unassumingly and then unexpectedly dives into phases such as cleavage, a bit of that unpredictable gastrulation, and later, the whole business of organ-building (organogenesis). Every phase plays its role, and usually, even a tiny shift can not only change visible traits but sometimes open a door to complications like congenital anomalies, which, in most cases, might even explain recurrent pregnancy loss (Hachem et al., 2017). Often, researchers discover these early signs bit by bit, linking them as they go to a broader view of development. Taking a wider view, identifying congenital quirks early is very vital for clinicians. It's not only something from a textbook—issues that arise during embryonic development can be affected by both genes and the environment, which can cause health problems. For example, a slight misstep during development might set the stage for defects like those seen in certain heart conditions; these disruptions can even trickle down into problems such as dysphagia or breathing difficulties due to odd structural abnormalities, such as a vascular ring (Hanneman et al., 2016). Most of the time, starting from the embryo's early days allows experts to manage and diagnose these conditions with greater skill. Exploring embryology involves many different areas, for example, genetics, reproductive medicine, and pediatric care. The more advanced preimplantation genetic testing becomes, the more likely it is to identify developmental disorders early, which helps with early and personalized interventions. With the advancement of new stem cell research, it is evident that exploring these early stages yields innovative ideas in regenerative medicine. All in all, by slowly peeling back those layers of embryological mystery, scientists and doctors are gradually building a more complete picture of human health, which, in turn, leads to improved prevention, diagnosis, and care strategies that can enhance quality of life (Figure 1.1).

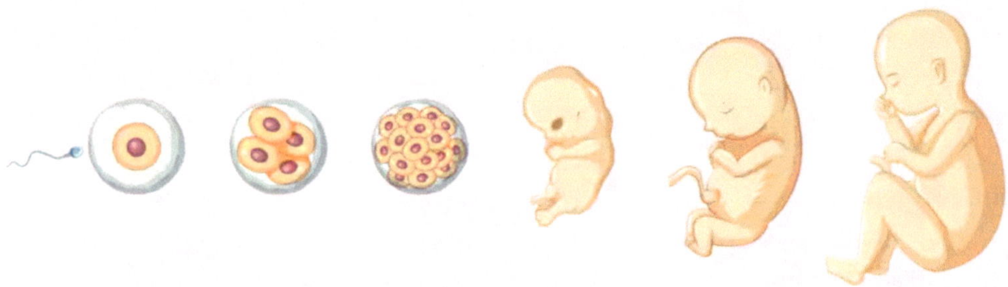

Figure 1.1. Embryology.

Source: https://cache.careers360.mobi/media/articles/uploads/froala_editor/images/2024/11/18/1731949248089.png.

Historical Background of Embryology

Embryology's early days somewhat resemble a patchwork of ideas that stretch back to ancient thinkers pondering the nature of life. Some of those early minds—like the Greeks—figured that something divine might be behind the beginnings of an embryo, and there was plenty of room for mystery. Then, things shifted during the Renaissance. Andreas Vesalius, for instance, started poking around with detailed anatomical studies, challenging the old, purely speculative ideas. His hands-on approach, along with others who followed, slowly shifted the field from dreamy philosophy into one grounded in close observation and real experimentation. By the 19th century, things took another turn. Microscopes burst onto the scene, letting scientists—not for the first time in their wildest imaginations—see the tiny building blocks of life at a whole new level. In most cases, this was a game-changer, and figures like Ernst Haeckel began to popularize ideas like recapitulation theory. Essentially, Haeckel argued that the early stages of an embryo tend to mirror its evolutionary past—a notion that, although not without its critics, managed to connect developmental twists with the story of evolution. His work, even if it sometimes receives mixed reviews, was pivotal in knitting embryology closer to the broader tapestry of biology. In the late 20th and early 21st centuries, researchers experienced a renaissance in the field of embryology. The Developmental Origins of Health and Disease (DOHaD) hypothesis emerged, suggesting that what happens early in life can significantly shape their health later on (generally speaking, the idea opens up whole new perspectives). Recent work has further developed these ideas, integrating developmental studies with other areas of biomedical research and even sparking close inter-field collaborations. Advances in stem cell techniques and organoid technology now enable scientists to grow mini, organ-like structures for applications ranging from drug testing to regenerative medicine experiments. Yet, all this progress raises ethical debates about using human embryos and lab-grown organoids—a conversation that continues to evolve (Annelien et al., 2017). All in all, these developments capture the complex, ever-changing nature of embryology and underscore its broad, interdisciplinary impact on contemporary science (Suzuki, 2017).

Importance of Embryology in Biological Sciences

Early on, development reveals a complex interplay of processes that demonstrate how living systems interact in unpredictable ways. Embryology isn't just about grasping how bodies usually form – it also helps us see when things might go sideways. Genetic quirks, environmental factors, or even subtle epigenetic shifts during critical moments can trigger congenital issues.

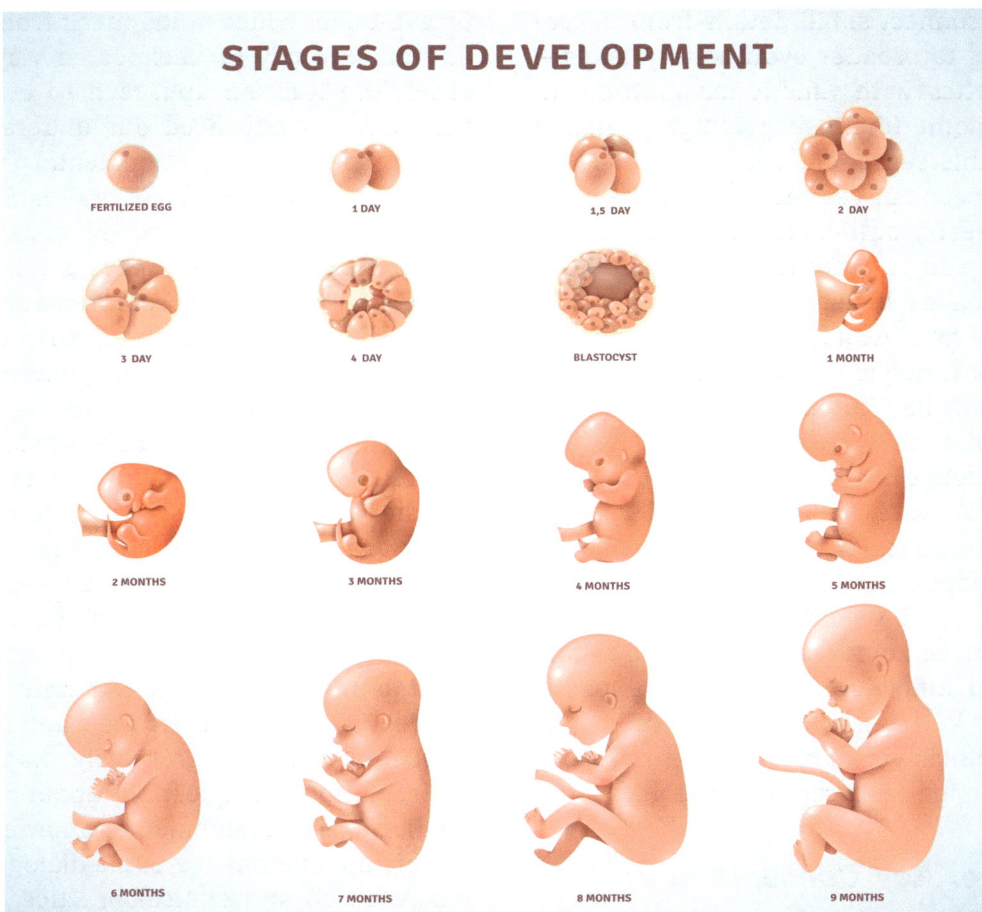

Figure 1.2. Embryology in biology.

Source: https://dcx0p3on5z8dw.cloudfront.net/Aakash/s3fs-public/inline-images/image001_36.png?S6wtCLE.N6pgzuLXa4WFTjo9dVTGuVGo.

By examining embryonic structures closely, scientists sometimes uncover clues for intervention or even prevention. This fundamental insight, in most cases, ultimately guides better diagnoses and treatments in medicine, proving time and again that embryology plays a significant role in advancing our biological and healthcare knowledge. Beyond its clinical edge, the field of embryology opens a window into the messy story of evolution. When experts compare how embryos grow in different species, they often spot that even minor shifts can lead to the rich variety of life we see now. It's like discovering hints of ancient genetic building blocks that have been refined over time to allow diversity to flourish. Examining these processes, researchers connect small details from micro-level changes to broader evolutionary leaps—mixing genetics with functional anatomy in a natural, sometimes surprisingly relaxed manner. In this sense, embryology works like a bridge between our genetic past and the ever-changing tapestry of life. Modern reproductive technologies add yet another twist to the tale. Methods such as *in vitro* fertilization (IVF) demonstrate how exploring embryology can lead to breakthroughs in reproductive care. As Sarah Franklin has noted in her work, these techniques not only yield successful results but also challenge our old ideas about kinship and genetics. Sure, they sometimes spark debates about ethics or new social norms, but they also deepen our understanding of how reproduction and genetics work. Thus, the interplay between embryological research and technological innovation continually expands our scientific knowledge, even if it occasionally requires rethinking what reproduction means in an ever-changing landscape (Figure 1.2).

Overview of Key Concepts in Embryology

Embryology begins with a single fertilized egg that gradually develops into a complete organism—a process driven by both our inherited genes and the cues from our surroundings. The idea of epigenesis sits at the heart of it; this concept suggests that our development comes not just from the genetic blueprint, but also from external factors, all mingled together in a kind of complex interplay. Back in the early 1900s, thinkers such as Thomas Hunt Morgan and his peers began poking at these ideas, blurring the lines between genetics and the questions of embryological change. Their early insights—sometimes a bit rough around the edges—laid the foundation for our current view on how embryos flexibly adjust over time to ever-changing environments (Costa et al., 2014). A different angle in this field is what folks call evolutionary developmental biology, or evo-devo, which weds ideas from evolution and embryology in unexpected ways. In most cases, the Russian approach to evo-devo, for instance, has advanced our understanding by demonstrating how developmental processes can influence evolutionary routes. Names like von Baer, Kowalevsky, and Mechnikoff keep cropping up as they built early case studies on how different species share common developmental traits. This back-and-forth comparison has slowly peeled back layers of morphogenesis—, how an organism determines its shape—and explained a great deal about why species branch out and diversify over time (Mikhailov et al., 2012). On the technological side, things have shifted significantly in embryology thanks to new tools and methods. Modern techniques—think genetic tweaking, advanced imaging, and deep molecular profiling—allow scientists to break apart what used to be an impenetrable puzzle, uncovering how cells decide on their roles and organs start to form. As we progressively map out these molecular details, questions about regenerative medicine and developmental disorders naturally bubble up. In many ways, the dialogue between lab research and clinical practice now seems like an ongoing conversation, one that promises fresh treatments for congenital issues and even age-related degeneration. These advances continue to keep embryology at the forefront of the intersection of current biology and medicine, steadily enriching the core knowledge of this vital field (Costa et al., 2014).

1.1. Stages of Embryonic Development

Embryonic development kicks off with a series of puzzling, almost haphazard steps that set everything in motion. Right after fertilization, the zygote starts splitting rapidly—a process known as cleavage—until a cluster of cells, typically referred to as the blastocyst, forms. This early burst is crucial; it prepares the embryo for later changes and helps establish a basic body plan. When that blastocyst eventually implants into the uterine wall, it sends out a bunch of signals to chat with the mother's tissues, which, in most cases, is key for getting nutrients and supporting further growth. If anything goes wrong in these initial, messy moments, major developmental issues can arise, so scientists thoroughly investigate these events. Understanding these early shifts, as odd as they might seem, lays the foundation for how tissues and organs eventually form—a matter that touches on both health and disease.

Then comes gastrulation, a pivotal stage where the embryo begins to rearrange itself in surprising ways. Suddenly, three main layers emerge—the ectoderm, mesoderm, and endoderm—each getting ready for its big role. Generally speaking, the ectoderm sets off to form the nervous system and skin, while the mesoderm starts work on muscles and the circulatory system, and the endoderm takes on inner organs like the lungs and liver. This whole reorganization, driven by precise cellular signals and gene cues, unfolds in a way that's both unpredictable and elegant. And yes, any slip-up here might lead to congenital anomalies, which underscores the importance of a deep dive into gastrulation for tackling developmental disorders. As the process progresses, organogenesis takes center stage. Here, the layers that were once clearly defined begin a new phase of differentiation and spatial coordination, organizing themselves into distinct organ systems. Take the heart, for example—what starts as a simple tube eventually undergoes complex, almost artful changes to become the vital organ we recognize today, illustrating just how interlinked different cell types can be. Regulatory players, such as signaling pathways and transcription factors, act as conductors in a symphony, ensuring that organs develop correctly and function smoothly in coordination with one another. Recognizing this phase is critical, as environmental factors or genetic quirks may disrupt these processes, influencing health outcomes later in life (Zegers-Hochschild et al., 2017; Yoshizaki et al., 2021) (Figure 1.3).

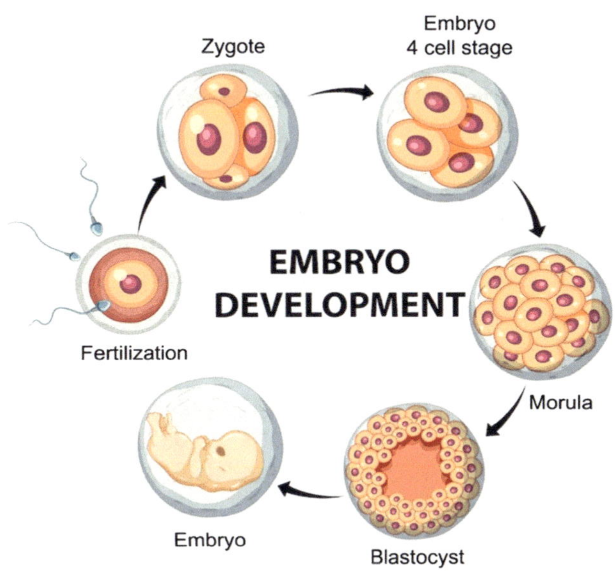

Figure 1.3. Stages of embryonic development.

Source: https://ferty9.com/wp-content/uploads/2025/04/Monsoon-Skin-Hair-Care-Tips-for-Kids-2023-03-28T192341.4121.png.

1.1.1. Fertilization and Zygote Formation

Fertilization jumps off a chain of events that truly shape an embryo. It starts when sperm meets egg; the sperm breaks through the egg's protective layers with a burst of enzyme release in what's called the acrosome reaction. That enzyme burst is crucial for allowing the sperm to reach the egg's cell membrane. Sometimes, paternal tweaks—such as changes in histones, for example, acetylation—can significantly alter the process, affecting chromatin decondensation and even the formation of the male pronucleus (Boitani et al., 2017).

In most cases, these subtle histone modifications ultimately affect the zygote's fate in ways that we're still trying to understand fully. After this initial encounter, the zygote quickly leaps into rapid cell divisions, a phase known simply as cleavage. One minute it's a single cell, the next it's a multicelled cluster that eventually shapes into a blastocyst ready to find shelter in the uterine lining. The young embryo relies on the nutrients stored in the egg—its built-in pantry—until it can access new supplies after implantation. Studies on plant embryos even suggest that nutrient management, the way nutrients are distributed within, plays a significant role as well (Chamberlin et al., 1993).

As the zygote begins to differentiate, determining when and where nutrients flow becomes a crucial part of setting the stage for later growth. The transition from zygote to early embryo involves significant morphological changes that facilitate preparation for implantation. The zygote doesn't just copy its genetic material—it rewrites its blueprint to carve out a unique identity, almost like reworking the recipe for life. Generally speaking, this whole remolding sparks a lot of ongoing research, with components like nGPx4 showing how paternal factors can affect what comes next (Boitani et al., 2017). Overall, the combination of genetic, epigenetic, and environmental cues makes this early developmental dance a fascinating, if sometimes complex, beginning to embryology (Figure 1.4).

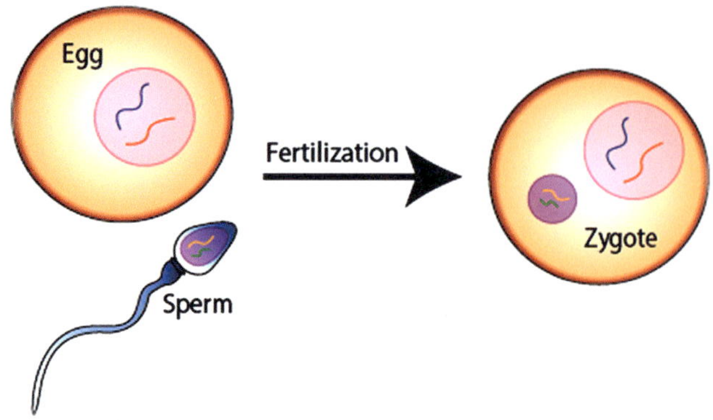

Figure 1.4. Fertilization and zygote formation.

Source: https://external-content.duckduckgo.com/iu/?u=https%3A%2F%2Fstudy.com%2Fcimages%2Fmultimages%2F16%2Ffertilization4590913850394814921.png&f=1&nofb=1&ipt=3fdf8cb0afd67e31973fdae2730065f1e8d335d7b7cbb0d15e99670607d74474.

1.1.2. Cleavage and Blastocyst Formation

Cleavage initiates early development in a manner that may seem somewhat surprising. Instead of growing larger, the single-celled zygote quickly splits into many smaller cells—a process that, though rapid and repetitive, keeps the original egg's resources intact while slowly switching on the embryo's genetic instructions. Temperature, nutrient levels, and even subtle local factors all tip the balance of these cell splits, with each division yielding little units called blastomeres that eventually rearrange themselves into what we call the blastocyst; this event, in most cases, sets up the embryo for later attachment to the uterine wall. As these divisions march along, the forming structure begins to diversify. The process eventually yields two groups: one, known as the inner cell mass (ICM), typically forms the embryo itself, while the other—the trophoblast—helps create the placenta and facilitates nutrient exchange. It's during this stage that a fluid-filled space, the blastocoel, starts to appear—a kind of internal cavity that plays a key role in keeping up growth and communication between the two cell types. Generally speaking, these unfolding steps highlight just how detailed and precisely timed early embryonic development truly is, reminding us that embryology is both a science and an art. Recent breakthroughs in reproductive technology, including various forms of assisted reproductive technology (ART), have shed new light on these early phases. For example, the ability to culture an embryo up to the blastocyst stage before attempting implantation means that clinicians can, in many cases, select embryos with the best prospects for success. This focus on the right timing and ensuring an optimal microenvironment tends to boost outcomes in fertility treatments. A solid understanding of the mechanisms at play during these early moments is crucial when addressing infertility challenges and guiding clinical practices. In most situations, the push to standardize terms and communicate clearly among healthcare professionals is seen as central to driving forward progress in both embryology and fertility care (Zegers-Hochschild et al., 2017) (Figure 1.5).

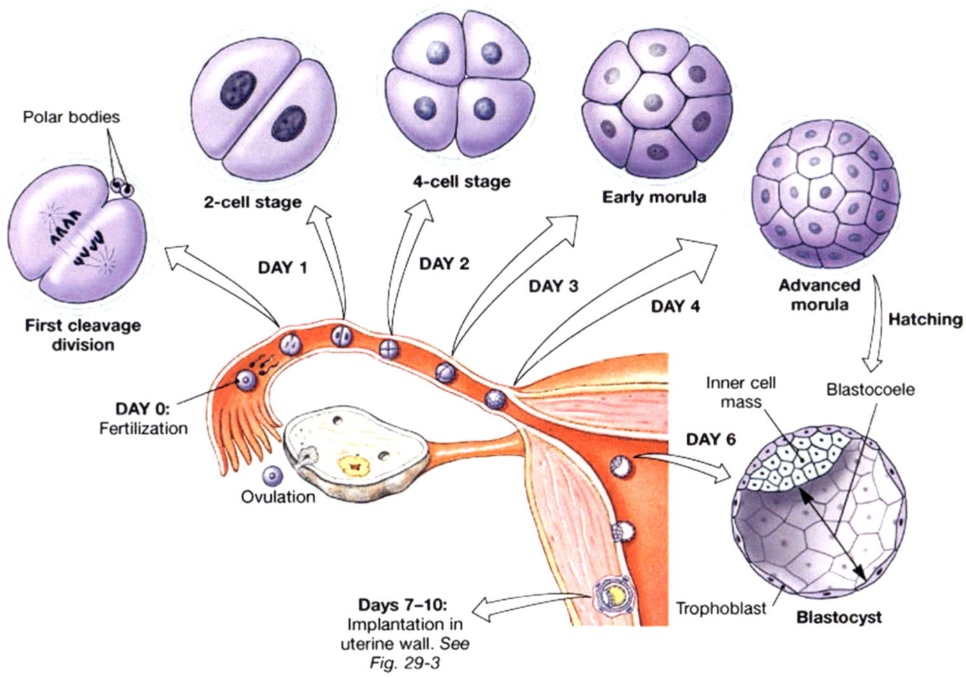

Figure 1.5. Cleavage and blastocyst formation.

Source: https://external-content.duckduckgo.com/iu/?u=https%3A%2F%2Fimage1.slideserve.com%2F2177966%2Fcleavage-and-blastocyst-formation-l.jpg&f=1&nofb=1&ipt=d1a14264a0aa81f4b7c891333599b5df16eb08da54f3a18e3edf8e45c537d014.

1.1.3. Gastrulation and Germ Layer Development

Early on in embryonic development, a lot goes on—and gastrulation turns out to be a big deal. At this stage, the embryonic disc reorganizes its cells, transforming from a relatively simple blob into a more complex structure with multiple layers. As the mesoderm and endoderm form, the way an embryo establishes its axis becomes crucial, influencing the development of many key structures that will later appear. Examining gastrulation offers a glimpse into how cells move and interact, particularly with signals from pathways such as the Wnt pathway, which play a significant role in determining a cell's fate. This complex, yet fascinating process lays down the framework of the organism and establishes the blueprint for processes such as organ formation and further differentiation. Cellular chatter and signaling networks play a significant role in germ layer development. Mesoderm, endoderm, and ectoderm—each layer starts to take on its identity by listening to a mix of growth factors and morphogens nudging them in different directions. As these layers develop, they pave the way for specialized tissues to form, affecting not only the body's shape but also its function. For example, getting the anterior-posterior axis right depends a lot on maintaining just the correct balance of these signaling molecules—a delicate act that reminds us how vital these biochemical networks are during gastrulation. Using 3D models in education can help students gain a better, more hands-on understanding of the shifting spatial and temporal patterns throughout this process (Hesterman et al., 2021). New lab techniques have opened up fresh ways to dive into gastrulation and the development of germ layers. Nowadays, *in vitro* models—such as embryoid bodies and gastruloids—provide researchers with a convenient setup to observe how early development occurs, especially when they modify the environment to observe changes in cell differentiation. Take, for instance, engineered microwell arrays, which help form clusters that mimic the epiblast, making it possible to study how Wnt signaling influences the early formation of neural progenitors (Girgin et al., 2023). These creative, sometimes unpredictable methods not only expand what we can study but also help fill in the gaps in our understanding. In many cases, they provide a new playground for exploring how genetic tweaks or even drug interventions might impact early growth, and they underscore the far-reaching applications of gastrulation research in disease modeling and regenerative medicine (Figure 1.6).

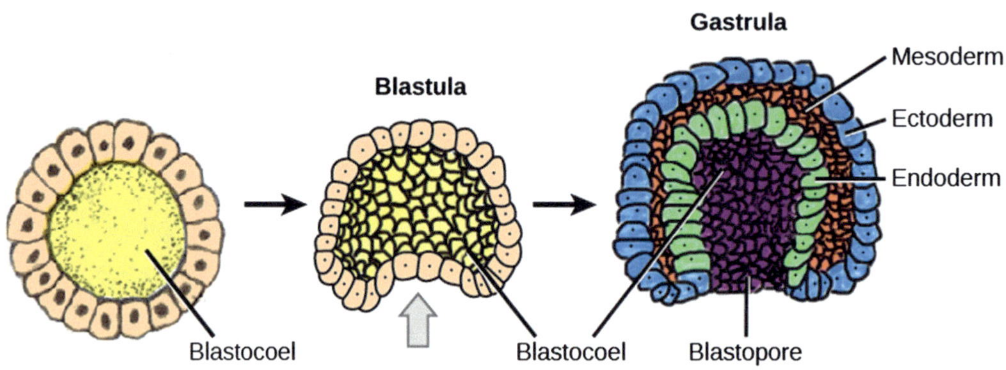

Figure 1.6. Gastrulation and germ layer development.

Source: https://stemcellthailand.org/wp-content/uploads/2014/10/3-germ-layers-Gastrulation.jpg.webp.

1.2. Cellular Mechanisms in Embryology

Embryogenesis isn't a linear, tidy process—it's more like a dynamic puzzle where early cell divisions and unexpected signals set the stage. Cells split and then start choosing paths almost on the fly, nudged by local cues. Morphogens, for example, are small molecules produced in specific locations that then spread out, forming gradients similar to faded watercolors and influencing neighboring cells in different directions. Research generally shows that even slight variations in these gradients can lead cells to develop into entirely different types, resulting in unique tissue patterns. In a way, these shifting signals help steer cells toward their eventual roles, gradually piecing together organ systems that mirror both inherited blueprints and the influence of their surroundings. Other crucial processes also come into play, and here, apoptosis—essentially programmed cell death—acts like a built-in cleanup crew, erasing damaged or surplus cells as development progresses. This selective removal ensures that the balance between new cell growth and necessary cell loss remains just right, which is key when forming things like limbs and organs. Then there are the familiar signaling routes, such as the Wnt and Notch pathways. In most cases, these pathways help keep everything on track, but if they slip out of line, it might lead to congenital changes. All of this illustrates how cells communicate with one another in subtle, sometimes unpredictable ways that underscore the overall complexity of early development. Beyond cell communication and cleanup, gene expression plays a starring role in the developmental drama. Transcription factors toggle genes on and off in ways that guide multipotent stem cells to evolve into specialized types. Here, both the genetic script and environmental hints blend to shape the final look of the organism. For instance, variations observed in situations like psoriatic arthritis demonstrate that even cells in similar settings can behave quite differently, suggesting that the embryonic context significantly influences gene outcomes. This intricate interplay remains one of developmental biology's big puzzles, as even the slightest misstep in these processes may sometimes lead to disorders later on (Figure 1.7).

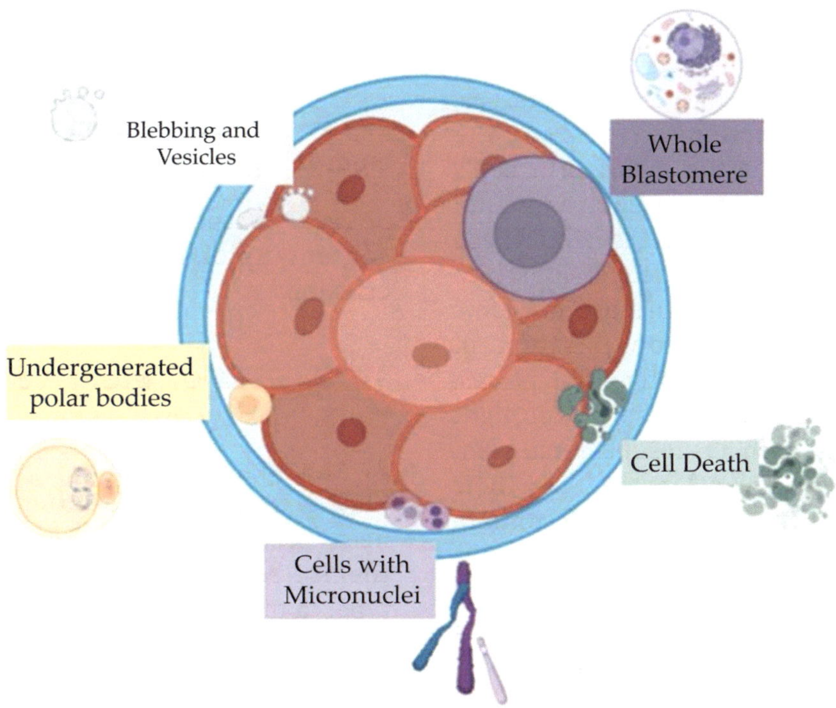

Figure 1.7. Cellular mechanisms in embryology.

Source: https://pub.mdpi-res.com/ijms/ijms-23-01349/article_deploy/html/images/ijms-23-01349-g001.png?1643337191.

1.2.1. Cell Division and Differentiation

Understanding cell processes lies at the heart of embryonic development. In the early stages, cells divide rapidly – employing both mitosis and meiosis – to gradually build a multicellular structure. The single zygote, for instance, undergoes several cleavage stages that split it into smaller units, known as blastomeres. This brisk multiplication sets the stage for later events when cells begin to branch out and acquire specific functions. Upon closer examination, it becomes apparent that a combination of regulatory signals and pathways governs this progression, ensuring, in most cases, that developing cells follow a generally orderly—but sometimes flexible—pattern. Embryonic cells don't just keep multiplying; they also start to specialize via differentiation. This shift from a uniform state to more defined types involves a host of changes in gene expression that transcription factors and various signaling cues help orchestrate. Through such specialization, a rich diversity of tissues and organs emerges, each tasked with functions critical to the organism's survival. The tug between a cell's inherent genetic blueprint and environmental hints plays a pivotal role in steering these lineage decisions. All in all, a deeper look into this process not only clarifies normal embryonic growth but also highlights how missteps in differentiation may lead to congenital issues. Recent studies have shed a greater spotlight on specialized cells, such as mesenchymal stem cells (MSCs), which are celebrated for their multipotency and their capacity to differentiate into various cell types under the right conditions. Ever since their discovery about 30 years ago, MSCs have garnered attention for their promise in regenerative medicine—largely due to their ability to modulate immune responses and promote tissue repair. Nowadays, researchers are busy unraveling the signaling mechanisms that govern the growth and diversification of MSCs, which neatly underscores their clinical potential. Grasping the basics of cell division and specialization not only deepens our grasp of embryology but also paves the way for new therapeutic strategies aimed at tackling a range of conditions, firmly positioning MSCs as key players in future biomedical advances (Yang et al., 2017; Mark et al., 2019) (Figure 1.8).

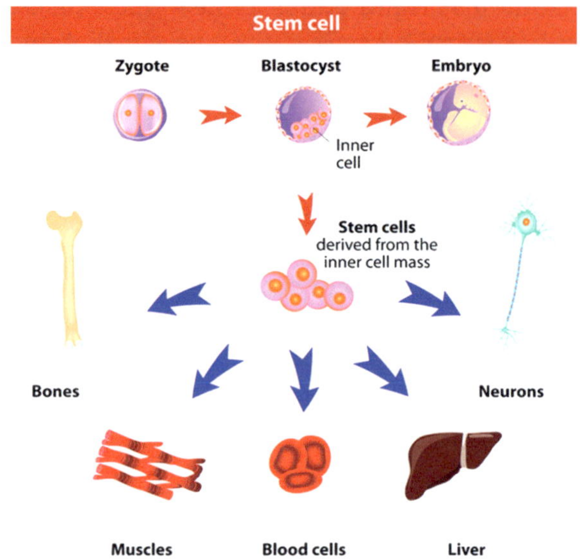

Figure 1.8. Cell division and differentiation in embryology.

Source: https://biologydictionary.net/wp-content/uploads/2020/04/Embryonic-stem-cells.jpg.

1.2.2. Role of Stem Cells in Development

At the heart of human growth, stem cells play a starring role—and not always in a neat, predictable way. These cells can renew themselves and shift into many specialized types, a trait that's vital for building and keeping our tissues going from early on in life through later years. Pluripotent cells, which can pretty much turn into any cell, kickstart every organ system in ways that feel almost like laying down an evolving blueprint. Meanwhile, adult stem cells maintain the engine by repairing and regenerating tissue, ensuring everything remains in balance. In most cases, getting to grips with these cellular maneuvers helps deepen our overall understanding of both development and the promise of regenerative medicine. A simple, linear process doesn't assemble complex structures in our bodies—they rely on a buzzing, often unpredictable mix of signals between cells. Take the gastrointestinal tract, for instance; its network of cells makes precise functioning possible, albeit in a somewhat messy way. Stem cell–generated organoids, offering a real three-dimensional glimpse into these interactions, reveal how cells sort themselves out and respond to the cues presented to them. These mini tissue models mimic the architecture and function of actual organs, illustrating not only the normal progression of development but also the abnormal deviations that can lead to conditions such as cancer or inflammation (Hautefort et al., 2022). Sometimes, one has to step back and notice how loosely connected ideas ultimately build up to form a more intricate, real-life structure. Then there's the twist of where these stem cells originate, which adds yet another layer of rugged charm to their potential. Whether a stem cell originates from an embryo or appears in adult tissue appears to shape its role in healing and repair. MSCs, for example, possess a natural ability to mitigate inflammation and modulate immune responses, thereby opening up new avenues for tackling inflammatory diseases (Mark et al., 2019). Their ability to slip into multiple cell types—coupled with a flair for immunomodulation—makes them a hot topic in the realm of regenerative therapies. As researchers continue to refine techniques to nudge and tailor the behavior of these cells, the dream of developing innovative treatments rooted in embryological insights steadily grows more tangible (Figure 1.9).

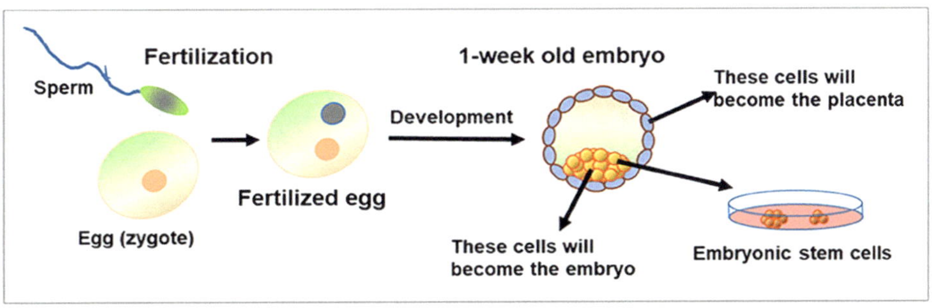

Figure 1.9. Role of stem cells in development.

Source: https://www.frontiersin.org/files/Articles/529612/frym-08-00032-HTML-r1/image_m/figure-1.jpg.

1.2.3. Apoptosis and Its Significance in Shaping Embryos

Cellular growth and differentiation in embryos occur under a tight kind of control that ensures complex organisms can form. Apoptosis, a type of programmed cell death, quietly removes cells that are extra or damaged—this isn't merely an act of elimination; it's a way to keep things organized. Removing unnecessary cells helps prevent abnormalities while ensuring that tissues and organs are arranged correctly. The tug-of-war between cell multiplication and cell removal is extremely delicate; even a slight shift might lead to developmental disorders or even tumors. Generally speaking, understanding how apoptosis regulates cells provides a clearer picture of embryological concepts such as tissue shaping and organ formation. In vertebrate embryos, consider the neural crest—a group of multipotent progenitor cells that are pretty remarkable in their flexibility and adaptability. These cells, which eventually form everything from sensory neurons to bits of facial cartilage, are guided by a complex gene network, and apoptosis plays a significant role in maintaining the numbers in check. Sometimes, it removes cells that don't belong or have become excessive, helping to keep both spatial and temporal order in development. As these cells migrate and change, the signals that tell them to stay or to become crucial—a fact that underscores the importance of apoptosis in building tissues that function properly (Sim Mões-Costa et al., 2015). There's more to apoptosis than just trimming away cells. It also connects deeply with the cellular signaling pathways vital for embryonic development. For instance, the endoplasmic reticulum, which is key to keeping a cell balanced, can malfunction and send stress signals (like the unfolded protein response) that trigger apoptosis. In the context of an embryo, this response ensures that cells unable to contribute appropriately to tissue formation or that have been stressed are removed. In most cases, understanding these cell-to-cell interactions reveals just how delicate the developmental balance is—and it raises interesting questions about what happens when apoptosis goes awry in congenital malformations and other developmental disorders (Almanza et al., 2018) (Figure 1.10).

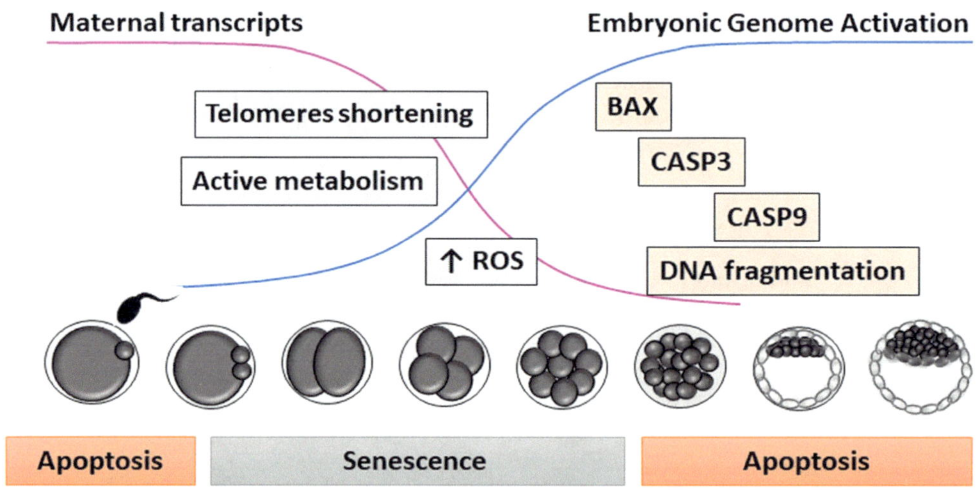

Figure 1.10. Apoptosis and its significance in shaping embryos.

Source: https://www.frontiersin.org/files/Articles/619902/fcell-08-619902-HTML/image_m/fcell-08-619902-g001.jpg.

1.3. Genetic Regulation of Development

Embryo 00development starts early on, driven by a delicate genetic mechanism that sets the pace for everything that follows. Specific genes—think of them as the conductors of a complex orchestra—turn on at just the right moments to guide what cells become, whether that's differentiating into specialized types or laying down the blueprint for organs and tissues. In many cases, factors like transcription activators and various signaling molecules come into action following unique sequences, almost as if they're improvising a tune rather than following a strict score. Experimental embryology has recently suggested that we may need more data-driven methods to elucidate these subtle cues—such as how patterns form and tissues self-organize in ways we still don't entirely understand (Busby et al., 2022). Researchers, using these approaches, are slowly unraveling the intricate dance of genetic signals that pushes embryos along their developmental path. On another note, the ethical side of tinkering with genetic blueprints is a whole other can of worms. With breakthroughs such as CRISPR-Cas9 making precise DNA tweaks a reality, questions about what's morally acceptable are coming to the forefront. Tools like these enable us to edit genes with incredible precision, but they also force us to confront concerns about the broader social and ethical implications of manipulating embryonic genes. There's been a lot of chatter about that 14-day limit on embryo research—a rule that, while set for good ethical reasons, might need another look given our new tech. Pushing research beyond those 14 days could provide deeper insights into development, but it also stirs debate about whether embryos nearing a point of independent function should be studied further (Appleby et al., 2018). To wrap things up, understanding how genes direct embryonic development is crucial—not just for advancing science, but also for maintaining our ethical compass. As the field evolves, combining cutting-edge genetic tools with classic research methods not only enhances our understanding of life's origins but also raises complex ethical questions. Lately, many in the field have been advocating for innovative regulatory measures that try to balance scientific curiosity with responsibility. Scientists, ethicists, and policymakers are gradually finding common ground, even if the conversation remains a bit messy at times; after all, progress isn't ever elegant. This open and sometimes unpredictable dialogue is what will ultimately help ensure that our strides in developmental biology remain both beneficial and ethically sound (Figure 1.11).

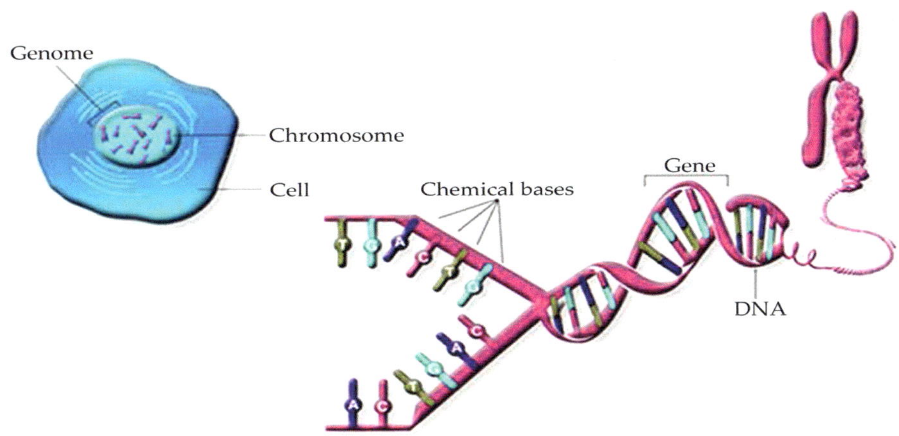

Figure 1.11. Gene regulation.

Source: https://external-content.duckduckgo.com/iu/?u=https%3A%2F%2Fcdn1.byjus.com%2Fbiology%2F2017%2F02%2F21110032%2FGene-Regulation.png&f=1&nofb=1&ipt=5fae3781659d930a45cf1df95948faf355b1bc91e61cb0ec1196e697963ac12e.

1.3.1. Role of Genes in Embryonic Development

Embryonic development begins as a complex and intricate process, governed by genes that act throughout the embryo. In those first early stages, something called zygotic genome activation shakes things up—maternal mRNAs start fading away, and suddenly, embryonic genes jump into action. Generally speaking, the switch from using the mother's stored instructions to the embryo's directions (that maternal-to-zygotic transition, or MZT) depends a lot on how various genes mix and match to keep tabs on cell division, differentiation, and metabolism. It's interesting that some genes—for example, those in the ubiquitin-proteasome pathway—play a significant role in clearing out proteins that, if they linger, might mess up the whole process. RNF114, an E3 ubiquitin ligase, has been shown to affect embryo viability by managing the breakdown of key players like TAB1, thus linking maternal factors with zygotic progression (Appleby et al., 2018). The way genes appear and disappear over time and space is crucial to establishing an embryo's body plan. Bone morphogenetic proteins (BMPs) and fibroblast growth factors (FGFs) are among the signals that prompt cells to assume specific roles and help initiate tissue formation. These cues guide stem cells into turning into specialized types—all while laying down the blueprint for the development of organ systems. And then there's gastrulation, a phase that essentially divides the embryo into three layers (the ectoderm, mesoderm, and endoderm) in ways that aren't always easy to predict. Grasping how these genes act and interact—even if it sometimes means repeating the same basic idea—sheds light on the nuts and bolts of embryogenesis and highlights potential spots where developmental disorders might creep in Appleby et al. (2018). It isn't just about form and differentiation; genetic regulation has a profound impact that can shape health well into the future. In most cases, if key developmental genes go off track—say, due to mutations or other dysregulations—the consequences can be severe, leading to birth defects or an increased risk of disease later in life. Odd pulses in gene expression during critical windows may disrupt normal organ formation, sometimes leading to malformations or impaired function. Research that ties together embryology and genetics has uncovered these links, pointing out that early gene interactions can leave lasting marks. As techniques like CRISPR become more refined, understanding exactly which genes do what in embryonic development provides new ways to reduce the risks associated with genetic disorders and enhance reproductive technologies—ultimately shifting how we approach both science and medicine (Yang et al., 2017) (Figure 1.12).

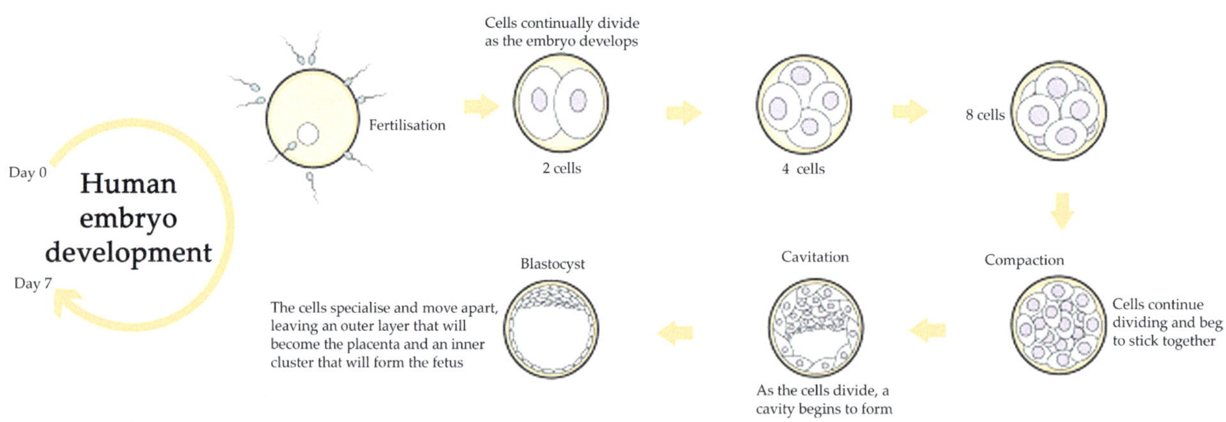

Figure 1.12. Gene is essential for human embryos.

Source: https://www.bournhall.co.uk/wp-content/uploads/Cas9-Final-002.png.

1.3.2. Genetic Mutations and Their Effects on Development

Embryonic development is a complex process, and genetic mutations introduce surprises that alter the way traits are expressed. Sometimes, these mutations affect significant developmental genes, disrupting how cells usually function and interact with one another. Take, for example, the changes in the Wnt signaling pathway; they've been linked to several developmental quirks. The Wnt pathway isn't just about pushing cells to multiply—it also helps decide what a cell will become, which is key when tissues and organs start forming. Such glitches often lead to congenital issues, highlighting the importance of keeping our genes intact during those early stages. Generally speaking, gaining a comprehensive understanding of this process requires integrating ideas from genetics, developmental biology, and clinical practice, which hints at new ways to treat these conditions. Cells have their ways of coping when stress builds up—one of them is the unfolded protein response (UPR). When genetic changes overload the endoplasmic reticulum's ability to fold proteins properly, the UPR jumps in to try to fix things. Sometimes, if the pressure just doesn't let up, that same process may even trigger programmed cell death—an extreme measure that shows just how tightly genetic mutations tie into whether a cell survives. The UPR affects many cellular pathways, maintaining a steady environment that supports crucial developmental steps while also relating to broader concepts of how cells communicate and collaborate during tissue formation. In other words, when mutations interfere with the UPR, they can cause developmental abnormalities that provide additional insights into the origins of congenital disorders and ultimately impact overall health. Genetic mutations have effects that go far beyond immediate cell behavior; they ripple out to shape wider developmental patterns and visible traits. Researchers often turn to model organisms, such as zebrafish and frogs, to observe how specific mutations unfold during different growth stages. These experiments highlight key molecules and pathways, such as the intricate Wnt cascade, that are fundamental to embryogenesis. Ongoing studies show that these pathways serve a dual purpose, supporting normal growth and even playing a role in the initiation of diseases and malformations. It turns out that genetic mutations can both disrupt and reveal the hidden workings of embryological development. Over time, a better understanding of these interactions may open the door to new approaches in preventing and treating developmental disorders, underscoring once again the central role genetics plays in shaping early life and its long-term outcomes.

1.3.3. Epigenetics and Its Influence on Embryology

Conrad Waddington coined the term "epigenetics" in the early 1900s, and ever since, scientists have been surprised at how gene expression can shift even when the DNA itself remains the same. This idea isn't just academic—epigenetics plays a significant role in early development, as the cell's molecular machinery regulates gene expression. DNA methylation and histone modifications, for example, quietly guide the embryo's first steps, ensuring that things like genomic imprinting work as intended; here, only one parent's allele is expressed during those critical preimplantation phases when cells splinter into different types, laying down the framework for later development (Huntriss et al., 2018). Such subtle control is key, even if it sometimes feels almost magical. A closer examination of epigenetic reprogramming during embryogenesis often yields insights into why developmental mishaps or reproductive hurdles arise. Generally speaking, the moments of gametogenesis and the early embryo are full of extensive retooling of a cell's epigenetic setup—a process that's vital for smooth fertilization and keeping the embryo viable. If these modifications go awry, problems such as congenital disorders or imprinting syndromes (for example, Beckwith-Wiedemann and Angelman syndromes) can occur. Interestingly, assisted reproductive technologies (ART) sometimes get a bad rap because they might inadvertently upset these delicate molecular balances; some studies have even hinted that ART may trigger off abnormal DNA methylation patterns, nudging up the risk of imprinting issues in offspring (Huntriss et al., 2018). Research into the connection between epigenetics and embryology continues to unearth surprises that could one day transform how we approach everything from normal development to targeted therapies. Advances in our grasp of how epigenetic markers tweak gene expression over time might lead to new approaches for treating infertility—or even help ease developmental problems linked to reproductive treatments. There's also growing chatter around stem cell–derived gametes and the ethical debates over rules like the 14-day limit for embryonic research, adding yet another twist to an already complex field. Ultimately, by unraveling these early regulatory shifts (and, yes, sometimes the details become complex), both researchers and clinicians can more effectively navigate the challenges of human reproduction and the associated health outcomes (Figure 1.13).

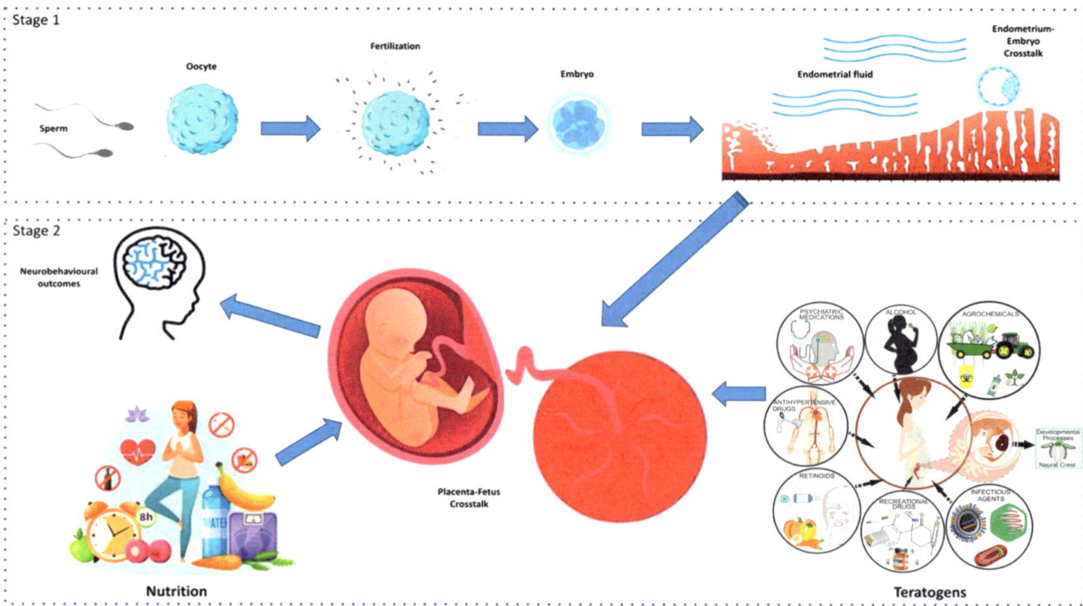

Figure 1.13. Epigenetics and its influence on embryology.

Source: https://media.springernature.com/lw1200/springer-static/image/art%3A10.1007%2Fs10815-022-02451-x/MediaObjects/10815_2022_2451_Fig1_HTML.png.

1.4. Comparative Embryology

Embryology has come a long way. It all began with early thinkers like Aristotle, who spent hours watching how animals grow and change. His texts, History of Animals and On the Generation of Animals, weren't perfect by today's standards, but they set out some of the very first ideas about how life kicks off and unfolds. Those early notes, scribbled down through close observation, laid a kind of rough map for grouping the natural world. Scientists are comparing how different species take shape—often spotting both shared features and quirky differences that hint at a common starting point. Building on those old ideas, researchers nowadays delve much deeper into the complex details using a comprehensive toolkit of molecular techniques. With new genomic and imaging techniques – high-powered methods that zoom in on life's raw materials – scientists study everything from chicks to mice to zebrafish to trace standard genetic blueprints. In most cases, finding these shared codes reveals that even minor tweaks can lead to significant changes in an organism's appearance and form. This kind of work, blending modern technology with age-old observations, effectively bridges the gap between what nature has been doing all along and the new ways we're now teasing apart the process. Anatomy museums also play a surprisingly significant role here. Museums—especially those in southern India (Venkatesh et al., 2016)—are packed with all sorts of specimens, including special exhibits on embryology and comparative anatomy. These places allow students to get up close with real-life examples of developmental stages, creating a tangible link between dry textbook theory and what's happening in nature. Sometimes the hands-on experience, even with some stray errors in labeling or a missing comma here and there, feels more authentic than any lecture. As education slowly shifts gears, incorporating digital and virtual park-like setups may further revamp these museums, solidifying their role in making the study of embryology more engaging and relevant in medical training (Figure 1.14).

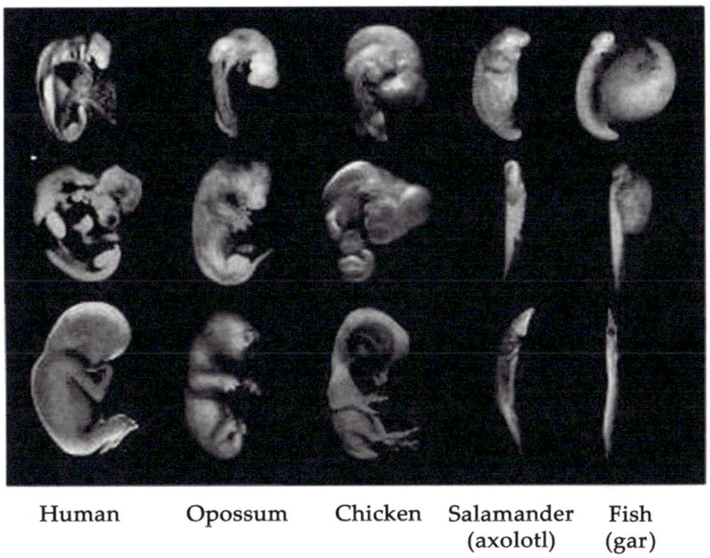

Figure 1.14. Comparative embryology.

Source: https://i.pinimg.com/474x/5b/f2/3d/5bf23d89d7369862e9e8183e328fbc2f.jpg.

1.4.1. Similarities and Differences Across Species

Embryonic development often tells a story of shared beginnings across diverse creatures. Many vertebrate embryos, for example, show early features like pharyngeal arches and a notochord—a sort of nod to an ancient, common lineage. These recurring traits aren't mere coincidences; they suggest that even as species branch off, fundamental processes such as cell differentiation and morphogenesis tend to persist across different lineages. It's interesting how these basic blueprints help us see that evolution often plays on the same deck of cards, linking life in ways that aren't always immediately obvious. At the same time, variations also make their mark, with timing often being the trickster. Heterochrony—that is, shifts in the pace or timing of growth—can manifest in two distinct forms. In some amphibians, for instance, a prolonged larval phase may lead to larger, more complex adults (what many call peramorphosis). In contrast, in other species, a tendency to retain juvenile traits into adulthood (pedomorphosis) becomes apparent. In most cases, these timing tweaks are influenced by environmental conditions or selective pressures, allowing each species to develop a unique strategy for thriving in its niche. Generally speaking, such shifts contribute considerably to the incredible diversity we see in nature. When one takes a step back and looks at the whole picture, the blend of shared features and distinct differences in embryological processes underscores a fascinating balance between maintaining familiarity and embracing innovation. Comparative embryology, as a discipline, enables us to gain insight into how evolution operates at both the cellular and molecular levels. Consider MSCs for a minute: even though they usually exhibit similar multipotency across species, each organism seems to add its little twist that suits its developmental needs. The extensive research on human MSCs—cited in over 55,000 publications—highlights their potential in tissue regeneration and clinical applications (Mark et al., 2019). By examining how these conserved traits interact with distinct developmental pathways, researchers are gradually mapping out the evolutionary landscape, thereby paving the way for innovative approaches in regenerative medicine and therapy.

1.4.2. Evolutionary Significance of Embryonic Development

Embryonic development isn't just about cells multiplying—it's a window into evolution itself. An egg starts as a tiny, single cell and then slowly develops into a whole organism; along the way, minor variations emerge that hint at ancient lineages.

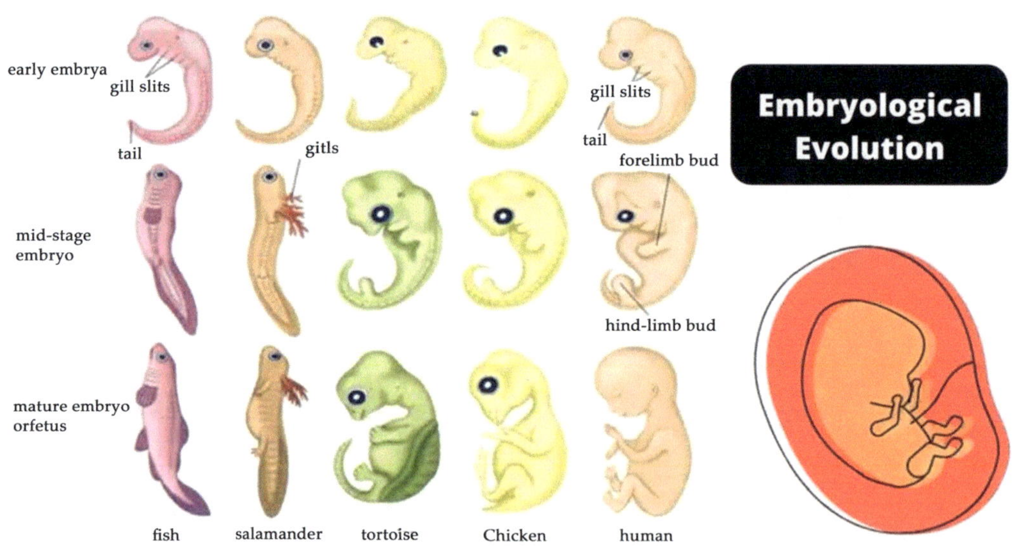

Figure 1.15. Evolutionary significance of embryonic development.

Source: https://biologynotesonline.com/wp-content/uploads/2024/03/Embryological-Evolution-1024x576.jpg.

Many species share a kind of "embryonic conservation," where similar early stages echo deep-rooted evolutionary ties. Take, for example, the work of A.O. Kowalevsky—his studies comparing early life phases in various creatures revealed a surprising continuity between invertebrates and vertebrates (Gilbert et al., 2002). This idea, broadly speaking, helped set the stage for what is now known as evolutionary developmental biology. Then there's the whole twist introduced by epigenetics. Back in the early 20th century, researchers such as Thomas Hunt Morgan began to notice that embryonic growth isn't just a straightforward genetic blueprint; extra layers of regulation also play a significant role. Mary Lyon's investigations, for instance, showed that epigenetic modifications can subtly alter heredity and lead to noticeable changes in traits across generations (Costa et al., 2014). In most cases, acknowledging these extragenetic factors helped shift developmental biology into new directions and expanded our understanding of how gene expression influences evolution. Examining these early developmental stages provides a unique living record of evolution, connecting molecular biology, genetics, and the art of development in unexpected ways. Early similarities among species can even serve as clues for piecing together phylogenetic relationships or understanding the events of speciation. In a messy yet fascinating way, embryology not only charts how life forms emerge but also reminds us to blend insights from different fields. This integrative approach ultimately deepens our grasp of life's complex—if sometimes unpredictably charming—nature (Figure 1.15).

1.4.3. Case Studies of Specific Organisms

Embryological development manifests in various surprising ways across different creatures. Take the zebrafish (*Danio rerio*) – its clear, fast-growing embryos have made it a favorite in labs. Scientists love watching these little fish because they allow them to see gene activity and even how environmental pressures influence the way embryos form; this can sometimes hint at why humans develop specific congenital issues. The simplicity of this organism allows researchers to capture those early cell movements in real time, setting a basic template that often applies to more complex beings. Plus, with so many genetic tools at hand, zebrafish keep on proving their worth when it comes to teasing apart the twists and turns of developmental patterns across different species. Then there's the Russian sturgeon (*Acipenser gueldenstaedtii*), which offers a distinctly different perspective on early life in the water. This fish stands out due to its prolonged gestation and a series of complex developmental stages. In most cases, recent studies suggest that everyday factors, such as temperature and salt levels, significantly influence whether the embryos will hatch properly.

Researchers also investigate how arsenic ends up in sturgeon fillets, even when using various processing techniques, and this type of work prompts us to consider the impact of human actions on aquatic development. All in all, these findings not only matter for aquaculture but also for a broader view of environmental contaminants and their impact on embryos in both marine and freshwater settings (Lidiya et al., 2024). Frogs, on the other hand, add another twist to the story. Their transformation journey, shifting from water-dwelling tadpoles to land-roaming adults, clearly shows how flexible development can be. Studies generally indicate that pressures such as habitat loss and pollution can impact tadpole growth, sometimes resulting in lower survival rates. By examining these early stages closely, scientists gain a better understanding of how environmental stressors affect growth and the entire metamorphosis process – a disruption that can ripple out to alter entire population dynamics and overall ecosystem health. With amphibians facing mounting challenges from climate change and shrinking habitats, tracking their development is more crucial than ever for conservation and building ecological resilience (Falconi et al., 2024).

1.5. Techniques in Embryological Research

Embryological research has taken a significant turn lately, exploring a range of methods that alter our understanding of early development. Lineage tracing enables scientists to track small groups of cells as they evolve over time—sometimes almost as if the cells are secretly revealing their plans—while gene editing with CRISPR/Cas9 provides a direct view of how specific genes influence growth. These techniques not only illuminate the pathways that build complex structures but also provide hands-on methods to influence cell fate. In most cases, these insights push the envelope for both basic science and potential treatments for congenital issues, melding biology with technology in a lively, if somewhat unpredictable, dance. Imaging techniques also play a significant role. Tools like confocal microscopy and live-cell imaging have allowed researchers, generally speaking, to catch the drama of life as it unfolds in real time. The resulting snapshots reveal surprising patterns of cell movement, unexpected shifts in differentiation, and quirky interactions during key moments of growth—sometimes even with a bit of redundancy that makes the story feel more natural. When these visuals are combined with precise measurements, the picture of tissue organization becomes a little less mysterious and more accessible, even if the flow isn't always perfectly smooth. Then there's the exciting spin brought by bioinformatics. High-throughput sequencing now provides scientists with a broad, almost panoramic view of gene expression during the earliest, formative stages of development. Computational models—even if they sometimes stray off on tangents—allow us to simulate various scenarios, enabling us to attempt to predict how these processes might unfold. This hybrid approach, which blends traditional techniques with the latest digital tools, is evident in studies such as those on chromaffin cell biology (Maneu et al., 2023) and (Haboubi, 2009). Generally speaking, by reconnecting historical insights with fresh data, researchers are slowly peeling back the layers of embryogenesis, revealing a complex tapestry that's as messy and fascinating as life itself (Figure 1.16).

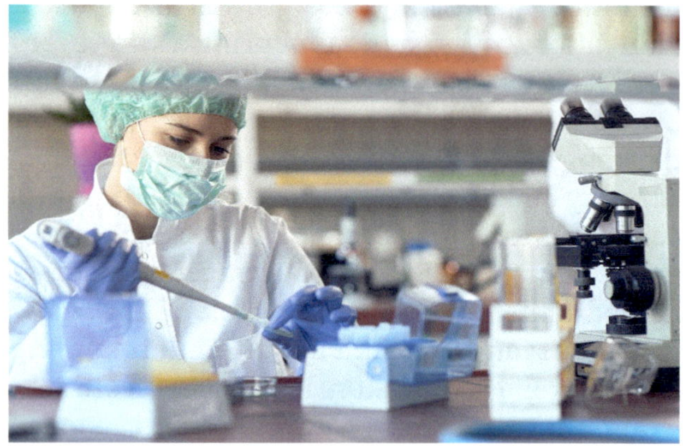

Figure 1.16. Embryological research.

Source: https://www.hamiltonthorne.com/wp-content/uploads/HamiltonThorne_ToxicologyResearch_330189630.jpg.

1.5.1. Imaging Techniques in Embryology

Imaging has significantly changed the way we view embryos. Researchers and clinicians now get to watch embryo development as it happens—no more waiting for a snapshot. Time-lapse microscopy and other high-resolution tools enable us to monitor embryos at every crucial moment, which is a significant advantage for procedures like IVF, where embryo quality is paramount. Traditional methods, however, often yield mixed results among embryologists, making it challenging to select the best candidate. In most cases, a more systematic and objective approach has emerged, underscoring the importance of clear and precise imaging in both the clinic and the lab (Khosravi et al., 2019). AI and machine learning have also entered the mix, upending how we assess embryos. By analyzing enormous piles of time-lapse images, these algorithms pick up on tiny, intricate features that hint at an embryo's viability—often doing a better job than old-school techniques (and sometimes even outsmarting individual embryologists). Take the new framework called STORK, which relies on deep neural networks; it has been impressively accurate in predicting blastocyst quality. This method provides a consistent and reproducible way to evaluate embryos, reducing the risk of multiple implantations and alleviating some ethical concerns associated with selection (Khosravi et al., 2019). Imaging's reach goes beyond IVF, stretching into stem cell research and tissue engineering in unexpected ways. 3D imaging, combined with genetic and molecular tests, provides fresh insights into developmental pathways and how stem cells behave in various settings. Sure, not every piece of the puzzle is solved yet—current methods still don't capture every nuance of these complex processes. The combination of imaging with regenerative medicine is especially intriguing when considering MSCs and their role in tissue repair. Researchers, even while juggling a few inconsistencies here and there, agree that imaging stays key in showing how MSCs evolve and boost developmental health, continually nudging the frontiers of regenerative therapy (Figure 1.17).

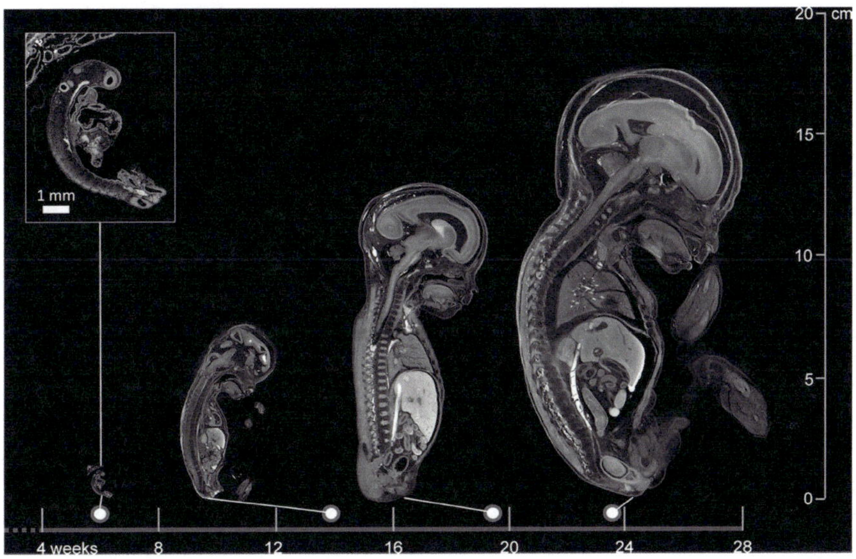

Figure 1.17. Imaging techniques in embryology.

Source: https://ars.els-cdn.com/content/image/1-s2.0-S1084952122000623-gr12.jpg.

1.5.2. Genetic Manipulation and CRISPR Technology

CRISPR-Cas9 and other gene-editing techniques have sparked a new perspective on what our ethical limits should be in the field of embryology. Gene edits are being carried out with the accuracy that was previously only imagined; researchers are now tackling genetic diseases that have persisted for generations. Yet, all this reminds us of past attempts at eugenics, when people tried to "improve" human traits. Some critics even say that playing with our genes might eventually lead to designer babies available only to the wealthy, which then could widen the gap between social classes. In most cases, it's clear that we must now rely heavily on ethical guidelines and regulations, especially since the inherent risks of gene editing may repeat mistakes from history, as mentioned in Melillo et al. (2017). When one steps back and looks at it, the effects of CRISPR run deeper than just medical breakthroughs—they brush up against questions of human rights and the rules that keep things in check. Advocates generally support the idea as a way to eliminate hereditary diseases, but a significant number of voices express concern about tampering with the human germline, leaving researchers somewhat unaccountable. Institutions like the National Academies of Sciences and Medicine have entered the conversation, attempting to establish ethical standards and research protocols to steer the ship in the right direction. Still, ideas on paper might not suffice; solid, enforceable laws are needed to properly balance scientific progress with ethical care, especially as our society's outlook on genetic enhancement continues to shift—something pointed out in Seitz et al. (2018). Looking ahead, it becomes increasingly complex to overlook the long-term implications of CRISPR on both embryological research and human evolution. Scientists are eager to unravel the mysteries of genetic engineering, and with that comes the enticing yet daunting prospect of shaping what future generations might become. Open discussions among a diverse group of stakeholders—from lab scientists to ethicists and everyday people—are crucial if we are to build a comprehensive understanding of the ethical terrain associated with gene editing. In this complex and unpredictable world of scientific innovation, the path forward must strike a balance between our drive to push boundaries and a sense of moral responsibility. After all, embracing new technologies shouldn't mean repeating the over-the-top quests for perfection seen in the past, as Melillo et al. (2017) so clearly hints (Figure 1.18).

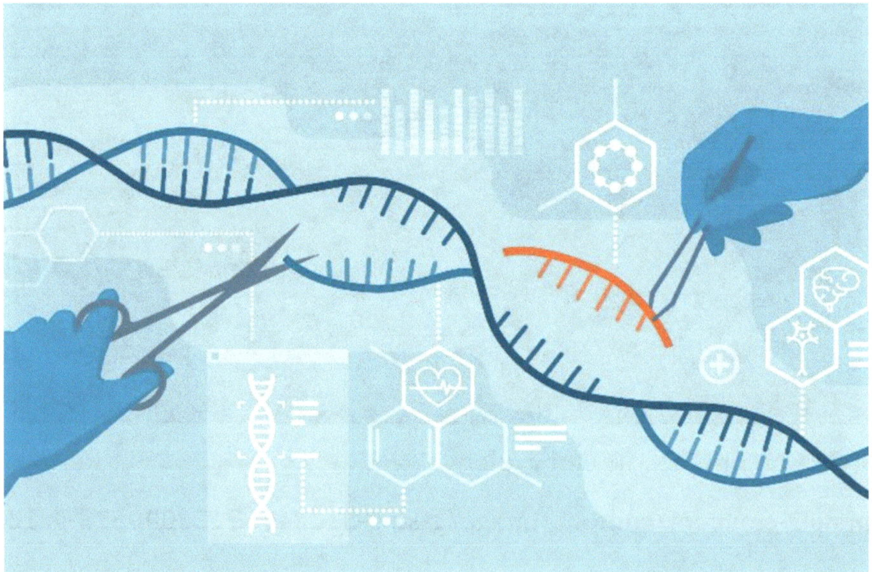

Figure 1.18. Genetic Manipulation.

Source: https://www.iberdrola.com/documents/20125/1527375/CRISPR-726x484.jpg/46cb36ee-b5e4-9ef6-47b1-2094abac7909?t=1642007315492.

1.5.3. Ethical Considerations in Embryological Research

Embryology's recent strides have sparked lively debates about working with human embryos. Scientists delve deeply into the intricacies of development and potential therapies, yet the moral implications continue to become more complex. It isn't only about the science; it's also about the unpredictable fallout when we start fiddling with life right from the get-go. Often, the heart of the debate lands on what embryos are and what rights they might hold—ideas that mix philosophical musings with religious beliefs in ways that hardly ever add up. Researchers and ethicists, in most cases, must juggle these varied viewpoints, repeatedly checking that their work remains true to both scientific honesty and the values society holds dear, all while keeping human dignity at the forefront. Then, things become even more complex when new techniques, such as artificial intelligence (AI), are introduced into embryological research. As Clark et al. (2024) casually point out, adding AI into the mix isn't as straightforward as it sounds—it stirs up issues about data transparency, autonomy, and the mysterious inner workings of algorithm-driven decisions. In embryology, where ethical lines are fine, using AI can trigger unexpected changes, raise concerns over consent, or even skew genetic data interpretation, leading to skewed outcomes. Generally speaking, ethical guidelines need to evolve in tandem with technological advances so that new methods don't inadvertently cross moral boundaries. This means researchers, policy makers, and ethicists must get ahead of the curve and sketch out frameworks that truly address the messy ethical terrain AI introduces, while safeguarding both research integrity and the rights of those involved. Furthermore, as ethical questions arise in embryological studies, the need for robust, comprehensive oversight becomes even clearer. Protecting the heart of good research, especially when its impact ripples throughout society, demands a kind of teamwork among scientists, ethicists, and regulatory bodies. The hands-on experiences shared by researchers—*see* Yang et al. (2024)—reveal just how complex it can be to maintain ethical practices amid shifting public expectations. This scenario encourages everyone to keep the conversation going, with continuous check-ins and occasional revisions of what "ethical" means as new challenges emerge. As progress in the field marches ahead, setting up solid oversight isn't just a bonus—it's downright necessary to ensure that scientific exploration remains both responsible and respectful, building the kind of trust and support that future innovations rely on.

1.6. Applications of Embryology

Biological research these days often revolves around understanding embryonic development – a process that has significant implications for medicine, agriculture, and other fields. Scientists are taking a hard look at how life begins, and single-cell sequencing has largely overturned old ideas. Instead of treating tissues as a single, large blob, these methods allow researchers to examine hundreds, sometimes millions, of cells simultaneously. This means that identifying which cell does what isn't just a neat trick—it might lead to new ways to address regenerative problems or childhood developmental issues, in most cases nudging us toward more effective therapies (Anaparthy et al., 2019). Even plants aren't left out of the mix. When folks study reproductive biology in plants, it's clear that embryology plays a key role far beyond animal development. Take the case of *Anoectochilus roxburghii*; looking at its seeds and embryos reveals surprising clues about when it flowers and fruits. Detailed shape and cell-structure studies indicate that its embryo undergoes rapid development, hinting at potential rapid germination adaptations. These observations not only enhance our understanding of plant reproduction but also serve as a gentle reminder of why conserving such vital flora is crucial for both biodiversity and practical farming (Li et al., 2019). And then there's the whole new world where early development meets genetic engineering. Techniques like CRISPR-Cas9 enable scientists to tweak genes with precision that was once unimaginable, opening up the possibility of organisms that behave just the way we'd like them to. In agriculture, such advances could mean crops that better handle the stresses of unpredictable weather, thus bolstering food security. Meanwhile, insights into how embryos begin development are starting to influence stem cell therapies, helping inform new regenerative treatments. All in all, this blend of old biological wisdom with modern technology is nudging us toward a future where medicine and agriculture are increasingly intertwined, driven by a deeper understanding of life's earliest stages (Anaparthy et al., 2019).

1.6.1. Implications for Reproductive Medicine

Breakthroughs in our understanding of embryology are transforming how patients receive care and how treatments are delivered. Doctors now have clearer ways to spot issues like PCOS, which means patients get care that's more on point. There's a mix of new guidelines, built on in-depth research, that weaves together complex data and patient voices (Teede et al., 2023). Often, these new guidelines prompt us to view things as a whole—not just the physical aspects but also mental well-being—hinting at the rise of personalized medicine. Tailoring care to each person's unique needs marks a significant shift in managing reproductive disorders, resulting in health systems and patient experiences that, generally speaking, improve over time. New tech is also turning the scene upside down. Take IVF, for example; using time-lapse technology (TLT) to pick embryos is a pretty big deal these days. Sure, TLT looks promising for bumping up IVF success rates, yet every lab needs to take a hard look at what it means to adopt such tools (Apter et al., 2020). Each IVF center must determine factors such as which morphokinetic factors are most essential and how to equip their teams accordingly. This shift towards data-driven, ever-evolving techniques demonstrates the ongoing effort to achieve better clinical outcomes, even if it means rethinking traditional approaches. Stepping back, the ripple effects of these changes are felt by society as a whole. Not everyone receives the same level of care, and treatment gaps still exist; therefore, there is a pressing need to explore how factors such as economic status, healthcare access, and education impact reproductive health (Teede et al., 2023). When researchers and clinicians tackle these challenging questions, the goal is to devise solutions that work for all, not just a select few. In most cases, a focus on inclusive research means that more folks stand to benefit from these medical advances—helping to boost public health and the overall quality of life for those facing reproductive challenges.

1.6.2. Role in Developmental Biology and Genetics

At the very beginning of embryonic life, genetic signals and subtle environmental cues mingle in ways that shape an organism's structure and function. Cells get nudged into specific roles while tissues form in a process that is as unpredictable as it is intriguing. For example, a mutation—such as a loss-of-function change in a gene like GRK2—can disrupt crucial pathways, including Hedgehog (Hh) and Wnt, sometimes leading to conditions like asphyxiating thoracic dystrophy (ATD) and other skeletal ciliopathies (Bosakova et al., 2020). In most cases, these genetic quirks remind us that understanding the regulators is crucial to understanding skeletal and organ development, hinting at possible routes for therapeutic intervention. Epigenetics adds another twist to the development story. It doesn't alter the DNA sequence; rather, it influences how genes behave. Various factors – such as what a mother experiences during pregnancy – can subtly alter a developing blueprint. For instance, animals exposed to prenatal stress might display long-lasting behavioral and physiological changes that echo through several generations. This type of intergenerational transmission illustrates the profound impact of epigenetic factors on development and the shaping of disease risks over time (Yehuda et al., 2018). Examining the broader picture in embryology, combining genetic blueprints with epigenetic fine-tuning provides fresh insights into both normal and abnormal growth. Gene expression relies on a blend of fixed instructions and environmental modifications that together define each cell's identity. When any part of this intricate system goes awry, developmental anomalies can emerge, urging us to consider the whole, intertwined process. Studying these interactions not only deepens our understanding of congenital disorders but may also uncover early biomarkers for intervention. In a sense, merging discoveries from genetics, epigenetics, and developmental biology paves the way for innovative treatments for genetic conditions originating in the embryonic stage, promising healthier futures (Bosakova et al., 2020) (Figure 1.19).

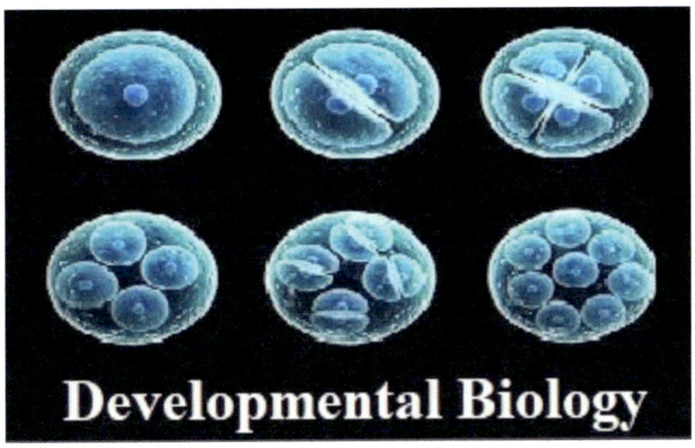

Figure 1.19. Role in developmental biology.

Source: https://thefactfactor.com/wp-content/uploads/2024/04/Developmental-Biology.jpg.

1.6.3. Contributions to Regenerative Medicine and Tissue Engineering

Embryology and regenerative medicine share quite a surprising bond—one that has quietly reshaped how we think about building tissues. People have noticed that early developmental processes, such as the way muscles form before birth, can inspire new ideas for repairing damaged tissues. For example, understanding the steps involved in muscle development in embryos has led researchers to new methods for growing skeletal muscle. iPSCs, teamed up with clever bioengineering tricks, seem to offer a promising route for creating muscle that works, even when genetics or major injuries throw a wrench into the works. This mix of ideas stretches the usual limits of medicine and—generally speaking—rekindles debates over the ethics of using stem cells from embryonic origins, pressing us to move forward carefully. Diving into axial progenitor biology often yields unexpected insights into tissue repair that involve multiple cell types. When one considers how the embryo builds its body axis (including the spinal cord, trunk muscles, etc.), a rough sketch emerges of how these progenitors might contribute to therapy. Recent lab advances have even made it possible to produce these cells *in vitro*, opening up opportunities for disease models and regenerative schemes. By roughly mimicking the environment of an embryo, techniques such as biofabrication and specific biophysical nudges help set the stage for the growth and transformation of these cells. This kind of approach not only surprises us with new ways to rebuild complex tissues but also hints that living organisms could one day better integrate these engineered pieces. When it comes to clinical applications, things start to get interesting. The concept of tuning the behavior of iPSCs through clever engineering advances the therapeutic landscape into new territory, particularly for conditions previously considered irreversible. In most cases, as researchers continue to tweak and test these methods, potential breakthroughs for degenerative diseases, injuries, and even some congenital issues seem increasingly within reach. Studies on the roles of muscle-resident cells keep reminding us just how intertwined embryological knowledge is with modern medical strategies. All these threads, woven together in unexpected ways, could eventually shift clinical practices toward more flexible, innovative approaches in tissue repair—underscoring, in no uncertain terms, the foundational role embryology still plays in advancing medical science.

SUMMARY

Embryology reveals that these early stages significantly influence the final form of an organism. Research continues to demonstrate that genes, cell interactions, and even the environment all interact in complex, sometimes chaotic ways—almost like a dance that's unpredictable yet vital. In most cases, these early cues aren't just minor details; they open up doors for medical breakthroughs. Take MSCs, for example—with more than 55,000 studies now examining their functions and mechanisms, their anti-inflammatory and immune-modulating properties appear to point toward a whole new realm in regenerative medicine (Mark et al., 2019). Looking back, the story of embryology unfolds through many surprising twists. Early researchers began by observing how shapes formed, and over time, their work evolved from basic morphology to more experimental and genetic insights. Phylogenetic trees—that is, those diagrams showing relationships among species—have become pretty important for understanding evolution, especially when one considers the latest findings on ancestral lineages. These clues not only help map out developmental routes but also shed some light on longstanding puzzles about evolutionary changes and their effects on how creatures are built, enriching discussion in both embryology and evolutionary biology (Casey et al., 2014). In conclusion, combining embryology with ideas from medicine and evolution effectively highlights the complexity of this field. As scientists continue to untangle the details of development, the conversation bridging basic science and practical therapy only deepens. MSCs, for instance, serve as a clear example of how our testing of embryologic fundamentals can lead to real-world applications, sparking hope for innovative treatments for a host of conditions. The way past discoveries blend with fresh, emerging possibilities points to an exciting future for both research and clinical practice. Ongoing exploration in this area promises not only to unravel the complexities of development but also to expand our overall understanding of life, reaffirming the essential role of embryological research in today's scientific landscape. Embryology continues to prove that integrating technology with everyday clinical work is more than just a modern trend—it's truly reshaping IVF as we know it. TLT is a great example, offering a new way to watch embryos grow and to make better picks when it comes to selection. ESHRE, the European Society of Human Reproduction and Embryology, has put out a bunch of guidelines for labs thinking about bringing TLT on board; generally speaking, they stress the need to check both the good and the bad sides of this approach and to pick the right morphokinetic factors from the start so that usage stays steady. Although these planned steps are intended to enhance IVF success, a clear, proven clinical benefit remains to be confirmed through further research (Apter et al., 2020). When one examines real-world tests and studies, one begins to see the various manifestations of TLT's impact. One intriguing investigation, for instance, utilizes deep learning models to assess the likelihood of pregnancy by analyzing fetal heart activity captured in time-lapse videos—a sign of our growing reliance on intelligent algorithms. This shift toward high-tech analysis is prompting researchers to delve into detailed morphogenetic clues that may reveal hidden patterns, ultimately guiding the selection of more viable embryos. In most cases, this blend of technology and embryology presents both clear opportunities and its set of challenges; ongoing studies are essential to refine these methods and ultimately help improve patient care (Trần Ngọc Đăng et al., 2019). Further chatter about emerging tech keeps spotlighting the ever-changing side of embryology. Bringing TLT into IVF labs isn't just about ramping up technical abilities—it also brings ethical questions, like how best to choose embryos, into sharper focus. By encouraging practitioners and patients—sometimes even in unexpected ways—to make informed choices, ESHRE's recommendations help foster a culture of transparency where access to accurate information truly informs reproductive decisions.

CLOSER LOOK:

IN VITRO FERTILIZATION (IVF)

IVF is a widely used ART that helps individuals and couples conceive a child when natural conception is difficult or impossible. The term "*in vitro*" refers to a process that occurs outside the body, typically in a laboratory setting. IVF involves several carefully coordinated steps. To generate a large number of mature eggs, the ovaries are first stimulated using hormonal medications. When the eggs are ready, a little surgical technique called follicular aspiration is used to remove them. A sperm sample is simultaneously taken from a donor or the male partner. To aid in fertilization, the recovered eggs and sperm are subsequently mixed in a regulated lab setting. In some cases, a technique called intracytoplasmic sperm injection (ICSI) may be used, where a single sperm is directly injected into an egg to improve chances of fertilization, particularly in cases of male infertility.

After fertilization, the resulting embryos are cultured for several days, usually three to five, to allow them to develop. Embryologists assess the quality of the embryos during this period and select the most viable one(s) for transfer. The selected embryo is then transferred into the woman's uterus through a simple and painless procedure. If implantation occurs, pregnancy proceeds just as it would naturally. In many cases, multiple embryos are created, and those not transferred can be frozen (cryopreserved) for future use. This offers additional chances of pregnancy without the need for repeated ovarian stimulation. IVF can be used in a variety of situations, including tubal factor infertility, endometriosis, unexplained infertility, age-related fertility decline, or genetic disorders that could be passed on to offspring. It also provides options for same-sex couples and single individuals seeking to become parents.

IVF has significantly evolved since the first successful birth through the procedure in 1978. Advances in hormone protocols, embryo freezing techniques, and genetic screening methods have all improved success rates and outcomes. Preimplantation genetic testing (PGT), for example, enables the screening of embryos for genetic abnormalities before implantation, thereby increasing the likelihood of a healthy pregnancy and reducing the risk of inherited diseases. Despite these advancements, IVF is not without its challenges. The process can be emotionally, physically, and financially demanding, with varying success rates depending on factors such as age, health, and fertility diagnosis. Certain women may encounter issues, including ovarian hyperstimulation syndrome (OHSS) or adverse effects from reproductive drugs. Additionally, ethical issues and laws differ from nation to nation, especially when it comes to the use of donor gametes or surrogates, surplus embryos, and embryo selection..

IVF is a powerful and increasingly accessible option for people facing fertility challenges, enabling millions around the world to build families. While it requires careful planning, medical support, and often emotional resilience, the technique continues to bring hope and joy to individuals who might otherwise be unable to conceive. Ongoing research and innovation are expected to improve further the safety, affordability, and effectiveness of IVF, making it an even more integral part of modern reproductive medicine in the years to come.

REFERENCES

1. Aitor Almanza, Carlesso, A., Chintha, C., Creedican, S., Doultsinos, D., Leuzzi, B., Luís, A., et al. (2018). Endoplasmic reticulum stress signaling–From basic mechanisms to clinical applications. *The FEBS Journal, 286*(2), 241–278. https://doi.org/10.1111/febs.14608.
2. Anaparthy, N., Ho, Y., Martelotto, L., Hammell, M., & Hicks, J. (2019). Single-Cell applications of Next-Generation sequencing. *Cold Spring Harbor Perspectives in Medicine, 9*(10), a026898. https://doi.org/10.1101/cshperspect.a026898Appleby, J., & Bredenoord, A. L. (2018). Should the 14-day rule for embryo research become the 28-day rule? *EMBO Molecular Medicine, 10*(9), e9437. https://doi.org/10.15252/emmm.201809437.
3. Apter, S., Ebner, T., Fréour, T., Guns, Y., Kovačič, B., Le Clef, N., Marques, M., et al. (2020). Good practice recommendations for the use of time-lapse technology. *Human Reproduction Open, 2020*. https://doi.org/10.1093/hropen/hoaa008.
4. Boitani, C., Esposito, V., Fiorenza, M. T., Fuso, A., et al. (2017). Involvement of sperm acetylated histones and the nuclear isoform of Glutathione peroxidase 4 in fertilization. https://core.ac.uk/download/141696214.pdf (accessed on 26 May 2025).
5. Bondareva, L. G., Rodionov, A. S., Sinitskaya, T. A., & Fedorova, N. E. (2024). Potential transformations of arsenic forms in fish during cooking processing: A case study of Russian sturgeon. *Toxicological Review*. https://www.semanticscholar.org/paper/97b69ea8cdf5b3a5e1357ac943ef253beb21ea9e (accessed on 26 May 2025).
6. Bredenoord, A. L., Clevers, H., & Knoblich, J. A. (2017). Human tissues in a dish: The research and ethical implications of organoid technology. *Science, 355*(6322), eaaf9414. https://doi.org/10.1126/science.aaf9414.
7. Busby, L., Saunders, D., Serrano Nájera, G., & Steventon, B. (2022). Quantitative experimental embryology: A modern classical approach. *Journal of Developmental Biology, 10*(4), 44. https://doi.org/10.3390/jdb10040044.
8. Chamberlin, M. A. (1993). *An anatomical, Ultrastructural, Autoradiographic, And Cytophotometric Study of Early Embryo, Endosperm, And Ovule Development in Soybean (Glycine max L. Merr)* [Doctoral dissertation]. https://core.ac.uk/download/38903230.pdf (accessed on 26 May 2025).
9. Clark, T., Caufield, H., Mohan, J. A., Al Manir, S., Amorim, E., Eddy, J. A., Gim, N., et al. (2024). AI-readiness for biomedical data: Bridge2AI recommendations. *bioRxiv*. https://www.semanticscholar.org/paper/a0bef9d5f188f4dde3535f98a90737dbcfe12397 (accessed on 26 May 2025).
10. Costa, R., & Frezza, G. (2014). Crossovers between epigenesis and epigenetics: A multicenter approach to the history of epigenetics (1901–1975). https://core.ac.uk/download/144472860.pdf (accessed on 26 May 2025).
11. Dunn, C. W., Giribet, G., Edgecombe, G. D., & Hejnol, A. (2014). Animal phylogeny and its evolutionary implications. *Annual Review of Ecology, Evolution, and Systematics, 45*, 371–395. https://doi.org/10.1146/annurev-ecolsys-120213-091627.
12. El Hachem, H., Crepaux, V., May-Panloup, P., Descamps, P., Legendre, G., & Bouet, P. E. (2017). Recurrent pregnancy loss: Current perspectives. *International Journal of Women's Health, 9*, 331–345. https://doi.org/10.2147/ijwh.s100817.

13. Falconi, M., & Grenni, P. (2024). Exchange of knowledge and the consolidation of culture for contamination management: Introduction to the RemTech Europe 2022 special series. *Integrated Environmental Assessment and Management.* https://www.semanticscholar.org/paper/6b8c61bc499c84861cb9d51e22a2d5aa386bdad3 (accessed on 26 May 2025).
14. Franklin, S. (2013). *Biological Relatives.* https://doi.org/10.1215/9780822378259.
15. Gilbert, S. F., & Mikhailov, A. T. (2002). From development to evolution: The re-establishment of the Alexander Kowalevsky Medal. https://core.ac.uk/download/73341688.pdf (accessed on 26 May 2025).
16. Girgin, M., Broguiere, N., Mattolini, L., & Lutolf, M. (2023). A new approach to generate gastruloids to develop anterior neural tissues. *Bio-Protocol, 13.* https://www.semanticscholar.org/paper/b80d7fe6d736c37648c05d92a667b66c22b501dc (accessed on 26 May 2025).
17. Haboubi, N. (2009). Colonic surgery for cancer: A new paradigm. *Colorectal Disease, 11.* https://www.semanticscholar.org/paper/a86272c4059b616b6b04d772e8be4be1b163894d (accessed on 26 May 2025).
18. Hanneman, K., Newman, B., & Chan, F. P. (2016). Congenital variants and anomalies of the aortic arch. *Radiographics, 37*(1), 32–51. https://doi.org/10.1148/rg.2017160033.
19. Hautefort, I., Poletti, M., Papp, D., & Korcsmáros, T. (2022). Everything you always wanted to know about organoid-based models (and never dared to ask). *Cellular and Molecular Gastroenterology and Hepatology, 14*(2), 311–331. https://doi.org/10.1016/j.jcmgh.2022.04.012.
20. Hesterman, R., Rose, S., LeFever, W., Stewart, R., Krone, M., Holihan, C., & Ackerman, K. M. (2021). Utilizing Playdoh in the classroom to construct a 3D model depicting cellular movements and tissue remodeling during human gastrulation, early organogenesis, and embryonic folding. *Journal of Microbiology & Biology Education, 22.* https://www.semanticscholar.org/paper/e0a5858ea5e8ff70791ffb224177b2ab906a37af (accessed on 26 May 2025).
21. Huntriss, J., Balen, A. H., Sinclair, K. D., Brison, D. R., & Picton, H. M. (2018). Epigenetics and reproductive medicine. *BJOG: An International Journal of Obstetrics & Gynecology, 125*(2), 150–160. https://doi.org/10.1111/1471-0528.15240.
22. Iberite, F., Gruppioni, E., & Ricotti, L. (2022). Skeletal muscle differentiation of human iPSCs meets bioengineering strategies: Perspectives and challenges. *npj Regenerative Medicine, 7,* Article 16. https://doi.org/10.1038/s41536-022-00216-9.
23. Kamath, V. G., Bhat, S., Asif, M., & Avadhani, R. (2016). Anatomy museums of southern India and medical education: An original research. *Indian Journal of Clinical Anatomy and Physiology, 3,* 45–49. https://www.semanticscholar.org/paper/eb85e1093273794595f258e97f4d29466d1b6214 (accessed on 26 May 2025).
24. Khosravi, P., Kazemi, E., Zhan, Q., Malmsten, J., Toschi, M., Zisimopoulos, P., Sigaras, A., et al. (2019). Deep learning enables robust assessment and selection of human blastocysts after *in vitro* fertilization. *npj Digital Medicine, 2,* Article 21. https://doi.org/10.1038/s41746-019-0096-y.
25. Knop, E., Knop, N., Millar, T. J., Obata, H., & Sullivan, D. A. (2011). The International Workshop on Meibomian Gland Dysfunction: Report of the Subcommittee on Anatomy, Physiology, and Pathophysiology of the Meibomian Gland. *Investigative Ophthalmology & Visual Science, 52*(4), 1938. https://doi.org/10.1167/iovs.10-6997c.

26. Kunova Bosakova, M., Abraham, S. P., Niţă, A., Hrubá, E., Buchtová, M., Taylor, S. P., Durán, I., et al. (2020). Mutations in GRK2 cause Jeune syndrome by impairing Hedgehog and canonical want signaling. *EMBO Molecular Medicine, 12*. https://doi.org/10.15252/emmm.201911739.

27. Li, Y., Meng, Z., Zhang, Y., Guo, S., & Lee, Y. (2019). Embryology of *Anoectochilus roxburghii*: Seed and embryo development. *Botanical Studies, 60*. https://www.semanticscholar.org/paper/eb31a74d7b15d141c4c5fbb86573f5e7cfd04a4e (accessed on 26 May 2025).

28. Maneu, V., Borges, R., Gandía, L., & García, A. G. (2023). Forty years of the adrenal chromaffin cell through ISCCB meetings around the world. *Pflügers Archiv–European Journal of Physiology, 475*, 667–690. https://www.semanticscholar.org/paper/96d0333335209b14b6de13bfd510486476250114 (accessed on 26 May 2025).

29. McNamara, K. J. (2012). Heterochrony: The evolution of development. *Evolution: Education and Outreach, 5*, 203–218. https://doi.org/10.1007/s12052-012-0420-3.

30. Melillo, T. R. (2017). *Gene Editing and The Rise of Designer Babies*. https://core.ac.uk/download/490695737.pdf (accessed on 26 May 2025).

31. Mikhailov, A. T. (2012). *Russian Comparative Embryology Takes Form: A Conceptual Metamorphosis Toward "Evo-Devo."* https://core.ac.uk/download/61920109.pdf (accessed on 26 May 2025).

32. Nielsen, M. R., Skougaard, M., Drachmann, C., Stisen, Z. R., Ditlev, S., Jessen, L. E., & Kristensen, L. E. (2025). Single-cell RNA sequencing highlights the influence of innate and adaptive immune response mechanisms in psoriatic arthritis. *Frontiers in Immunology, 15*. https://www.semanticscholar.org/paper/e9c4695e5e51d615c0118d374041f5959616d5e2 (accessed on 26 May 2025).

33. Pittenger, M. F., Discher, D. E., Péault, B., Phinney, D. G., Hare, J. M., & Caplan, A. I. (2019). Mesenchymal stem cell perspective: Cell biology to clinical progress. *npj Regenerative Medicine, 4*, Article 22. https://doi.org/10.1038/s41536-019-0083-6.

34. Seitz, J. D. (2018). *Striking a Balance: Policy Considerations for Human Germline Modification*. https://core.ac.uk/download/149274299.pdf (accessed on 26 May 2025).

35. Simões-Costa, M., & Bronner-Fraser, M. (2015). Establishing neural crest identity: A gene regulatory recipe. *Development, 142*, 242–257. https://doi.org/10.1242/dev.105445.

36. Somoza, R. A., Welter, J. F., Correa, D., & Caplan, A. I. (2014). Chondrogenic differentiation of mesenchymal stem cells: Challenges and unfulfilled expectations. *Tissue Engineering Part B: Reviews, 20*, 596–608. https://doi.org/10.1089/ten.teb.2013.0771.

37. Suzuki, K. (2017). The developing world of DOHaD. *Journal of Developmental Origins of Health and Disease, 9*, 266–269. https://doi.org/10.1017/S2040174417000691.

38. Teede, H., Tay, C. T., Laven, J. J. E., Dokras, A., Moran, L. J., Piltonen, T., Costello, M., et al. (2023). Recommendations from the 2023 International Evidence-Based Guideline for the Assessment and Management of Polycystic Ovary Syndrome. *The Journal of Clinical Endocrinology & Metabolism, 108*(9), 2447–2469. https://doi.org/10.1210/clinem/dgad463.

39. Trần Ngọc Đăng, Cooke, S. A., Illingworth, P., & Gardner, D. K. (2019). Deep learning as a predictive tool for fetal heart pregnancy following time-lapse incubation and blastocyst transfer. *Human Reproduction, 34*, 1011–1018. https://doi.org/10.1093/humrep/dez064.

40. Wiese, K. E., Nusse, R., & van Amerongen, R. (2018). Want signaling: Conquering complexity. *Development, 145*(12), dev165902. https://doi.org/10.1242/dev.165902.

41. Wymeersch, F. J., Wilson, V., & Tsakiridis, A. (2021). Understanding axial progenitor biology *in vivo* and *in vitro*. *Development, 148*(11), dev180612. https://doi.org/10.1242/dev.180612.

42. Yadegari, J. G., Khalaf, A., Oladi, A., Shahbazi, A., & Mahmoudvand, H. (2025). *In vitro, in vivo*, and cellular mechanisms of *Astragalus onobrychis* L. extract against protoscoleces and hydatid cysts of *Echinococcus granulosus*. *Frontiers in Pharmacology, 16*, Article 1285393. https://www.semanticscholar.org/paper/56cd82293c6dff532b6471270ca69a57a2a0840a (accessed on 26 May 2025).

43. Yang, S. I., & Kang, T. S. (2024). A narrative inquiry of the experiences with family cutoffs: Focusing on a couple of Christian counselors. *Korean Association for Learner-Centered Curriculum and Instruction*. https://www.semanticscholar.org/paper/987ca84090427ea1bd92a1c4334f19e3efaf50ee (accessed on 26 May 2025).

44. Yang, Y., Zhou, C., Wang, Y., Liu, W., Liu, C., Wang, L., Liu, Y., et al. (2017). The E3 ubiquitin ligase RNF114 and TAB1 degradation are required for maternal-to-zygotic transition. *EMBO Reports, 18*, 205–216. https://doi.org/10.15252/embr.201642573.

45. Yehuda, R., & Lehrner, A. (2018). Intergenerational transmission of trauma effects: Putative role of epigenetic mechanisms. *World Psychiatry, 17*, 243–257. https://doi.org/10.1002/wps.20568.

46. Yoshizaki, K., Kimura, R., Kobayashi, H., Oki, S., Kikkawa, T., Mai, L., Koike, K., et al. (2021). Paternal age affects offspring via an epigenetic mechanism involving REST/NRSF. *EMBO Reports, 22*(1), e51524. https://doi.org/10.15252/embr.202051524.

47. Zagris, N. (2022). Aristotle (384–322 BC): The beginnings of embryology. *The International Journal of Developmental Biology, 66*(1–3), 5–8. https://www.semanticscholar.org/paper/ce0e6d801c1dd2c978bdc18fb4ef794d4d1e3d75 (accessed on 26 May 2025).

48. Zegers-Hochschild, F., Adamson, G. D., Dyer, S., Racowsky, C., de Mouzon, J., Sokol, R. Z., Rienzi, L., et al. (2017). The International Glossary on Infertility and Fertility Care, 2017. *Fertility and Sterility, 108*(3), 393–406. https://doi.org/10.1016/j.fertnstert.2017.06.005.

49. Zegers-Hochschild, F., Adamson, G. D., Dyer, S., Racowsky, C., de Mouzon, J., Sokol, R. Z., Rienzi, L., et al. (2017). The International Glossary on Infertility and Fertility Care, 2017. *Human Reproduction, 32*(9), 1786–1801. https://doi.org/10.1093/humrep/dex234.

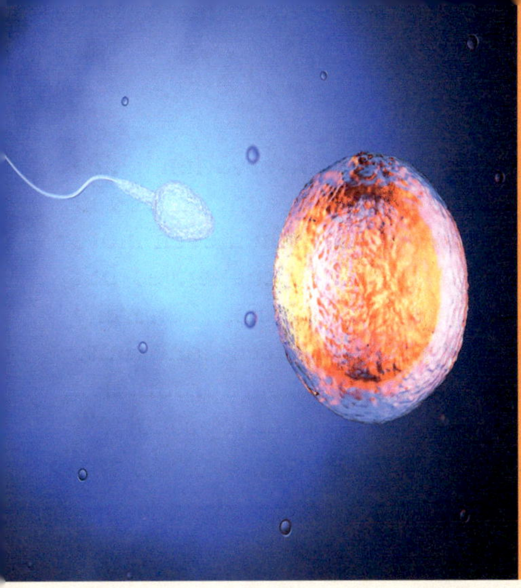

Chapter 2
GAMETOGENESIS

Contents

Introduction

Organisms produce gametes through a process that's crucial for maintaining species. Gametogenesis, as it's often called, isn't just a neat term—it's the mix of different cell splits and tweaks that eventually form sperm and eggs in animals, or pollen and ovules in plants. Understanding how gametogenesis works is crucial not only in biology but also in medicine and agriculture, where factors such as reproductive health and crop success are of paramount importance. Looking at those genetic and molecular details, it isn't some distant theory; it's a lively mix of cell activities and environmental factors that shape how reproduction goes down. At the heart of this matter lies the clear difference between meiosis and mitosis. Meiosis, for instance, is the process that cuts the chromosome number in half, and this step is huge for mixing genes. This mixing-up—thanks to independent assortment and crossing over—generates a significant amount of genetic variation. Over time, organisms have adapted these processes under the pressure of evolution, resulting in diverse strategies across species. This isn't only a topic for biology books; it also touches on challenging issues like conservation, since maintaining species depends on robust reproduction and good genetic health. Recent strides in reproductive technology, such as in vitro fertilization (IVF) and gene editing, have shed even more light on why gametogenesis is so essential. These advances may solve some fertility challenges, but they also spark debates about manipulating genes and the conservation of our species. Generally speaking, it's crucial to consider how both internal factors and external influences contribute to gametogenesis. Luxton et al. (2024) highlight the ecological aspects of these reproductive strategies, while Wendisch et al. (2024) examine how environmental shifts can influence reproductive patterns in different species. All in all, gametogenesis proves to be a blend of biology, ecology, and technology—a multifaceted subject that warrants a closer examination as we confront ongoing challenges to biodiversity and healthcare (Figure 2.1).

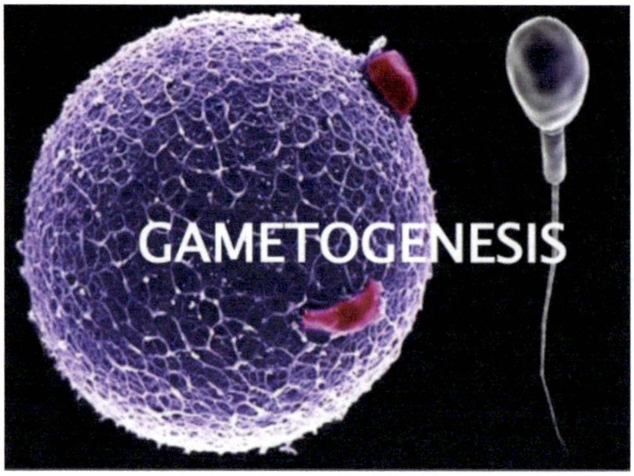

Figure 2.1. Gametogenesis.

Source: https://www.onlinebiologynotes.com/wp-content/uploads/2017/03/gametogenesis-1-638.jpg.

Definition of Gametogenesis

Creating the cells that kick off reproduction in living beings isn't a simple affair—it's a detailed process that keeps species going. Known as gametogenesis, this journey splits into two main paths: one for males (spermatogenesis) and one for females (oogenesis). It all starts when primordial germ cells (PGCs) morph into gametes that eventually come together in fertilization to spark new life. Along the way, there are several stages—first a round of mitosis, then meiosis—that ensure these gametes end up with only half the usual genetic material. In most cases, this drop in chromosome number is crucial for preserving genetic balance over generations, allowing a species' lineage to continue while maintaining a balanced genetic pool. Besides its prominent biological role, the language surrounding gametogenesis has broadened to encompass more aspects of reproductive health as well. Various groups have recently set out to standardize definitions, aiming to clarify communication among doctors, researchers, and patients. For example, the International Committee for Monitoring Assisted Reproductive Technologies has published glossaries that nail down key terms about fertility and infertility, generally speaking, to clear up any confusion about reproductive tech and care. Initiatives like these serve as a reminder that precise language matters—a small word mix-up can lead to significant misunderstandings about treatments and outcomes. Additionally, these efforts aim to encompass a broad range of conditions that impact reproductive abilities, ultimately providing a more comprehensive understanding of gametogenesis in human health. How we sort and understand gametogenesis has a profound impact on both evolutionary biology and medical science. When scientists delve into the intricacies of gamete formation, advances in genetic testing and environmental sampling often reveal new insights into reproductive processes, which in turn broaden our understanding of evolutionary relationships among eukaryotic organisms. Discoveries of new groups and genera further highlight the natural diversity of gametogenesis across species. This expanding body of knowledge not only shapes evolutionary theory but also lays the groundwork for tackling fertility issues in the clinic. All in all, developing a standardized glossary of terms related to infertility and fertility care seems essential—it helps researchers, healthcare providers, and patients get on the same page, paving the way for better interventions and a clearer overall understanding of reproductive health and gametogenesis as a whole (Zegers-Hochschild et al., 2017; Sina et al., 2018).

Importance in Sexual Reproduction

Gamete formation is at the heart of how organisms maintain their genetic diversity and develop properly. DNA methylation, which undergoes dynamic remodeling, especially during male gametogenesis, plays a significant role here. Research on rice, for example, shows that methylation shifts occurring immediately after meiosis appear to reveal a finely tuned system that primes sperm for fertilization. When scientists investigated the role of enzymes like CMT3a and CMT3b, they discovered that these proteins are closely linked to regulating gene expression and managing transcription factors essential for the proper functioning of gametes. This careful epigenetic balancing act helps create a solid blueprint for the genetic makeup of coming generations, generally supporting the idea that such variation is essential for evolution and adaptation (Li et al., 2024). Alongside these epigenetic changes, a complex network of biochemical pathways adds layers to the complexity of gamete production. Mitochondrial adrenodoxins—often called ADXs—handle key electron transfers that eventually influence steroid formation, a vital process for both male and female gametogenesis. In plants especially, the ADX–ADXR–P450 shuttle appears indispensable for developing female gametes and even for starting embryogenesis. Observations indicate that certain steroids, such as homocastasterone, are, in most cases, critical for gametophyte viability. When this hormonal pathway goes off track, as seen in some genetic mutants, damaging traits can emerge. Such evidence suggests that steroid biosynthesis is a broadly conserved process, underlining its importance in reproductive success across species (Bellido et al., 2022). In a tangled interplay, genetic, epigenetic, and biochemical factors combine in ways that drive successful sexual reproduction. This multifaceted network ensures that gametes form correctly and function as they should, affecting everything from fertilization to early embryo growth. When examining how molecular pathways engage during gametogenesis, it becomes clear that enhancing reproductive fitness depends on improving both gamete quality and overall viability. These mechanisms aren't isolated; they interact rather loosely, emphasizing that sexual reproduction holds deep evolutionary significance. The way organisms adjust their reproductive tactics to environmental shifts shows that gametogenesis isn't just about propagating species—it actively fuels genetic diversity, a cornerstone of natural selection. All in all, these processes transcend mere reproduction, capturing something fundamental about life itself (Bellido et al., 2022; Li et al., 2024) (Figure 2.2).

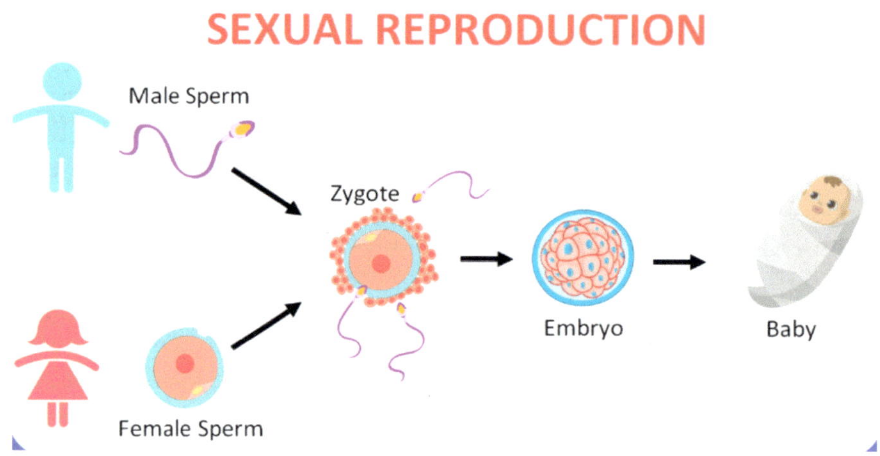

Figure 2.2. Sexual reproduction.

Source: https://cdn.teachoo.com/8f5e1dff-cbda-4ffc-9dbe-ac370561db6d/sexual-reproduction---teachoo.png.

Overview of the Process in Different Organisms

Many creatures undergo gametogenesis in their unique ways, each reflecting distinct reproductive strategies and evolutionary adaptations. Take flowering plants, for example—species like St. Johns wort (*Hypericum perforatum*) don't always follow a single playbook. Generally speaking, their gametogenesis can flip between sexual and asexual routes. In *H. perforatum*, there's this neat trick called apomixis, where somatic cells in the ovule's nucellus somehow develop into unreduced embryo sacs. It's almost as if the plant's imitating the regular sexual process without actually going through it. Studying how *H. perforatum* handles gametogenesis not only unpacks its tangled genetic network but also hints at how both sexual and asexual paths may be intertwined. This insight, in most cases, could eventually help steer agricultural practices towards blending apomictic traits into vital crops through genetic tweaks (Barcaccia et al., 2015). Looking at animal gametogenesis, it is primarily driven by meiosis—an essential process that generates genetic diversity. Here, things split into phases, such as spermatogenesis, which produces large numbers of nimble sperm, and oogenesis, the process that results in just a few large, nutrient-rich oocytes. These events, occurring in the male and female gonads, respectively, mirror the evolutionary push that often prioritizes quality over sheer numbers, especially in species where female reproduction tends to invest more in each gamete. Plus, hormones—like gonadotropins and various sex hormones—play a significant role by fine-tuning the timing and development of these cells. In effect, this hormonal network adds a layer of complexity that underpins reproduction across many animal groups, a nuance that highlights the adaptive nature of these processes particularly well (Verween et al., 2007). Looking beyond individual species, examining gametogenesis across different groups not only clarifies how reproduction works, but also reveals broader environmental consequences. In aquatic realms, for instance, organisms like corals tend to synchronize their reproductive cycles with natural signals—such as lunar phases and specific water temperatures—ensuring that spawning occurs at just the right moment for optimal fertilization outcomes. It's a vivid example of how external cues can shape reproductive success. Furthermore, research into biofouling in industrial systems reveals that these reproductive cycles can have a ripple effect on community dynamics, influencing species interactions in unexpected ways. Understanding these relationships could lead to more innovative strategies for managing invasive species—take the larval stages of *Mytilopsis leucophaeata* in cooling systems, for example—which, in turn, helps tackle both ecological and industrial challenges. All in all, combining reproductive strategies with environmental factors highlights the need for ongoing, in-depth exploration of gametogenesis (Verween et al., 2007).

2.1. Types of Gametogenesis

Sexual reproduction depends on producing gametes, and this happens in so many different ways across living things. Take animals—most species tend to have two major routes. On one hand, males push out sperm continuously throughout most of their lives through a process called spermatogenesis. On the other hand, females develop oocytes in a limited number of cycles, which naturally ends up meaning fewer gametes overall. This uneven rate of production often influences how species approach reproduction; for example, investing in fewer but larger gametes can increase the chances that the offspring will thrive. Generally speaking, these differences suggest the evolutionary forces at work that subtly shape the process of gametogenesis in various organisms. Plants, however, tell a different story. Instead of the more straightforward animal process, they mix things up with something called alternation of generations. Essentially, a diploid sporophyte initiates the process by producing haploid spores through meiosis, and then these spores develop into male and female gametophytes. These gametophytes go on to produce gametes that, once fused, restore the diploid condition in the zygote. It's interesting—and somewhat complex—to observe how regulatory mechanisms determine cell fate during this division and differentiation, highlighting the intricate interactions between genetic programming and environmental cues. In most cases, these adaptations not only facilitate successful reproduction but also enhance genetic variation and population resilience in changing conditions (Huang et al., 2024). Then there's the whole matter of hybridization, which adds an extra twist. In some amphibians, for instance, these mixing events can unexpectedly alter population structures and the overall genetic composition. Consider water frogs like *Pelophylax epeiroticus* and *P. kurtmuelleri*; research indicates that hybrids in these species exhibit unique and sometimes puzzling reproductive strategies. The data generally suggest that while hybridization happens at a relatively low rate, the reproductive barriers remain strong, nudging us to avoid simplistic ideas about gamete formation across different species. Additionally, hybridization can generate new genetic combinations, enriching the gene pool and making populations more adaptable over time. All in all, digging into these nuances is essential for a real grasp of evolutionary dynamics in our diverse biological world (Papežík et al., 2025) (Figure 2.3).

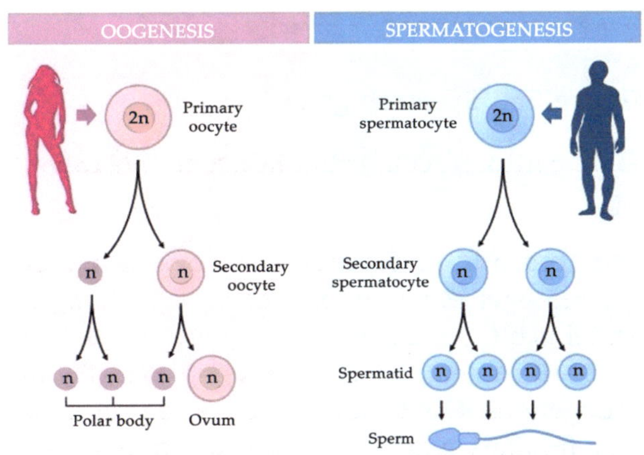

Figure 2.3. Types of gametogenesis.

Source: https://old-ib.bioninja.com.au/_Media/gametogenesis_med.jpeg.

2.1.1. Spermatogenesis

Deep in the maze of seminiferous tubules within the testes, a series of unexpected changes kick off what many might call a wild cellular ride. It all begins when PGCs start to develop, with spermatogonia multiplying through mitosis until some of them unexpectedly shift into becoming primary spermatocytes. Suddenly, these primary cells jump into meiosis—a step that cleverly cuts the chromosome count from diploid to haploid. Before long, the secondary spermatocytes divide into spermatids, small cells that eventually develop into fully mature spermatozoa. This ever-unfolding cascade, with its mix of molecular signals and cellular chit-chat, generally ensures that the sperm produced are robust and ready for the next step.

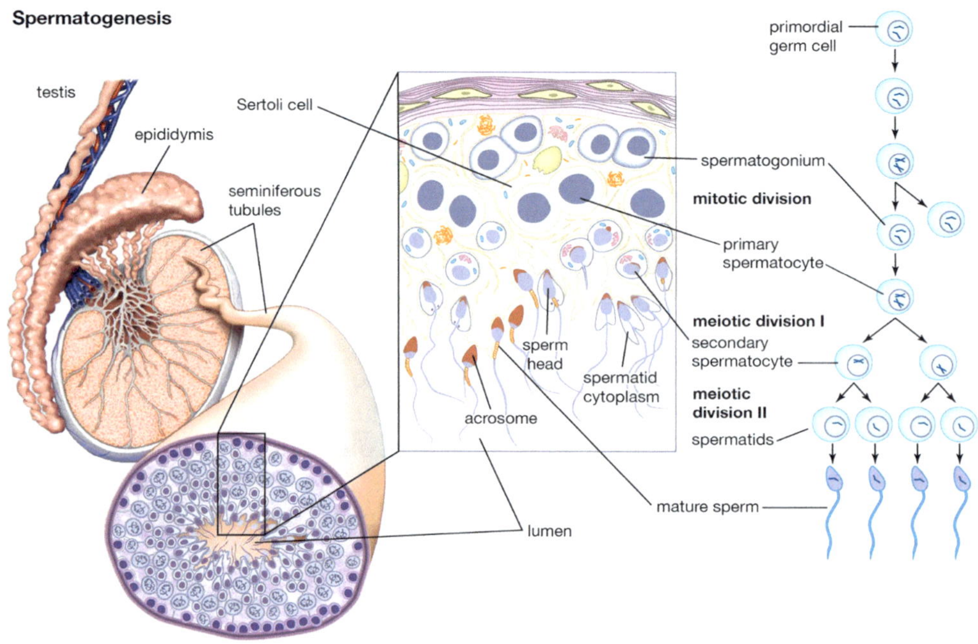

Figure 2.4. Spermatogenesis.

Source: https://cdn.britannica.com/49/135449-050-D1730B7E/spermatogenesis-human-anatomy.jpg.

More recently, researchers have begun to focus on specific RNA molecules that may be influencing spermatogenesis in unexpected ways. Long non-coding RNAs, for instance, aren't busy coding for proteins but instead seem to affect gene expression in unexpected corners. Take lncRNA Gm2044 in mice—it's been flagged as a key player, diving into complex networks and acting like a competing endogenous RNA to subtly modulate protein production vital for sperm development. In most cases, such findings suggest that transcriptional and post-transcriptional processes are pretty tangled, each looping back into the other in ways we're still trying to understand fully. It's hard to miss the role of mitochondria in all this—these tiny powerhouses keep the energy flowing for sperm viability and movement. Mitochondrial translation, paired with the fine-tuning of ribosomal regulation, has emerged as a critical component in enabling sperm to function correctly. Some studies even suggest that RNA-binding protein complexes, such as AMG-1/SLRP-1, play a role in maintaining mitochondrial homeostasis during the complex process of sperm formation. Then there's that delicate balance between energy production and metabolic function, which seems to influence how energetically sperm can navigate toward fertilization directly. All in all, this intricate dance between mitochondrial dynamics and spermatogenesis demonstrates the profound interdependence of these cellular processes, leaving ample room for further exploration in reproductive biology (Figure 2.4).

2.1.2. Oogenesis

Oogenesis is a key part of forming gametes—it's all about the growth and change of oocytes. This process begins during the early embryonic stages and continues well into a female's reproductive years, with hormones and cellular signals engaging in a dynamic back-and-forth. Cells start as PGCs and then, through events such as repeated cell divisions and the twists of meiosis, they gradually take shape into mature oocytes, assisted by nearby somatic cells that help chaperone the formation of ovarian follicles. In most cases, modern molecular biology, using model organisms, has shed some light on the gene controls behind these steps.

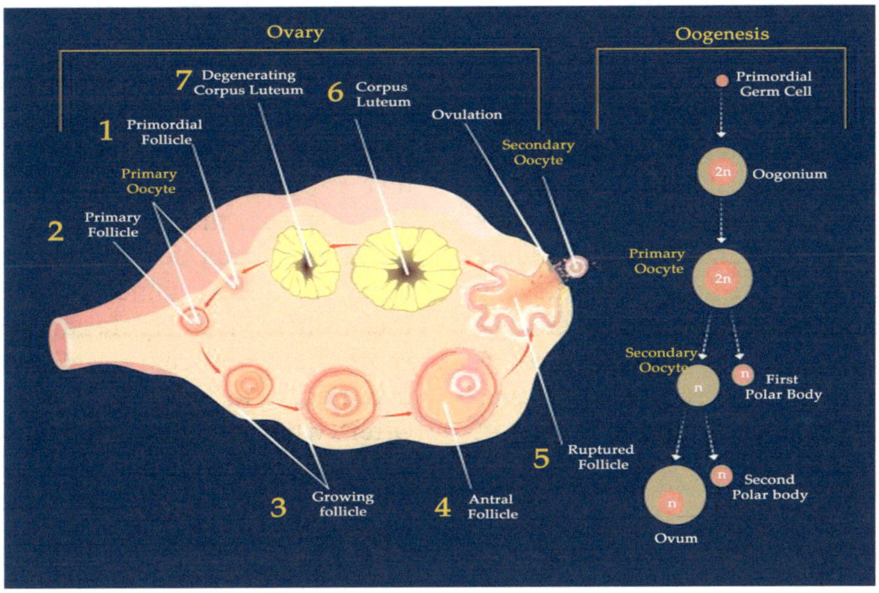

Figure 2.5. Oogenesis.

Source: https://external-content.duckduckgo.com/iu/?u=https%3A%2F%2Fcdn1.byjus.com%2Fwp-content%2Fuploads%2F2017%2F02%2F130.png&f=1&nofb=1&ipt=5457c3c1f8633bd8d88b1063cbadcaee82c5650fac448ffa15cfc06ee90b8683.

For example, work with *Platynereis dumerilii* has revealed that some genes stick around unchanged, hinting at the deep evolutionary roots of oocyte development (Ribeiro et al., 2025). Delving deeper into oogenesis, some researchers have suggested the possibility of mimicking this complex process in a laboratory. Recent experiments using induced pluripotent stem cells have even managed to coax cells into acting like functional oocytes—showing, generally speaking, the impressive potential of stem cell tech. Interestingly, when scientists mixed human PGC-like cells with mouse somatic cells, they identified several hurdles that still need to be addressed for reliable oocyte formation. These lab-based methods not only open up new opportunities for reproductive health advancements but also stir up ethical and practical debates. Different species and culture systems are being tested, as researchers attempt to clear the roadblocks and establish new approaches to understanding mammalian gametogenesis. All this work consistently underscores the integral role of folliculogenesis in the overall picture (Jang et al., 2024). Folliculogenesis, by creating the proper microenvironment, is essential for an oocyte to mature properly. Inside the ovary, there's a dynamic, sometimes unpredictable, interplay between somatic cells and developing oocytes—each influenced by a mix of hormonal feedback loops. The follicle structure—primarily built from granulosa and theca cells—supports not only the growth of the oocyte but also its eventual release during ovulation. Even a slight slip in this delicate interaction can lead to issues like infertility. Recently, new laboratory techniques, such as fine-tuning *in vitro* reconstitution to create xenogeneic follicles, have begun to bridge gaps in our understanding of gametogenesis. Being able to develop fully mature oocytes in this way expands the possibilities in reproductive biology, offering fresh avenues for investigating fertility and development, even if it sometimes leaves us with more questions than answers (Jang et al., 2024) (Figure 2.5).

2.1.3. Differences Between Male and Female Gametogenesis

Gametogenesis shows how males and females approach reproduction in their unique ways. In males, it's pretty much a never-ending process—they keep on making sperm all the time, churning out gametes continuously. For example, in creatures like *Corallium japonicum* detailed histological work uncovered gene signals hinting at rapid gamete maturation and a heavy sperm output. On the other hand, females take a resource-intensive route, producing fewer but larger gametes. Generally speaking, this type of investment is crucial for mixing up genes and facilitating fertilization, as seen in many organisms. Understanding these mixed strategies provides insight into the evolutionary pressures that shape reproduction, while also revealing the intricate complexities of sexual differentiation in gametogenesis. A key element that sets male from female gametogenesis is the way genes and physical traits are expressed for each sex. In brown algae such as *Saccharina japonica*, noticeable differences emerge at both the gametophyte and gamete stages. Researchers discovered that roughly 37.53% of the genes expressed during the gametophyte phase are sex-biased, with an apparent tilt toward male genes in mature gametophytes. Those male-biased genes are associated with important traits, such as sperm motility and the formation of cell walls. Meanwhile, female gametes tend to exhibit gene activity associated with egg recognition and storage. This type of variable gene expression doesn't just support success at the gamete level—it also suggests that evolutionary pressures may be driving each sex toward more specialized functions during gametogenesis. The effects of these differences ripple far beyond individual reproductive outcomes, influencing population dynamics and the overall survival of species. Often, when females focus on developing their oocytes, the result is higher parental care and better resource allocation, which enhances the chances of offspring viability. In contrast, males, by producing enormous amounts of sperm, may trigger competitive behaviors that sway mating outcomes. Observations in *Corallium japonicum* and other species further back up these dynamics, with discoveries of sex-specific gene expressions during key developmental stages. Identifying the genes that regulate these processes opens up new avenues for conservation efforts and deepens our understanding of reproductive strategies across species. Taking a closer look at how male and female gametogenesis differ not only highlights core biological principles but also informs broader ecological and evolutionary studies in this field.

2.2. The Process of Spermatogenesis

Spermatogenesis happens in the seminiferous tubules inside the testes. It all starts with diploid spermatogonia—those stem cells that divide mitotically—to eventually give rise to primary spermatocytes. Right then, these primary spermatocytes undergo meiosis, transforming into haploid secondary spermatocytes and later into spermatids. Hormones such as testosterone and follicle-stimulating hormone (FSH) generally regulate the overall progress of the process, while Sertoli cells in the surrounding microenvironment provide support at every step. Understanding these early stages proves key when looking into male fertility and tackling reproductive disorders, even if the details can get a bit tangled along the way. In more recent times, researchers have turned to *in vitro* approaches that mimic the natural setting of the testes. Using stem cells as a starting point, scientists are now attempting to replicate the whole spermatogenesis journey outside the human body. There are innovative methods available—such as organ-on-chip (OoC) technology—that recreate the testicular environment by simulating both cellular interactions and fluid dynamics. In most cases, these techniques not only help break down the complex dynamics of cell-to-cell communication but also hold promise for treating male infertility. The idea that viable spermatozoa can emerge from induced pluripotent stem cells is both exciting and, frankly, a bit revolutionary. Ultimately, delving into the intricacies of spermatogenesis is far more significant than its fundamental biological implications. Detailed insights into the cellular and molecular mechanics directly shape new strategies in assisted reproductive technologies (ART). For example, combining *ex vivo* culture systems with modern bioengineering tools might offer alternatives for those with compromised fertility. Recent studies, for instance, have demonstrated that dynamic culture conditions, combined with custom-made scaffolding, can enhance both cell survival and maturation. As these technologies evolve – yes, even with a few bumps along the way – the prospects for effective ART solutions look brighter than ever, tying fundamental research tightly to tangible clinical advances (Figure 2.6).

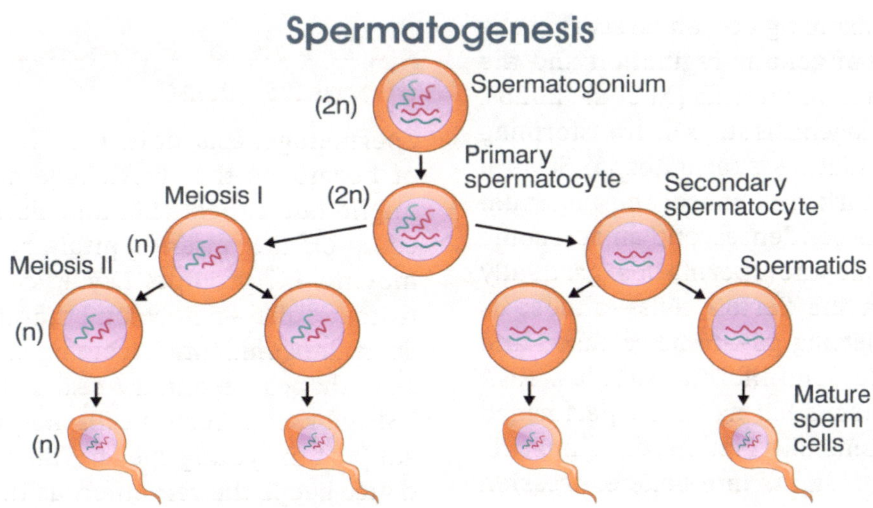

Figure 2.6. The process of spermatogenesis.

Source: https://www.vedantu.com/question-sets/01c6c929-ae8f-4227-8681-36bb0e29eae67589302375809982065.png.

2.2.1. Stages of Spermatogenesis

Spermatogenesis isn't a straight-line process—it's a series of unfolding stages that collectively shape sperm cells for reproduction. It all starts with spermatogonia, the stem cells located in the seminiferous tubules, which multiply through regular mitotic divisions. Then, in an unexpected twist, some of these cells switch roles and become primary spermatocytes, which then enter the first meiotic division. During this phase, genetic material is mixed in a way that generally boosts diversity. Additionally, mechanisms such as NAE1-mediated neddylation help maintain balance; if these controls fail, infertility may result (Xi et al., 2025). Things get even more dynamic as the cells advance. Primary spermatocytes undergo meiosis I, splitting into two secondary spermatocytes that each carry half the usual genetic load—timing is crucial here. These secondary cells enter meiosis II, dividing into four spermatids and advancing the process toward becoming full-fledged gametes. Accurate chromosome crossovers are essential during these steps, and if the stabilization of recombination intermediates slips up, it can lead to major defects. Nae1-SKO male mice have demonstrated difficulties in this delicate balancing act, underscoring the interdependence of genetic regulation and the orderly progression of meiosis (Xi et al., 2025). Eventually, spermiogenesis steps in, transforming spermatids into mature spermatozoa. Several visual changes mark this phase: the flagellum forms, the nucleus condenses, and an acrosome develops, all while the spermatids gradually break away from the Sertoli cells—almost as if they're finally letting go—to be released into the lumen of the seminiferous tubules. RNA sequencing studies, such as those performed on model organisms like Platynereis dumerilii, provide valuable insights into gene expression patterns associated with both spermatogenesis and oogenesis. In most cases, these findings enhance our understanding of germ cell development and even suggest the evolutionary conservation of key genes, laying the groundwork for broader research into gamete formation across species (Figure 2.7).

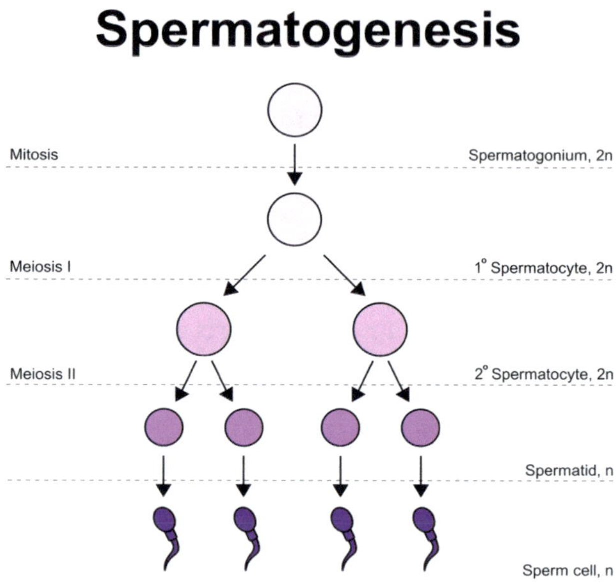

Figure 2.7. Stages of spermatogenesis.

Source: https://upload.medbullets.com/topic/116008/images/spermatogenesis%20-%20moises%20dominguez.jpg.

2.2.2. Role of Hormones in Spermatogenesis

Spermatogenesis, at its core, is a wild interplay of hormones that work together in ways one might not expect. LH and FSH, for instance, come off the anterior pituitary and get things moving. LH prompts Leydig cells to crank out testosterone—a hormone that not only nudges spermatogonia into becoming mature sperm but also shapes secondary sexual features—while FSH works on Sertoli cells, helping them better support the young sperm. This whole hormonal dance keeps the seminiferous tubules balanced, and when it gets thrown off, reproductive problems can crop up, highlighting just how essential these signals are. Testosterone isn't just there for show either; it wears several hats during sperm development. Generally speaking, it modulates the production of proteins that sperm cells need. Take cadherins, for example. These proteins help cells adhere to one another, migrate, and maintain the integrity of the seminiferous epithelium's architecture. One protein in particular, N-cadherin, plays a crucial part in preserving the blood-testis barrier, and testosterone levels influence its activity. This relationship between hormones and structural proteins suggests a broader picture—how cellular structure and function might be altered, inviting further exploration. Hormones also set the pace and timing of the whole spermatogenic cycle. Feedback loops that involve testosterone and inhibin work together to control the secretion of gonadotropins, striking a balance that's key for proper sperm production. Some evidence even suggests that higher testosterone levels may boost sperm count, whereas too much estrogen, on the flip side, might impair development. Environmental factors, stressors, and other disruptions can upset these delicate hormonal pathways, making the process highly sensitive to change. In most cases, understanding these nuanced hormonal influences is vital for addressing male fertility issues. It could guide future therapeutic advances in reproductive health—especially as modern challenges add extra layers of complexity to the field (Figure 2.8).

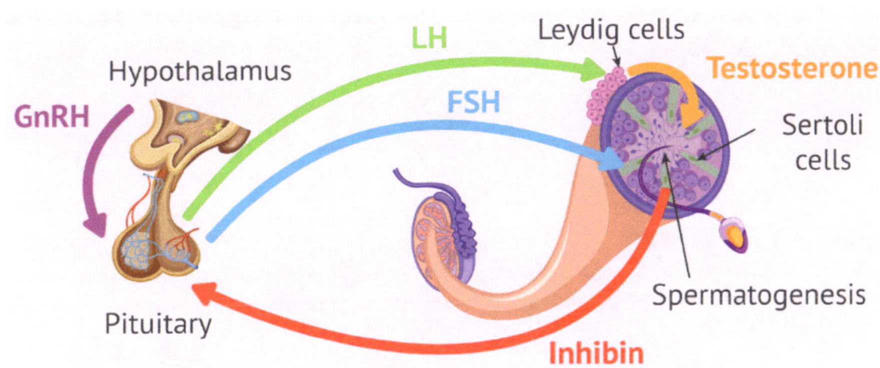

Figure 2.8. Hormonal regulation of spermatogenesis.

Source: https://www.invitra.com/en/wp-content/uploads/2014/07/regulation-hormonal-spermatogenesis.png.

2.2.3. Duration and Location of Spermatogenesis

Spermatogenesis is key to reproductive biology, happening mainly in the testes' seminiferous tubules. This process begins with spermatogonial stem cells and progresses through a series of steps that, in a typical human, span approximately 64 to 72 days—during which millions of sperm are produced daily. It's amazing how each part of this cycle, happening in different zones of the tubules, renews the sperm supply and hints at various local environmental impacts. The fact that production takes place in such a dedicated setting underlines how important both the timing and the site are for successful fertilization. Inside these tubules, the layout is rather unique: Sertoli cells, Leydig cells, and germ cells all mingle at different development stages. Sertoli cells, for instance, are essential for nurturing young sperm by providing nutrients and vital signals, while Leydig cells send hormonal cues that shape the entire activity. Sometimes, these cells even communicate in unexpected ways—an interaction that creates a critical microenvironment, since the germ cells are susceptible to disruptions. This very localized set-up doesn't just help the sperm mature; it also acts as a sort of shield, guarding against potential reproductive issues. Recent studies have started to tease out the role environmental factors play in this delicate process. Exposure to endocrine-disrupting chemicals (EDCs), for instance, can throw a wrench into the works by messing with hormone signals, which in turn can push down semen quality. Research generally suggests that there's been a worrisome drop in sperm quality paired with a bump in male reproductive disorders, especially in industrialized areas over the last several decades. All these points to just how critical it is to grasp both the timing and the location of spermatogenesis, since these sperm-making cells, particularly vulnerable to xenobiotics like xenoestrogens, demand ongoing study and attention (Géraldine Delbès et al., 2006; Diamanti et al., 2009).

2.3. The Process of Oogenesis

Female egg production occurs through a process called oogenesis, which begins even before birth. It begins with tiny PGCs that appear early and migrate to the forming ovaries. Once there, they multiply and, over time, shift into primary oocytes—but here's the twist: each one pretty much halts in prophase I of meiosis until a hormonal signal later, during either the menstrual or estrous cycle, nudges it back into action.

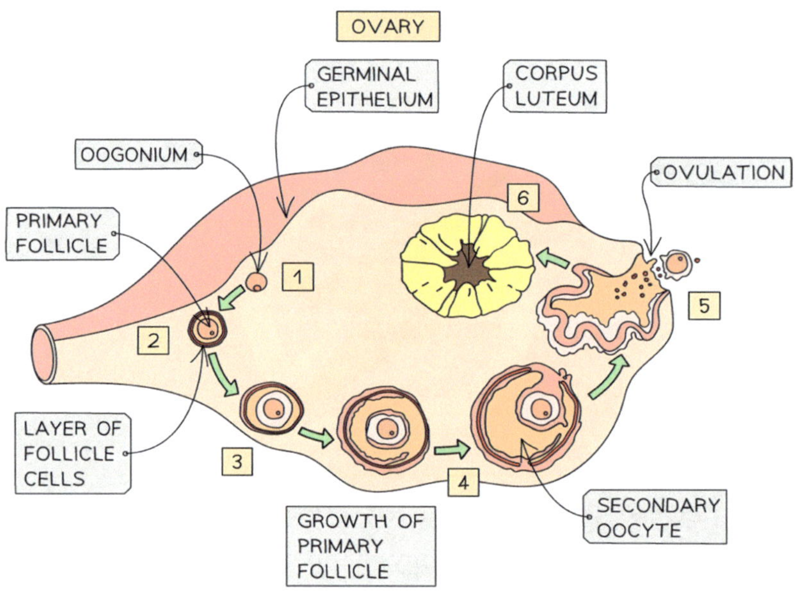

Figure 2.9. The process of oogenesis.

Source: https://www.tutoroot.com/blog/wp-content/uploads/2022/10/oogenesis-1.png.

This pause is crucial; it helps ensure that, in most cases, a mature egg is released periodically so that genes can pass on to the next generation. As the egg continues its journey toward maturity, a combination of larger body processes and specific molecular cues takes effect. Around each primary oocyte, follicles gather; these little structures supply vital nutrients and signals (sometimes even redundant cues) to guide its progress. FSH, for example, plays a significant role by pushing the growth of granulosa cells and helping to form a fluid-filled pocket known as an antrum. Recent studies, in most cases, point to long noncoding RNAs as subtle regulators that might tweak follicle development and enhance the egg's competence. However, exactly how they do so remains an active research question (Wichman et al., 2017). On top of that, a delicate balance between gene expression and environmental factors profoundly influences fertility outcomes. Levels of various microRNAs (miRNA) appear to shift at different stages of oocyte development, thereby offering precise—but not always perfectly consistent—checks and balances along the way. In zebrafish, for instance, specific germ plasm miRNAs have been identified that appear to facilitate the initiation of these key PGCs and promote overall gamete development (Zhang et al., 2017). All this suggests new directions for examining how eggs mature, indicating that both genetic programming and external signals are part of a complex, intertwined process affecting reproductive health (Figure 2.9).

2.3.1. Stages of Oogenesis

Oogenesis begins as a complex, multistep process. PGCs first split to become oogonia, which then start collecting all kinds of cytoplasmic materials—a sort of preparation phase for later changes. At this point, these oogonia gradually morph into primary oocytes, and that's when meiosis is set into motion. Interestingly, these oocytes pause in prophase I until ovulation occurs. Generally speaking, this long pause can open the door for de novo mutations to occur early in the process, mutations that may later affect offspring in unexpected ways (Rocío Acuña-Hidalgo et al., 2016). Primary oocytes soon become part of a larger picture through follicular development. Instead of following a neat, step-by-step plan, these cells embed within ovarian follicles, which provide a mix of essential hormones and a supportive microenvironment. Gonadotropins play a significant role here, stimulating follicle growth and, by extension, influencing the quality and quantity of oocytes. Then, somewhat unpredictably, the shift happens: primary oocytes turn into secondary ones at ovulation as meiosis resumes and reaches metaphase II. For the most part, however, the oocyte holds off on finishing meiosis unless it meets a sperm. All in all, the endgame of oogenesis comes together in a remarkably fine-tuned way. Once fertilization occurs, the secondary oocyte completes meiosis rapidly, resulting in a mature ovum paired with a polar body; this division of cytoplasmic components appears designed to support early embryonic life. It's interesting how this cyclic process in females stands in stark contrast to the more continuous rhythm of spermatogenesis, each following its quirky blueprint for reproduction. These nuances not only shed light on fertility challenges but also point toward possible interventions when genetic mishaps—like de novo mutations arising in gametes—come into play (Michael, 2015) (Figure 2.10).

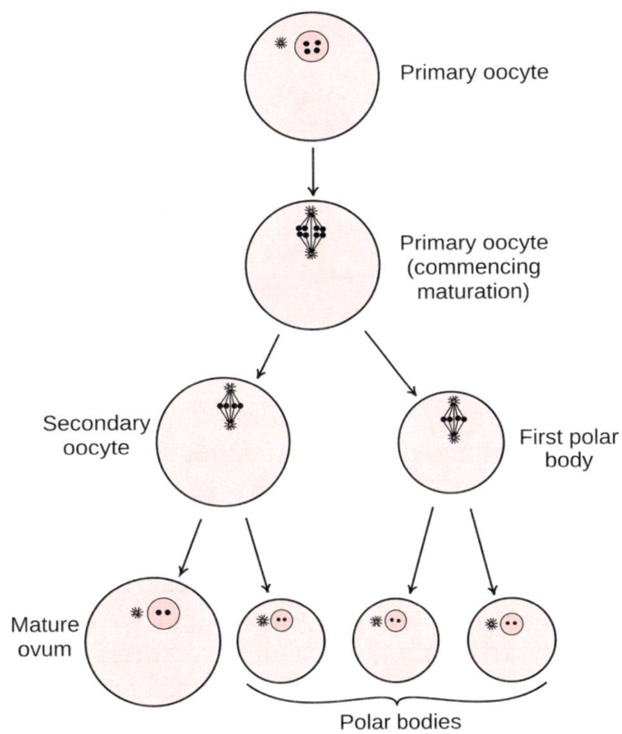

Figure 2.10. Stages of oogenesis.

Source: https://upload.wikimedia.org/wikipedia/commons/thumb/4/44/Gray5.svg/260px-Gray5.svg.png.

2.3.2. Hormonal Regulation of Oogenesis

Developing oocytes is no simple feat—it relies on a tight hormonal dance that makes everything work. Nuclear receptors are the key figures here, and recent findings suggest that Hormone receptor 4 (Hr4) plays a crucial role in *Drosophila* oogenesis. Hr4 plays a significant role not only in the ovary but also in tissues like muscles, where it helps maintain germline stem cells and promotes follicle growth. When Hr4 isn't doing its job, more GSC dropouts and stunted follicle formation are seen, which drives home how intertwined hormonal signals are with oogenesis. In most cases, examining the inner workings of nuclear receptors like Hr4 can provide insight into the complex mechanisms that regulate female gametogenesis (Lesley et al., 2021).

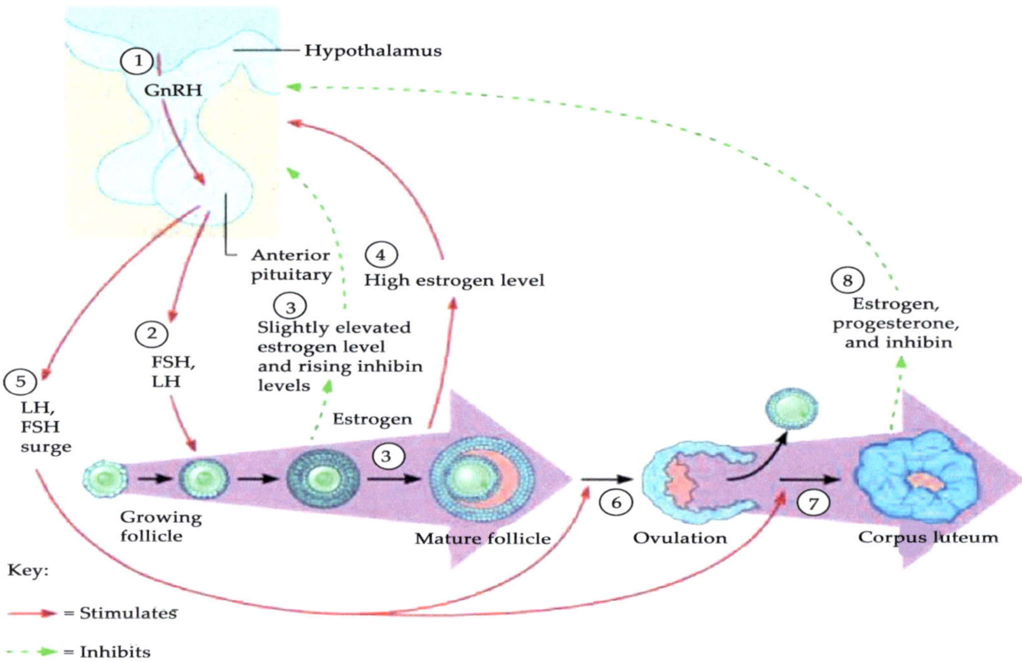

Figure 2.11. Hormonal regulation of oogenesis.

Source: https://external-content.duckduckgo.com/iu/?u=https%3A%2F%2Fimage.slidesharecdn.com%2Fhumandevbio-141002060804-phpapp02%2F95%2Fhuman-developmental-biology-11-638.jpg%3Fcb%3D1412230222&f=1&nofb=1&ipt=79b09450a8074397a294ec787b33efde52f23d5dcaa73fa6b358abe0973e86a3.

Hormones run the show in oogenesis beyond just quick genetic tweaks—they bring along a host of environmental and body-wide signals. Take estrogen and progesterone, for example. Although we usually associate them with vertebrates, these hormones also play a significant role in maturing oocytes and regulating follicle dynamics. They not only boost follicle growth but also help regulate the ovulation schedule. Often, when environmental cues (like shifts in temperature or light) come into play, they tip the hormonal balance and end up affecting reproductive success. Examining how various hormonal signals interact with ovarian structures provides a more comprehensive and nuanced understanding of gametogenesis—a perspective that's particularly useful when considering evolutionary adaptations in reproductive strategies (Ubeda-Manzanaro et al., 2016). In aquaculture and fisheries, the way hormones regulate oogenesis is crucial for managing and safeguarding fish stocks. Hormones, in conjunction with environmental factors such as temperature and day length, can influence spawning behaviors and impact gametogenesis in fish. Research on genes like Brdt—touted as a regulator in this process—suggests the need for a closer examination of their roles during oocyte development across various aquatic species. Grasping these subtle hormonal influences not only helps improve reproductive outcomes but also shapes better plans for species conservation in today's changing environments. All in all, the complex interplay of hormones and gametogenesis continually reminds us why ongoing, in-depth research in this area is so essential (Ubeda-Manzanaro et al., 2016) (Figure 2.11).

2.3.3. Comparison of Oogenesis to Spermatogenesis

Gametogenesis doesn't follow one strict rule—it works in its quirky ways for each sex. Males keep producing sperm non-stop; their bodies are busy in the seminiferous tubules where germ cells are always on call, and each round of division typically wraps up by churning out four mature sperm cells. Females, by comparison, start life with a limited stash of oocytes, so their process is more of a cycle. Every month, one primary oocyte is selected to resume its division, but it halts at metaphase II until a fertilization spark arrives. This difference in timing and numbers generally illustrates how evolution has tailored each reproductive strategy to the body's needs in humans and other mammals. When one looks closer at cell division and differentiation, the splits between these two methods become even more apparent. In most cases, spermatogenesis transforms one diploid spermatogonium into four haploid sperm cells through two rounds of meiosis, a strategy that relies on sheer numbers and genetic diversity.

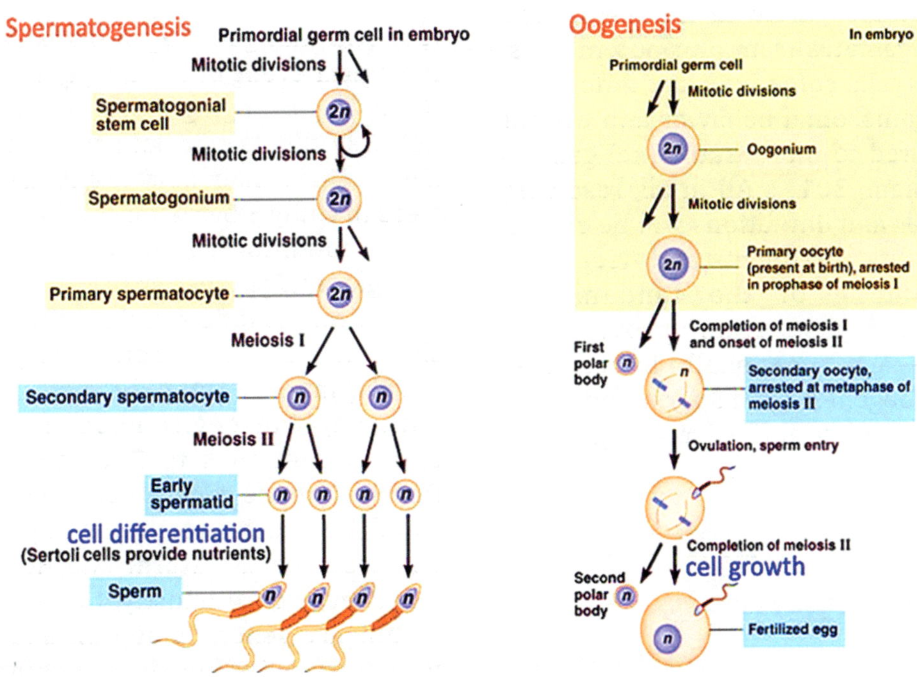

Figure 2.12. Difference between spermatogenesis and oogenesis.

Source: https://www.vedantu.com/seo/content-images/a2523eeb-f508-4243-b1dc-8039db5bb707_1..png.

In contrast, oogenesis takes a less equal route—its asymmetric splits produce a single, hefty ovum while shunting away extra cytoplasm into polar bodies, which eventually get discarded. This lopsided approach, although it may seem odd, ensures the ovum contains the right resources for development after fertilization. Essentially, these differences—one emphasizing quantity and the other quality—highlight adaptive strategies that influence fertility and success. Research still suggests that many details of how these processes operate remain unclear and require further *in vivo* and *in vitro* investigation (Stuart, 2014). Recent progress in reproductive technologies and genetic research has begun to reveal how these natural processes might be manipulated or even recreated outside the body. Even though scientists have managed to generate functional gametes in the lab, noticeable gaps remain between these *in vitro* creations and their naturally produced counterparts. Such gaps raise some pretty pivotal questions about genetic soundness and the subtle epigenetic cues at play. Studies indicate that while it's possible to get gametes from pluripotent cells, these lab-made cells sometimes act differently in terms of chromosomal behavior and overall viability compared to more traditional gamete production (Boiani, 2017). All in all, resolving these differences and limitations will be crucial to refining fertility treatments and deepening our understanding of the fundamental biology behind reproduction, providing a more nuanced—and occasionally imperfect—picture of how oogenesis and spermatogenesis contribute to the process (Figure 2.12).

2.4. Genetic Variation in Gametogenesis

Gametogenesis is, in many ways, a complex process that contributes significantly to the genetic diversity observed in nature. When cells set out to become gametes, they undergo meiosis. In this process, events like crossing over and independent assortment occur, much like a card shuffle, yielding a diverse array of unique allele combinations. It's this natural remixing that boosts diversity, not just in how organisms look, but also in how they navigate environmental challenges. Often, slight shifts in reproductive strategies emerge in response to local stressors, hinting that the very act of gametogenesis hides a lot of adaptive potential. Across species, the way genetic variation unfolds during gametogenesis tends to be linked to each organism's background - its history and the environment it inhabits. Take, for example, findings from studies on *Diphasiastrum digitatum* in the Eastern U.S. Here, it turns out that water regimes and other environmental factors matter a great deal more than mere geographic separation. Generally speaking, shifts in habitat or climate don't just scramble the rules; they steer genetic divergence in unexpected ways, opening up challenges and, at times, fresh evolutionary avenues.

It shows that gametogenesis isn't just a sterile biological event but is deeply interwoven with the living, changing world around us. And it's not only plants that join the genetic shuffle—animals have their story to tell. Research on larch trees in chilly Siberia, for example, suggests that harsh conditions, such as blistering cold and drought, nudge these species into making subtle yet crucial genetic tweaks. In most cases, such shifts help fine-tune both their physiology and development, equipping them better to deal with ongoing environmental stress. As our climate continues to fluctuate unpredictably. Delving into the genetic details of gametogenesis could be crucial to predicting which species will weather the storm and how biodiversity might evolve. Ultimately, this link between an organism's genetic blueprint and its ecological backdrop underlines just how intertwined life truly is (Figure 2.13).

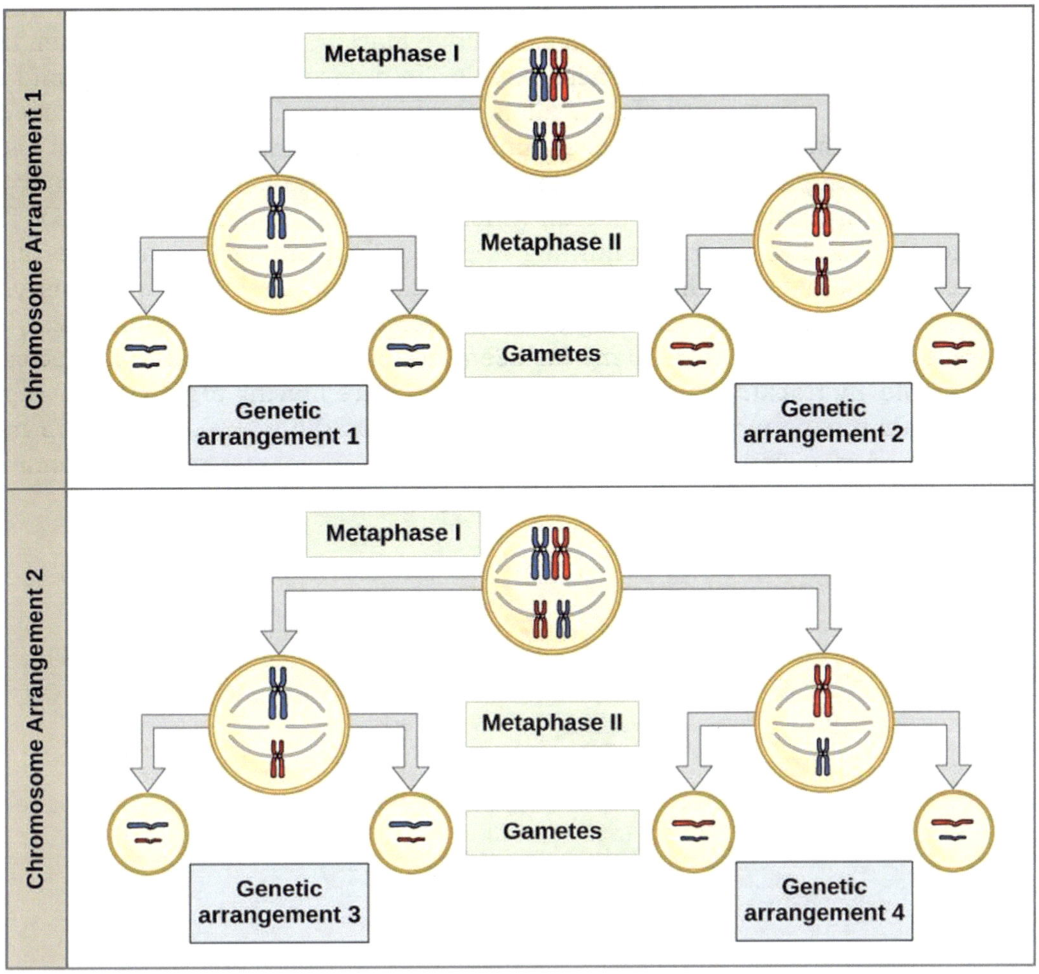

Figure 2.13. Genetic variation in gametogenesis.

Source: https://files.mtstatic.com/site_44 63/15921/0?Expires=1746679019&Signature=l19tIdE1qI7jhDFafh4D4TI7SZM8pRlu9DC1LT1ScyG AC14yqrHs0DJotwBImjeL GaYPfPbTEB5uOTwHISYGiz7TWSaW Gv2c 3eBzSkVft3YdgMh mL6AmeIPY~lc5we VOSXxhWegprX~E9aJ4vk4xv- a293w6I8ezQw2ale~OLFQ_&Key-Pair-Id=APKAJ5Y6AV4GI7A555NA.

2.4.1. Meiosis and Its Role in Genetic Diversity

Meiosis fuels genetic diversity by mixing up genes in creatures that reproduce sexually. It begins with two rounds of cell division—each time resulting in gametes that contain only half the chromosomes of the parent. This "halving" isn't just about reducing numbers; it reorders genetic material via crossing over and independent assortment, giving rise to new gene blends in offspring. Some research suggests that, in most cases, the balance between sexual and asexual reproduction matters when it comes to overall diversity. For example, studies with yeast show that when meiotic events are rare, the genome's variation tapers off, which underlines meiosis's key role in generating genetic variety (Ollivier et al., 2025). Looking a bit deeper into the process reveals that the mechanics of meiosis are tied up with how genes are regulated and diversified. Take histone modifications, for instance—they play a significant role in homologous recombination and influence the creation of crossovers. In *Arabidopsis*, active marks, such as H3K4me3, tend to appear near sites where recombination occurs. These tweaks help chromosomes line up and segregate correctly, while also sparking the mix of new allele combinations through crossing over. In many cases, mutants that lack these modifications exhibit abnormal chromosome behavior and reduced fertility. Generally speaking, understanding these biochemical details sheds light on how meiosis enhances both genetic diversity and the overall fitness of species (Singh et al., 2025). The effects of meiosis extend well beyond a simple shuffling of genes. That mix of genetic material is crucial for natural selection, enabling populations to adapt to changing environments. This variety can make a real difference—sometimes assisting communities to bounce back from stress, and other times, if the process falters or is infrequent (as seen in some facultative sexual species), leaving them more vulnerable. By tracking these trends, researchers are piecing together how reproductive strategies and genetic mixing work together to shape the incredible spread of life. In most cases, this is why the role of meiosis in creating gametes and driving genetic diversity remains a topic of ongoing academic discussion (Ollivier et al., 2025) (Figure 2.14).

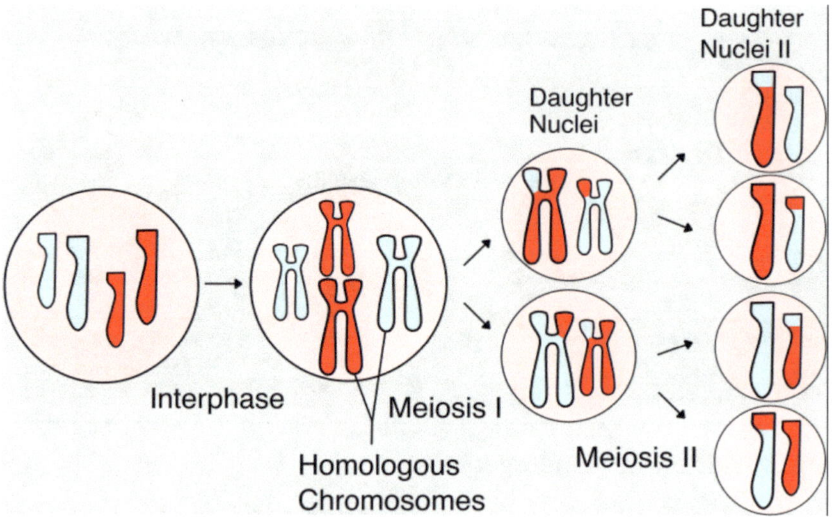

Figure 2.14. Meiosis and its role in genetic diversity.

Source: https://upload.wikimedia.org/wikipedia/commons/thumb/9/96/Meiosis_Overview_new.svg/800px-Meiosis_Overview_new.svg.png.

2.4.2. Crossing Over and Independent Assortment

Gametogenesis isn't just a sterile process of reproduction—it's where gene-swapping kicks off a whole mix of outcomes. In prophase I, homologous chromosomes pair up and then exchange small DNA fragments, a process known as crossing over. This swap, which typically creates new allele combinations, often increases the genetic diversity of the gametes. In most cases, this increased variability gives a population a bit of extra resilience, helping it adjust when the environment suddenly shifts. Although crossing over is a well-known phenomenon, its intricate details can sometimes lead to unpredictable genetic twists that, in a way, are crucial to evolution. In doing so, crossing over not only enriches the gene pool but also nudges the evolutionary path of species in unexpected directions. Then there's independent assortment—a mechanism that also has its quirky role. During metaphase I, the chromosomes line up in a somewhat random order, meaning that maternal and paternal bits end up getting shuffled together in surprising ways. For instance, in species with many chromosomes, the number of possible mixes is almost endless, resulting in offspring that sport distinct phenotypes. In most cases, this kind of randomness can even influence which traits are expressed, contributing to both genetic stability and adaptability. When alleles separate on, it creates room for novel genetic makeups that are crucial for a species to adapt to shifting circumstances. Combining these two processes effectively sets the stage for a dynamic genetic landscape. They aren't merely about swapping genetic pieces—these processes serve as the building blocks for a population's evolutionary success, delivering a unique blend of traits in each new generation. This unique mosaic, after all, can mean the difference between thriving and struggling in environments that change quickly or push competition to the limit. Generally speaking, as these mechanisms unfold, they help lay the foundation for both the individual's ability to adapt and the species' broader evolutionary journey. Ultimately, this unpredictable interplay highlights the crucial role genetic diversity plays in enabling life to continue evolving, despite its sometimes chaotic nature (Figure 2.15).

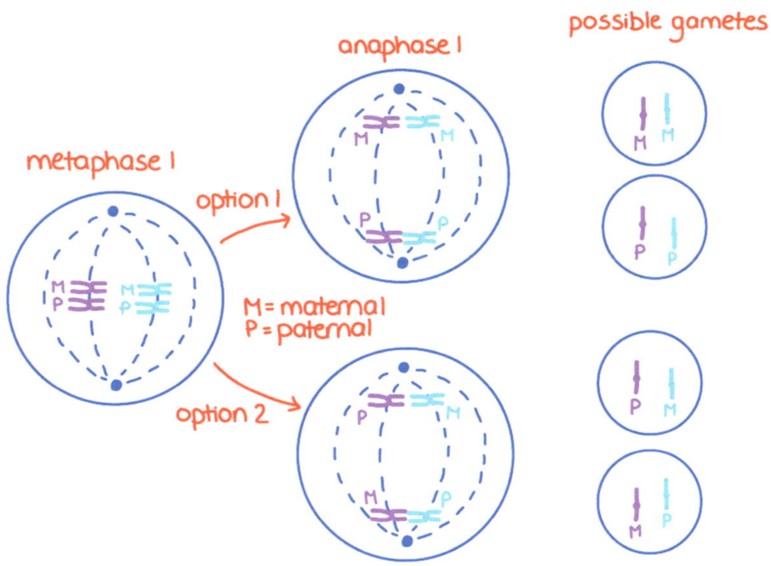

Figure 2.15. Crossing over and independent assortment.

Source: https://i0.wp.com/zhtutorials.com/wp-content/uploads/2024/04/Independent-assortment.png?fit=911%2C670&ssl=1.

2.4.3. Implications for Evolution and Adaptation

Gametogenesis—it's at the heart of how species reproduce, and the mix of steady genetic systems and more flexible traits seems to shape evolutionary wins. Plants, for instance, sometimes show a firm side in the architecture of their reproductive parts, yet they can also adjust rather unexpectedly when faced with changes outside. This curious blend—stable structure on one hand and adaptive reaction on the other—helps them juggle resources during gamete formation, which in most cases boosts their overall fitness. When one looks a bit closer at these processes, one starts to see why many believe that much of evolution hinges on just how changeable developmental routes can be (Li et al., 2025). Interestingly, this insight not only deepens our understanding of how plants manage reproduction but also sparks ideas for agricultural tweaks, potentially improving crop yields and resilience by fine-tuning genetics to meet specific challenges. Evolution doesn't play out only within a single species—it ripples through entire populations and even shapes diversity broadly. In many cases, adaptations like gametogenesis reveal how organisms counter pressures such as food shortages, shifting weather patterns, or habitat disturbances. Take animal species: strategies like calorie restriction (CR) highlight how the body's processes might reconfigure metabolism under stress, prioritizing survival while still leaving room for reproduction when times improve. This ability to subtly adjust reproductive output in response to environmental cues reveals a clear link between gamete production and broader ecological survival strategies; in effect, energy-saving tactics and efficient cellular operations become crucial for maintaining populations in a changing world (Kumar, 2025). When creatures navigate the complex, ever-changing environment around them, the evolutionary importance of gametogenesis becomes apparent. The inherent blend of rigidity and adaptability in reproductive strategies enables many species to flourish in vastly different habitats over the long term. Peeking into the workings behind gamete development reveals clues at both microscopic and larger, system-wide levels. Indeed, exploring the genes that lend stability, as well as those that permit flexibility, not only builds a framework for understanding evolutionary shifts but also feeds directly into methods for boosting crop resilience and sustainability in farming. All in all, this back-and-forth dance of adaptation and evolution appears critical for withstanding environmental stress, reinforcing that deep, intricate relationship between gametogenesis and evolutionary mechanisms (Li et al., 2025).

2.5. Disorders Related to Gametogenesis

Studies examining gamete formation have shown that when development goes off track, various disorders can emerge. Sometimes gamete creation gets disrupted, which can lead to issues like cryptorchidism—when a male's testicles fail to settle where they should. Some research even hints that if expectant mothers are exposed to chemicals like BPA and parabens, it might raise the odds of this condition. For example, high BPA levels in a mother's blood early on have been linked with both birth-related and later-developing cases, as noted in Benjamin et al. (2020). Grasping these links is pretty essential since it points out a growing worry about environmental toxins messing with reproductive health, especially when a fetus is most at risk. There's also a broader spectrum of male reproductive issues tied to gamete production that seem to be on the rise. Research suggests that exposure to endocrine disruptors can disrupt normal testicular development, leading to abnormal changes in genital tract formation. These problems can show up in different ways – like a shorter gap in the anogenital area or even a smaller penile length – and have been repeatedly connected to maternal chemical exposure during pregnancy. Some studies, however, encounter challenges such as small sample sizes or other confounding factors that make drawing firm conclusions somewhat difficult. All in all, identifying these problems underscores the need for more in-depth research into how the environment influences gametogenesis, not just for immediate issues but also for potential effects across generations. Furthermore, the ripple effects of these developmental mishaps extend far beyond reproduction; they also impact maternal and child health overall. The way a mother's health interacts with her chemical exposures demonstrates the need for comprehensive strategies to mitigate these risks. Generically speaking, recent analyses point out striking disparities in maternal mortality rates, which are often swayed by social and demographic factors that later affect reproductive outcomes. Upping access to quality reproductive care—along with stricter regulations on harmful exposures—is essential for mitigating these kinds of risks. Addressing these intertwined challenges may not only improve reproductive outcomes but also contribute to achieving broader health goals worldwide, as seen in the ongoing efforts highlighted in Kassebaum et al. (2017).

2.5.1. Infertility Issues in Males and Females

Infertility is a heavy challenge many couples face—it blends biology, everyday life habits, and even what's in our environment. Gametogenesis, the process that forms eggs and sperm, is crucial for our reproductive health, yet when something goes wrong—say, when PGCs don't create or migrate as they should—the whole process can break down. Bad habits like poor nutrition, substance abuse, or constant stress throw hormones off balance, adversely affecting both sperm creation and egg production.

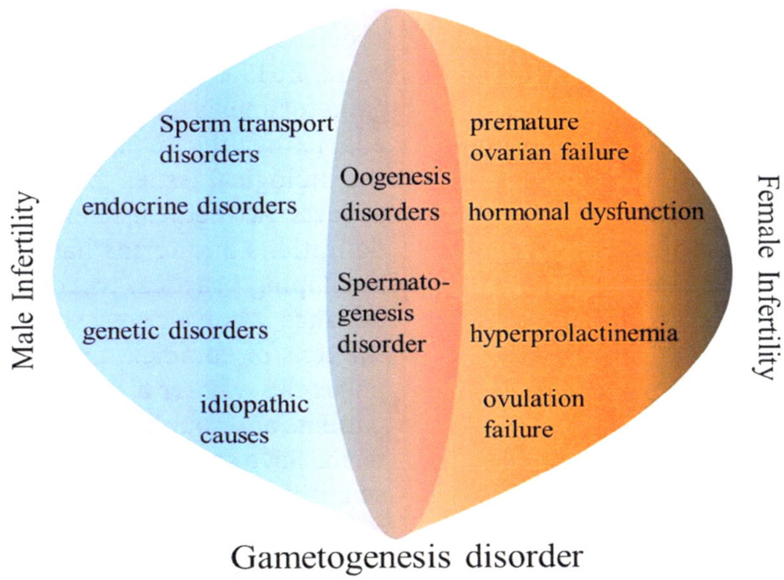

Figure 2.16. Infertility issues in males and females.

Source: https://www.researchgate.net/publication/354509598/figure/fig1/AS:1066581257891840@1631304196048/Main-causes-of-infertility.png.

Generally speaking, understanding how these processes falter is key if we're going to address infertility effectively. It isn't just a personal struggle either; infertility comes with a heavy emotional load and is increasingly seen as a public health puzzle that needs more research and public awareness. Various factors contribute to its rise – congenital quirks and the side effects of cancer treatments (like chemotherapy and radiation) can weaken germ cell health, thereby messing with an individual's ability to conceive. Recent studies, delving into the molecular workings behind gametogenesis, suggest possible new therapies. For instance, emerging reproductive tech might allow for preserving germ cells before treatments even start—keeping the door open for future parenthood. In most cases, this mixed approach reminds us that tackling infertility means looking at both biological challenges and the social, even psychological, repercussions. Taking a broader look, understanding gametogenesis in all its messy details has become essential. Rather than focusing solely on basic cell production, one must also consider how local signals—paracrine and autocrine cues—guide germ cell development. Environmental toxins, everyday dietary choices, and a host of external pressures can disrupt the delicate balance necessary for proper gametogenesis. Current literature even suggests that combining our insights on germ cell dysfunction with socio-behavioral adjustments may pave the way for more effective fertility strategies. By addressing both the inner workings of our bodies and the outside influences, the scientific community can open doors to fresh treatment options and stronger support systems, ultimately helping couples pursue their dreams of starting a family and fostering a healthier society (Figure 2.16).

2.5.2. Genetic Disorders Arising from Gametogenesis

Gametogenesis sits at the core of reproduction, passing on genetic material while occasionally messing up in ways that lead to disorders. Mistakes in forming gametes can sometimes spawn genetic quirks—think Down syndrome, Turner syndrome, or even Klinefelter syndrome. Often, these issues crop up because chromosomes don't split as expected during meiosis, leaving some gametes with an odd number. When such gametes meet at fertilization, the resulting zygote ends up with an unusual chromosomal mix that can significantly disrupt development and overall health. Generally speaking, understanding how gametogenesis unfolds is crucial for identifying these issues and developing strategies to mitigate their impact in reproductive medicine. Genetic disorders emerging from gametogenesis have far-reaching effects that ripple out beyond the health of a single person. They can upend family dynamics and even shift societal structures, bringing along challenges like physical disabilities, bumps in cognitive abilities, and emotional strains that hit everyone involved. In many cases, the long-term burden on healthcare—from ongoing treatments to therapies and special education—can be pretty heavy. Plus, there's the social stigma that sometimes comes bundled with these disorders, which can isolate affected individuals or lead to discrimination. For these reasons, there has been a growing push to establish more explicit definitions around infertility and fertility care—a consensus-driven glossary now helps bridge the gap between patients, healthcare providers, and researchers (Zegers-Hochschild et al., 2017). Clearing up the language around gametogenesis and its related genetic disorders enables healthcare professionals to address both the biological issues and the deeper emotional aspects. As medical science advances, updating definitions and terms has played a crucial role in shaping practical treatment approaches. For instance, when we start seeing infertility through the lens of complex gametogenic anomalies, it paves the way for a more supportive setting for patients and couples. Efforts to standardize these terms have shown promise, not only sharpening scientific debate but also ensuring that people affected by these conditions receive care that encompasses every aspect of their well-being (Zegers-Hochschild et al., 2017). All in all, this broad and flexible approach underscores the need for ongoing research and adaptation in our understanding of gametogenesis.

2.5.3. Environmental Factors Affecting Gametogenesis

The connection between the environment and gametogenesis is central to how species reproduce. Temperature, for instance, plays a significant role in steering the metabolic processes that build gametes. In many marine bivalves, even small temperature changes can tweak reproductive hormones and affect gonadal formation. One study on the turkey-wing mussel – a reliable example in most cases – showed that temperature swings throughout the seasons have a profound influence on the metabolic buildup leading to spawning. In winter, lower temps often bring on a kind of pause in gonadal development, underscoring temperature as a significant factor for timing and efficiency in gametogenesis. These seasonal patterns compel species to adjust their reproductive strategies, enabling them to enhance their potential while conserving energy (Sarkis et al., 1992). Food availability is another key player that impacts gametogenesis by affecting how energy and vital nutrients are stored. When the turkey-wing mussel faces a lean food supply during essential growth spells, there isn't enough nutrient storage to support gamete production. Interestingly, these mussels sometimes manage to survive nutritional stress by tweaking their metabolism—a subtle but telling sign of the link between their surroundings and reproductive output. Seasonal shifts in food supply can dictate when gametogenesis occurs, and over time, organisms have evolved varied strategies to take advantage of plentiful resources while enduring challenging times, ensuring their ongoing survival (Sarkis et al., 1992). Internal biological rhythms, combined with external environmental cues, add yet another layer of complexity. Many organisms have developed molecular mechanisms that enable them to sense shifts in their environment and adjust their reproductive timing accordingly. Research on blue mussels, for example, generally indicates that changes in light and temperature can influence so-called clock genes, which then help regulate their reproductive cycles. This kind of coordination—though it may seem subtle—is crucial for synchronizing gamete release with the optimal conditions for fertilization. Matching internal timing to external signals enables these creatures to capitalize on favorable moments, which is especially important in today's rapidly changing climate, where even minor disruptions could disrupt gametogenesis and impact overall ecosystem health.

2.6. Advances in Gametogenesis Research

Gametogenesis is a topic that's receiving a fresh look these days, with scientists finding that epigenetic tweaks—such as DNA methylation and histone modifications—appear to be more important than previously thought. Instead of sticking to the usual textbook explanations, researchers now note that these changes help determine which genes get switched on during both sperm and egg development, and, consequently, can affect the quality of the gametes. It turns out that everyday choices—what one eats, how stressed one is—might subtly alter these marks, hinting that lifestyle counts when it comes to reproduction. In most cases, this new perspective has shifted the field's perspective on infertility, opening up promising new therapeutic ideas (Safti et al., 2024). At the same time, there has been a growing interest in how DNA damage influences gametogenesis. Maintaining DNA integrity is crucial for producing healthy gametes, making factors such as aging, oxidative stress, and exposure to toxins significant concerns for oocyte quality. Some studies show that even minor breaches in DNA integrity can lead to problems with fertility and even cause embryos to fail. Researchers are, in many cases, exploring ways to enhance the natural repair mechanisms in oocytes—an approach that could be a game changer for women battling diminished ovarian reserve or other fertility issues (Xiu-Xu et al., 2024). Sometimes the complexity of these mechanisms surprises many in the field, which means there's still plenty to explore. And it doesn't stop there. Advances in our understanding of gametogenesis are spilling over into broader issues of reproductive health, especially in ART. By piecing together how gametes develop step by step, experts are gaining insights that might streamline techniques like IVF. When genetic and epigenetic studies merge in real-world medical practices, it could lead to improved methods for selecting the most viable gametes and enhancing overall success rates. Researchers from molecular biology to reproductive medicine are increasingly drawn to this interdisciplinary approach, which, generally speaking, makes the field ripe for innovation. As science continues to evolve, turning these fresh insights into everyday clinical strategies becomes increasingly crucial for tackling the challenges of infertility (Safti et al., 2024; Xiu-Xu et al., 2024) (Figure 2.17).

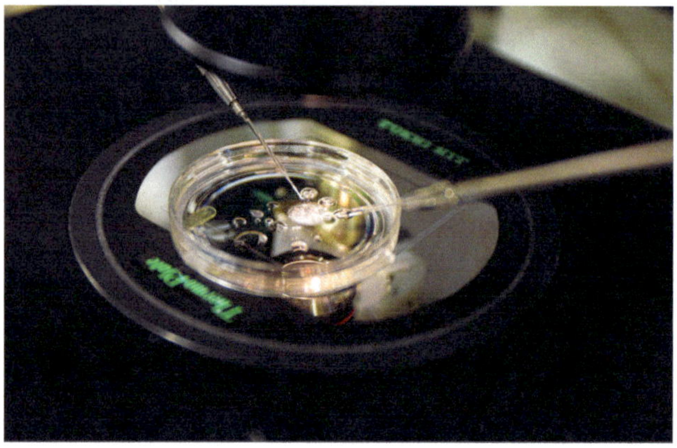

Figure 2.17. Gametogenesis Research.

Source: https://s3.amazonaws.com/cms.ipressroom.com/296/files/20242/20240305+Haploid+study+-+Mitalipov3.jpg.

2.6.1. Stem Cell Research and Gametogenesis

Recent stem cell breakthroughs have unlocked some truly innovative ways to mimic the natural process of gamete formation—even if it's all happening in a laboratory setting. Scientists in the field of *in vitro* gametogenesis (IVG) are working to transform pluripotent stem cells into functional gametes, a development that could significantly transform fertility treatments and reproductive technology. For example, some studies have successfully produced mice that came from two mothers or two fathers, demonstrating that these lab-created gametes can indeed lead to successful reproduction. This kind of progress offers hope not only in tackling infertility—especially for same-sex couples and women facing age-related fertility decline—but also sets the stage for applications in conservation and even genetic disorder prevention (Cho et al., 2023). Gametogenesis is a complex puzzle where every step, from cell multiplication to differentiation, matters—a fact that makes stem cell technology all the more valuable. Recent work in *in vitro* spermatogenesis (IVS) has revealed just how intricate this process can be. Scientists are often challenged by the need to recreate the particular environment of the testes that supports cell growth and maturation. To overcome this, many researchers have turned to instruments such as bioreactors and microfluidic systems, which help establish conditions that closely mimic what occurs in living tissues. Additionally, advances in tissue engineering are gradually opening up new avenues for studying spermatogenesis under laboratory conditions, thereby enhancing both basic research and potential clinical applications aimed at improving male fertility (Cho et al., 2023). On the other hand, while stem cell-derived gamete technology holds immense promise, it also raises a host of ethical questions that require careful consideration. The idea of using induced pluripotent stem cells to generate viable gametes naturally raises issues about what this could mean for human-assisted reproduction. Even though these developments may one day alter our entire perspective on reproduction, the prevailing view is that, for now, applying such techniques to humans is hindered by moral and safety concerns. Experts generally agree that significant biological and technical hurdles remain, suggesting that using these methods in reproductive medicine may be a long way off—likely not for at least a decade. It seems only prudent to start grappling with these ethical challenges now, ensuring our debates keep pace with the rapid advances in gametogenesis.

2.6.2. Assisted Reproductive Technologies (ART)

Reproductive medicine has been changing a lot lately, and assisted reproduction is feeling that shift in surprising ways. New methods like IVF first gave real hope to people who struggled with infertility—suddenly, there were more options on the table. This breakthrough not only expanded our understanding of conceiving a child, but it also helped reveal how reproductive cells develop, shedding light on the delicate interplay of hormones and genetic signals at play. In most cases, examining how ART relates to the natural process of gamete formation reveals the intricate connection between these biological details, and researchers are now shifting toward developing treatments that align more closely with individual health profiles (Megibl, 2024). Fertility approaches, including techniques like intracytoplasmic sperm injection (ICSI), continue to evolve, proving especially useful for overcoming specific male infertility issues, and they tend to lift overall chances of pregnancy. It's interesting—these strategies not only improve outcomes for couples facing challenges but also open doors for a broader range of people, such as same-sex couples and single individuals who want to start a family. Using donor gametes or even surrogacy, these newer methods blur the lines of traditional family concepts, making the idea of parenthood a much broader, more inclusive notion. Social, ethical, and legal dilemmas are now part of the conversation as we grapple with the implications of these changes for reproductive autonomy and family formation (Chen et al., 2023). Beyond improving individual reproductive outcomes, ART is carving out its role in the arena of reproductive genetics. Genomic research is providing us with fresh insights into congenital conditions and other reproductive disorders—insights that may lead to improved pre-implantation genetic screening, enabling the selection of embryos unlikely to carry certain inherited issues. These genetic breakthroughs don't just affect individual cases; they may also influence public health strategies related to reproduction. Blending scientific, ethical, and societal views, this steadily broadening approach makes it clear that advances in assisted reproduction support not only individual families but also the long-term well-being of future generations (Chen et al., 2023; Megibl, 2024) (Figure 2.18).

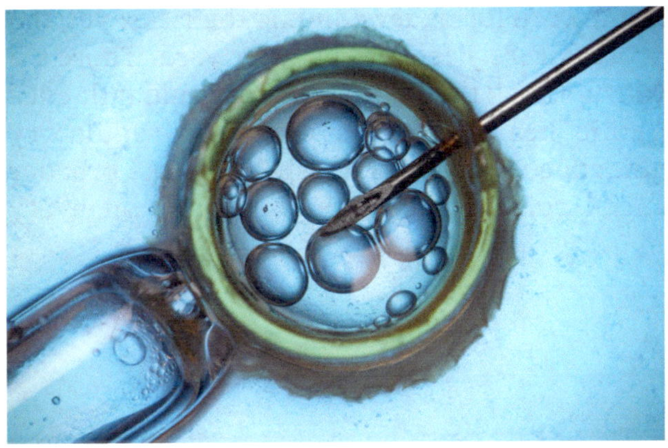

Figure 2.18. Assisted reproductive technology.

Source: https://medlineplus.gov/images/AssistedReproductiveTechnology_share.jpg.

2.6.3. Ethical Considerations in Gametogenesis Research

Gametogenesis research has surged in recent years, sparking a host of ethical quandaries that aren't easily pinned down. Researchers are now tinkering with embryo genetics, and—a curious twist—this raises a divide between changes that affect a person's overall health versus those that fundamentally shape who they are (Sparrow, 2021). It seems like altering genetic material isn't just about fixing health issues; it can, quite unexpectedly, redefine a person's identity. One may find that determining whether these interventions impact an individual's future autonomy or merely their immediate well-being has become a moral tug-of-war. And then there's the non-identity challenge, which leaves us asking if it's ever right to bring a person into existence under conditions that might not offer them a clear benefit. On a different note, exploring male reproductive toxicity throws a whole new batch of ethical puzzles into the mix. Scientists, while examining the impact of various chemicals, find themselves in a tricky balancing act—pursuing scientific inquiry without jeopardizing male reproductive health. They identify critical key traits of potential toxicants (Arzuaga et al., 2019) and use these clues to establish a framework for understanding the risks; yet, the process rarely feels straightforward. There's a constant risk that these findings could influence public health policies or shape regulatory guidelines, and, generally speaking, the broader social consequences weigh heavily on every decision made along the way. Then there's the matter of informed consent—a fundamental cornerstone in this kind of research. It isn't enough to just run the experiments; participants need to be informed about what's at stake, including the procedures involved, potential risks, and all possible outcomes when their gametes are manipulated or their genes are tweaked. This insistence on clarity, even if it is a bit messy at times, underlines the notion that real transparency allows people to make truly informed choices about their involvement in studies that might affect not only their reproductive futures but also the lives of generations to come. Ethical oversight, whether it stems from specific regulations or institutional boards, must safeguard these interests while still allowing innovation to progress—a balance that remains as challenging as it is necessary.

SUMMARY

Gametogenesis offers a glimpse into the very nuts and bolts of reproduction—revealing clues not just for biology buffs but also for practical applications in fields like medicine and conservation. The way germ cells grow and change reveals some fundamental life principles, yet it also suggests new approaches for enhancing fertility. For example, tinkering with *in-vitro* methods might revamp treatments for those facing infertility and even boost genetic diversity among at-risk species. Environmental factors, too, appear to influence gamete quality, providing additional insights into how to enhance reproductive success in both humans and wildlife. All told, these scattered insights suggest we need to keep poking around in the cellular details to get what's going on. Next-generation sequencing now enters this scene, opening doors to understanding gene behavior in ways we never thought possible. Generally speaking, using this high-speed technology allows scientists to piece together gene networks that steer germ cell formation, identifying pathways that quietly regulate fertility. It not only digs deep into our internal blueprints but also helps flag biomarkers tied to reproductive challenges. This new tech, by informing precision medicine in reproductive health (Satam et al., 2023), nudges a slow but steady transformation in how we view gametogenesis and the broader realm of reproductive research. Drawing insights from ecology and evolution, the study of gametogenesis weaves an unexpected thread between cellular detail and the broader environmental context. Natural stresses and energetic limits, for instance, can directly affect how gametes form and survive—giving us a rough sketch of how species might either adapt or falter as ecosystems shift. Researchers, by examining these bioenergetic pressures and assorted stressors, gradually build a picture of population resilience under real-world pressures. This not only enriches our basic biological understanding but also steers conservation strategies that desperately need to adapt in our rapidly changing world (Inna, 2013). Gametogenesis initiates the transformation of simple germ cells into the key players—sperm and eggs—that enable sexual reproduction. Instead of following a neat, predictable plan, this process juggles meiosis to shuffle genes and mix up the genetic deck, ensuring diversity in a way that feels almost spontaneous. Hormones from areas like the hypothalamus and pituitary, in most cases, help shape the course of events; this hormonal push and pull, essential for maintaining balance, influences traits such as how well sperm swim and how robust an egg develops. Recent work, which delves into both cell-level details and overall body responses, now offers clues that may explain some infertility issues. In a sense, every discovery not only opens doors for better reproductive treatments but also hints at broader benefits for regenerative medicine, making the in-depth study of gametogenesis a key pursuit. Creating functional gametes depends on a series of interdependent cellular happenings that don't follow one strict order. Meiosis plays a starring role by splitting homologous chromosomes into single sets—a move that preserves our genetic blueprint across generations. Then there's the genetic recombination aspect, that casual yet crucial remixing of DNA, which increases genetic diversity and fuels evolution. Some studies even suggest that the immediate environment surrounding developing gametes—the microenvironment—can unpredictably alter how these cells mature. Factors such as oxidative stress or even slight hormonal imbalances may, at times, disrupt gamete quality, a nuance that keeps researchers on their toes. By probing these influences further, scientists hope to snag specific biomarkers and eventually design targeted interventions to boost fertility outcomes in clinical settings. The study of gametogenesis, however, isn't confined to cellular biology—it extends into developmental biology and broader medical fields. Insights from this area often inform therapeutic strategies for various reproductive disorders and contribute to the treatment of cancers associated with germ cell issues.

CLOSER LOOK

PLATYNEREIS DUMERILII

Platynereis dumerilii is a marine annelid worm widely used as a model organism in developmental biology, neurobiology, and evolutionary studies. Belonging to the class Polychaeta, this segmented worm is found in shallow coastal waters, particularly in the Northeast Atlantic and the Mediterranean Sea. Its popularity in scientific research stems from its relatively simple anatomy, transparent larval stages, and well-characterized life cycle, which make it particularly suitable for microscopic observation and experimental manipulation. *P. dumerilii* has become a valuable system for studying ancestral traits of bilaterians—organisms with bilateral symmetry—due to its position in the evolutionary tree as a slow-evolving species that retains many features of the last common ancestor of most animals. Because of this, it is an essential comparative model for comprehending the development of the nervous system, gene regulation, and photoreception..

The life cycle of *Platynereis dumerilii* includes both sexual and larval stages, beginning with external fertilization, where eggs and sperm are released into the seawater. Fertilized eggs develop into trochophore larvae, which are free-swimming and ciliated, allowing researchers to observe early developmental processes such as gastrulation and organ formation. These larvae later metamorphose into juvenile worms and eventually mature into sexually reproductive adults. One of the key features of this species is its strong phototactic behavior, accompanied by the presence of various light-sensitive structures, including simple eyes (ocelli) and photoreceptor cells in the brain and trunk. This has made *P. dumerilii* particularly useful for studying the evolution and function of light detection and circadian rhythms. It also responds to lunar cycles in the wild, synchronizing reproduction with the phases of the moon, which provides insights into chronobiology and the response to environmental cues.

In molecular biology, *P. dumerilii* has been instrumental in studying gene expression patterns, particularly those related to Hox genes and other conserved developmental regulators. The transparency of its embryos allows for *in vivo* imaging of gene activity and cell lineage tracing. Researchers have also used it to study the development of the nervous system, thanks to its relatively simple yet well-organized neural architecture, which includes a ventral nerve cord and a brain with distinct regions. It has also helped elucidate the evolution of neurotransmitters and sensory systems, offering parallels to both invertebrate and vertebrate species. Recent advances in genomic tools, including CRISPR/Cas9 gene editing and transcriptomics, have further enhanced the utility of *P. dumerilii* as a model organism.

Platynereis dumerilii serves as a bridge between traditional invertebrate models, such as *Drosophila*, and vertebrate systems, including zebrafish and mice, making it invaluable for comparative evolutionary studies. Its primitive yet informative biological features provide a window into ancestral developmental pathways and gene networks conserved across animal species. As molecular techniques continue to evolve, this marine worm will likely remain a cornerstone of research into evolution, development, and neurobiology, shedding light on the deep genetic and physiological connections that unite diverse life forms.

REFERENCES

1. Acuña-Hidalgo, R., Veltman, J. A., & Hoischen, A. (2016). New insights into the generation and role of de novo mutations in health and disease. *Genome Biology, 17*, Article 241. https://doi.org/10.1186/s13059-016-1110-1.
2. Adl, S. M., Bass, D., Lane, C. E., Lukeš, J., Schoch, C. L., Смирнов, A. B., Agatha, S., et al. (2018). Revisions to the classification, nomenclature, and diversity of eukaryotes. *Journal of Eukaryotic Microbiology, 66*(1), 4–119. https://doi.org/10.1111/jeu.12691.
3. Arzuaga, X., Smith, M. T., Gibbons, C. F., Skakkebæk, N. E., Yost, E. E., Beverly, B., Hotchkiss, A. K., et al. (2019). Proposed key characteristics of male reproductive toxicants as an approach for organizing and evaluating mechanistic evidence in human health hazard assessments. *Environmental Health Perspectives, 127*(9), 096001. https://doi.org/10.1289/ehp5045.
4. Galla, G., Vogel, H., Sharbel, T. F., & Barcaccia, G. (2015). De novo sequencing of the Hypericum perforatum L. flower transcriptome to identify potential genes that are related to plant reproduction sensu lato. *BMC Genomics, 16*(1). https://doi.org/10.1186/s12864-015-1439-yBellido, A., Distéfano, A., Setzes, N., Cascallares, M. M., Oklestková, J., Novák, O., Ramirez, J., et al. (2022). A mitochondrial ADXR–ADX–P450 electron transport chain is essential for maternal gametophytic control of embryogenesis in *Arabidopsis. Proceedings of the National Academy of Sciences of the United States of America, 119*. https://www.semanticscholar.org/paper/49aa8591d80ac02ebbac95c799af0d7bd2501564 (accessed on 26 May 2025).
5. Bharti, D., Tikka, M., Lee, S. Y., Bok, E. Y., Lee, H. J., & Rho, G. J. (2021). Female germ cell development, functioning and associated adversities under unfavorable circumstances. *International Journal of Molecular Sciences, 22*, 1979. https://doi.org/10.3390/ijms22041979.
6. Bharti, D., Tikka, M., Lee, S. Y., Bok, E. Y., Lee, H. J., & Rho, G. J. (2021). Female germ cell development, functioning and associated adversities under unfavorable circumstances https://doi.org/10.20944/preprints202101.0307.v1.
7. Boiani, M. (2017). Call for papers: *In vitro*-generated germ cells—facts and possibilities. *Molecular Human Reproduction, 23*(1), 1–3. https://www.semanticscholar.org/paper/bde8f9ef9728b79149c5b5a52b494f899fb5d0d4 (accessed on 26 May 2025).
8. Chang, Z., Miao, L., & Wang, P. (2025). Mitochondrial ribosome regulation drives spermatogenesis and male fertility. *Biology of the Cell, 117*(2), e12007. https://www.semanticscholar.org/paper/893cc98a714d05cca8d3f47b532579f58f8edc13 (accessed on 26 May 2025).
9. Chapman, E. C. (2019). *The Molecular Basis of Circadian and Seasonal Rhythms in The Blue Mussel Mytilus edulis*. https://core.ac.uk/download/556180898.pdf (accessed on 26 May 2025).
10. Chen, X., Shi, H., Li, C., Zhong, W., Cui, L., Zhang, W., Geng, L., et al. (2023). The effect of SARS-CoV-2 infection on human embryo early development: A multicenter prospective cohort study. *Science China Life Sciences*. https://www.semanticscholar.org/paper/363b46cd44ce427112d1908df7858ce16307273d (accessed on 26 May 2025).
11. Cho, I. K., & Easley, C. A. (2023). Recent developments in *in vitro* spermatogenesis and future directions. *Reproductive Medicine, 4*(3), 215–232. https://doi.org/10.3390/reprodmed4030020.
12. Cho, I., & Easley, C. A. (2023). Recent developments in *in vitro* spermatogenesis and future directions. *Reproductive Medicine*. https://www.semanticscholar.org/paper/511ad42dd6ac3d42cff02c0dbbcecfdfcd612df2 (accessed on 26 May 2025).

13. Delbès, G., Levacher, C., & Habert, R. (2006). Estrogen effects on fetal and neonatal testicular development. *Reproduction, 132*(4), 527–538. https://doi.org/10.1530/rep.1.01231.

14. Diamanti-Kandarakis, E., Bourguignon, J. P., Giudice, L. C., Hauser, R., Prins, G. S., Soto, A. M., Zoeller, R. T., et al. (2009). Endocrine-disrupting chemicals: An Endocrine Society scientific statement. *Endocrine Reviews, 30*(4), 293–342. https://doi.org/10.1210/er.2009-0002.

15. Fisher, B. G., Thankamony, A., Mendiola, J., Petry, C., Frederiksen, H., Andersson, A., Juul, A., et al. (2020). Maternal serum concentrations of bisphenol A and propyl paraben in early pregnancy are associated with male infant genital development. *Human Reproduction*. https://www.semanticscholar.org/paper/d9315dce4540661e6571834d22a551fed267546c (accessed on 26 May 2025).

16. Griswold, M. D. (2015). Spermatogenesis: The commitment to meiosis. *Physiological Reviews, 96*(1), 1–17. https://doi.org/10.1152/physrev.00013.2015.

17. Hojsgaard, D. (2018). Transient activation of apomixis in sexual neotriploids may retain genomically altered states and enhance polyploid establishment. *Frontiers in Plant Science, 9*, 230. https://doi.org/10.3389/fpls.2018.00230.

18. Horer, S., Feichtinger, M., Rosner, M., & Hengstschläger, M. (2023). Pluripotent stem cell-derived *in vitro* gametogenesis and synthetic embryos—It is never too early for an ethical debate. *Stem Cells Translational Medicine, 12*, 569–575. https://www.semanticscholar.org/paper/9b3f2c8d7e055f7bdf12a927389cdf5d53856b8e (accessed on 26 May 2025).

19. Huang, X., & Sun, M. X. (2024). Cell fate determination during sexual plant reproduction. *The New Phytologist*. https://www.semanticscholar.org/paper/24e007a450b68a0140f395ab9f66de8c0b19b296 (accessed on 26 May 2025).

20. Jang, S. W., Kim, Y. R., Han, J. H., Jang, H., & Choi, H. W. (2024). Generation of mouse and rat xenogeneic ovaries *in vitro* for production of mouse oocyte. *Animal Cells and Systems, 28*(4), 303–314. https://www.semanticscholar.org/paper/d33b4eea44a2d5b5d5d8a3290059b3d7c9143bb4 (accessed on 26 May 2025).

21. Kassebaum, N., Barber, R., Bhutta, Z., Dandona, L., Gething, P., Hay, S., Kinfu, Y., et al. (2017). Global, regional, and national levels of maternal mortality, 1990–2015: A systematic analysis for the Global Burden of Disease Study 2015. *Obstetrical & Gynecological Survey*. https://www.semanticscholar.org/paper/1a5d8e3f695a549252b3b8e229440e1eb70f74b0 (accessed on 26 May 2025).

22. Kumar, A. (2025). Evolutionary implications and health consequences of calorie restriction: A review. *Asian Journal of Research in Zoology*. https://www.semanticscholar.org/paper/7fbc601f2d38bc9aac071b97c5e97df725f71c1d (accessed on 26 May 2025).

23. Kyryk, V. (2024). Stem cell therapy for cardiac regeneration: Key points. *Cell and Organ Transplantology*. https://www.semanticscholar.org/paper/6a1b536f3691ad0d162e4187a4a2e2ffd1507b5f (accessed on 26 May 2025).

24. Li, P., An, Z., Xu, N., Li, J., Li, Q., & He, C. (2025). Phenotypic plasticity and stability in plants: Genetic mechanisms, environmental adaptation, evolutionary implications, and future directions. *Plant, Cell & Environment*. https://www.semanticscholar.org/paper/44e86d1f6a16ca82ef3d9b20ac73961ad8a7bdf3 (accessed on 26 May 2025).

25. Li, X., Zhu, B., Lu, Y., Zhao, F., Liu, Q., Wang, J., Ye, M., et al. (2024). DNA methylation remodeling and the functional implication during male gametogenesis in rice. *Genome Biology, 25*. https://www.semanticscholar.org/paper/e9f0aaf0ccaaa8b7cf4794e2993f7c4040f451cb (accessed on 26 May 2025).

26. Luxton, S., Smith, G. S., Williams, K. J., Ferrier, S., Bond, A. J., & Prober, S. (2024). An introduction to key ecological concepts, financial opportunities, and risks underpinning aspirations for nature positive. *Bioscience, 74*(5), 450–466. https://www.semanticscholar.org/paper/b0c920d49a771423336d6ddbb89994c4e881b37d (accessed on 26 May 2025).

27. Megibl, H. R. (2024). New horizons in understanding and developing treatments for human reproductive physiology. *International Journal of Pharmaceutical and Bio-Medical Science*. https://www.semanticscholar.org/paper/4bb7dd1099ef008971b1655b38e4b8987f8e1885 (accessed on 26 May 2025).

28. Meucci, S., Kruse, S., Haupt, S., Stoof-Leichsenring, K., Krutovsky, K., Bernhardt, N., Harpke, D., et al. (2025). Biological processes underlying genetic adaptation of larches to cold and dry winter conditions in Eastern Siberia. *Ecology and Evolution, 15*. https://www.semanticscholar.org/paper/e090933c273d3cfe8c2054b9d45e76e18867265f (accessed on 26 May 2025).

29. Nowicki, M., Houston, L. C., Boggess, S., Huff, M., Staton, M. E., & Trigiano, R. (2025). Integrative analysis of *Diphasiastrum digitatum* Holub: Unveiling genetic variation and ecological adaptations for sustainable ecosystem management. *Ecology and Evolution, 15*. https://www.semanticscholar.org/paper/b68a8bf185ff74b59d2b64774736df94bfb8a5c8 (accessed on 26 May 2025).

30. Ollivier, L., Charlesworth, B., & Pouyet, F. (2025). Beyond recombination: Exploring the impact of meiotic frequency on genome-wide genetic diversity. *bioRxiv*. https://www.semanticscholar.org/paper/a1cc38010da3f61b8f408b74fefabb6334b7eae4 (accessed on 26 May 2025).

31. Papežík, P., Aschengeschwandtnerová, S., Benovics, M., Dedukh, D., Doležálková-Kaštánková, M., Choleva, L., Javorčík, A., et al. (2025). A pattern of hybridization and population genetic structure of two water frog species (Ranidae, Amphibia) in the southwestern Balkans. *Zoological Scripta*. https://www.semanticscholar.org/paper/dfd6cdbef94348cd2a9ea5422fbdf3e71f7a293d (accessed on 26 May 2025).

32. Pepino, M. M. C., Manalili, S. E., Sekida, S., Mezaki, T., Okumura, T., & Kubota, S. (2024). Gene expression profiles of Japanese precious coral *Corallium japonicum* during gametogenesis. *PeerJ, 12*. https://www.semanticscholar.org/paper/4641094d5cd53c34ee87615a3b7e0e00ed742c6e (accessed on 26 May 2025).

33. Piprek, R. P., Kloc, M., Mizia, P. C., & Kubiak, J. Z. (2020). The central role of cadherins in gonad development, reproduction, and fertility. *International Journal of Molecular Sciences, 21*, 8264. https://doi.org/10.3390/ijms21218264.

34. Piprek, R. P., Kloc, M., Mizia, P. C., & Kubiak, J. Z. (2020). The central role of cadherins in gonad development, reproduction and fertility. *Preprints*. https://doi.org/10.20944/preprints202010.0037.v1.

35. Ribeiro, R. P., Null, R. W., & Özpolat, B. D. (2025). Sex-biased gene expression precedes sexual dimorphism in the agonadal annelid *Platynereis dumerilii*. *Development*. https://www.semanticscholar.org/paper/8d77b33cb60a70dc0439dd0748d9fe3e4836245a (accessed on 26 May 2025).

36. Saftić Martinović, L., Mladenić, T., Lovrić, D., Ostojić, S., & Dević Pavlić, S. (2024). Decoding the epigenetics of infertility: Mechanisms, environmental influences, and therapeutic strategies. *Epigenomes, 8*(3), 34. https://doi.org/10.3390/epigenomes8030034.

37. Sarkis, S. C. (1992). *The Turkey-Wing Mussel, Arca Zebra: Aspects of its Ecology, Reproduction and Physiology in Bermudan Waters* [Master's thesis, University of Bermuda]. CORE. https://core.ac.uk/download/29818746.pdf.

38. Satam, H., Joshi, K., Mangrolia, U., Waghoo, S., Zaidi, G., Rawool, S., Thakare, R. P., et al. (2023). Next-generation sequencing technology: Current trends and advancements. *Biology, 12*(7), 997. https://doi.org/10.3390/biology12070997.

39. Sharma, S., Venzac, B., Burgers, T. C. Q., Le Gac, S., & Schlatt, S. (2020). Microfluidics in male reproduction: Is *ex vivo* culture of primate testis tissue a future strategy for ART or toxicology research? *Molecular Human Reproduction, 26*(3), 179–192. https://doi.org/10.1093/molehr/gaaa006.

40. Singh, A. K., Chowdary, K. A., & Shen, W. (2025). SDG8 and HUB2 depositing euchromatin histone marks play important roles in meiosis and crossing-over regulation. *The Plant Journal: For Cell and Molecular Biology, 121*(3), e17241. https://www.semanticscholar.org/paper/8a6fbf04464c50200cbfe36488fb5238132cbe7b (accessed on 26 May 2025).

41. Sokolova, I. M. (2013). Energy-limited tolerance to stress as a conceptual framework to integrate the effects of multiple stressors. *Integrative and Comparative Biology, 53*(4), 597–608. https://doi.org/10.1093/icb/ict028.

42. Sparrow, R. (2021). Human germline genome editing: On the nature of our reasons to genome edit. *The American Journal of Bioethics, 22*(1), 4–15. https://doi.org/10.1080/15265161.2021.1907480.

43. Stuart, D. (2014). Sorting out meiosis. *Cytometry Part A, 85*, 369–370. https://www.semanticscholar.org/paper/2ecab16a788cc678eca6dda860f3923bf095ab6a (accessed on 26 May 2025).

44. Tang, A., Zhang, X., Dinh, M., & Cambria, E. (2024). Prompted aspect key point analysis for quantitative review summarization. *arXiv*. https://www.semanticscholar.org/paper/ed73a37eb5200c4864e622947c4299886cdfe7a1 (accessed on 26 May 2025).

45. Ubeda-Manzanaro, M., Ortiz-Delgado, J., & Sarasquete, C. (2016). The bromodomain testis-specific gene (Brdt) characterization and expression in gilthead seabream, *Sparus aurata*, and European seabass, *Dicentrarchus labrax. European Journal of Histochemistry (EJH), 60*. https://www.semanticscholar.org/paper/91db17ea85882c8577d4277ef6ea373711ff0166 (accessed on 26 May 2025).

46. Verween, A. (2007). *Biological Knowledge as A Tool for An Ecologically Sound Biofouling Control: A Case Study of The Invasive Bivalve Mytilopsis leucophaeata in Europe* [Doctoral dissertation, University of Ghent]. CORE. https://core.ac.uk/download/55809652.pdf (accessed on 26 May 2025).

47. Weaver, L. N., & Drummond-Barbosa, D. (2021). Hormone receptor 4 is required in muscles and distinct ovarian cell types to regulate specific steps of *Drosophila* oogenesis. *Development, 148*. https://www.semanticscholar.org/paper/d8c41d9107a86a54065f90a40a0408ac5634beb2 (accessed on 26 May 2025).

48. Weedall, G. D., & Hall, N. (2014). Sexual reproduction and genetic exchange in parasitic protists. *Parasitology, 142*(S1), S120–S127. https://doi.org/10.1017/S0031182014001693.

49. Wendisch, M., Crewell, S., Ehrlich, S., Herber, A. B., Kirbus, B., Lüpkes, C., Mech, M., et al. (2024). Overview: Quasi-Lagrangian observations of Arctic air mass transformations–introduction and initial results of the HALO–$(\mathcal{AC})^3$ aircraft campaign. *Atmospheric Chemistry and Physics.* https://www.semanticscholar.org/paper/0b5321cfff1fdb9fc3b3a1447189499c8e324e40 (accessed on 26 May 2025).

50. Wichman, L., Somasundaram, S., Breindel, C., Valerio, D. M., McCarrey, J. R., Hodges, C. A., & Khalil, A. M. (2017). Dynamic expression of long noncoding RNAs reveals their potential roles in spermatogenesis and fertility†. *Biology of Reproduction, 97*(3), 313–323. https://doi.org/10.1093/biolre/iox084.

51. Xi, Y., Gong, C., Zhang, Z., Zhu, F., Zhang, Y., Tang, Y., Yan, L. H., et al. (2025). NAE1-mediated neddylation coordinates ubiquitination regulation of meiotic recombination during spermatogenesis. *Theragnostic, 15*(11), 3122–3142. https://www.semanticscholar.org/paper/c2d73e475fa9d9d51166b51741f2be3758e72a36 (accessed on 26 May 2025).

52. Xu, X. H., Wang, Z., Lv, L., Liu, C., Wang, L., Sun, Y., Zhao, Z., et al. (2024). Molecular regulation of DNA damage and repair in female infertility: A systematic review. *Reproductive Biology and Endocrinology, 22*, Article 41. https://doi.org/10.1186/s12958-024-01273-z.

53. Zegers-Hochschild, F., Adamson, G. D., Dyer, S., Racowsky, C., de Mouzon, J., Sokol, R. Z., Rienzi, L., et al. (2017). The international glossary on infertility and fertility care, 2017. *Fertility and Sterility, 108*(3), 393–406. https://doi.org/10.1016/j.fertnstert.2017.06.005.

54. Zegers-Hochschild, F., Adamson, G. D., Dyer, S., Racowsky, C., de Mouzon, J., Sokol, R. Z., Rienzi, L., et al. (2017). The International Glossary on Infertility and Fertility Care, 2017. *Human Reproduction, 32*(9), 1786–1801. https://doi.org/10.1093/humrep/dex234.

55. Zhang, J., Li, Y., Luo, S., Cao, M., Zhang, L., & Li, X. (2021). Differential gene expression patterns during gametophyte development provide insights into sex differentiation in the dioicous kelp *Saccharina japonica*. *BMC Plant Biology, 21*. https://www.semanticscholar.org/paper/ba977d5d622f835e93fef72eb0d18f86a16c4820 (accessed on 26 May 2025).

56. Zhang, J., Liu, W., Jin, Y., Jia, P., Jia, K., & Yi, M. (2017). MiR-202-5p is a novel germ plasm-specific microRNA in zebrafish. *Scientific Reports, 7*, Article 2290. https://doi.org/10.1038/s41598-017-07675-x.

57. Zhu, Q., Sun, J., An, C., Li, X., Xu, S., He, Y., Zhang, X., et al. (2024). Mechanism of LncRNA Gm2044 in germ cell development. *Frontiers in Cell and Developmental Biology, 12*. https://www.semanticscholar.org/paper/92733180054e2ad19304182d62caceac54b84b61 (accessed on 26 May 2025).

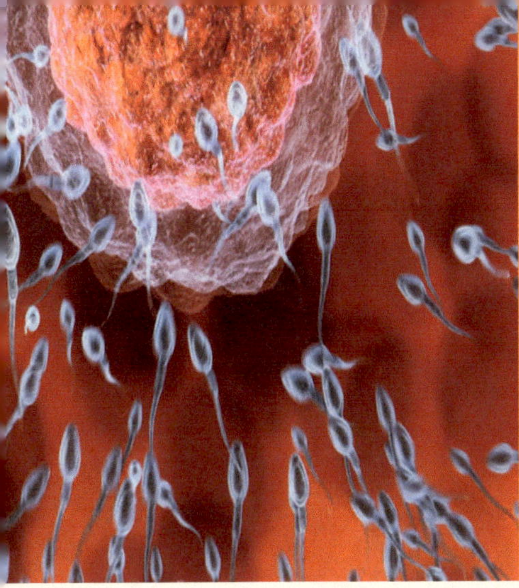

Chapter 3
FERTILIZATION

Contents

Introduction

Life starts on the cellular level – a spark in tiny, unseen places that sets reproduction and growth in motion. Fertilization, for example, isn't just two gametes coming together; it jumps off a whole cascade of interactions where genetic bits from two different organisms mix in sometimes unexpected ways. Researchers have probed these phenomena using tools from molecular biology, genetics, and evolutionary ideas, attempting to unravel a complex network of events. Grasping these basics gives us a glimpse into how living things persist and adapt to their surroundings – a fact that matters in everything from farming practices to medicine. Taking a closer look reveals that the sperm meeting the egg isn't just a random encounter – it's regulated by a host of specific proteins and signaling methods that steer what happens next. Breakthroughs in microscopy and biochemistry have enabled scientists to capture these events in real time, revealing that successful fertilization depends on a complex interplay of factors that sometimes unfolds in a surprising rhythm. There's also that twist with oxidative stress: too much oxidant exposure can damage cells, yet a little bit is just what's needed to set off key redox signals. This fine-tuned balance effectively confirms that cellular environments must be precisely set for reproduction to function correctly (Sies et al., 2017). Beyond the science, fertilization touches on debates that run deep in society today. With advances like *in vitro* fertilization (IVF) and gene editing on the rise, ethical questions about the moral status of embryos and what future generations might inherit get way too complex. People discuss topics such as informed consent for reproductive methods and the long-term implications of these new technologies. These debates shape both public policy and individual decisions. Ultimately, understanding how fertilization works not only enhances our grasp of biology but also sparks conversations about ethics and humanity's progress, making this subject an extensive and multifaceted exploration (Figure 3.1).

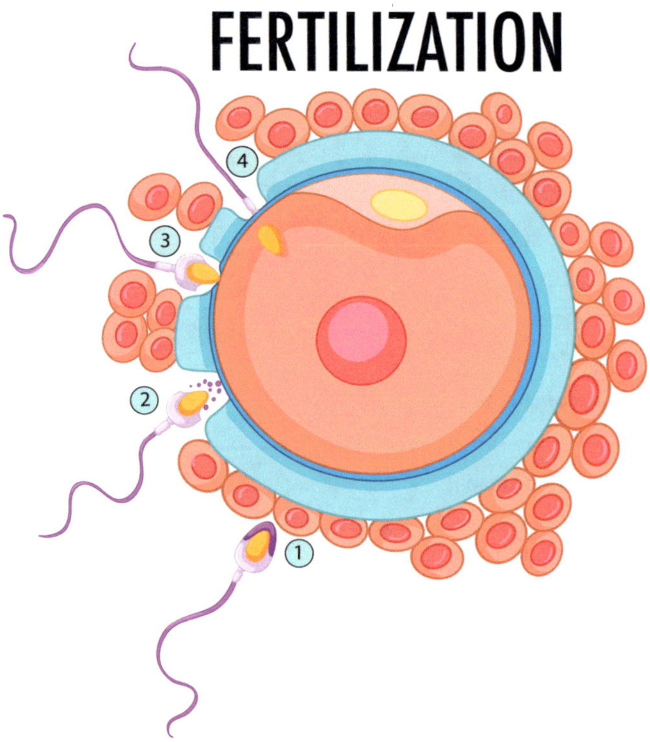

Figure 3.1. Understanding fertilization.

Source: https://ivfturkey.com/wp-content/uploads/2024/01/ui2j_pgz6_220218-scaled.jpg.webp.

Definition of Fertilization

Fertilization kicks off the whole reproductive process when male and female gametes get together—it's by no means just textbook jargon. In most cases, that union sparks the creation of a zygote, which then embarks on a remarkable, if intricate, journey toward forming a whole organism. The process isn't solely about the collision of gametes; it involves subtle physiological and molecular shifts that twist the simple act into something far more complex. Although these definitions may sound like academic buzzwords, they have a significant impact on how we approach fertility and even shape reproductive medicine. Recent discussions among experts suggest that clarifying our terminology can lead to more effective treatments and more apparent scientific progress. Looking deeper, a clear picture of fertilization matters beyond the lab—it ripples into health debates and even everyday discussions about society's challenges with fertility. Generally speaking, when we nail down the language, it's not just about what happens at the cellular level, but also about influencing clinical practices and public policy. There have been efforts to standardize the terms used across medical, scientific, and even casual conversations, partly because unclear language can obscure the fact that not every case of infertility is tied to a single disease (Richardson et al., 2023). This layered perspective, although it may seem repetitive at times, is key for both doctors and families trying to navigate the often complex world of reproductive health. There's also an environmental side to all this—fertilization isn't isolated from the world around it. At times, one might even say that the way gametes connect reflects broader links between nature and society. As human influences extend beyond ecological limits, disturbances in ecosystems can inadvertently alter fertility rates in many species (Richardson et al., 2023). It's quite fascinating: changes in the environment reverberate back on how organisms reproduce, which means that understanding fertilization today requires integrating insights from biology, environmental science, and public policy. Overall, a well-rounded approach helps us see that reproductive health issues are woven into both our natural world and the fabric of our daily lives.

Importance in Reproduction

Reproduction in mammals is a wild mix of hormones and body signals that work together—often in surprising, irregular ways—to make fertilization possible. In females, the ovaries produce hormones that initiate the menstrual cycle, which typically involves the gradual maturation of the egg over time. Then, as ovulation happens, the egg makes an unexpected journey over to the fallopian tubes, where—most times—fertilization takes place. It's like nature arranges a meet-up between sperm and egg in just the right setting to give birth to a zygote. Once that union occurs, the new zygote shifts into a kind of travel mode, heading toward the uterus, where a welcoming lining and a mix of hormones help it settle in; however, the process can sometimes feel a bit unpredictable. Understanding how these events unfold not only provides insight into human reproduction but also reveals clues about potential issues that may affect fertility; clearly, this warrants more in-depth research in reproductive biology and treatment options (Franc et al., 2022). Tiny microbial communities living in our reproductive systems play a crucial role in keeping things running smoothly, often in surprising ways. In both seminal and vaginal fluids, these little critters help maintain a balance that can influence sperm strength, movement, and even the entire fertilization process itself. The exchange of microbes during sexual reproduction—there occurs a natural microbial swap—which ends up shaping the landscape of fertility. Recent studies indicate that this process, in most cases, works much like random particle diffusion, affecting the evenness of these communities and possibly even smoothing the path for sperm movement and survival. In a way, these findings bridge the gap between the world of microbes and the broader context of reproductive biology, suggesting that there's still much to explore about how these relationships may impact fertility and our understanding of sexual reproduction (Ma, 2022). Reproduction reaches far beyond biological mechanics; it touches on health, family planning, and even our roles in society. Creating a new life is not just essential for species survival; it also plays a crucial role in shaping our emotions and the bonds within communities, with all the complex emotions that come with it. Advances in reproductive technology offer fresh hope for tackling infertility, though they also stir up ethical debates about autonomy and the changing shape of family ties. With a steadily evolving grasp on reproductive health—bolstered, in most cases, by breakthroughs in bioengineering and broad-based models—we're now looking at more personalized treatments that could boost the chances of a successful pregnancy. All things considered, as we navigate these complex and fascinating realms of reproduction, it becomes increasingly important to have candid and informed discussions about these advances and their implications for society as a whole (Franc et al., 2022) (Figure 3.2).

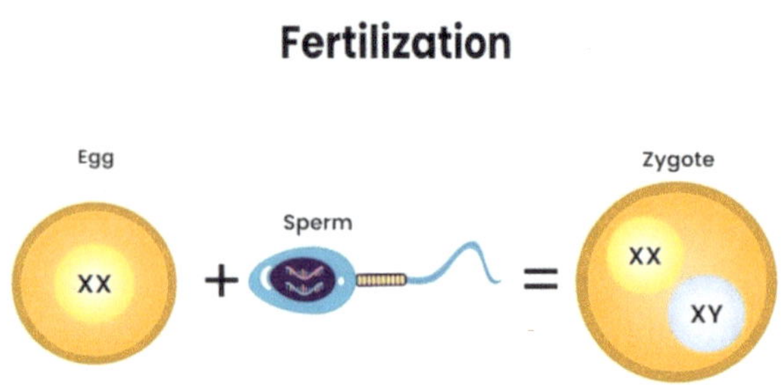

Figure 3.2. Fertilization importance in reproduction.

Source: https://external-content.duckduckgo.com/iu/?u=https%3A%2F%2Fimg.freepik.com%2Fpremium-vector%2Ffertilization-fusion-two-haploid-gametes-form-diploid-zygote-human-reproduction_530733-2144.jpg&f=1&nofb=1&ipt=ab3eee2b2ab98424b5469d52f8adca6a96a0f76a1075dc4da10e998c21b33402.

3.1. Types of Fertilization

Fertilization in nature comes in many flavors, each revealing a bit more about how species have adapted to their surroundings. Many water-dwelling creatures, like certain fish and amphibians, let their eggs and sperm float out into the environment—a process that happens outside the female body. Often, these events are triggered by cues such as temperature shifts or the phases of the moon; it's a method that enhances genetic diversity, yet it also comes with risks, such as predators or unexpected weather disrupting the process. In contrast, most land animals use internal fertilization. Here, sperm find refuge inside the female reproductive tract, creating a much safer environment and, in many cases, a better chance for offspring to survive. Moving deeper into reproductive biology, researchers have been paying close attention to epididymosomes—tiny vesicles from the epididymis that help get sperm ready for action. As sperm travel along, they pick up proteins and other molecules from these vesicles, which tweak their protein profiles and overall functionality. It's an intriguing adaptation; the proteins, some of which are key for mobility and successful fertilization, seem to fine-tune the whole process. In most cases, these findings underscore the sophistication of internal fertilization, with male reproductive systems playing a crucial role—a fact that recent studies have been eager to highlight. Examining fertilization from a broader perspective, the topic extends beyond simple biology—it also reveals insights into larger evolutionary trends. The various methods, whether external or internal, reveal a great deal about how organisms adapt to diverse ecological niches. For instance, understanding these differences can shed light on patterns in genetic diversity, shifts in population dynamics, and even correlations with cancer susceptibility (Joshua, 2022). Additionally, recognizing the cellular and systemic differences between the sexes that optimize reproductive outcomes suggests a deeper level of adaptation. Ongoing research continues to unravel these complexities, emphasizing that in biological and medical studies—including oncology, where sex differences matter—a nuanced view of fertilization strategies is essential (Barrachina et al., 2022).

3.1.1. External Fertilization

Many aquatic creatures initiate reproduction by releasing their gametes directly into the water. Eggs and sperm are let out nearly simultaneously—kind of a natural gamble to boost the chances they'll meet. Water conditions, such as temperature, salinity, and oxygen levels, significantly impact whether those gametes can remain viable long enough to perform their function. Researchers have noticed that some species even put on a sort of mating dance to help keep the timing in check. Sure, this method works well in vast, open water, although it also leaves gametes dangerously exposed to predators and unpredictable environmental changes. A bunch of fish and amphibians rely on external fertilization, and in doing so, they help keep the whole aquatic ecosystem buzzing with life. Their spawning events tend to align with natural cues—often lunar cycles or seasonal shifts—which demonstrates just how closely they are tied to their surroundings. This connection isn't just about the eggs and sperm meeting; it also influences the population dynamics in these watery habitats. In the 2018 edition of The State of World Fisheries and Aquaculture, it's noted that managing these populations properly is a key part of reaching overall environmental goals. Generally speaking, blending hands-on ecological insights with a concern for social fairness seems to support both species preservation and community well-being. At the same time, there's growing concern about how climate change and habitat degradation are disrupting all of this. Warmer temperatures and shifting waters might disturb the delicate timing needed for fertilization. Additionally, more pollutants—such as excess nutrients from agricultural runoff—could further compromise gamete viability and disrupt the health of entire ecosystems. Given these challenges, examining the process of external fertilization in greater detail is crucial for developing effective conservation strategies. As pointed out in the impacts of climate change on aquatic biodiversity, we need an approach that covers both natural and socio-economic angles. This type of layered understanding is crucial for helping species that rely on external fertilization remain resilient as their environment continues to evolve (Figure 3.3).

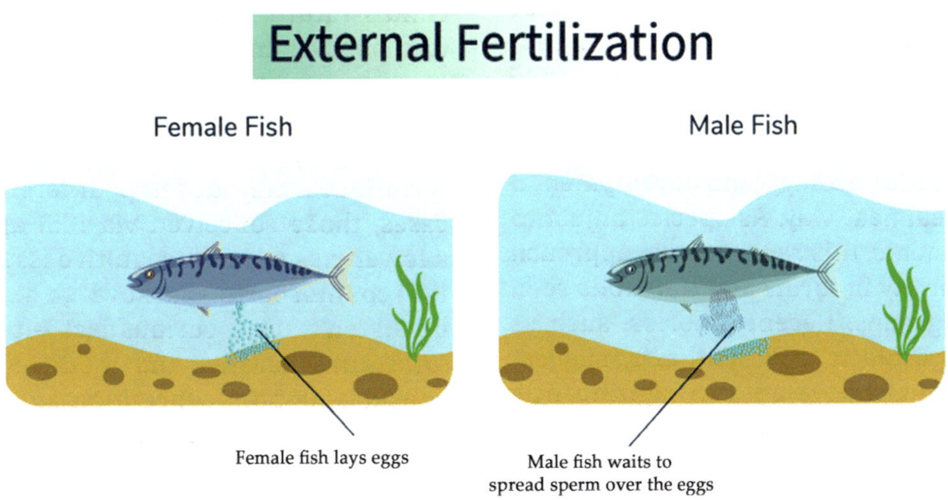

Figure 3.3. External fertilization.

Source: https://media.geeksforgeeks.org/wp-content/uploads/20240318174409/External-Fertilization.png.

3.1.2. Internal Fertilization

Reproductive strategies have evolved in ways that profoundly impact how species persist and adapt to change. Internal fertilization—think of it as sperm being delivered straight into the female tract—offers a kind of safe space for embryos to start, which boosts the odds of things working out. It's convenient on land, where exposing delicate gametes to the harsh outdoors can disrupt their development. In fact, by keeping fertilization sheltered and under control, this method illustrates how evolution, nature, and reproduction intersect; it's a topic that even evolutionary biologists find crucial (Kyrou et al., 2018).

What's even more interesting is the range of unique body tweaks that come up with internal fertilization. Take mammals, for instance; they have features like a uterus that not only acts as a nurturing spot but also allows gestation to last a bit longer, giving embryos more time to develop. This extra care often means that offspring have a better shot at surviving. Additionally, with sperm competition playing a role, a variety of adaptations have evolved in both male and female roles—shaping not only physical traits but also behaviors that help species manage their overall reproductive strategy (Kyrou et al., 2018). Looking at the big picture, internal fertilization ties together ideas from genetics, ecology, and developmental biology in a real neat way. As species adjust to their environments, this reproductive approach nudges the variety in forms and functions seen across many groups. Recent theories, such as the extended evolutionary synthesis, suggest that how animals develop can significantly influence evolution; here, internal fertilization isn't simply about making a baby—it's a complex interplay of genes and surroundings working together. Studying this process, then, provides a richer, albeit sometimes messy, insight into how organisms and their environments evolve and change over time (Kevin et al., 2015) (Figure 3.4).

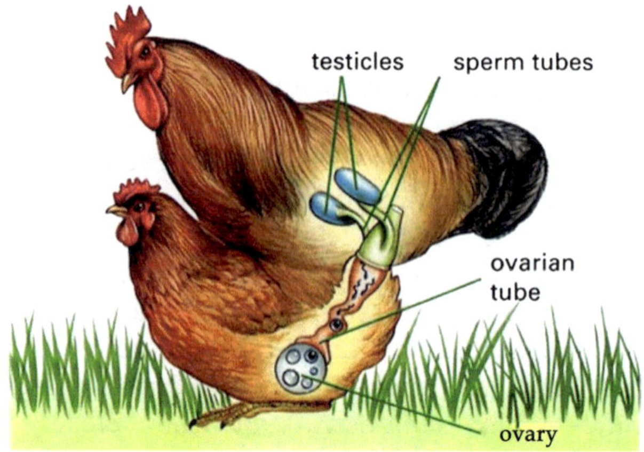

Figure 3.4. Internal fertilization.

Source: https://external-content.duckduckgo.com/iu/?u=https%3A%2F%2Fimages.collegedunia.com%2Fpublic%2Fimage%2Fc6509bd56f874e0feea94a732680212b.png&f=1&nofb=1&ipt=e32647764489aa7a61d9db9c6b8f42897c5da037466e1f1a1ab176691d924b14.

3.1.3. Comparison of Both Types

Assisted reproduction brings up more than just success rates—it shows us that the ways we try to overcome infertility can also shape a child's future. IVF and ICSI, for example, are two popular methods that, while both aiming to help parents conceive, don't seem to affect later development in precisely the same way. Studies indicate that children born using these techniques may develop differently; in many cases, those conceived via ICSI appear to face a lower risk of neurocognitive issues than their IVF counterparts (Surkova et al., 2025). This detail isn't just a curious fact—it matters a lot for future parents and medical teams when considering both conception and the potential effects on a child's mental and emotional growth. When it comes to preparing for embryo transfer, the details become a bit more complex. The state of the endometrium plays a significant role in whether a pregnancy takes hold, and there are two general methods to manage it: the natural cycle (NC) and the artificial cycle (AC). Surprisingly, research suggests that NC tends to give higher biochemical pregnancy rates than AC. To illustrate, one study found that women undergoing frozen-thawed embryo transfers experienced a 89.5% rate with NC, whereas AC only reached approximately 53.4% (Tyagitha et al., 2024). This means that choosing the right kind of endometrial setup isn't just a minor technical detail—it has a real impact on outcomes. It calls for careful thought from healthcare providers, tailoring methods to individual needs. Peeling back another layer, the situation isn't as binary as just "success" or "no success." Picking between IVF and ICSI, and even deciding on how to prepare the endometrium, reveals a more nuanced connection between method choice and results. Even though clinical pregnancy rates may remain relatively stable across different endometrial approaches, the increase in biochemical markers during natural cycles suggests a more supportive environment for early implantation (Tyagitha et al., 2024). In most cases, ongoing research is slowly unraveling how these decisions might affect not only immediate outcomes but also the long-term development of children. Future studies could offer deeper insights and lead to refined strategies that enhance the overall efficacy of these assisted reproductive techniques.

3.2. The Process of Fertilization

Fertilization marks the beginning of the journey toward creating a new life; it's when a sperm and an egg come together to form a zygote. Before that happens, there's a busy mix of chemical signals and cell chats that set the stage for the encounter. Sperm must navigate their way through the female tract, overcoming hurdles such as thick cervical mucus and the push-pull of uterine contractions. When they finally get to the egg, they switch into high gear with a change called capacitation. This process enhances their mobility and modifies their outer layer, enabling them to trigger the necessary reaction to break through the egg's protective casing. In most cases, any trouble with sperm quality—perhaps because of environmental factors like endocrine disruptors—can mess up fertilization or lead to odd embryo development, which shows how vital male reproductive health is (Santiago et al., 2024). Once a sperm enters, the egg responds almost immediately, undergoing a series of rapid changes that secure the event. At that moment, the oocyte finishes its second division to become a fully mature ovum and sends off chemicals that keep other sperm from barging in. This speedy reaction not only locks in the right mix of genes but also fires up the cellular machinery needed for what comes next.

Research has shown that specific proteins in both sperm and egg play a significant role in this process—variations in these proteins appear to be linked to the efficiency of fertilization (Santiago et al., 2024). It seems these interactions can be influenced, to some extent, by how the system handles environmental toxins. Then there's the curious case of taste receptors, which adds a whole new twist to the story. These receptors aren't just for enjoying food—they've been found in sperm cells and ovarian tissues too. Scientists believe that taste receptors, especially TAS2Rs, might help steer the conversation between sperm and egg, increasing the odds of successful fertilization. Some studies show that these receptors appear in the cell layers surrounding the egg, affecting not only its maturation but also influencing sperm movement and performance. They might even pick up chemical cues that guide sperm like a natural GPS toward the egg. By examining the mechanisms of these TAS2Rs closely, researchers aim to unravel the intricate details of fertilization and refine assisted reproductive techniques, ultimately enhancing fertility outcomes (Figure 3.5).

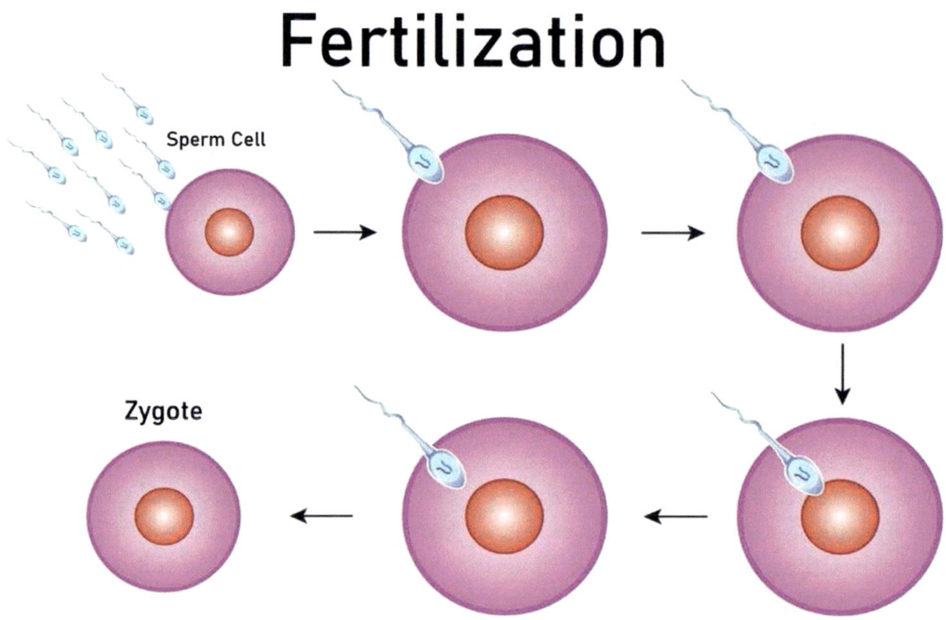

Figure 3.5. Fertilization process.

Source: https://external-content.duckduckgo.com/iu/?u=https%3A%2F%2Fstatic.vecteezy.com%2Fsystem%2Fresources%2Fpreviews%2F032%2F311%2F950%2Fnon_2x%2Ffertilization-process-with-step-by-step-sperm-egg-and-zygote-rendering-cell-design-vector.jpg&f=1&nofb=1&ipt=2157fe7ef9e79f3581694325375 87f2cbfd86a9757af80443baeedbd6f405a23.

3.2.1. Gamete Formation

Gamete formation kicks off life's wild dance—it's the moment when two individuals mix their genetic codes to spark something entirely new. In most sexually reproducing species, germ cells first switch gears and dive into meiosis, churning out haploid gametes (sperm for males and oocytes for females), and in doing so, they cut the chromosome count in half. This halving is crucial, as it sets everything up so that when fertilization occurs, the complete chromosomal set is restored. It isn't just about the numbers, though; even the nitty-gritty molecular details—like how the acrosome (that little structure on sperm's acrosome) gets built up—play a central role. Recent work on mammalian fertilization highlights the importance of the intricate interplay between cell structure and function (Victoria et al., 2021). As gametes mature, a host of cell organelles seem to join an impromptu jam session, obvious when sperm start forming their acrosomes. The process isn't a smooth, one-step affair; it kicks off in what many call the Golgi phase and progresses toward full-blown maturity in a series of steps that can feel somewhat unpredictable. Throughout these stages, parts of the cell—such as the endoplasmic reticulum and trans-Golgi network—collaborate under the influence of several genes, which generally work to keep the process on track even when things seem a little disorganized. This entire, yet beautifully coordinated, molecular process makes it clear: gamete formation isn't just a warm-up act, but a finely tuned sequence of milestones that pave the way for fertilization success (Xiong et al., 2021). Ultimately, the maturing gametes must perfectly synchronize with the timing of fertilization to complete reproduction. A standout moment is the acrosome reaction—a key event that lets the sperm breach the egg's protective layers. This biochemical cascade isn't some random flash in the pan; it's the grand finale of all those preparatory acts that came before. On top of that, teasing apart how genes quietly regulate these steps opens promising avenues for tackling infertility and boosting reproductive technologies. All in all, diving deeper into gamete formation reveals both its complex intricacies and its almost poetic precision, confirming its central role in the broader reproductive journey—from the initial union through to subsequent development (Victoria et al., 2021) (Figure 3.6).

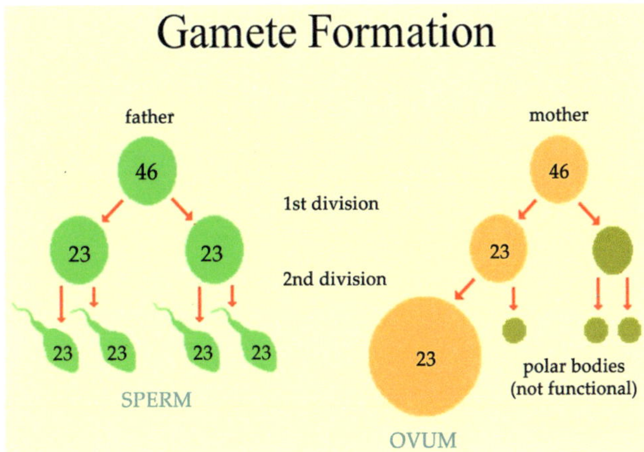

Figure 3.6. Gamete formation.

Source: https://external-content.duckduckgo.com/iu/?u=http%3A%2F%2Fibiologia.com%2Fwp-content%2Fuploads%2F2019%2F07%2FGameteFormation.jpg&f=1&nofb=1&ipt=1334b4c91754a2ee6e0ba1bb85d357992be3320d141611227526bbd741df3510.

3.2.2. Fusion of Sperm and Egg

Fertilization begins when a sperm and an egg unite, triggering a series of events that ultimately lead to the formation of a new life. This isn't just a simple merge—it's a subtle dance of molecules doing their part. The sperm's journey isn't straightforward either; it first prepares itself (what most people call capacitation) and then undergoes the acrosome reaction, during which it releases enzymes to break through the egg's outer coat. Tiny exosomes filled with seminal plasma proteins also play a part here, quietly boosting the sperm's chances of success. Research, for example, has highlighted that proteins involved in everything from initial recognition to the actual membrane fusion are key players in this union (Yu et al., 2023). The egg, on its end, doesn't sit idly by. It uses specific proteins on its surface—and on the sperm's—to sort out the right partner for the job. As the sperm's acrosome reaction unfolds, a burst of hydrolases and other enzymes helps soften the egg's protective layer, making room for a close connection. In most cases, these protein cues appear precisely when needed, forming a network that gently guides the recognition process. A recent study even highlighted that specific differentially expressed proteins play a central role in the synchronization of sperm and egg during fertilization (Ethan et al., 2018). Once the membranes finally merge, the story takes a whole new turn inside the cell. That merger sparks internal signals—most notably, a sudden surge of calcium—which not only wraps up the egg's meiotic processes but also stops extra sperm from jumping in. This calcium spike, generally speaking, acts as a green light for early embryonic development while keeping the whole process neat and controlled. Understanding these internal shifts is vital, especially when even minor disruptions can lead to fertility problems or issues with embryo development (Yu et al., 2023) (Figure 3.7).

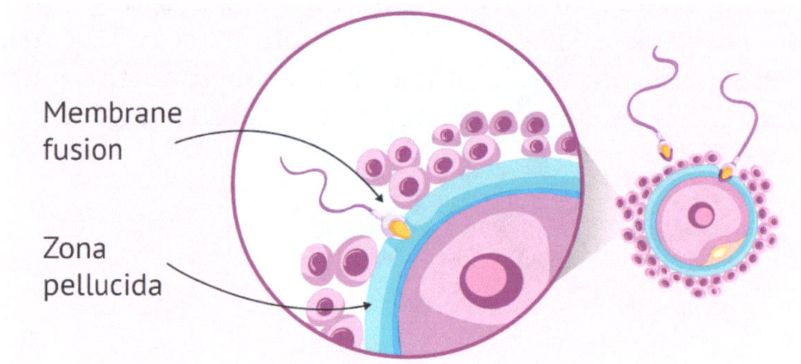

Figure 3.7. Fusion of egg and sperm membranes.

Source: https://www.invitra.com/en/wp-content/uploads/2018/11/fusion-of-egg-and-sperm-membranes.png.

3.2.3. Zygote Development

Shortly after fertilization, the zygote embarks on an unexpected journey of change. It's first move? Rapid, almost frantic cell divisions called cleavage, where the single cell splits repeatedly without increasing in size. Despite the constant overall dimensions, more and more cells cram in until what we call a morula takes shape. Equally intriguing is how sperm metabolism—its energy-yielding processes—suddenly matters a great deal, not just for sparking fertilization but also for guiding both the zygote and the growing embryo along the right path. In most cases, research suggests that the energy functions of sperm extend their influence well beyond the initial union, subtly affecting the father's biological contribution and setting the stage for successful implantation and healthy pregnancy outcomes (Abruzzese et al., 2024). Around five to six days post-fertilization, that dense morula morphs into something new—a blastocyst. This transformation is marked by the emergence of a fluid-filled cavity, known as the blastocoel. Here, cells start to find their niche: those nestled in the inner cell mass (ICM) will eventually build the embryo proper, while the outer trophoblasts step into their key role in forming the placenta. The female reproductive tract isn't just in the background, either; it provides a supportive setting that smooths the molecular chatter crucial for letting the blastocyst stick to and eventually invade the endometrial lining. Essentially, the maternal environment and early embryonic development have to come together in a delicate, almost unscripted dance (Francés-Herrero et al., 2022). As the blastocyst readies itself for implantation, it encounters a host of challenges—both from the mother's immune defenses and physical barriers within the uterus. The whole process depends on a tricky mix of hormonal cues and a receptive uterine lining that's been properly primed to let the blastocyst adhere and slowly break into the endometrium. Even minor changes in this finely tuned system can throw off fertility. Researchers, in most cases, are examining these interactions to pinpoint potential therapeutic targets while deepening their understanding of reproductive health. When one looks at zygote development from fertilization onward, it not only clarifies how early human life takes shape but also opens doors to improved assisted reproductive techniques that might ultimately ease infertility issues (Francés-Herrero et al., 2022; Abruzzese et al., 2024) (Figure 3.8).

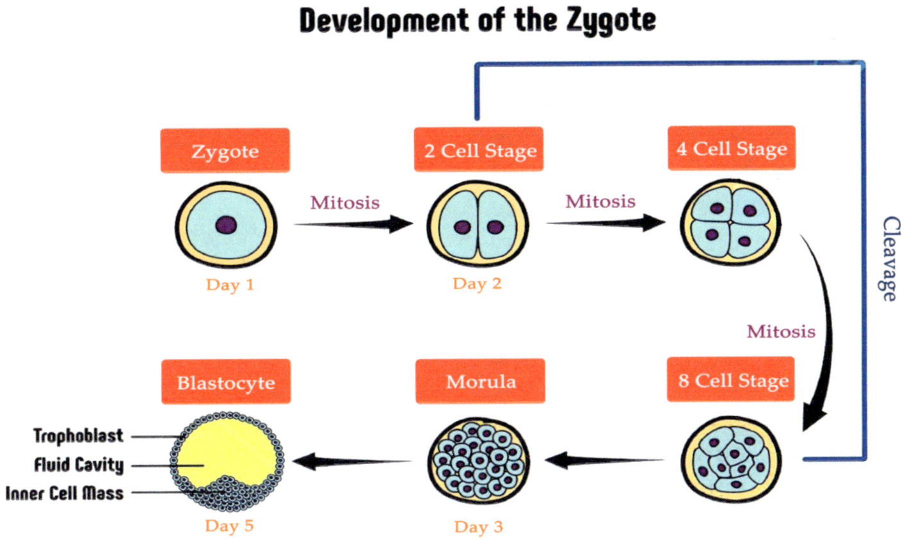

Figure 3.8. Development of the zygote.

Source: https://external-content.duckduckgo.com/iu/?u=https%3A%2F%2Fthumbs.dreamstime.com%2Fz%2Fdevelopment-zygote-diagram-including-all-stages-cell-mitosis-cleavage-morula-blastocyte-day-wise-medical-science-92185014.jpg&f=1&nofb=1&ipt=bc8cca85b41603bfe0008ea8878508c03d4d6f7adc3147c7f5d793945ebbb64c.

3.3. Factors Affecting Fertilization

When it comes to fertilization, the setting matters—what's in the soil can help or throw things off. One might say that having enough of the basic nutrients (nitrogen, phosphorus, potassium) is key; these elements boost plant health and naturally encourage more pollen and better ovule formation. On the other hand, substances like heavy metals and pesticides can stress the plant's internal processes. Research generally shows that metals such as cadmium and lead, for example, trigger biological stress that hinders flowering and pollination success (Alengebawy et al., 2021). Additionally, pesticide residues may disrupt the delicate balance among soil microbes, potentially harming the plant's reproductive outcomes. In short, the mix of plenty or scarcity in nutrients along with toxic substances essentially sets the stage for whether fertilization succeeds. There's also the factor of living interactions—plants don't reproduce in isolation. Pollination, a critical step in fertilization, leans heavily on the presence of specific pollinators. When these important insect visitors decline due to habitat loss or chemical exposure, many plants suffer a significant impact. Research often reveals that a diverse range of insect species is essential for pollination and maintaining genetic diversity in plant populations. Additionally, microplastics in the environment can exacerbate the issue by serving as both physical stressors and carriers of harmful chemicals that may harm pollinator health (Campanale et al., 2020). All of this demonstrates that the web connecting plants, their insect partners, and the surrounding environment is remarkably complex and necessitates conservation approaches that encompass multiple angles. It's not just outside influences that matter; what's going on inside the plant counts too. Reproductive parts, such as flowers and ovules, depend on receiving sufficient water and the proper temperatures. For instance, drought conditions can cause flowers to fall off or reduce ovule viability, significantly reducing fertilization chances. At the same time, the plant's hormones guide its reproductive processes. When these hormonal signals become disturbed—say, by a buildup of heavy metals that alters hormone levels (Alengebawy et al., 2021)—the timing and overall success of reproduction suffer. Taking into account both these internal mechanisms and the external pressure from the environment gives us a fuller picture of how plants manage to reproduce, even if the whole process is a delicate balancing act.

3.3.1. Environmental Conditions

Considering agriculture, climate, soil quality, and local conditions, they interact in ways that can impact crop performance. Nowadays, fertilization methods often capitalize on these natural influences to maximize the benefits of nutrient applications. When soils are poor or when weather goes extreme, vital elements like nitrogen, phosphorus, and potassium may not be as available as they should be – and that, in turn, limits plant growth while urging farmers to try new fertilization approaches. For example, a foliar application method can sometimes enhance the way plants absorb nutrients, especially under challenging conditions. Some studies suggest that blending foliar nano-chitosan-NPK with plant growth-promoting rhizobacteria (PGPR) can lead to better yields and also reduce environmental pollution (Gadallah et al., 2023). Overall, it appears that our ecological setting and the way we apply fertilizers are closely intertwined. Different fertilization methods can influence both the yield and quality of crops – a factor that depends significantly on surrounding conditions. Take cherry tomatoes, for instance; here, nutrient management proves pivotal in many greenhouse setups. Research, generally speaking, shows that slight tweaks in fertilization treatments can make a big difference in growth, yield, and even fruit quality. In many cases, incorporating organic components like humic acid provides a balanced approach that supports both the plant's productivity and its nutritional content.

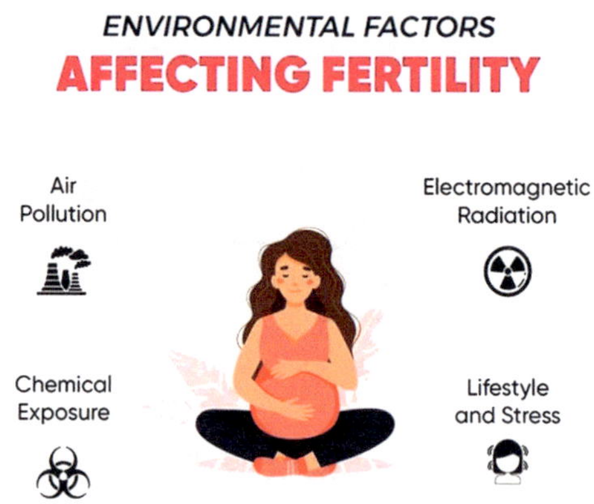
ENVIRONMENTAL FACTORS
AFFECTING FERTILITY
Air Pollution
Electromagnetic Radiation
Chemical Exposure
Lifestyle and Stress

Figure 3.9. Environmental factors.

Source: https://scontent.fdel11-1.fna.fbcdn.net/v/t39.30808-6/492357792_122 72 91086072232_2079460735212720815_n.jpg?stp=dst-jpg_p526x296_tt6&_nc_cat=110&ccb=1-7&_nc_sid=127cfc&_nc_ohc=r0VzO3jzsGsQ7kNvwGz3zSm&_nc_oc=AdnBJQzHzE7MwjWBcxej5b_20w5K7iGk3TM361fJ0ZRWE_ODCvH321r1vQFQMG7Fdu16JxIJPV5M3tPJbYdoIskl&_nc_zt=23&_nc_ht=scontent.fdel11-1.fna&_nc_gid=F7VRGahOkzH-rZ_6l-4u2g&oh=00_AfLju6KkSxOIGroSH8YKkHV0OvUBVzjjNCNTVnmjCuahZA&oe=6822227C.

The way nutrients interact with varying greenhouse environments demonstrates that a well-tailored fertilization strategy can overcome even the most challenging growing conditions (Nie et al., 2023). It's also important to consider how fertilization practices affect the environment. Mistakes, such as improper application, can cause fertilizer runoff, which may lead to issues like waterway eutrophication—a threat to aquatic ecosystems. Researchers, in most cases, recommend methods that help curb nutrient loss, especially when the soil conditions aren't ideal. Techniques such as using combined NCS-NPK with PGPR not only tend to boost crop production but also play a part in protecting the environment. These insights, overall, underline that sustainable farming depends on respecting the inextricable link between fertilization practices and ecological health (Gadallah et al., 2023) (Figure 3.9).

3.3.2. Genetic Compatibility

Fertilization isn't merely about two gametes merging, but more about whether their genetic blueprints click. Different organisms show us that when genetic make-ups mix, there's a hidden dance of evolutionary trial and error. For example, several species depend on unique gene signals to nudge the fertilization process in the right direction—this way, the offspring end up being hardy and well-suited for their surroundings. That blend of genetic details and reproductive quirks opens up a broad, intriguing field of study, one where the right match isn't just crucial within one species but might even bridge the gap between different ones.

Flowering plants bring their twist to the table. In these cases, the meeting of pollen and pistil acts as a kind of bouncer at the door of fertilization. Many angiosperms lean on something called the self-incompatibility (SI) mechanism—a neat trick to avoid inbreeding while keeping the gene pool lively. Interestingly, these pollen–pistil encounters shift considerably across various plant families; in some instances, the rules about which pollen grain gets to fertilize are almost like a game with ever-changing regulations. Recent molecular studies, particularly those examining the Asteraceae family, have shed light on a range of strategies that enhance reproductive success in diverse environments (Alexandra et al., 2011). A host of evolutionary pressures drives these gene-matching systems, urging species to adapt to survive. Generally speaking, when compatible genes come together, they increase heterozygosity, which in turn enhances overall fitness and helps populations withstand environmental fluctuations. In most cases, this enhanced survival tells us more about how adaptable organisms can be—even influencing how sex determination processes play out across diverse taxa (Bachtrog et al., 2014). As researchers unravel the complex interactions between genes and reproduction, they gain a clearer understanding of how genetic compatibility not only enhances individual outcomes but also influences the evolving tapestry of life and the resilience of entire ecosystems (Figure 3.10).

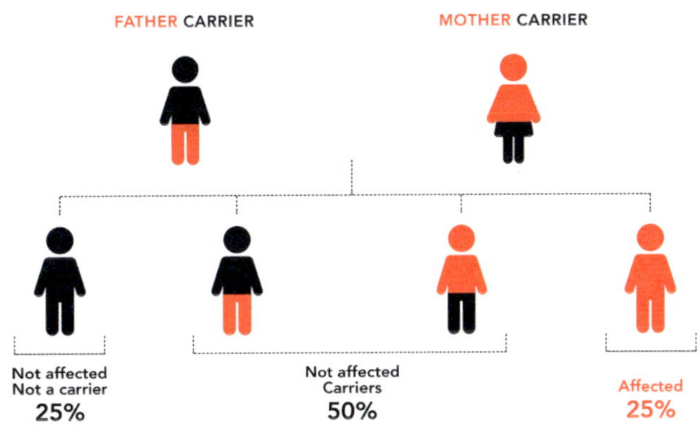

Figure 3.10. Genetic compatibility.

Source: https://www.institutobernabeu.com/wp-content/uploads/2021/06/TCGen-scaled.jpg.

3.3.3. Timing and Synchronization

Fertilization hinges on getting its timing right—a sort of raw, unscripted interplay of life's events. There is a brief window of time during which sperm can function and the female ovulation moment, and these must occur nearly concurrently, almost by chance. It isn't just a narrow meeting of gametes; nature seems to weave this timing into a broader ecological rhythm. In some species, when reproductive cycles synchronize, it not only boosts the odds of mating but also maintains genetic diversity, which in most cases helps populations weather environmental fluctuations. The way timing and this offbeat synchronization work together can be seen as a core driver behind reproductive success and evolutionary tweaks that increase an organism's odds of thriving.

Outside of this immediate get-together of gametes, the clockwork of fertilization reverberates through nature in surprising ways. Seasonal shifts and local weather quirks tend to shape reproductive cycles—organisms have wedded their timing to resource availability for their young. For instance, when climate change messes with these cycles, it might throw off not only animal breeding seasons but also crop yields, fueling debates in today's agricultural discussions. Additionally, as weather patterns gradually shift, the resulting unpredictability in these reproductive windows can sometimes make species more vulnerable to pests and diseases. All of this signals a need for adaptive strategies that take those environmental fluctuations into account, even if the dance remains unpredictable at times.

Digging deeper, the precise moment of fertilization turns out to be a big deal for how embryos later develop. Research generally suggests that even slight shifts in timing can lead to significant differences in embryo health, as crucial steps like cell division and specialization depend on a precise start. A minor slip-up here might pave the way for developmental changes or reduced overall viability. This entire scenario highlights that both the mechanics of fertilization and the environmental signals that prompt it are crucial for initiating life. As noted in numerous detailed discussions about modern farming practices, understanding these nuanced dynamics can help shape more effective interventions to cope with a changing climate, potentially offering a more resilient approach to fertility in both natural and managed settings (Skend Sžić et al., 2021; Dadlani et al., 2023).

3.4. Fertilization in Different Organisms

Sexual reproduction isn't a one-size-fits-all process. Sperm and egg jump into action in ways that depend on where and how an organism lives. Take many water-dwelling creatures, like fish and amphibians—they drop eggs into the water, and nearby sperm give them a chance to meet, even though nature's risks, such as predators and unpredictable surroundings, are lurking around. On land, creatures such as mammals opt for a more secure route by keeping fertilization inside the female's body, which, in most cases, creates a controlled space for the embryo to grow. Life tends to mix up its approach to make sure reproduction gets a good shot no matter the environment.

Fertilization extends far beyond the mere meeting of sperm and egg; a complex array of hidden cellular and molecular steps is involved. Consider flowering plants, for example—double fertilization occurs. One sperm unites with an egg to form the zygote, while another joins with two polar nuclei to produce the triploid endosperm that feeds the baby plant. In some invertebrates, such as sea urchins, a cascade of chemical cues draws sperm toward the egg, sparking the vital union. Generally speaking, these procedures repeat themselves in various forms, and they truly open a window into the intricacies of how life continues to build itself. The way fertilization has evolved bears huge weight on biodiversity and survival. As climates shift and habitats shrink under the pressure of human activity, species sometimes have to change their playbook. Certain frogs, for instance, can switch between laying eggs externally and resorting to more internal methods, showing off a kind of reproductive flexibility that's hard not to admire. Meanwhile, breakthroughs in molecular biology and genetics are steadily revealing the key proteins and gene players that drive these processes. Such insights not only help untangle puzzles about fertility in both medicine and farming, but they also guide ongoing conservation efforts (Peter et al., 2022; Perveen et al., 2024) (Figure 3.11).

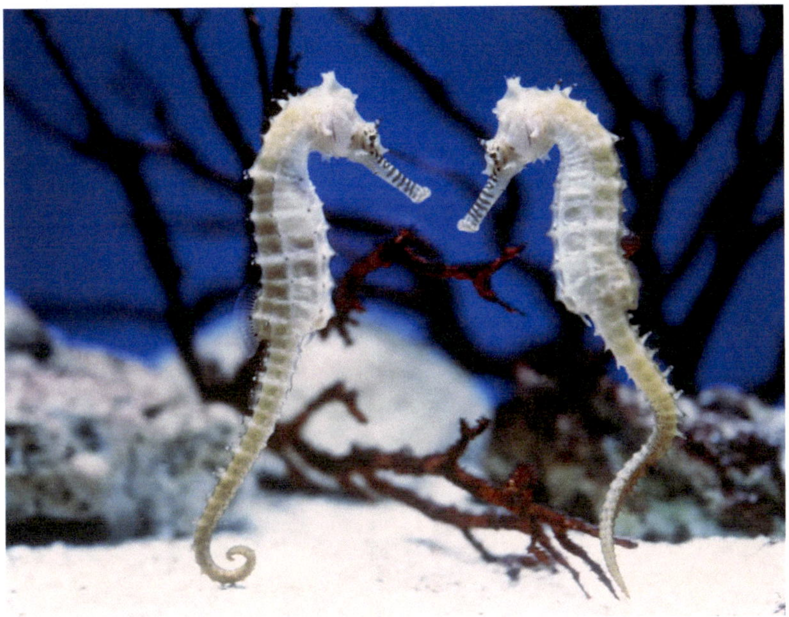

Figure 3.11. Fertilization in Different Organisms.

Source: https://media.hswstatic.com/eyJidWNrZXQ iOiJjb250ZW50Lm hzd3N0YXRpYy5jb20iLCJrZXkiOiJna WZcL3dlaXJkcmVwcm8tb3JpZy5q cGciLC JlZGl0cyI6eyJyZXN pemUiOnsid2lkdGgiOiIxMjAwIn19fQ==.

3.4.1. Fertilization in Plants

Plant fertilization is vital to a plant's ability to reproduce and keep its species going. It all starts when pollen grains—carrying the male gametes—are formed and then reach a receptive flower's stigma. Once there, the pollen triggers germination by creating a tube that serves as a guide for the sperm cells on their way to the ovule. Inside that ovule, one sperm merges with an egg cell to form a zygote, while its partner teams up with two polar nuclei and ends up making a triploid endosperm, which in most cases feeds the developing embryo. All these steps work together in a kind of unpredictable dance that not only boosts genetic variety but also paves the way for seed creation, meaning new plants can eventually grow. Environmental factors also play a role, often in unexpected ways. Nutrient levels and competition, for instance, can alter reproductive outcomes and even influence the number of species that thrive in an area. Several studies have suggested that nitrogen (N) deposition can disrupt plant diversity by altering species composition and competitive interactions (Pan et al., 2011). In grassland areas, higher nitrogen often prompts plants to invest more aboveground, while those better suited to underground growth are sidelined. This uneven effect raises alarms about biodiversity loss – responses to fertilization aren't uniform across the board. As human-driven nitrogen inputs infiltrate more plant communities, understanding how these shifts relate to fertilization becomes crucial for safeguarding biodiversity and managing our ecosystems. Recent work generally suggests that we need to set firm limits for nitrogen deposition

(Bobbink et al., 2010). With rising nitrogen levels in the air posing a serious threat, it's essential to see how they affect both fertilization and overall ecosystem health. In most cases, the thresholds that researchers identify help shape policy moves aimed at reducing nitrogen loads, especially where ecosystems are most sensitive. This idea—that fertilization, nutrient inputs, and species competition are all tangled together— calls for a broad, thoughtful approach to looking after nature. Sustainable practices that encourage real biodiversity are crucial now more than ever, especially as ecosystems face mixed pressures from human actions and shifting climate trends, ensuring that plant communities can keep on thriving for future generations (Figure 3.12).

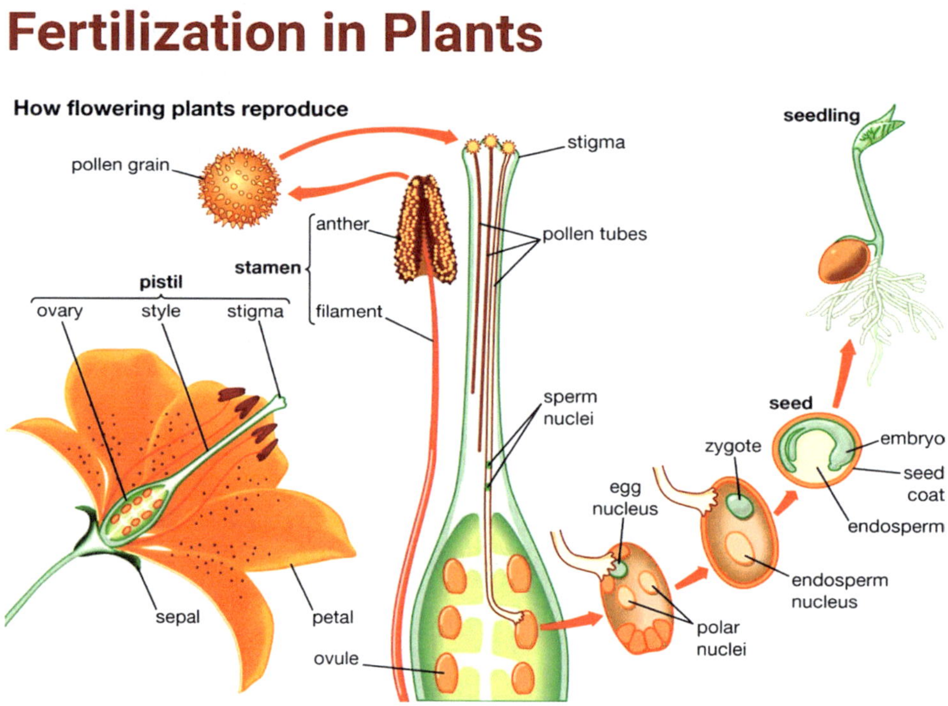

Figure 3.12. Fertilization in plants.

Source: https://microbenotes.com/wp-content/uploads/2022/04/Fertilization-in-Plants.jpeg.

3.4.2. Fertilization in Animals

Fertilization in animals is a complex process that initiates reproduction in unexpected ways. It all starts when a sperm meets an egg—a meeting steered by a jumble of chemical messages and tiny structural tweaks. Proteins like those in the CRISPR family get involved by helping the sperm move and the egg recognize its partner. In several species, these proteins appear repeatedly, performing various functions to initiate processes. Then there's a group known as CAP superfamily proteins, which seem to fine-tune ion channels in reproductive cells, nudging the necessary changes for the egg and sperm to work together properly and initiate early embryo development (Gaikwad et al., 2020). Understanding these basics often opens the door to insights into fertility issues and overall reproductive health across many animals. When fertilization carries on, the sperm's entry triggers a series of cell responses that are anything but just a simple warm-up. This step isn't merely about preparing the egg—it's crucial to ensuring fertilization succeeds. A kind of protein handshake happens between the sperm and the egg, a match-up that almost feels tailor-made. Recent studies hint that if these signals get a bit mixed up, fertility troubles might follow, suggesting that those tiny molecular exchanges hold more weight than we sometimes think. With exciting tools like CRISPR/Cas9, researchers are now poking around in the non-coding parts of DNA, curious if tweaking these regions can shift reproductive outcomes. By fiddling with gene regulation linked to fertilization, there's potential to bump up reproduction rates in a variety of animal species (Li et al., 2018). The whole process culminates in the creation of a zygote that quickly begins to divide and take shape. This fast start lays out the blueprint for all future development. So, proper fertilization isn't just crucial for a single species—it underpins the rich tapestry of life itself. Investigations into the roles and evolutionary histories of CAP proteins add another layer to this picture, revealing how different animal groups have developed their ingenious reproductive strategies. In many cases, this evolutionary spin reveals how fertilization helps maintain balance in nature, guiding species as they adapt in diverse ways. As ongoing research delves deeper into these molecular details, it promises new avenues for addressing reproductive health challenges and enhancing the survival of both individual organisms and entire species (Gaikwad et al., 2020) (Figure 3.13).

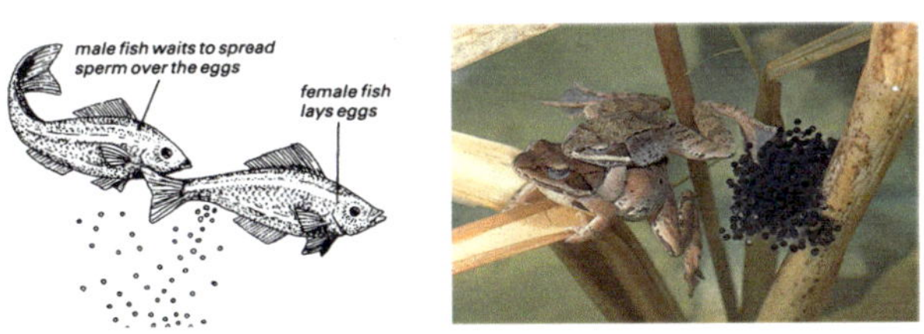
male fish waits to spread sperm over the eggs
female fish lays eggs

Figure 3.13. Fertilization in animals.

Source: https://thm-monocle-interactive.s3.amazonaws.com/fJ2HVPbbSI%2FExternal+Fertilization.png.

3.4.3. Unique Adaptations in Various Species

Different species have developed some ingenious ways to increase their fertilization odds. Take amphibians, for example – females release eggs into the water while nearby males add sperm; it's a straightforward tactic that appears to increase the likelihood that eggs and sperm will meet when water is present. In contrast, many land-living creatures, such as reptiles and mammals, have adopted the more cautious approach of internal fertilization, which serves as a protective measure for their developing young against nature's unpredictable hazards. These reproductive moves, repeated over time in various ecosystems, remind us why understanding reproductive ecology is crucial to understanding how life diversifies and adapts under different pressures, ultimately maintaining offspring viability and long-term survival. Temperature swings and other environmental challenges have prompted species to develop their ingenious solutions. For instance, many plants have fine-tuned the timing of their flowering and fertilization so that they coincide with the ideal climatic window—this usually results in better pollination success. Some studies suggest that high-temperature (HT) stress can significantly impair plant fertility and overall development, ultimately reducing crop yields worldwide (Hasanuzzaman et al., 2013). In response, many plants have evolved a range of biochemical tricks—such as triggering heat-sensitive gene expression—to help mitigate the adverse effects of HT. Generally speaking, these shifts highlight the dynamic interplay between our changing environment and the diverse ways species manage to continue reproducing. The harsh, ever-changing environment also pushes various organisms to develop resilient reproductive tactics. Aquatic beings, for example, often go all out by releasing vast quantities of eggs and sperm into open water—a bit like spreading one's bets in a very unpredictable lottery. This approach, though risky, sometimes tips the balance in favor of successful fertilization amid turbulent conditions. And, as climate change reshapes habitats in unexpected ways, species are forced into continual reproductive tweaks. All of these interactions, complete with their messy, natural repetitions, serve as a reminder of how ecological pressures and evolutionary challenges are tightly woven into the ongoing story of life.

3.5. Assisted Reproductive Technologies (ART)

Reproductive medicine has come a long way, reshaping infertility treatments thanks largely to leaps in Assisted Reproductive Technologies (ART). Couples who once struggled with natural conception now find a whole set of tools at their disposal—tools that range from the well-known IVF to newer, more intricate techniques like advanced genetic screening. Updates in lab methods are constantly needed, as shown by resources like the World Health Organization's Laboratory Manual for the Examination and Processing of Human Semen (Wang et al., 2022a). In most cases, these innovations are not just technical upgrades but life-changing advancements that help many families on their journey toward parenthood. It's striking how ART, once just a fanciful idea in scientific discussions, now practically creates life in the lab. Take, for instance, the breakthroughs of Robert Edwards and Patrick Steptoe. Their groundbreaking work in the 1970s—and that first IVF success in 1978—transformed what was once highly theoretical into a daily clinical reality. Their collaboration boosted further research and, admittedly, sparked ethical debates about reproductive rights and the limits of technology. Newer methods, such as the twin advances of cryopreservation and genetic screening of embryos, have further elevated success rates (Maryna Petrushko et al., 2021). ART isn't simply about helping conception; it plays a key role in sustaining reproductive health. These days, many couples generally see these reproductive techniques as essential resources rather than desperate last resorts. With innovations like preimplantation genetic diagnosis, hopeful parents can now choose embryos that are free from certain hereditary conditions—cutting down on the risk of genetic diseases. This mix of everyday medical advances and high-tech screening not only reflects progress in science but also forces society to rethink ethical nuances, as we come to terms with these powerful choices. Assisted reproduction continues to evolve, bringing fresh possibilities and a somewhat complex, yet profoundly human, renegotiation of what it means to overcome infertility (Maryna Petrushko et al., 2021; Wang et al., 2022a) (Figure 3.14).

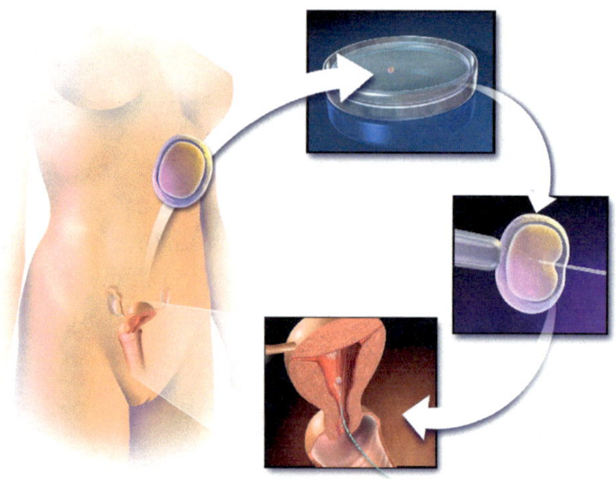

Figure 3.14. Assisted reproductive technology.

Source: https://upload.wikimedia.org/wikipedia/commons/d/db/Blausen_0060_AssistedReproductiveTechnology.png.

3.5.1. In Vitro Fertilization (IVF)

Reproductive technology has advanced significantly—IVF now plays a crucial role in helping people start families. With IVF eggs are fertilized outside the body, offering renewed hope for couples facing infertility. One tricky part is how embryos are selected since their quality can determine whether implantation succeeds. Recently, advanced algorithms and deep learning have been applied to examine microscopic images at several key stages of development. For instance, new scoring methods have achieved 96.1% accuracy, thanks to Graph Convolutional Networks (Perumal et al., 2024). All in all, these breakthroughs appear to indicate improved IVF outcomes and healthier beginnings for future parents.

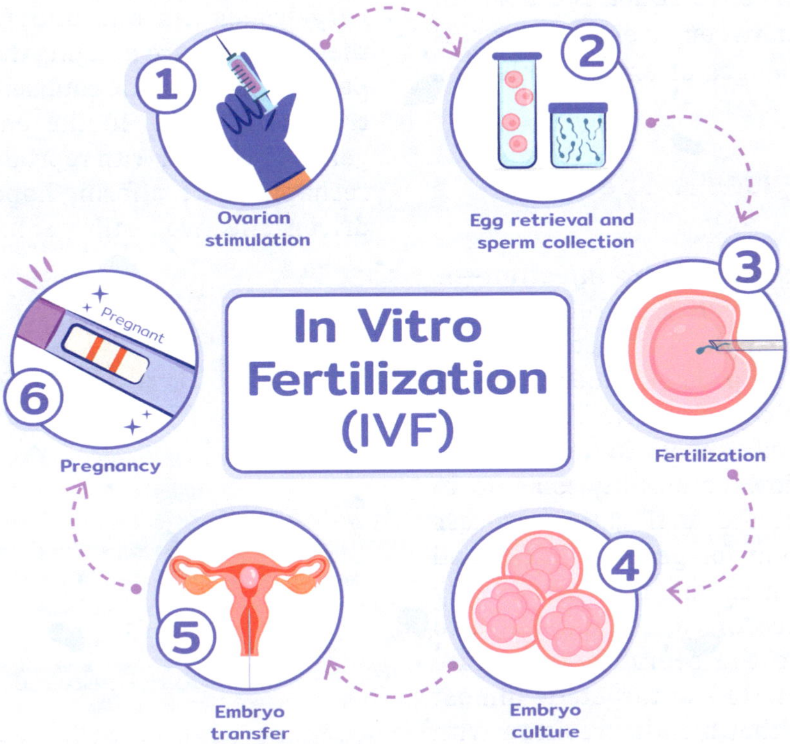

Figure 3.15. IVF (*In Vitro* fertilization).

Source: https://credenceivf.com/wp-content/uploads/2024/06/27596569_7082964.jpg.

Traditionally, embryo selection in IVF relied on subjective looks—embryologists using methods like the Istanbul scoring system to guide them. This hands-on approach sometimes creates inconsistency, especially when multiple embryos share similar traits. To smooth out these bumps, researchers are now turning to machine learning models that categorize embryos into viable and non-viable groups, while also taking into account patient age and developmental stage. Early findings suggest that these systems achieve an overall accuracy of approximately 65%, along with improved sensitivity rates (Charnpinyo et al., 2023). In most cases, this shift provides a more reliable method for determining which embryos to transfer, potentially enhancing pregnancy success. The mix of AI and reproductive tech is reshaping the IVF landscape, but it also stirs up some ethical questions. Deep learning can help rank embryos more objectively, yet that raises debates over reducing life to a set of numbers and even the risk of hidden biases creeping in. Sure, improved success rates are exciting, but there's still concern over what exactly counts as a "good" embryo and whether algorithmic decisions might oversimplify things. It's a complex picture that calls for ongoing, sometimes messy, discussions among doctors, ethicists, and society at large. Ultimately, maintaining an open conversation is crucial for striking a balance between scientific progress and the moral challenges of embryo selection (Figure 3.15).

3.5.2. Intracytoplasmic Sperm Injection (ICSI)

ICSI—intracytoplasmic sperm injection—is a breakthrough in assisted reproduction. It works by placing a single sperm straight into an egg, which can help when older methods like IVF just aren't cutting it. This direct technique often gives a boost in cases where sperm counts are low or motility isn't up to par; it smooths out the fertilization process and even leaves room for genetic checks and selection. In many cases, this method not only increases the chance of conception but also appears to enhance the overall success rate in ART procedures. It's a targeted, almost hands-on approach that blends precision with innovation in modern reproductive medicine. That said, ICSI isn't without its concerns. Some recent studies suggest that children conceived this way might, in most cases, have a slightly higher chance of neurodevelopmental challenges—think cerebral palsy, intellectual disability, or even autism spectrum disorder (Djuwantono et al., 2020). These findings, in general, suggest the need for extra monitoring as the child grows, allowing parents and doctors to remain vigilant. Many experts argue that a solid informed consent process and thorough counseling are essential when choosing ICSI, since solving immediate infertility issues might come with longer-term considerations that aren't entirely straightforward. Genetic and biological factors also play a crucial role in determining the effectiveness of ICSI. Emerging research suggests that mutations in specific genes may contribute to certain fertilization failures and other complications in ART procedures (Xue et al., 2022). Spotting these genetic oddities doesn't just help improve success rates—it also paves the way for treatments that target these very issues. As our understanding deepens, these insights are nudging the field toward more personalized genetic counseling and finely tuned treatment plans. In the end, the merging of genetic research with reproductive technology is reshaping ART, offering hope for more science-driven, effective fertility solutions (Figure 3.16).

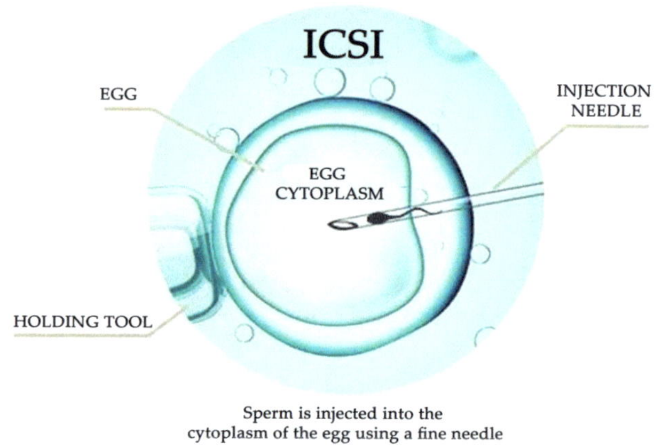

Figure 3.16. Intracytoplasmic sperm injection (ICSI).

Source: https://www.pfcla.com/hs-fs/hubfs/Pfcla%20Assets/Image/intracytoplasmic-sperm-injection-icsi-procedure-min.webp?width=502&height=357&name=intracytoplasmic-sperm-injection-icsi-procedure-min.webp.

3.5.3. Ethical Considerations

Modern fertilization techniques—especially IVF—have become a lot more complicated and stir up some pretty tricky ethical issues. IVF isn't just a straightforward medical service anymore; over time, it's shifted into realms shaped by social currents, like what folks now call "planned" oocyte cryopreservation. This change, generally speaking, raises questions about delaying parenthood and the social nudges that lead many women toward fertility preservation. In turn, these motivations can spark debates about informed consent and even the creeping commercialization of reproductive choices. There's also that concern where financial interests get too cozy with reproductive technology, sometimes pushing vulnerable people into expensive procedures without a clear grasp of the related health risks. Then again, when IVF becomes industrialized, a new set of entirely different ethical challenges arises. Clinics are adding on extra procedures—some not fully vetted—and some of these add-ons have unexpectedly been linked to a drop in live birth rates, something hardly seen until recently. Now, practitioners find themselves in a difficult spot; they must decide which treatments truly benefit patients versus those that might be profit-driven ventures. It isn't just about technical expertise—doctors are expected to offer choices that are backed by solid, evidence-based information while also protecting patient autonomy. In most cases, striking that balance between breakthrough innovation and genuine patient wellbeing is vital. And if we zoom out a bit further, the ethics of fertilization intersect with broader societal concerns. Accessibility and fairness play significant roles here since advanced reproductive tech isn't available to everyone. This gap can even lead to a sort of two-tier system in reproductive healthcare, which naturally raises fundamental questions about justice in medicine. It prompts us to consider how ethical frameworks should evolve—frameworks that demand greater transparency in practice and ensure that advancements benefit all individuals, regardless of their socioeconomic status. Addressing these complex, interwoven ethical issues will be key to fostering a future in reproductive technology that's both responsible and inclusive.

3.6. Implications of Fertilization

Fertilization weaves into the fabric of our environment in ways that affect more than just plant growth. It connects with broad ecological systems, influencing everything from the productivity of our farmlands to the overall health of nature. Nitrogen fixation, for example, is a crucial part of this process—and novel approaches, such as bioelectrochemical nitrogen fixation (e-BNF), are opening up new ways to enhance nitrogen levels in soil. Research shows that the bacterium *Pseudomonas stutzeri* A1501 can produce ammonium through unexpected, innovative routes that circumvent the usual problems caused by chemical inhibitors and costly catalysts. Furthermore, microorganisms in some cases harness extracellular electron donors. This discovery not only fine-tunes nitrogen fertilization but also hints at the possibility of leveraging native soil microbes to advance farming practices. In most cases, such breakthroughs could lead to higher crop yields with reduced dependency on synthetic fertilizers, nudging us toward a more sustainable agricultural future (Chen et al., 2020). The way ecosystem services interconnect is crucial for understanding the broader impacts of fertilization. Boosting crop production might sound beneficial, yet if one ecosystem service is pushed to its maximum—say, agricultural yield—it can unintentionally weaken others, such as biodiversity or the natural rhythm of nutrient cycling. Studies generally suggest that overemphasizing a single service can lead to a decline in ecological balance. And while this interconnectedness may seem somewhat complex, understanding it becomes increasingly urgent as modern farming practices face growing scrutiny for their environmental impact. Researchers, by mapping these ties (sometimes in an almost offhand manner), help shape sustainable land management methods that favor overall ecosystem health, repeating the importance of considering numerous, interrelated environmental aspects (Elena et al., 2009). Technological advances and ecological intricacies now prompt us to view fertilization as something that extends beyond simple agricultural benefits. Achieving sustainable fertilization appears to be a balancing act—one that must juggle boosting crop output while keeping ecosystems intact. Techniques like e-BNF, for example, offer an opportunity to reduce chemical inputs and promote natural soil fertility; however, a cautious approach is necessary because transitioning to these methods can lead to significant changes in farm infrastructure and necessitate new educational efforts for farmers. By integrating lessons from microbial research with insights on ecosystem services, policymakers can, in most cases, develop frameworks that support more sustainable fertilization practices. Ultimately, aligning farming methods with a deeper ecological understanding may guide us toward an agricultural landscape that is both robust and more environmentally friendly (Elena et al., 2009; Chen et al., 2020).

3.6.1. Impact on Biodiversity

Fertilization can shake up the natural web of life—its effects on soil biodiversity aren't always obvious at first glance. Long-term use of fertilizers alters how soil creatures organize themselves, and these critters are crucial for maintaining many vital ecosystem functions. Generally speaking, studies show that adding organic matter tends to boost the overall performance of soil, linking soil life tightly with the health of the entire ecosystem. At times, the subtle reactions of these groups hint at shifts in the ecosystem's balance, especially since the quirky mix of different ecological clusters helps sustain core soil functions. When one looks closer, it becomes clear that fertilization not only alters soil health but also has a ripple effect on overall biodiversity in land systems (Wang et al., 2022b). Nitrogen input into plant communities adds another twist to this story. Meta-analytic reports often note that increasing nitrogen levels results in significant losses—not only in species richness but also in the abundance of particular species. These declines, which can worsen with higher temperatures and extended study periods, demonstrate that biodiversity responses are closely tied to their context.

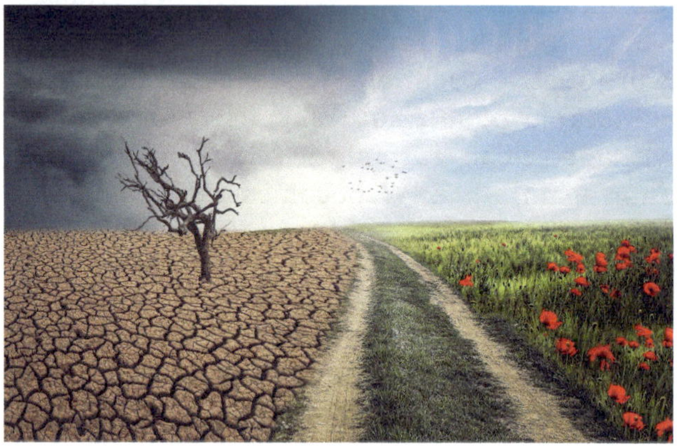

Figure 3.17. Soil biodiversity.

Source: https://external-content.duckduckgo.com/iu/?u=https%3A%2F%2Fscx2.b-cdn.net%2Fgfx%2Fnews%2Fhires%2F2021%2Fclimatechange.jpg&f=1&nofb=1&ipt=5550aa6694d79fd8cda1d4cbce1348bef424544b2dde26ac88c9ffbbf35dabf8.

For example, legumes tend to be particularly sensitive to excess nitrogen, a detail that highlights how fertilization can affect some community members more significantly than others. All in all, the cascading effects of these nutrient changes extend well beyond short-term crop gains, prompting us to consider broader implications for biodiversity (Midolo et al., 2018). Fertilization practices extend into a broader ecological context, prompting us to consider ecosystem management in a more comprehensive light. Ecosystem multifunctionality relies on a diverse mix of both soil organisms and plant communities; often, our modern agricultural practices inadvertently chip away at the very resilience that ecosystems depend on. There's a pressing need to adopt sustainable fertilization methods—ones that weigh ecosystem health and biodiversity alongside productivity goals. As we try to balance farming needs with environmental care, the insights we gather from these complex relationships can point us toward more responsible land management. Ultimately, prioritizing long-term ecological health may necessitate reevaluating and adjusting our use of fertilizers within a broader environmental context (Wang et al., 2022b) (Figure 3.17).

3.6.2. Role in Evolution

Fertilization isn't merely a simple joining of sperm and egg—it turns out to be a pretty wild stage for evolution. Right after mating, females often take a backseat role that turns out not to be so passive at all; they influence which sperm gets the chance to fertilize the egg. This secret maneuver, known in everyday terms as cryptic female choice, occurs behind the scenes and significantly influences the genetic mix and reproductive outcomes. Eberhard's early work, for instance, suggests that when females have a say, sperm selection can swing dramatically, altering who ends up as the dad and nudging sexual selection along unforeseen paths. With today's technology constantly improving, scientists can now observe that these choices emerge at several points—whether during sperm storage or at the very act of fertilization—making the whole process far more complex than it might seem at first glance (Renée et al., 2017). Switching over to another scene, some flowering plants have taken a different route by shifting from outcrossing to self-fertilization. In many cases, these plants have developed built-in mechanisms that favor self-pollination, which not only alters their genetics but also affects their ecology and even their appearance. As a result, selfing tends to lead to a decrease in genetic diversity compared to crossbreeding plants. Researchers, by sifting through molecular differences among closely related species, have started to uncover what drives these various shifts. Sometimes, though, the fuzzy picture created by linked selection makes it hard to pinpoint just how much the need for reproductive assurance drives selfing. All of this suggests that when different fertilization strategies are combined with evolutionary pressures, one ends up with a unique adaptive capacity that warrants a closer examination of both ecological and genomic details (Spencer et al., 2014). At its core, fertilization does much more than secure the next generation—it also lays the groundwork for maintaining genetic diversity and helping species adapt over time. Whether it's through the subtle control in cryptic female choice or the sweeping changes brought by self-fertilization, the act of fertilization turns out to be split into many unexpected roles. On one hand, hidden female choice gives us a glimpse into how females can quietly tip the scales in choosing particular sperm; on the other, self-fertilization shows just how significant a shift can be triggered when a species opts to go it alone. Taken together, these complex dynamics remind us that the way organisms mate isn't isolated—it's closely intertwined with how evolution itself unfolds, deepening our understanding of both mating systems and the lasting changes in plants and animals alike (Spencer et al., 2014; Renée et al., 2017).

3.6.3. Consequences of Fertilization Failure

Unsuccessful fertilization isn't just a personal hurdle—it ripples out into emotional and social life, too. Couples struggling with infertility often end up dealing with heavy stress, like anxiety, depression, and sometimes that nagging sense of not being enough. The social stigma tied to these challenges might even intensify those feelings, so many end up keeping quiet about their struggles. On top of that, repeated issues with conception often drive up healthcare bills with extra treatments, therapies, and those complicated assisted reproduction options.

All that emotional and financial weight can put a strain on relationships—occasionally even sparking marital conflicts or breakups. Generally speaking, as research continues to uncover the connection between mental well-being and reproductive health, it's becoming increasingly clear that understanding fertilization failures is vital for both doctors and society at large (Cicinelli et al., 2021). There are physical signs that often accompany these emotional struggles. For instance, many women might notice their menstrual cycles becoming irregular or experience ovulatory problems; sometimes, conditions like polycystic ovary syndrome (PCOS) rear their head, complicating later attempts at conceiving. Sometimes, the failure to conceive can even signal that something else might be off—maybe a hormonal imbalance or an anatomical issue that needs a closer look. Some recent studies have also pointed to chronic endometritis as a potentially significant factor hindering implantation, which warrants attention (Critchley et al., 2020). When one considers how reproductive health and the condition of the endometrium are so closely intertwined, it seems clear that addressing these physiological challenges is crucial to achieving better fertility outcomes and overall health. Then there's the broader societal picture. Fertilization troubles highlight a real need for better reproductive education and more accessible resources. With fertility treatments becoming more common these days, many are finally realizing just how complex reproductive health can be, and that has sparked calls for fair access to fertility care—especially since many socioeconomic and demographic groups aren't on equal footing. Awareness campaigns and educational programs, even when they sometimes repeat the same info, can help clear up misconceptions about infertility and pregnancy, making it easier for folks to talk about these issues openly. By fostering a more inclusive conversation, society may finally chip away at the stigma surrounding fertility problems, encouraging individuals to seek proper support, which could ultimately enhance their chances of successful conception in the future (Critchley et al., 2020; Cicinelli et al., 2021) (Figure 3.18).

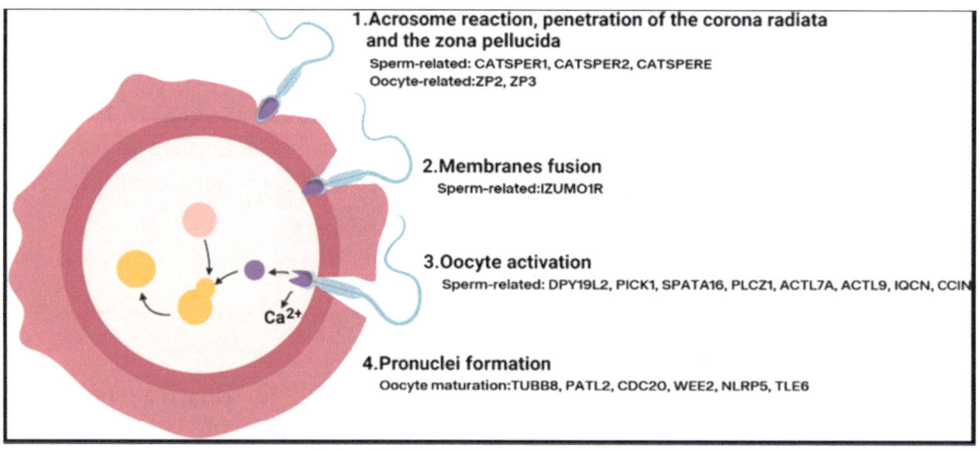

Figure 3.18. Fertilization process and genetic causes of fertilization failure.

Source: https://www.researchgate.net/publication/371411715/figure/fig1/AS:11431281177278454@1690424194713/Fertilization-process-and-genetic-causes-of-fertilization-failure.png.

SUMMARY

Fertilization isn't a simple matter it's a complex interaction of many factors working together in ways that can often surprise us. In plants, for example, the shape of a flower and the timing of its growth can widely influence what happens after a bloom; sometimes, the changes that follow anthesis directly steer fertilization outcomes. Take *Marathrum rubrum* (Guzmán-Merodio et al., 2024)—its reproductive organs seem to respond almost instinctively to specific environmental nudges and developmental signals, and even a small glitch in this balance might lower a species' fitness or survival, ultimately shaking up local biodiversity. When we switch the focus to human male reproduction, the picture gets another layer of complexity due to our endocannabinoid system (ECS). Emerging studies generally indicate that components like the CB1 receptor play a surprisingly significant role in how sperm move and function – key elements for achieving fertilization. There's mounting evidence that, in most cases, if the ECS is disrupted, sperm quality and overall fertility can decline (Maccarrone, 2013). This suggests that examining these biochemical pathways is crucial when considering interventions or lifestyle changes aimed at enhancing reproductive health; furthermore, it indicates that everyday exposures and choices may subtly influence these vital processes. Our expanding understanding of fertilization makes it clear that life's reproductive success, whether in aquatic plants or human biology, is a result of a complex interplay between environmental cues and internal mechanisms. The unexpected combination of floral design in water plants with the biochemical rhythms that control sperm function reveals just how layered and unpredictable reproduction can be. Recognizing these intertwined effects opens up fresh chances to guide conservation efforts (Guzmán-Merodio et al., 2024) and refine human reproductive health practices (Maccarrone, 2013) – a reminder that in our ever-changing world, there's always more to learn about the delicate art of fertilization. Fertilization doesn't come down to one simple factor—it's a mix of biology and clinical history all jumbled together. The state of the uterus stands out as a big deal; conditions like endometriosis can throw a wrench into things. Some studies suggest that women with a history of endometriosis might get lower live birth rates when they go through IVF with oocyte donation. A systematic review and meta-analysis, for example, found that even though the adverse effect is relatively modest, registry data showed statistical significance, hinting that uterine receptivity is something not to be ignored. Doctors, in most cases, need to dig into a patient's reproductive background because those details might point them to the best way to handle IVF and bump up treatment success. New developments in cellular and tissue science have started to shake up reproductive medicine in unexpected ways. Researchers are now examining stem cells from angles that extend beyond the reproductive organs—sometimes even revisiting aspects of cardiovascular health. Generally speaking, focusing on safer, more accessible stem cell sources and experimenting with how to cultivate them more effectively is becoming a priority. For instance, tissue-specific progenitors taken from the myocardium might help mend underlying issues that affect fertility due to overall systemic health. In most cases, this broader idea—that improving overall body wellness can enhance reproductive potential—adds a new layer to how we think about effective fertilization strategies in clinical settings. Then there's the evolving field of stem cell therapy, which is slowly but surely hinting at even more combined treatment options. Researchers and clinicians are testing different stem cell types together, hoping that combining these approaches can offer real benefits, especially in challenging reproductive cases. Indeed, questions about the optimal method or dosage for these cells frequently arise, and further research is undoubtedly necessary before we can definitively settle the matter.

CLOSER LOOK

HETEROZYGOSITY

Heterozygosity is a genetic term that refers to the presence of two different alleles at a specific gene locus in an organism's genome. In diploid organisms, such as humans, each individual inherits two copies of each gene—one from each parent. When these copies, or alleles, are different, the individual is said to be heterozygous at that locus. In contrast, if both alleles are the same, the individual is homozygous. Heterozygosity plays a crucial role in genetics, evolution, and population biology, as it is a key measure of genetic variation within a population. High levels of heterozygosity are often associated with greater genetic diversity, which is essential for the adaptability and survival of a population. This diversity can enhance an organism's ability to resist diseases, adapt to environmental changes, and maintain healthy reproduction. In population genetics, average heterozygosity is used as an indicator of a population's genetic health, with higher values suggesting a rich gene pool and lower values potentially indicating inbreeding or genetic drift.

At the molecular level, heterozygosity can affect phenotypic traits in different ways, depending on the nature of the gene and its alleles. In some cases, one allele may be dominant and mask the effects of the other, recessive allele, so the heterozygous genotype displays the dominant trait. In other instances, incomplete dominance or codominance can result in a phenotype that is intermediate or a combination of both alleles. This genetic variability is fundamental to Mendelian inheritance and has important implications for understanding hereditary diseases. For example, carriers of certain genetic disorders, such as cystic fibrosis or sickle cell anemia, are heterozygous for a mutated gene but may not exhibit symptoms because the normal allele compensates for the defective one. In some cases, such as with the sickle cell trait, heterozygosity can even confer a survival advantage, as individuals who are heterozygous for the sickle cell allele have a degree of resistance to malaria—a classic example of balancing selection in evolutionary biology.

Heterozygosity is also essential in plant and animal breeding programs, where maintaining or increasing genetic variation is necessary for long-term sustainability and improvement of species. Breeders often select heterozygous individuals to promote hybrid vigor, also known as heterosis, where the offspring of genetically diverse parents exhibit improved growth, fertility, or resilience compared to their inbred counterparts. In conservation biology, measuring heterozygosity helps identify endangered populations at risk of inbreeding depression, which can lead to reduced fitness and increased susceptibility to disease. Genetic tools such as microsatellite markers and SNP (single-nucleotide polymorphism) analysis are commonly used to assess heterozygosity levels across genomes, providing valuable data for managing and conserving biodiversity.

Heterozygosity is a fundamental concept in genetics that reflects the genetic diversity within individuals and populations. It influences evolutionary potential, disease resistance, and overall fitness. Whether in the context of medical genetics, evolutionary theory, or conservation efforts, understanding heterozygosity helps scientists and researchers appreciate the intricate balance of genetic variation that sustains life and allows species to adapt and thrive in changing environments.

REFERENCES

1. Abruzzese, G. A., Sanchez-Rodriguez, A., & Roldan, E. R. S. (2024). Sperm metabolism. *Molecular Reproduction and Development, 91*(10). https://doi.org/10.1002/mrd.23772Adewusi, A. O., Asuzu, O. F., Olorunsogo, T., Olorunsogo, T., Adaga, E. M., & Daraojimba, D. O. (2024). AI in precision agriculture: A review of technologies for sustainable farming practices. *World Journal of Advanced Research and Reviews, 21*(1). https://doi.org/10.30574/wjarr.2024.21.1.0314.
2. Alengebawy, A., Abdelkhalek, S. T., Qureshi, S. R., & Wang, M.-Q. (2021). Heavy metals and pesticides toxicity in agricultural soil and plants: Ecological risks and human health implications. *Toxics, 9*(3), 42. https://doi.org/10.3390/toxics9030042.
3. Allen, A. M., Thorogood, C. J., Hegarty, M., Lexer, C., & Hiscock, S. J. (2011). Pollen–pistil interactions and self-incompatibility in the Asteraceae: New insights from studies of *Senecio squalidus* (Oxford ragwort). *Annals of Botany, 108*(4), 687–698. https://doi.org/10.1093/aob/mcr147.
4. Bachtrog, D., Mank, J. E., Peichel, C. L., Kirkpatrick, M., Otto, S. P., Ashman, T.-L., Hahn, M. W., et al. (2014). Sex determination: Why so many ways of doing it? *PLoS Biology, 12*(7), e1001899. https://doi.org/10.1371/journal.pbio.1001899.
5. Barrachina, F., Battistone, M. A., Castillo, J., Mallofré, C., Jodar, M., Breton, S., & Oliva, R. (2022). Sperm acquire epididymis-derived proteins through epididymosomes. *Human Reproduction, 37*(4), 651–668. https://doi.org/10.1093/humrep/deac015.
6. Barrett, S. C. H., Arunkumar, R., & Wright, S. (2014). The demography and population genomics of evolutionary transitions to self-fertilization in plants. *Philosophical Transactions of the Royal Society B: Biological Sciences, 369*(1648), 20130344. https://doi.org/10.1098/rstb.2013.0344.
7. Bennett, E. M., Peterson, G., & Gordon, L. (2009). Understanding relationships among multiple ecosystem services. *Ecology Letters, 12*(12), 1394–1404. https://doi.org/10.1111/j.1461-0248.2009.01387.x.
8. Bobbink, R., Hicks, K., Galloway, J. N., Spranger, T., Alkemade, R., Ashmore, M. R., Bustamante, M., et al. (2010). Global assessment of nitrogen deposition effects on terrestrial plant diversity: A synthesis. *Ecological Applications, 20*(1), 30–59. https://doi.org/10.1890/08-1140.1.
9. Bronstein, M. M., Bruna, J., LeCun, Y., Szlam, A., & Vandergheynst, P. (2017). Geometric deep learning: Going beyond Euclidean data. *IEEE Signal Processing Magazine, 34*(4), 18–42. https://doi.org/10.1109/msp.2017.2693418.
10. Campanale, C., Massarelli, C., Savino, I., Locaputo, V., & Uricchio, V. F. (2020). A detailed review study on potential effects of microplastics and additives of concern on human health. *International Journal of Environmental Research and Public Health, 17*(4), 1212. https://doi.org/10.3390/ijerph17041212.
11. Charnpinyo, N., Suthicharoenpanich, K., Onthuam, K., Engphaiboon, S., Chaichaowarat, R., Suebthawinkul, C., & Siricharoen, P. (2023). Embryo selection for IVF using machine learning techniques based on light microscopic images of embryo and additional factors. In *2023 45th Annual International Conference of the IEEE Engineering in Medicine & Biology Society (EMBC)*. https://www.semanticscholar.org/paper/e744e0379b139aedbfcbf5db22a16b453b2d39ad (accessed on 26 May 2025).

12. Chen, S., Jing, X., Yan, Y., Huang, S., Liu, X., Chen, P., & Zhou, S. (2020). Bio electrochemical fixation of nitrogen to extracellular ammonium by *Pseudomonas stutzeri*. *Applied and Environmental Microbiology, 87*(21), e01998–20. https://doi.org/10.1128/aem.01998-20.
13. Cicinelli, E., Cicinelli, R., & Vitagliano, A. (2021). Antibiotic therapy for chronic endometritis and its reproductive implications: A step forward, with some uncertainties. *Fertility and Sterility, 115*(6), 1445–1446. https://doi.org/10.1016/j.fertnstert.2021.03.025.
14. Critchley, H., Babayev, E., Bulun, S. E., Clark, S., Garcia-Grau, I., Gregersen, P. K., Kilcoyne, A., et al. (2020). Menstruation: Science and society. *American Journal of Obstetrics and Gynecology, 223*(5), 624–664. https://doi.org/10.1016/j.ajog.2020.06.004.
15. Dadlani, M., & Yadava, D. K. (2023). *Seed Science and Technology*. https://doi.org/10.1007/978-981-19-5888-5.
16. Degner, E. C., Ahmed-Braimah, Y. H., Borziak, K., Wolfner, M. F., Harrington, L. C., & Dorus, S. (2018). Proteins, transcripts, and genetic architecture of seminal fluid and sperm in the mosquito *Aedes aegypti*. *Molecular & Cellular Proteomics, 18*(Suppl 1), S6–S22. https://doi.org/10.1074/mcp.ra118.001067.
17. Deneke, V. E., & Pauli, A. (2021). The fertilization enigma: How sperm and egg fuse. *Annual Review of Cell and Developmental Biology, 37*, 391–414. https://doi.org/10.1146/annurev-cellbio-120219-021751.
18. Djuwantono, T., Aviani, J. K., Permadi, W., Achmad, T. H., & Halim, D. (2020). Risk of neurodevelopmental disorders in children born from different ART treatments: A systematic review and meta-analysis. *Journal of Neurodevelopmental Disorders, 12*, Article 23. https://doi.org/10.1186/s11689-020-09347-w.
19. Firman, R. C., Gasparini, C., Manier, M. K., & Pizzari, T. (2017). Postmating female control: 20 years of cryptic female choice. *Trends in Ecology & Evolution, 32*(5), 368–382. https://doi.org/10.1016/j.tree.2017.02.010.
20. Food and Agriculture Organization of the United Nations. (2018). *The State of World Fisheries and Aquaculture 2018*. https://doi.org/10.18356/8d6ea4b6-en.
21. Francés-Herrero, E., Lopez, R., Hellström, M., de Miguel-Gómez, L., Herraiz, S., Brännström, M., Pellicer, A., et al. (2022). Bioengineering trends in female reproduction: A systematic review. *Human Reproduction Update, 28*, 798–837. https://www.semanticscholar.org/paper/f1fdcf06660108a22e328d776a52ec11fc09a42e (accessed on 26 May 2025).
22. Francés-Herrero, E., Lopez, R., Hellström, M., de Miguel–Gómez, L., Herraiz, S., Brännström, M., Pellicer, A., et al. (2022). Bioengineering trends in female reproduction: A systematic review. *Human Reproduction Update, 28*, 798–837. https://doi.org/10.1093/humupd/dmac025.
23. Gadallah, A. E. M., Arafa, A. S., Yahia, W. M. B., Badawy, S., & Rabeh, H. (2023). Cotton productivity and fiber quality improvement by nano chitosan-NPK fertilizer integrated with plant growth promoting rhizobacteria application in North Delta of Egypt. *Alexandria Science Exchange Journal*. https://www.semanticscholar.org/paper/6f765d4d489f51e27f65f9f7cfbd5e5227c74b1a (accessed on 26 May 2025).
24. Gaikwad, A., Hu, J., Chapple, D. G., & O'Bryan, M. K. (2020). The functions of CAP superfamily proteins in mammalian fertility and disease. *Human Reproduction Update, 26*(6), 689–723. https://doi.org/10.1093/humupd/dmaa016.

25. Gatta, P. P. (2022). *The State of World Fisheries and Aquaculture 2022*. FAO eBooks. https://doi.org/10.4060/cc0461en.

26. Guzmán-Merodio, D., Luna-Ramos, R., Núñez-Farfán, J., Collazo-Ortega, M., & Márquez-Guzmán, J. (2024). The reproductive biology of *Marathrum rubrum* Novelo & C. T. Philbrick: Morphological and anatomical changes during flower development. *Botanical Sciences*. https://www.semanticscholar.org/paper/de9a25068e04a94cfddaa2400554a0959849f618 (accessed on 26 May 2025).

27. Hasanuzzaman, M., Nahar, K., Alam, M. S., Roychowdhury, R., & Fujita, M. (2013). Physiological, biochemical, and molecular mechanisms of heat stress tolerance in plants. *International Journal of Molecular Sciences, 14*(5), 9643–9684. https://doi.org/10.3390/ijms14059643.

28. Intergovernmental Panel on Climate Change. (2015). *Climate Change 2014: Synthesis Report*. https://doi.org/10.59327/ipcc/ar5-9789291691432.

29. Kyrou, K., Hammond, A., Galizi, R., Kranjc, N., Burt, A., Beaghton, A., Nolan, T., et al. (2018). A CRISPR–Cas9 gene drive targeting doublesex causes complete population suppression in caged *Anopheles gambiae* mosquitoes. *Nature Biotechnology, 36*(11), 1062–1066. https://doi.org/10.1038/nbt.4245.

30. Kyryk, V. (2024). Stem cell therapy for cardiac regeneration: Key points. *Cell and Organ Transplantology*. https://www.semanticscholar.org/paper/6a1b536f3691ad0d162e4187a4a2e2ffd1507b5f (accessed on 26 May 2025).

31. Laland, K. N., Uller, T., Feldman, M. W., Sterelny, K., Müller, G. B., Moczek, A. P., Jablonka, E., et al. (2015). The extended evolutionary synthesis: Its structure, assumptions and predictions. *Proceedings of the Royal Society B: Biological Sciences, 282*(1813), 20151019. https://doi.org/10.1098/rspb.2015.1019.

32. Li, M., Liu, X., Dai, S., Xiao, H., & Wang, D. (2018). High efficiency targeting of non-coding sequences using CRISPR/Cas9 system in tilapia. *G3: Genes, Genomes, Genetics, 9*(1), 287–295. https://doi.org/10.1534/g3.118.200883.

33. Luddi, A., Semplici, B., Luongo, F. P., Governini, L., Ponchia, R., Morgante, G., Leo, V., et al. (2021). O-217 Bitter taste receptors expression in human follicular cells: New perspectives in female fertility. *Human Reproduction*. https://www.semanticscholar.org/paper/b36703ccb0370d259c38e2eb297d1cc74b319714 (accessed on 26 May 2025).

34. Ma, Z. (2022). Microbiome transmission during sexual intercourse appears stochastic and supports the Red Queen hypothesis. *Frontiers in Microbiology, 12*, 789983. https://doi.org/10.3389/fmicb.2021.789983.

35. Maccarrone, M. (2013). Endocannabinoids as markers of sperm quality: Hot spots. *Frontiers in Endocrinology, 4*, Article 133. https://www.semanticscholar.org/paper/c4d0e805005333332d529f72a93970520480de7c (accessed on 26 May 2025).

36. Midolo, G., Alkemade, R., Schipper, A. M., Benítez-López, A., Perring, M. P., & de Vries, W. (2018). Impacts of nitrogen addition on plant species richness and abundance: A global meta-analysis. *Global Ecology and Biogeography, 28*(4), 398–413. https://doi.org/10.1111/geb.12856.

37. Nie, J., Li, Y. H., Yang, X., Zheng, J., Xie, Y., & Shi, L. (2023). Effect of fertilization treatment on growth, yield, fruit quality, and nutrition accumulation of cherry tomato. *Applied Ecology*

and Environmental Research. https://www.semanticscholar.org/paper/68b363f4379362a69d2df3ff65c85adf8c117b1e (accessed on 26 May 2025).

38. Paffoni, A., Casalechi, M., de Ziegler, D., Cicinelli, E., Somigliana, E., Viganò, P., & Vitagliano, A. (2024). Live birth after oocyte donation *in vitro* fertilization cycles in women with endometriosis. *JAMA Network Open, 7*(1). https://www.semanticscholar.org/paper/9e5e06926ee74c10317395c6da4dc7628e1cbc22 (accessed on 26 May 2025).
39. Pan, Q., Bai, Y., Wu, J., & Han, X. (2011). Hierarchical plant responses and diversity loss after nitrogen addition: Testing three functionally-based hypotheses in the Inner Mongolia grassland. *PLoS ONE, 6*(9), e20078. https://doi.org/10.1371/journal.pone.0020078.
40. Perumal, V., Balaraman, A. R., Balaraman, D. V., & Rajasekar, S. J. S. (2024). Embryonic quality assessment using advanced deep learning architectures utilizing microscopic images of blastocysts. In *2024 46th Annual International Conference of the IEEE Engineering in Medicine and Biology Society (EMBC)*. https://www.semanticscholar.org/paper/f44013d6f64084506509c3867b2b731a38ba338e (accessed on 26 May 2025).
41. Perveen, H., & Weeds, J. (2024). Protein sequence classification using natural language processing techniques. *bioRxiv*. https://www.semanticscholar.org/paper/531c8b0cd5bca9171f8f3a02c1b54febfe3344f9 (accessed on 26 May 2025).
42. Petrushko, M., Piniaiev, V., & Yurchuk, T. (2021). The history of assisted reproductive technologies: From prohibition to recognition. *History of Science and Technology, 11*(2), 315–328. https://doi.org/10.32703/2415-7422-2021-11-2-315-328.
43. Richardson, K., Steffen, W., Lucht, W., Bendtsen, J., Cornell, S., Donges, J. F., Drüke, M., et al. (2023). Earth beyond six of nine planetary boundaries. *Science Advances, 9*(17), eadh2458. https://doi.org/10.1126/sciadv.adh2458.
44. Rubin, J. B. (2022). The spectrum of sex differences in cancer. *Trends in Cancer, 8*(4), 303–315. https://doi.org/10.1016/j.trecan.2022.01.013.
45. Santiago, J., Simkova, M., Silva, J., Santos, M. A. S., Vítků, J., & Fardilha, M. (2024). Bisphenol A negatively impacts human sperm microRNA and protein profiles. *Exposure and Health*. https://www.semanticscholar.org/paper/c1c432a416b840d4275c53fb2c35f6e1afed48a7 (accessed on 26 May 2025).
46. Sies, H., Berndt, C., & Jones, D. P. (2017). Oxidative stress. *Annual Review of Biochemistry, 86*, 715–748. https://doi.org/10.1146/annurev-biochem-061516-045037.
47. Skendžić, S., Zovko, M., Pajač Živković, I., Lešić, V., & Lemić, D. (2021). The impact of climate change on agricultural insect pests. *Insects, 12*(5), 440. https://doi.org/10.3390/insects12050440.
48. St. Peter, F., Vadrev, S. M., & Soufan, O. (2022). R400: A novel gene signature for dose prediction in radiation exposure studies in humans. *Semantic Scholar*. https://www.semanticscholar.org/paper/d8eb48a7abde1bf39d8d998e2479338c8dbe56f1 (accessed on 26 May 2025).
49. Surkova, K. L., & Zvereva, N. V. (2025). The development of higher mental functions of children born with intracytoplasmic sperm injection, compared with *in vitro* fertilization. *Психология и Психотехника*. https://www.semanticscholar.org/paper/65b26f7705f626aea75ed888e8e39a42d2d951b5 (accessed on 26 May 2025).

50. Tyagitha, G. A., Nuryanto, K., Pratama, G., Maidarti, M., Harzif, A., Sumapraja, K., Lestari, S. W., et al. (2024). Comparison of natural versus artificial cycles for endometrial preparation prior to frozen embryo transfer. *Universal Medicina*. https://www.semanticscholar.org/paper/84539300f7306e003b509bf6d1ea10b33e36fafa (accessed on 26 May 2025).

51. von Schondorf-Gleicher, A., Mochizuki, L., Orvieto, R., Patrizio, P., Caplan, A. S., & Gleicher, N. (2022). Revisiting selected ethical aspects of current clinical *in vitro* fertilization (IVF) practice. *Journal of Assisted Reproduction and Genetics, 39*, 591–604. https://doi.org/10.1007/s10815-022-02439-7.

52. Wang, C., Mbizvo, M. T., Festin, M., Björndahl, L., & Toskin, I. (2022a). Evolution of the WHO "Semen" processing manual from the first (1980) to the sixth edition (2021). *Fertility and Sterility, 117*(2), 237–245. https://doi.org/10.1016/j.fertnstert.2021.11.037.

53. Wang, Y., Chen, P., Wang, F., Han, W., Qiao, M., Dong, W., Hu, C., et al. (2022b). The ecological clusters of soil organisms drive the ecosystem multifunctionality under long-term fertilization. *Environment International, 161*, 107133. https://doi.org/10.1016/j.envint.2022.107133.

54. Xiong, W., Shen, C., & Wang, Z. (2021). The molecular mechanisms underlying acrosome biogenesis elucidated by gene-manipulated mice. *Biology of Reproduction, 105*(4), 789–807. https://doi.org/10.1093/biolre/ioab117.

55. Xue, Y., Cheng, X., Xiong, Y., & Li, K. (2022). Gene mutations associated with fertilization failure after *in vitro* fertilization/intracytoplasmic sperm injection. *Frontiers in Endocrinology, 13*, 1086883. https://doi.org/10.3389/fendo.2022.1086883.

56. Yu, K., Xiao, K., Sun, Q., Liu, R., Huang, L., Zhang, P., Xu, H., et al. (2023). Comparative proteomic analysis of seminal plasma exosomes in buffalo with high and low sperm motility. *BMC Genomics, 24*, Article 91. https://doi.org/10.1186/s12864-022-09106-2.

57. Zegers-Hochschild, F., Adamson, G. D., Dyer, S., Racowsky, C., de Mouzon, J., Sokol, R. Z., Rienzi, L., et al. (2017). The International Glossary on Infertility and Fertility Care, 2017. *Fertility and Sterility, 108*(3), 393–406. https://doi.org/10.1016/j.fertnstert.2017.06.005.

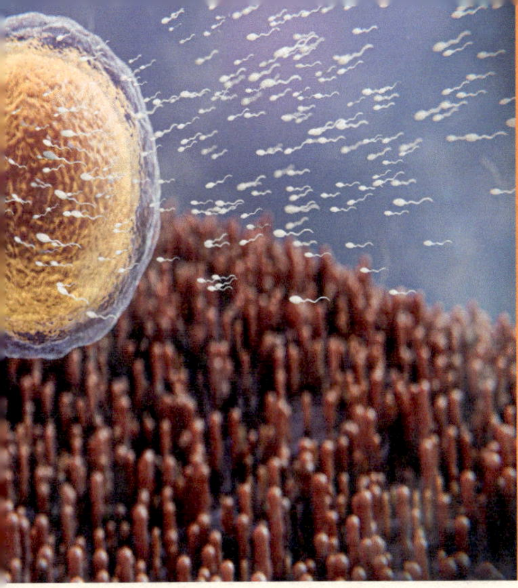

Chapter 4

CLEAVAGE AND BLASTOCYST FORMATION

Contents

Introduction

Shortly after fertilization, human growth kicks off with a burst of transformation in the early embryo. What happens next is a layered, sometimes unexpected journey—starting with events like cleavage and the eventual formation of the blastocyst, which, in many ways, lays down the groundwork for all that follows. We now see that figuring out these early steps isn't just a matter for developmental biology; it also helps tackle many of the fertility issues doctors face today. Conversations on embryology have evolved over time, particularly as standardized language has emerged to help researchers, clinicians, and even patients communicate effectively. In one big push, experts agreed on a list of 283 terminologies related to infertility and fertility care, aiming to bring a more unified approach to how we talk about these topics. This clearly demonstrates how effective communication in prenatal care can impact treatment decisions and patient understanding, providing an important backdrop for studying both cleavage and the formation of the blastocyst. The zygote doesn't hang around as a solo cell for long—it splits repeatedly in a process we call cleavage, quickly evolving into a collection of cells that eventually shape the blastocyst. At this stage, things are happening fast: a series of key, rapid cell divisions unfolds, each one carefully timed and coordinated. As these new cells, the blastomeres, begin to assume their roles, they form two distinct groups: one set that will become the inner cell mass (ICM) and another that develops the outer layer, both of which are essential for later development. Research generally indicates that these early stages are characterized by dynamic changes, where even subtle environmental cues or shifts in cellular signals can tip the balance toward different outcomes. Updated fertility glossaries now push for sharper definitions so that conditions affecting cleavage—and by extension, the health of the blastocyst—can be understood more clearly. Such clarity is vital not only for medical practitioners but also for the people dealing with fertility challenges, as it helps them make better-informed choices about their reproductive options. Cleavage and blastocyst formation aren't just isolated biological events; they ripple out into the broader fields of reproductive medicine and health policy. When science and clinical practice meet—often in unexpected ways—it becomes easier to address various infertility issues seen across different groups. The fresh glossary of terms, for instance, plays a vital role in setting a common language, one that brings a more cohesive feel to discussions about infertility and its treatments. Efforts like these are crucial in our global community, where fertility disparities persist, and where clear, albeit sometimes imperfect, communication can truly make a difference in both research and patient care. Ultimately, gaining a solid understanding of the intricacies of cleavage and blastocyst formation is crucial, prompting us to continue the conversation and collaborate to achieve better reproductive health outcomes for everyone (Figure 4.1).

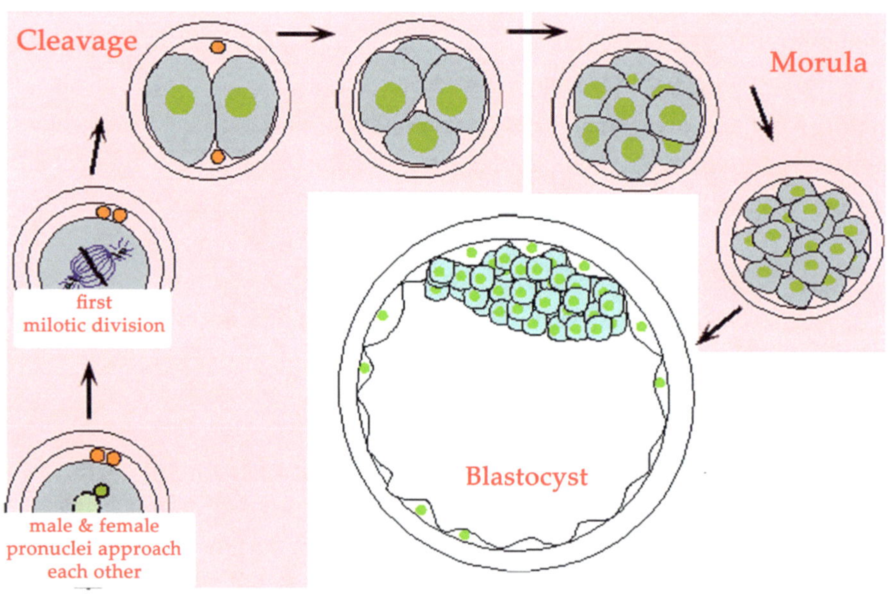

Figure 4.1. Cleavage and blastocyst formation.

Source: https://external-content.duckduckgo.com/iu/?u=https%3A%2F%2Fwww.histology.leeds.ac.uk%2Ffemale%2Fassets%2Fflash%2Fembryonic2004_static.jpg&f=1&nofb=1&ipt=7f6caab880efbaf17e87cecb4cbfc2163a1d7ee5512e06f5f225669fac6b085f.

Definition of Cleavage in Embryonic Development

Early on, embryonic development begins with some remarkable cell events that essentially set the stage for everything to follow. Right after fertilization, there's this burst of dividing—what folks call cleavage—that turns a single zygote into what we refer to as a blastula. It's wild: instead of getting bigger, the egg splits up into a bunch of tiny cells, known as blastomeres, keeping the overall size nearly the same. This rapid-fire splitting, without much growth in between, lays down the basic blueprint needed for later cell specialization and the overall shape of the developing embryo. As these divisions keep happening, the little cells don't just stick together randomly. Depending on the species and even the egg type, they end up arranging themselves in surprising ways. For example, in amphibians, one often sees a nearly perfect radial layout—a neat, almost petal-like symmetry. In contrast, in other creatures, the cells might twist into spiral or even discoidal patterns. Generally speaking, these different arrangements play a significant role in how cells eventually decide their fates. At the same time, various signaling pathways begin firing, nudging the process along toward forming a more organized structure—the blastocyst—which eventually prepares for its transition to the uterine lining. Besides the bustling activity of cleavage, another key player shows up: the extracellular matrix, or ECM. Think of the ECM as a dynamic, 3-D scaffold that not only props up the embryo but also guides essential cell activities like migration and differentiation. Collagen, glycoproteins, and other ECM components mix with the dividing cells, influencing exactly where each one is positioned and how it performs. Even the overall organization of this matrix can influence the shift from rapid cell division to proper blastocyst formation, which is crucial for determining the future developmental course. In most cases, if these early cleavage patterns go awry, it can spell trouble, leading to less viable embryos or even genetic defects. Therefore, understanding these interactions is crucial for improving fertility treatments and advancing developmental biology research (Viotti, 2020) (Figure 4.2).

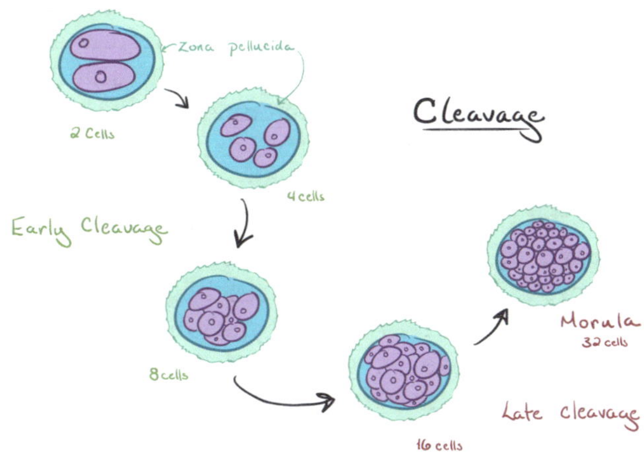

Figure 4.2. Cleavage in embryonic development.

Source: https://cdn.kastatic.org/ka-perseus-images/00d8fac6b7ca6f6e1f0f0f7963f6e2354ea0f50b.svg.

Importance of Blastocyst Formation

Right after fertilization, the zygote begins to split in a rapid and frenzied manner—a process known as cleavage. Oddly enough, these quick divisions don't make the embryo any larger; instead, they lay down an early blueprint by gearing cells up for different jobs. As more cells get active, things suddenly shift: the structure morphs into a blastocyst, where an inner clump of cells (destined to become the fetus) emerges alongside an outer layer that eventually forms the placenta. In most cases, a well-formed blastocyst is key; if this step falters, implantation might not take hold, or the embryo could be lost early on. The blastocyst's overall quality tends to mirror its chances for successful implantation and further development. Recent work—generally speaking—has highlighted telomere length as a biological indicator of embryo quality. Research shows that telomere lengths noticeably increase from the cleavage phase to the blastocyst stage (Achi et al., 2010), suggesting that the cellular environment is more supportive of growth at this stage.

This boost in telomere length isn't just about tracking cellular aging; it also reflects the embryo's capacity for further division and differentiation. In a way, the genomic stability and developmental efficiency seen in the blastocyst are closely wedded to how viable the embryo turns out to be. Even metabolism gets in on the act during these early transformations. Instead of simply churning out energy, the embryo's metabolic processes begin to steer cell fate, tweak DNA methylation, and even stir up reactive oxygen species (ROS)—yes, it's a bit of a mixed bag. If these metabolic routines deviate slightly from the intended path, the consequences can be severe, potentially disrupting proper development and leading to implantation failure or disorders (Lewis et al., 2015). As researchers continue to peel back the layers of this metabolic mystery, they hope that a better understanding of the interplay between metabolism and blastocyst quality will spark advances in assisted reproduction and embryo selection methods. In short, understanding these underlying dynamics might help predict who's more likely to implant successfully and, ultimately, boost overall fertility treatment outcomes.

4.1. The Process of Cleavage

Right after fertilization, cleavage starts in a surprisingly messy way—cells divide rapidly without much growth, turning one fertilized egg into a bunch of smaller ones. These little blastomeres split apart under a jumble of genetic cues and chemical signals. Getting this division spot-on is crucial because even a slight error can throw the following stages off track. Researchers have observed that when cells are either displaced or discarded during this phase, it can significantly impact how well the embryo develops later on (Coticchio et al., 2021). In a sense, every single cleavage event is essential; the way cells arrange themselves early on lays the groundwork for turning into a blastocyst. Then there's the issue of compaction.

As cells start to stick together more closely, they form a type of clumped, cohesive structure. This isn't just a random physical shuffle—it actually builds the basic framework needed for later cell differences to crop up. Sometimes, though, not all cells join in and end up with a partly compacted morula, where a few cells are left out. It turns out that this uneven mix isn't just about appearances; it can significantly impact the embryo's potential and its subsequent development. Studies generally show that embryos with only partial compaction tend to have lower rates of blastocyst formation and overall viability, suggesting that the local cell environment is a significant factor (Agnieszka et al., 2016).

Exploring these early steps of cleavage and compaction goes beyond mere scientific curiosity—it has real-world perks, especially for assisted reproductive technologies (ART). With time-lapse imaging these days, embryologists can watch the tiny motions and timings in ways that weren't possible before, spotting clear ties between how cells split and the health of the embryo. This deeper look helps clinicians refine which embryos are most suitable for in vitro fertilization (IVF), thereby boosting success rates. Plus, understanding how slight changes in cleavage might affect pregnancy rates means patient care can become more nuanced. All in all, while the early stages of embryo development are intricate and a bit unpredictable, they also hold the key to improving reproductive health and pushing forward biomedical science (Coticchio et al., 2021) (Figure 4.3).

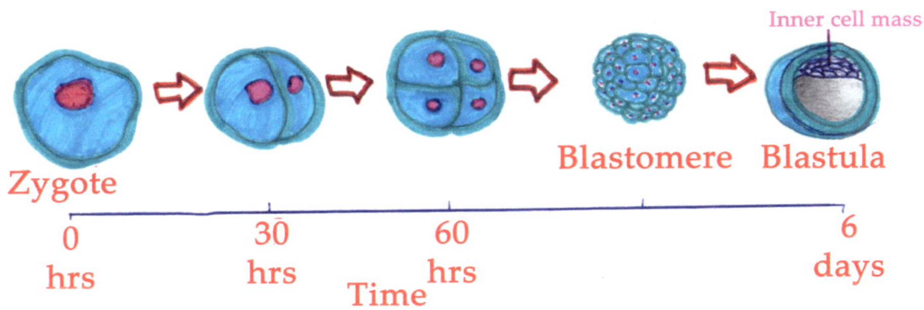

Figure 4.3. Cleavage process.

Source: https://fasciainfo.wordpress.com/wp-content/uploads/2015/04/cleavage-process.png.

4.1.1. Description of Cleavage Stages

Embryonic development begins with a series of events that we typically group under the term cleavage. Once fertilization occurs, the zygote starts rapidly splitting—those fast, sometimes almost simultaneous cell divisions turn one lone cell into a cluster. Approximately 30 hours after fertilization, the first division occurs, resulting in the formation of two blastomeres. It's fascinating how these divisions not only happen so quickly but also neatly divide up the original cytoplasm, making each new cell smaller even though the overall size of the embryo barely changes. With each new round of division, the embryo undergoes subtle shape shifts that, in most cases, lay the groundwork for later processes such as differentiation and compaction; this dynamic underlines the layered complexity of early development. In the first few days after fertilization, further surprising changes occur. As the cleavage goes on, the little blastomeres start bonding more closely—almost as if they're conversing—to eventually form what we call a morula by about day three. At this stage, one typically sees between 16 and 32 cells closely packed together, held by sticky, adhesive forces that build a kind of makeshift network. In that tight ball, several signaling routes get activated, nudging the embryo slowly toward the blastocyst phase. The morula, with its crowded arrangement, sets the stage for the formation of the blastocoel—a fluid-filled cavity that makes the blastocyst stand out. This clumping and repeating process of compaction is crucial, as it ultimately leads to the emergence of different cell groups, including those destined to become the trophoblast and the ICM. By roughly day five, the embryo reaches the blastocyst stage, and things start shifting in a significant way. The transformation from a morula to a blastocyst sees the blastocoel forming, which then helps the embryo expand and get ready to attach to the uterine lining. What we're looking at here is a shift away from those extremely rapid early divisions toward a more organized, complex structure that combines cell specialization with noticeable shape changes. At this juncture, cells deep within the inner mass begin to show signs of picking different cell types, while the outer layer forms into what's known as the trophectoderm. This outer group will eventually play a significant role in implantation and placentation. Generally speaking, understanding this pivot sheds light on improvements in ART; innovations such as vitrification have improved the cryopreservation success rates for embryos at this critical stage (Rienzi et al., 2016). Furthermore, when researchers evaluate blastocyst morphology, they repeatedly find that individual cell traits can predict implantation outcomes, challenging some of our longstanding ideas in embryology (Capalbo et al., 2014) (Figure 4.4).

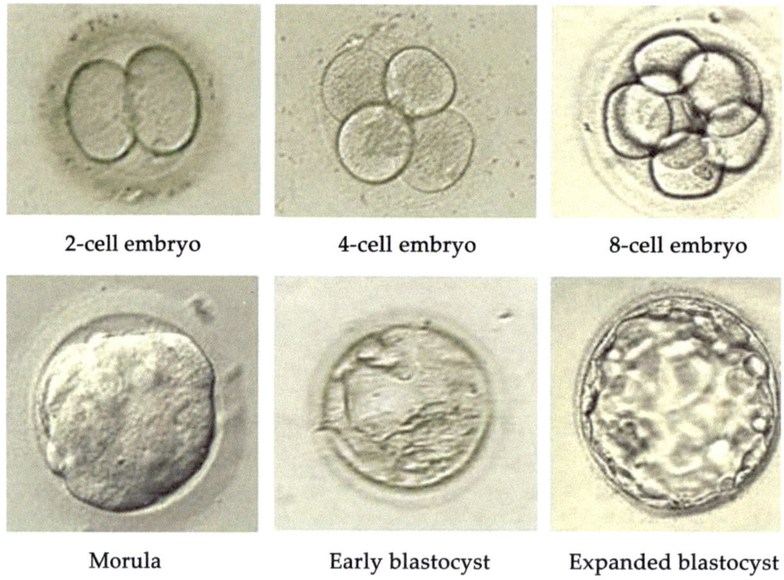

Figure 4.4. Cleavage stages.

Source: https://www.eugonia.com.gr/[template_url]/photos/450px/140-grouped.jpg.

4.1.2. Types of Cleavage Patterns (e.g., Holoblastic Versus Meroblastic)

Early in development, embryos exhibit different ways in which cells divide, which significantly shape how tissues ultimately form. Think about holoblastic cleavage – a process where, say, frogs and sea urchins have their fertilized egg completely divide into many tiny, almost equal-sized cells called blastomeres. This splitting gives each cell a fair share of the cytoplasm and other goodies, letting them interact and "communicate" with one another as the embryo develops. It's crucial, as these initial moves lay the groundwork for building specialized structures in the growing embryo (Pierre-François Lenne et al., 2020). Then there's meroblastic cleavage, which occurs in animals with eggs rich in yolk, such as birds and reptiles. In these cases, only a small patch of the egg – one that barely has any yolk – actually gets divided, while the big yolk blob stays untouched primarily. That tiny region forms what's known as a blastodisc, resting on top of the yolk, which ends up with a unique and slightly unpredictable cell layout that later needs to work well together. The real challenge is that the cells have to juggle their signals and cues in a tight spot next to all that yolk. Generally speaking, this kind of split shows off a natural compromise between sharing resources and pushing cell growth along (Pierre-François Lenne et al., 2020). Examining both approaches side by side opens up an evolutionary window into multicellularity. Over time, as creatures adapted to their surroundings, the distinction between holoblastic and meroblastic modes proved to be closely tied to survival tactics in various habitats. A mix of chemical traits and mechanical forces drives these cell divisions, and that, in turn, helps build the complex structures we see in multicellular life. Even when mammalian blastocyst formation is considered, those early cell interactions are setting the stage. Ongoing research, with its unique quirks and imperfect details, continues to reveal the critical importance of these division styles in the long, complex story of life (Liebich et al., 2020) (Figure 4.5).

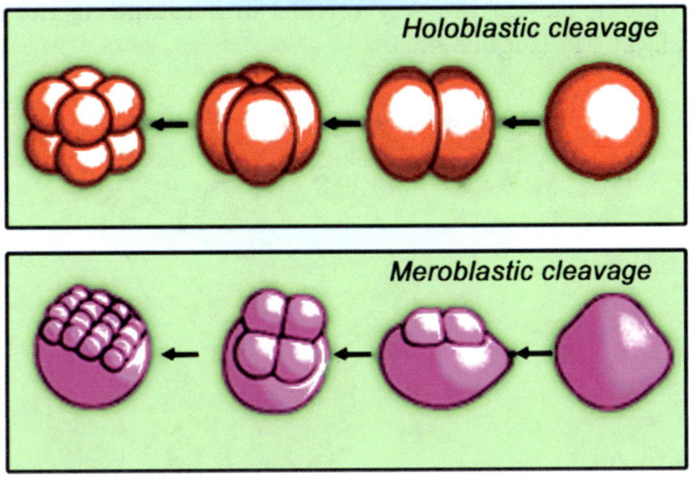

Figure 4.5. Types of cleavage patterns.

Source: https://external-content.duckduckgo.com/iu/?u=https%3A%2F%2Fwww.vedantu.com%2Fquestion-sets%2F96c870d7-7b93-4bf7-a1af-7c693cfb2a5188598736140051028l4.png&f=1&nofb=1&ipt=b9189c88b533881c49edd1e744124513bd8f25a9bbdf346b2c4d540c38fb112f.

4.1.3. Role of Cleavage in Cell Division and Growth

Early on in embryogenesis, cleavage – those quick, successive cell divisions right after fertilization – sets the stage. The zygote, undergoing a sort of dramatic transformation, quickly divides into many small cells, yet the overall size remains about the same. In most cases, this process distributes both resources and genetic material to each blastomere, helping the embryo transition into the blastocyst stage. Timing is everything; even slight irregularities in how these divisions occur can trigger developmental changes, such as aneuploidy, which highlights the crucial importance of getting the cell splits right (Barker et al., 2014). Cell interactions during this time also come into play, loosely assembling the embryo's earliest layers and nudging lineage specification along. The physical forces at work – the pushes and pulls as cells divide – end up playing a big part in holding together the embryo's structure and function. The way cells line up and interact, without a strict playbook, guides the formation of key tissues, such as the trophectoderm and endoderm. Generally speaking, when researchers use computational modeling, they're gradually uncovering an intricate tug-of-war between genetic cues and mechanical influences. For example, the precise positioning of cells, along with their varied adhesion traits, appears to significantly influence how robustly the endoderm forms, suggesting that the physical layout is just as important as the genetic instructions in early development (Jedrusik et al., 2011). As cleavage marches on, hitting the blastocyst phase turns out to be a serious turning point. This is when features such as the blastocoel and the ICM start to appear, marking a new chapter in embryonic growth. Not only does the pattern of cell division decide the embryo's physical makeup, it also tweaks the timing for gene expression needed for the following stages. There's a sort of symbiotic push-and-pull between mechanical forces and genetic signals—cell positioning and movement even seem to help orchestrate ICM formation. Observing these nuances, researchers suggest that both the formation of the blastocoel and the way cells maneuver around are vital pieces of the puzzle. All in all, this blend of physical and genetic factors effectively highlights the layered, multifaceted nature of early embryonic development, paving the way toward understanding the subtleties of blastocyst formation (Jedrusik et al., 2011) (Figure 4.6).

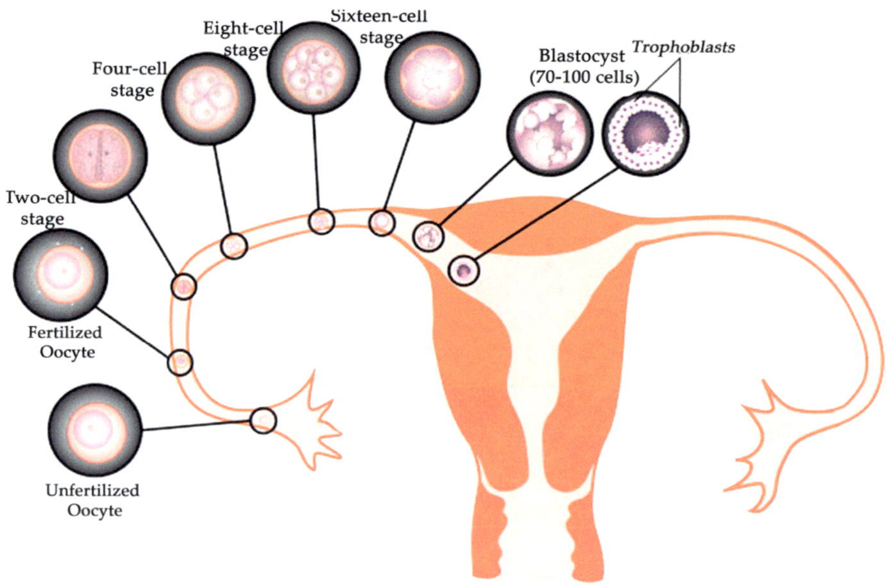

Figure 4.6. Cell cleavage.

Source: https://ars.els-cdn.com/content/image/3-s2.0-B9780128012383644756-f64475-01-9780128118993.jpg.

4.2. Cellular Mechanisms in Cleavage

Cellular coordination during cleavage initiates the remarkable journey from a fertilized egg to a fully developed multicellular embryo. At this early stage, cells divide rapidly without significant overall growth, so the pathways responsible for chromosome sorting and cell survival must be precise. A substantial part of this process is handled by NEK2—a serine/threonine protein kinase that facilitates the progression of cells through mitosis. In most cases, messing with NEK2 slows down cleavage and even stunts blastocyst formation. When NEK2 is inhibited, unusual cell cycle patterns emerge, triggering increased DNA damage and a spike in cell death, which ultimately disrupts the formation of key mitochondrial structures necessary for energy and early survival (Se-Jeon et al., 2024). There's also Myo-Inositol (Myo-Ins), adding another twist to these early events. Myo-Ins works somewhat like an antioxidant and is vital for maintaining the redox balance steady during these hectic rounds of cell division. Some experimental work suggests that adding extra Myo-Ins can significantly enhance blastocyst formation and improve the viability of dividing embryos. For example, around 20 mM of Myo-Ins increases intracellular glutathione levels while lowering ROS – a clear indication of healthier cells and reduced apoptosis. This regulation of oxidative stress is crucial, as higher markers of mitochondrial function in Myo-Ins-treated embryos point to a better adaptation to the intense metabolic demands of early development (Jawad et al., 2024). Mixing everything, the interaction between different signaling routes and cell functions underlines the complexity of early embryonic development. The link between NEK2 and the Wnt/β-catenin pathway, for instance, is significant since the latter is central to gene regulation during both cleavage and blastocyst formation. When NEK2 activity drops, β-catenin and its target genes follow suit, disturbing key developmental processes. This scenario highlights the importance of these interconnected pathways in maintaining genome integrity and ensuring orderly cell division. So, gaining an understanding of these cellular mechanisms not only sheds light on the intricacies of cleavage and blastocyst formation but may also reveal new avenues for intervention when developmental issues arise (Se-Jeon et al., 2024) (Figure 4.7).

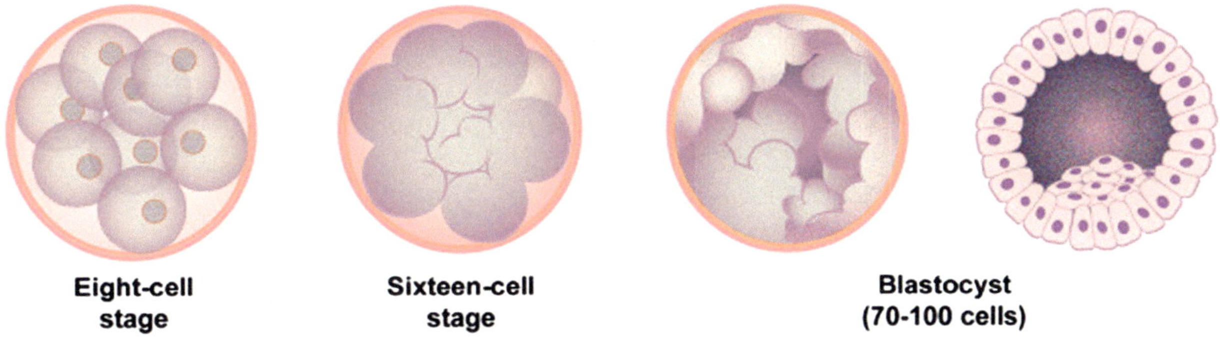

Figure 4.7. Cellular mechanisms in cleavage.

Source: https://ars.els-cdn.com/content/image/3-s2.0-B9780128012383644756-f64475-02-9780128118993.jpg.

4.2.1. Role of Mitosis in Cleavage

Embryonic development hinges on how cells grow and split—a process that's far from random. Mitosis kicks everything off right after fertilization, acting as the engine that drives a lone zygote to divide repeatedly, eventually forming a cluster of cells. This burst of division forms a blastocyst, which sets the stage for implantation and the later creation of the placenta. Even small slips in this process can mess up the embryo's structure and function, so keeping things in perfect order is key. Cell division isn't just a simple split; it's a finely tuned series of events that shapes how embryonic cells end up. Take the protein NEK2, for instance. When NEK2 gets held back, things go awry—cleavage slows down and blastocyst formation takes a hit. In studies on porcine embryos, blocking NEK2 resulted in unusual changes in the nucleus, accompanied by spikes in DNA damage and cell death. Generally speaking, these observations highlight how minor disruptions in mitosis can have a profound impact, dramatically affecting embryo viability (Se-Jeon et al., 2024). On top of that, there's a constant back-and-forth between mitosis and cell signaling. The Wnt/β-catenin pathway, known to regulate cell growth and differentiation, demonstrates how external signals can influence the inner workings of a cell during these early stages. In a sort of twist, when NEK2 is inhibited, it not only slows down mitosis but also cuts back on β-catenin and its related targets—altering decisions essential for trophoblast development. This interplay, with its cascade of effects on placentation and embryonic health, underscores the delicate balance required for proper cleavage and the formation of a robust blastocyst (Kn Möfler et al., 2019) (Figure 4.8).

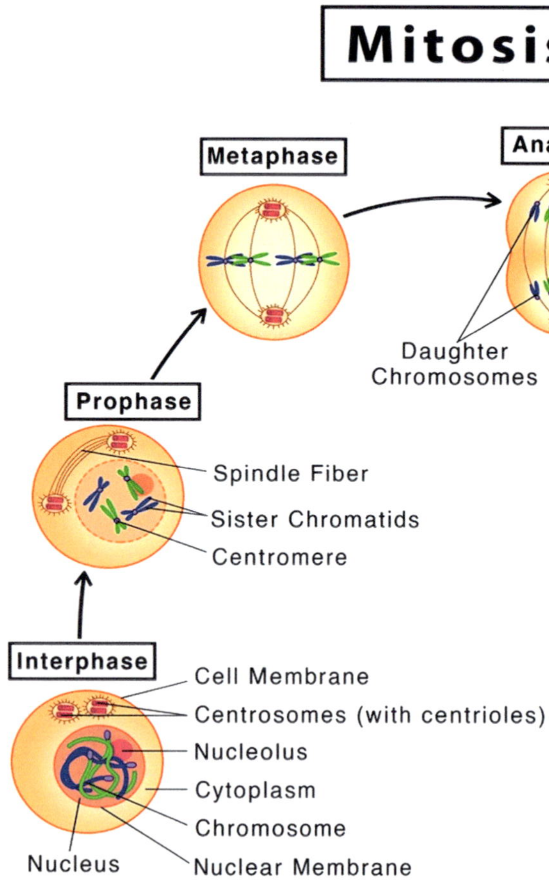

Figure 4.8. Role of mitosis in cleavage.

Source: https://microscopiaiwm.wordpress.com/wp-content/uploads/2023/12/mitosis-phases-diagram.jpg?w=950.

4.2.2. Cytoplasmic Factors Influencing Cleavage

Cleavage initiates a pivotal phase in early embryonic development immediately after fertilization, when cells begin to divide almost as if on autopilot. Genes do have their say, but what's inside the cell matters a lot too—proteins, mRNAs, and various little organelles all help set up the cell's inner layout and push the mechanics needed for division. Take, for example, how the placement of maternal mRNAs can lead to an uneven spread of these crucial elements; this unevenness gently nudges what path the daughter cells might follow later on. In most cases, the back-and-forth between the zygotic blueprint and the mother's contributions ends up forming the very framework of the embryo. Inside the cell, things get even more interesting when these cytoplasmic actors also fine-tune the timing and rhythm of the splits. Generally speaking, proteins like cyclins and cyclin-dependent kinases (CDKs) work like conductors, coordinating the steps of the cell cycle. At the same time, ions and small molecules blend into the mix as messengers. This type of coordination helps ensure that divisions occur precisely when they should, paving the way for proper blastocyst formation—even if a misstep here can lead to unusual cleavage patterns that shed light on developmental biology and issues with infertility (Zegers-Hochschild et al., 2017). The story doesn't stop at just dividing cells, either. The inner flow of the cytoplasm and the strength of the cell's internal scaffolding play a significant role in maintaining a cell's shape and managing the small shifts that occur during division. Additionally, the maternal environment—consider the unique blend found in the oocyte's cytoplasm—can significantly influence later events, such as how cells determine their roles. It seems fairly clear that aligning everyone on the same page with definitions and terms could greatly facilitate collaboration among researchers, clinicians, and policymakers as they tackle the complex world of reproductive sciences and developmental issues (Zegers-Hochschild et al., 2017).

4.2.3. Genetic Regulation During Cleavage

Mammalian embryogenesis unfolds with a maze of careful steps—especially noticeable during cleavage, when the zygote splits rapidly. It isn't just a simple matter of adding more cells; there's a hefty dose of genetic control that cues cells into finding their roles.

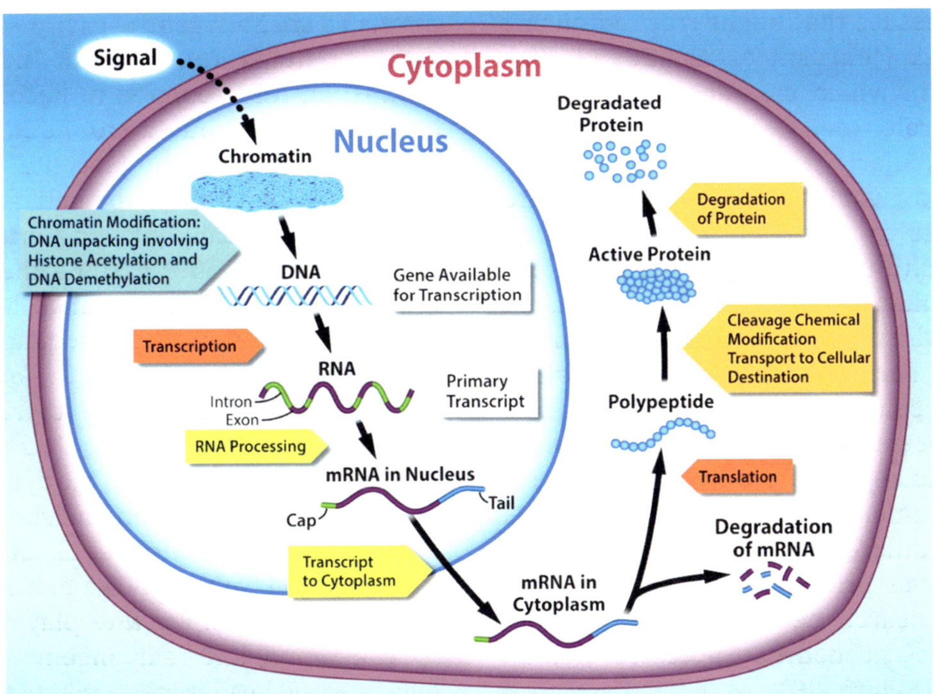

Figure 4.9. Genetic regulation during cleavage.

Source: https://louis.pressbooks.pub/app/uploads/sites/26/2022/04/84-1024x768.png.

Gene activity and physical forces appear to work in tandem here, nudging cells into specific locations and maintaining their health. Nowadays, computer models give us a glimpse into this complex network of processes, suggesting that where a cell ends up may alter its genetic signals, or sometimes the other way around. These insights, in many cases, shine a light on how the trophectoderm and endoderm form, setting the stage for a proper structure needed for implantation and further growth (Jedrusik et al., 2011). As cleavage continues, the inner workings that shape embryo form begin to stand out more clearly. Cells line up roughly along what we call the animal-vegetal and embryonic-abembryonic axes, and this alignment appears to be driven by a tendency to minimize elastic energy. It raises the question: do cells naturally steer themselves into these patterns, or is it more about external pressures giving them a slight push? Some studies generally suggest two possibilities for the formation of the endoderm layer: either an internal directional force steers the cells, or pressure from the blastocoel gently molds them into place. Figuring out these dynamics not only deepens our understanding of basic early development but also lays the groundwork for exploring issues that might crop up during embryogenesis (Jedrusik et al., 2011). The environment in which cleavage occurs plays a significant role, too. Recent breakthroughs in IVF—particularly those using enclosed, isolator-based workstations—demonstrate the importance of mimicking a natural setup for embryo culture. These controlled systems have been linked with noticeable boosts in developmental success, with more embryos reaching the blastocyst stage and sporting healthier cell counts. All in all, such findings emphasize that external conditions significantly impact genetic regulation during cleavage; a stable environment helps ensure that cells multiply and differentiate correctly. This sort of insight proves priceless, both in the clinic and at the research bench, illuminating the delicate balance needed for successful human reproduction (Figure 4.9).

4.3. Transition from Cleavage to Blastocyst

The change kicks in when early embryonic growth shifts from rapid cleavage to forming what we call a blastocyst—a moment loaded with changes in how cells act and settle down. In the cleavage phase, the embryo rapidly divides into a series of tiny cells, known as blastomeres, without significant growth in size. Research shows these splits bring about a mix of cell behaviors; sometimes cells move differently or express genes in unexpected ways. When scientists isolate medaka blastomeres, they often observe unusual behaviors, such as abortive division or even cell fusion – a hint that the usual rules of cell growth don't equally govern every single cell. This jumble of activity paves the way for blastocyst formation, during which cells begin to differentiate and organize more purposefully for the steps ahead (Li et al., 2010). Somewhere along cleavage, a key transformation happens. The embryo begins to develop a shallow, central cavity – the blastocoel – which helps shuffle cells into two rough groups: an ICM destined to become the future embryo and an outer trophoblast layer that gets ready to form the placenta. At this point, cells begin to commit to their fates, with the inner cells typically growing into the embryo while the outer ones assume their supportive roles. Researchers, for instance, have examined telomere length as a quality gauge; they found that telomeres shrink from the oocyte through the cleavage process, only to rebound when the blastocyst takes shape. This subtle shift in telomere length underlines the dynamic nature of early cell development and marks quality during this critical period (Achi et al., 2010). All in all, the transition from cleavage to blastocyst neatly illustrates the complex interplay of cell division, specialization, and rearrangement that unfolds during early development. What starts as a loose collection of blastomeres eventually becomes a tightly organized blastocyst, with each cell seemingly taking on a role—and sometimes even repeating actions—in ways that surprise us. The lessons learned from observing individual blastomeres at work deepen our understanding of basic developmental biology and may even lead to new insights in reproductive technology and regenerative medicine. Telomere length, acting as a quality signal for the embryo, adds yet another twist that highlights the importance of this shift in both natural and assisted reproduction contexts. Ultimately, understanding these processes thoroughly can significantly enhance our comprehension of development and contribute to improved reproductive health outcomes (Achi et al., 2010; Li et al., 2010).

4.3.1. Timing of Transition in Mammalian Development

Early mammalian development begins with a series of shifts that significantly shape what comes next. The zygote divides rapidly, and—almost unexpectedly—a process called cleavage unfolds. This isn't about the embryo getting bigger overall; it's more about creating more cells through a series of organized splits. In no particular order, this phase suddenly lays down the basis for the blastocyst, where cells begin to branch off into distinct groups: one that forms the ICM and another that makes up the trophoblast.

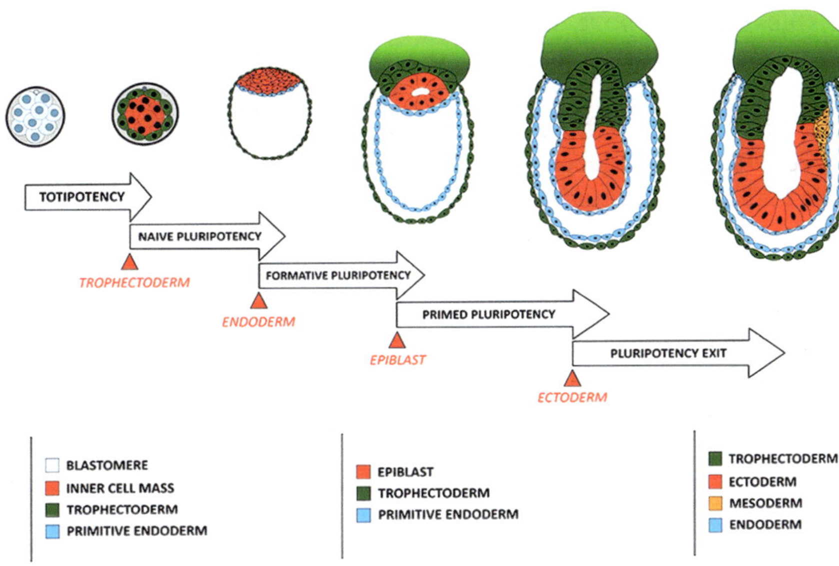

Figure 4.10. Timing of transition in mammalian development.

Source: https://www.frontiersin.org/files/Articles/639244/fcell-09-639244-HTML/image_m/fcell-09-639244-g001.jpg.

When one looks closely at the timing behind these events, one notices that even slight changes can mess with how cells decide their roles—sometimes throwing off implantation or other later processes. Generally speaking, studies have suggested that these early steps aren't just mechanical routines; they're also influenced by molecular signals that may, in a roundabout way, trigger rejuvenation processes, aligning with broader discussions about aging and development as seen in the ground zero model (Vadim, 2020). Switching gears from cleavage to blastocyst formation, metabolism suddenly takes on a starring role. New research suggests that specific metabolic pathways are crucial in determining cell fate—essentially, whether a cell continues to divide, changes its function, or enters a state of rest. At this point, getting the balance right between glycolysis and mitochondrial energy production becomes a big deal; emerging evidence shows there's a link between a cell's energy state and its eventual identity. In most cases, this type of metabolic reprogramming is crucial for establishing the optimal environment for the blastocyst to develop and eventually implant. It's almost as if the interplay of energy and behavior adds extra layers to our understanding of development—echoing, in an oddly familiar way, some of the rejuvenation processes we see in pluripotent stem cells (Shyh et al., 2013). The timing of these developmental shifts also seems to align with larger evolutionary ideas, such as the phylotypic stage—a brief period during which many embryos appear remarkably similar, as if they're all following an ancient blueprint with fewer disruptions. When these changes take effect, they activate biological mechanisms that support smooth morphogenesis and proper cell differentiation, while simultaneously attempting to minimize cellular damage. It's interesting to note that, although the early rejuvenation process may extend through these stages, it eventually gives way to aging-related events as development progresses. In a somewhat contradictory yet natural fashion, early embryogenesis ultimately balances rejuvenation efforts alongside a path that ultimately leads to aging—a continuum stretching from that initial state to full maturity (Vadim, 2020) (Figure 4.10).

4.3.2. Morphological Changes During the Transition

Embryonic development takes a significant turn when the process transitions from cleavage into what is known as a blastocyst. Right after fertilization, the zygote starts splitting rapidly into small, irregularly shaped cells called blastomeres. These tiny cells combine into a clump that later reshapes into a blastocyst, featuring a central cluster of inner cells alongside a surrounding layer of trophoblast cells. This isn't merely a change in cell arrangement; it also gets the embryo ready to attach to the uterine wall. In most cases, maintaining a consistent cell layout is crucial to future viability, and both genetic cues and environmental factors play their roles—even if sometimes they're somewhat unpredictable. During this period, a host of cellular processes jump in to help reorganize everything for the next stage. One striking event is the formation of the blastocoel – a fluid-filled space that appears as the ICM starts pulling away from the outer trophoblast cells. This change in structure is crucial because it creates the kind of layout needed for the upcoming developmental maneuvers. Meanwhile, specific genes that control cell signaling, adhesion, and differentiation begin to get more active, essentially steering the future fates of these embryonic cells.

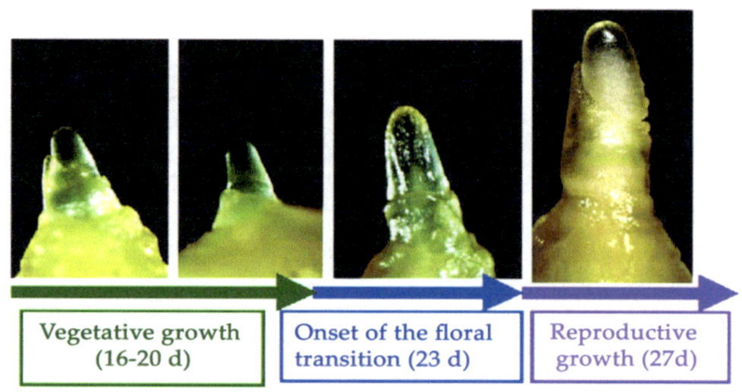

Figure 4.11. Morphological changes during the transition.

Source: https://www.researchgate.net/profile/Michael-Muszynski/publication/51576458/figure/fig1/AS:669214679515141@1536564621602/morphological-changes-of-the-shoot-apical-meristem-during-the-floral-transition-of-the.png.

Digging into these cellular and molecular shifts reveals that both internal and external influences can maintain or disrupt this delicate order—proving that early development is both dynamic and occasionally messy. The ripple effects of these shape changes persist well beyond the early stages, influencing later events such as implantation and placentation. Research generally suggests that even slight disruptions during the cleavage-to-blastocyst transition can lower embryo quality, potentially leading to poorer implantation outcomes and adverse long-term effects. Factors like oxidative stress, for instance, can damage the cells' structure and function, highlighting the critical importance of maintaining a solid cellular environment (Jae-Yoon et al., 2020). A shared, standardized vocabulary for these processes has also been established, which helps researchers and clinicians communicate more clearly—ultimately guiding interventions in ART (Zegers-Hochschild et al., 2017) (Figure 4.11).

4.3.3. Significance of the Transition for Implantation

Cleavage and blastocyst formation mark a key phase in early development, setting the stage for implantation. The embryo moves from its initial cell, splits into a more organized blastocyst, switching up both its shape and functions in ways that boost its ability to stick to the uterine lining. This isn't just about a rapid surge in cell numbers or changing roles—it also demands that cell divisions happen right on schedule. Early on, those first cleavage events are especially prone to error; frequent changes in the cell cycle can lead to developmental missteps or even cell death, which compromises overall viability. Getting a handle on these early dynamics is crucial, as they lay the groundwork for a successful implantation and later fetal growth (Bettegowda et al., 2011). When considering embryonic development as a whole, the cell cycle must shift smoothly from one phase to the next, maintaining a delicate balance between cell multiplication and specialization. In most cases, making the jump from somatic cell traits to those needed during embryonic cleavage is crucial. Studies generally show that when this shift isn't quite up to snuff—as seen in some somatic cell nuclear transfer (NT) embryos—it can drag out the cell cycle and even lead to cleavage arrests. This slowdown disrupts the timely formation of a blastocyst, which is crucial for a successful implantation. At the same time, the embryo's energy demands spike while it uses less of the key amino acids needed for growth, further hindering proper development (Varshavsky et al., 2012). Once the blastocyst starts to form, two main parts emerge: the ICM and the trophoblast. Each part plays its vital role in the implementation. This split helps the embryo adhere to the uterine wall and eventually invade the endometrium—a crucial step in initiating nutrient exchange and support. Examining the molecular level, such as shifts in gene expression and the role of programmed cell death, provides insights into why things sometimes go awry. For instance, the controlled cell death observed in the ICM appears to act as a quality control mechanism, ensuring only the best cells survive for implantation. Overall, these nuances highlight the complexity of the blastocyst stage and underscore the importance of proper transitions for successful implantation and subsequent fetal development (Bettegowda et al., 2011).

4.4. Formation of the Blastocyst

The journey begins with a fertilized egg unexpectedly splitting into smaller parts. Early on, the cell division—done in a not-so-perfect way—yields little blastomeres that later clump together into something we call the blastocyst. This isn't just cells gathering; it's a mix of genetic cues and environmental nudges that push each cell toward its fate and help them stick together. Generally speaking, a smooth cleavage dance is key, and even minor missteps during this phase can profoundly affect the embryo's future viability (Budrewicz et al., 2024). Cells soon begin to assume different roles in a process known as cellular specialization. The inner group, which is destined to develop into the embryo, compacts and forms the groundwork for later tissues. At the same time, the outer layer—the trophoblast—is busy preparing for implantation and nutrient transfer. Strangely enough, when early cell divisions show glitches, like unexpected spindle movements, it can result in extra nuclei or fragments emerging that might weaken the blastocyst's overall structure (Ono et al., 2024). In most cases, this early cell environment plays a considerable role, steering the fate of the little embryo in ways that aren't always predictable. The blastocyst stage isn't a final destination; it's more like the launching pad for critical decisions about implantation and further development. Successful formation relies on a careful balance of gene activity and cell signals, which essentially guide both cell multiplication and differentiation. At the same time, errors during cleavage—sometimes leading to aneuploidy—can be seen later as developmental glitches. Interestingly, even embryos with changes in early cell division sometimes manage to form a functioning blastocyst, although their implantation capabilities may be slightly off-kilter. This resilience, albeit imperfect, demonstrates the dynamic and adaptable nature of early development, while underscoring the significant influence of those initial moments (Budrewicz et al., 2024) (Figure 4.12).

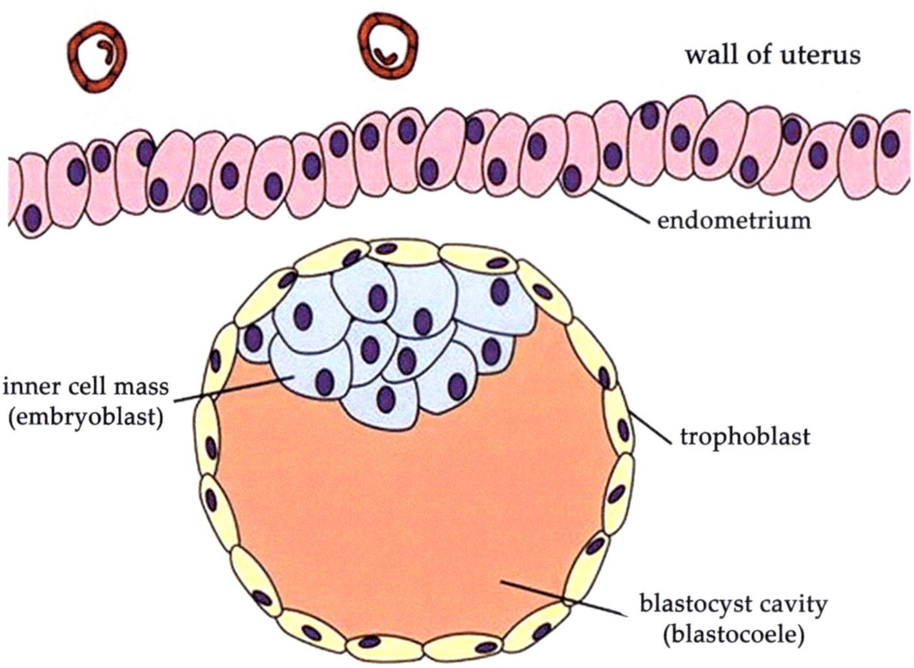

Figure 4.12. Formation of the blastocyst.

Source: https://upload.wikimedia.org/wikipedia/commons/9/9e/Diagram_of_Blastocyst_stage.png.

4.4.1. Structure of the Blastocyst (Inner Cell Mass and Trophoblast)

The shift from the morula to the blastocyst marks a significant change—cells begin to assume distinct roles. Two different groups suddenly get active: deep inside, there's a tight-knit cluster commonly called the ICM, and on the outside, there's the trophoblast. The ICM, packed with stem cells that can become almost any tissue, is pretty much set to form the embryo itself. On the other hand, the trophoblast wraps around the outside and typically assumes the role of anchoring the blastocyst to the uterus. In many cases, these two groups, although different, work together at this early stage to initiate placenta formation and establish the support systems essential for fetal growth.

As the blastocyst moves forward, the behavior of the trophoblast becomes intriguingly complex. Suddenly, it isn't just a simple outer shell; it splits into two main types: the cytotrophoblasts and the syncytiotrophoblast. The cytotrophoblasts – basic single-nucleus cells – serve as early precursors, while the syncytiotrophoblasts merge, forming a multinucleated layer that invades the uterine lining. This invasive capacity, which at times may seem somewhat aggressive, is crucial because it establishes the vital connections between mother and fetus necessary for nutrient transfer and waste removal.

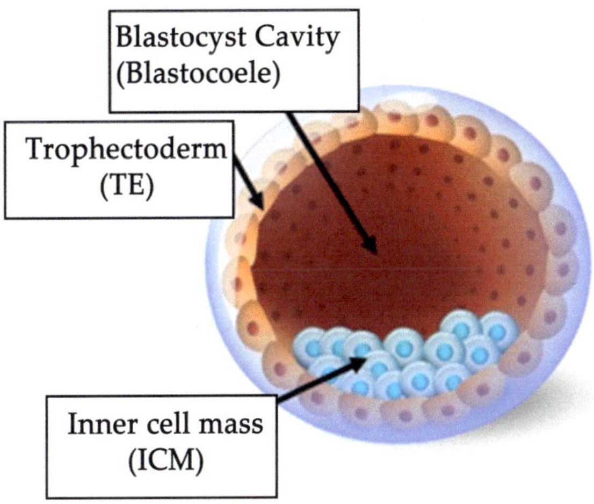

Figure 4.13. Structure of the blastocyst.

Source: https://external-content.duckduckgo.com/iu/?u=https%3A%2F%2Fwww.researchgate.net%2Fpublication%2F359928665%2Ffigure%2Fdownload%2Ffig2%2FAS%3A11479204348887O5%401650696967475%2FThe-human-blastocyst-The-structure-comprises-two-differentiated-cell-types-and-a-central.png&f=1&nofb=1&ipt=701061335707f2db857c09f4154f2c563bec070b37bf60300049eff49b57b02d.

The lively back-and-forth between these cells and the uterine tissues essentially sets the stage for a successful pregnancy and lays the groundwork for later placental functions. It's hard to overstate the importance of the ICM, which truly is the backbone of the developing organism. Through a process of cellular "conversation" involving signaling pathways and molecular mechanics, these cells gradually determine their future roles, ultimately forming the diverse tissues and organs we observe. Recent research, in most cases, has begun to map out these processes – shining a light on pathways like Wingless and Notch that play a crucial role in steering both trophoblast actions and cell fate decisions. Generally speaking, these findings highlight an intricate balance needed for proper placentation, with disturbances potentially linking to complications such as miscarriage or preeclampsia. A deep, albeit sometimes complex, understanding of how the ICM and trophoblast interact within the blastocyst remains essential for deciphering the code behind successful embryonic development (Kn Möfler et al., 2019; Griselda et al., 2020) (Figure 4.13).

4.4.2. Processes Involved in Blastocyst Formation

Starting with a single cell, the path to a blastocyst is hardly a straight shot. It begins with the zygote rapidly dividing—a process often called cleavage—that turns one cell into a small cluster known as the morula, usually holding around 16 to 32 cells. At this stage, the cells begin to shift around in ways that feel almost improvised, laying the groundwork for what comes next. A significant moment occurs when the cells start to clump together, a process known as cellular compaction. This closer contact sets the stage for later division into the parts that form the embryo and its supporting tissues. In many cases, studies (Coticchio et al., 2021) indicate that if this compaction process goes awry—say, with some cells left out or oddly shifted—the overall quality and number of resulting blastocysts can be compromised, posing challenges especially in assisted reproductive settings. As the morula moves into the blastocyst stage, things start to get interesting with two distinct cell groups emerging. The innermost group, the ICM, is destined to become the embryo, while the outer layer, known as the trophoblast, handles implanting into the uterine lining. This division isn't random at all; it relies on a mix of cell signals and mutual "conversations" that steer each cell toward its role. Morphokinetic studies, generally speaking, reveal that even minor changes during or after compaction can seriously affect the blastocyst's ability to develop correctly. For instance, research shows that if the morula doesn't compact uniformly—resulting in cases where cells become excluded or even get pushed aside—the chance of forming high-quality blastocysts diminishes, complicating the outcomes of embryo transfer procedures (Coticchio et al., 2021). Then there are the influences of external factors, which are often overlooked. Harmful exposures affecting sperm can ripple all the way through and alter early development. Research on the protein profiles of sperm exposed to environmental toxins has revealed shifts in protein expression that are crucial for both successful fertilization and early embryonic development. Fertilization with compromised sperm tends to result in slower cleavage and even blastocysts showing genetic irregularities, underscoring just how vital sperm health is in these early stages. This interplay between external stressors and sperm quality highlights the fragile and complex nature of early embryonic development, reminding us that even minor upstream changes can lead to significant downstream consequences (Figure 4.14).

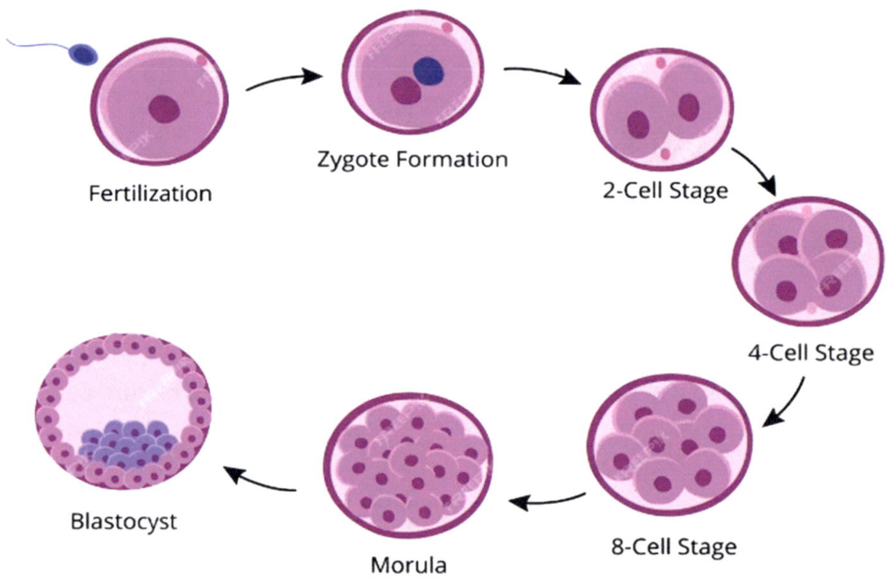

Figure 4.14. Processes involved in blastocyst formation.

Source: https://www.fertilicaivf.com/images/Blastocyst.webp.

4.4.3. Comparison of Blastocyst Formation in Different Species

Blastocyst formation marks the initiation of a crucial phase in early embryonic development; species differ significantly in how this stage unfolds. Variation here provides hints about evolution—different reproductive needs and environmental challenges appear to have nudged each species in a unique direction. Take humans, for example. The blastocyst in our species exhibits some metabolic characteristics not observed in other mammals. Research generally points out that embryos that aren't viable tend to have higher levels of mitochondrial DNA (mtDNA), hinting at a link between mtDNA quantity and embryo health. Mitochondrial condition may play a significant role in whether a blastocyst successfully implants (Fragouli et al., 2015). This nuance helps us understand why human embryogenesis follows a different path compared to other species that may carve out their developmental routes. Looking deeper, the molecular side of blastocyst formation mixes what's familiar with what's distinct across species. One study using single-cell RNA sequencing has shed light on notable differences between human and mouse embryos. In most cases, human epiblasts express unique markers, such as the transcription factor KLF17—a feature that is not easily observed in mice. The activation of key signaling pathways, such as TGF-β, tends to be more pronounced in human embryos, which in turn affects how cells adhere to pluripotency or begin to differentiate. Interestingly, while certain factors in mice are confined to specific lineages, their human counterparts don't always follow this neat pattern, suggesting a divergence in how cell lineages are established (Blakeley et al., 2015). These subtle differences in gene activity and signaling remind us that embryonic development is a complex, ever-changing process. These developmental twists extend beyond basic biology and permeate practical fields such as assisted reproduction. As we learn more about species-specific methods of forming the blastocyst, the implications for clinics offering IVF are becoming increasingly difficult to ignore. For example, biomarkers linked to mtDNA levels may eventually refine the selection of embryos, potentially increasing implantation rates and overall pregnancy success. Comparative studies between humans and mice also help shed light on why some embryos fail to implant or develop issues such as aneuploidy. This kind of insight is exciting because it not only deepens our understanding of developmental biology but also opens new doors for optimizing reproductive techniques in clinical settings (Fragouli et al., 2015). Ultimately, untangling these differences yields both richer scientific insights and practical benefits for reproductive health practices.

4.5. Role of the Blastocyst in Development

Blastocyst formation stands out as one of the key milestones in early mammalian development—when a loose cluster of cells transforms into a more organized, functional structure necessary for implantation and subsequent growth. In many cases, a burst of cellular events (differentiation, compaction, and so on) occurs almost simultaneously, nudging cells into distinct roles. The built-in layout enables the ICM to converse, in its way, with the surrounding trophectoderm; this natural back-and-forth is essential for the embryo to interact with its maternal environment. It's this kind of cellular chatter that paves the way for the uterine attachment and kicks off the nutrient exchange, setting up what we'd call the fetal-maternal interface—a critical foundation for further development. All in all, these intercellular dynamics form the groundwork for everything that follows in embryogenesis. As the structure takes shape, specific proteins and cellular mechanisms get intertwined in steering its development. The expression patterns of particular kinases—namely ROCK1 and ROCK2, which are part of those Rho-associated coiled-coil protein families—illustrate the biochemical shifts during this stage. Generally speaking, ROCK1 is highly active during the early cleavage stages, coordinating cell movements before its levels drop noticeably by the time the blastocyst emerges; meanwhile, ROCK2 increases, especially within the trophectoderm. This switch suggests that ROCK2 may be crucial in driving cell differentiation and supporting the signaling processes essential for implantation and tissue development. In a way, this uneven expression reveals the molecular intricacies behind blastocyst formation and underscores the fine-tuning needed for a viable embryo (Zhang et al., 2014). Beyond serving as a passive structure, the blastocyst actively engages in several biochemical signaling pathways to prepare itself for implantation. For example, early-stage embryos treated with specific inhibitors show that halting the ROCK pathways tends to stall development immediately after cleavage—a clear indication of how critical these molecular players are. It's interesting to note that signaling molecules, such as lysophosphatidic acid, can even enhance formation rates, providing a glimpse into how external factors may influence developmental outcomes. This mix of inherent molecular mechanisms and outside cues paints the blastocyst as a dynamic, responsive entity that continuously negotiates between its internal state and the maternal environment during these pivotal early phases (Kersten et al., 2016) (Figure 4.15).

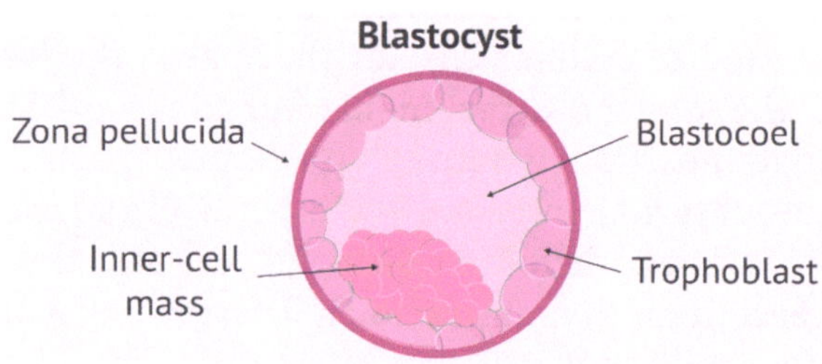

Figure 4.15. Role of the blastocyst in development.

Source: https://external-content.duckduckgo.com/iu/?u=https%3A%2F%2Fbabygest.com%2Fen%2Fwp-content%2Fuploads%2F2019%2F10%2Fblastocyst-development.png&f=1&nofb=1&ipt=c982b962d404d5eb62bf915b7f8c136a70ee456f3cfa123323559ea246254c13.

4.5.1. Functions of the Inner Cell Mass (ICM)

Early in development, the ICM makes its debut as a cluster of versatile, pluripotent cells that kick off the future growth of the embryo. Right after the embryo undergoes cleavage and becomes a blastocyst, these cells begin to differentiate—splitting into two groups that eventually form the epiblast and the hypoblast. Each group contributes in its way to building both embryonic and extra-embryonic structures, and this early division essentially sets up the main principal body axes and even initiates the movement of the embryonic membranes. The ICM's inherent flexibility even allows it to adjust on the fly to the embryo's surroundings during early gestation, which is crucial for overall smooth development. When the blastocyst implants in the uterine wall, the ICM isn't just there to hand out cells; it also sends out signals that nudge the nearby maternal tissue into action. There's a lot of evidence showing that it releases various signaling molecules that help trophoblast cells multiply and move—both of which are key for proper implantation. At the same time, the ICM has to strike a delicate balance between renewing itself and branching off into specialized cells, a juggling act that is essential for the embryo's optimal development. In most cases, if the ICM's functions become out of whack, it can lead to developmental glitches and less efficient implantation, with maternal factors such as age playing a role in how well everything holds together (Ezoe et al., 2023). Examining the broader context of blastocyst formation, the ICM plays a pivotal role in ensuring a healthy pregnancy and robust embryonic development. Its job isn't limited to differentiation; it's also busy crafting the local environment. For instance, the ECM it produces helps cells communicate and manages nearby stem cell niches, which are vital for ongoing development. Some recent studies suggest that when the ICM misfires, gene expression patterns can become disrupted, potentially compromising the embryo's overall developmental competence. All in all, as researchers continue to investigate the ICM's functions, it becomes increasingly clear that understanding its biology is crucial for advancing reproductive technologies and addressing infertility issues on a global scale (Zegers-Hochschild et al., 2017) (Figure 4.16).

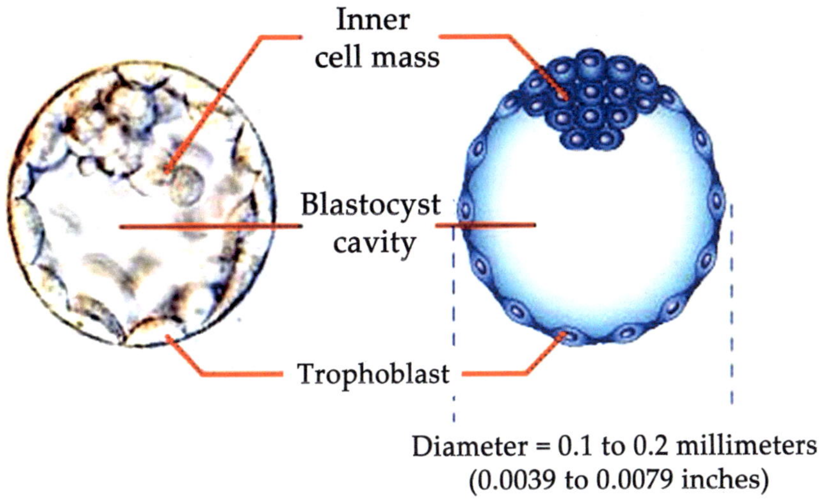

Figure 4.16. Blastocyst inner cell mass (ICM).

Source: https://external-content.duckduckgo.com/iu/?u=http%3A%2F%2Fwww.biologyjunction.com%2Fimages%2Flooklike.jpg&f=1&nofb=1&ipt=5fda4707420e8e7c50587b268386a7d37afe52d4e5f97ec4b119024b9f9277d9.

4.5.2. Role of the Trophoblast in Implantation

Embryonic development and maternal physiology mix in unexpected ways—trophoblast cells often steal the show during implantation. This stage follows cleavage and the formation of the blastocyst, and suddenly, the trophoblast shifts into a range of cell types that seem vital for establishing a pregnancy. In a way, these cells don't just help the blastocyst nestle into the uterine lining; they also kick off critical signaling paths that allow the mother's body recognize the pregnancy. This process is particularly evident when different cell types, such as the cytotrophoblast and syncytiotrophoblast, emerge and change during the peri-implantation period, highlighting a dynamic process crucial for anchoring the embryo within the uterus (Jiang et al., 2019). Trophoblast function isn't a one-note affair either. Their ability to "talk" to maternal tissues proves crucial for both a steady implantation and the building of placental structures. The ECM, for example, undergoes significant changes due to the trophoblast's influence, which encourages cells to adhere and migrate into the uterine tissue. They also release a host of signaling molecules that modulate the maternal immune response, thereby reducing the risk that the embryo might be rejected. Interestingly, trophoblasts exhibit specific markers that trigger reactions in the endometrium, which is crucial for creating an environment that welcomes the implanted blastocyst. Generally speaking, these interactions are closely tied to maternal health and the overall success of implantation (Dissanayake et al., 2022). As implantation progresses, trophoblasts display a surprising ability to adapt, often adjusting to the conditions they encounter. In this process, they shift into different states that lead to the creation of specialized structures—crucial for nutrient transfer and gas exchange, both of which are fundamental for embryonic growth. Their continued multiplication and transformation help reinforce the developing embryo's hold on maternal tissue, forming the basis of placental architecture while securing essential growth factors for the fetus. In many cases, the trophoblast serves as a crucial bridge between embryonic development and the mother's body's adaptation, underscoring its indispensable role in this intricate implantation process (Jiang et al., 2019) (Figure 4.17).

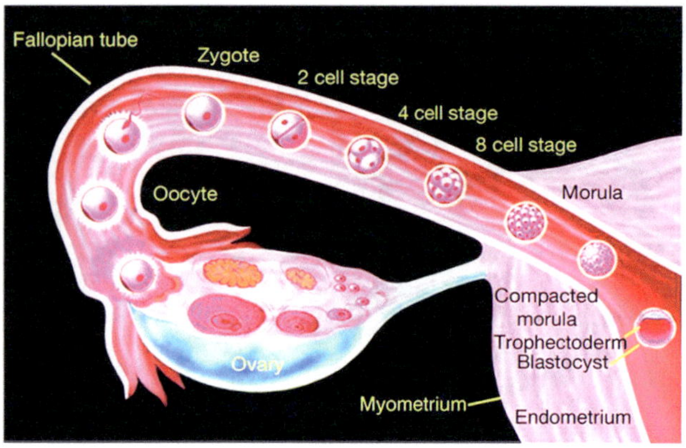

Figure 4.17. Role of the trophoblast in implantation.

Source: https://external-content.duckduckgo.com/iu/?u=https%3A%2F%2Fdm5migu4zj3pb.cloudfront.net%2Fmanuscripts%2F22000%2F22991%2Fmedium%2FJCI0422991.f1.jpg&f=1&nofb=1&ipt=7d0eb9942d466ccfe5914430aa0725ec5459414bedb15d85eb0418fe896c39b3.

4.5.3. Importance of Blastocyst in Establishing Pregnancy

Switching from cleavage to the blastocyst phase marks a turning point in early embryonic development—it's where things start to get interesting for a pregnancy. Around five days after fertilization, a blastocyst appears, featuring a central cell clump that will eventually be the embryo and an outer trophoblast layer that sort of "shakes hands" with the uterus. This separation is crucial, as the inner cells develop into the embryo proper. At the same time, the trophoblast facilitates the blastocyst's attachment to the uterine lining, establishing the maternal-fetal connection necessary for exchanging nutrients and waste. In a way, the blastocyst's knack for implanting and chatting with maternal tissues heavily influences whether a pregnancy will work out, making it a major player in reproductive biology. Quality matters a lot here, too—studies generally suggest that a blastocyst's condition can impact implantation rates and overall pregnancy success. IVF breakthroughs have prompted individuals to select only the best blastocysts, with indicators such as a clearly defined ICM often being seen as a green light for viability. On the other hand, any glitches during early cleavage can disrupt the process (Giancani et al., 2020). And it isn't just about structure; biochemical and hormonal factors also play a role. Take melatonin, for instance—better known for its role in sleep—it also appears to enhance oocyte quality and facilitate the blastocyst's settlement by mitigating oxidative stress and fine-tuning key signals (Carlomagno et al., 2018). This blend of hormonal cues with cell development shows just how many elements have to come together, linking the embryo's growth with the mother's overall health in a pretty intricate way.

4.6. Factors Affecting Cleavage and Blastocyst Formation

Early embryonic growth is a complex process, guided by a combination of factors that determine how cells divide and ultimately form a blastocyst. A key part of this puzzle is the egg cell's quality—oocytes carry a weight that can steer an embryo's future. In many studies, eggs activated by parthenogenesis tend to fall short, often resulting in fewer cells in the blastocyst (Chen et al., 2018). At the same time, there's generally a noticeable spike in Xist—the long noncoding RNA that, in simple terms, quiets one of the X chromosomes—which sometimes hints that something's off with the usual cell division routine, ultimately leading to a less robust blastocyst. In most cases, understanding the molecular basis of oocyte quality is essential to enhance embryo viability, whether in animal research or ART. The hormonal backdrop also plays a significant role during those early stages. Progesterone and estrogen, for example, are busy moderating a range of bodily processes—

affecting how receptive the uterus is and how smoothly an embryo can implant. Their levels help set the pace for cell divisions and keep the embryo's development on track. Interestingly, the timing between fertilization and ovulation is also critical; even a slight delay can disrupt normal cellular processes, leading to abnormal developmental paths. There's now, generally speaking, a kind of agreed-upon terminology in fertility care that makes it easier for clinicians and researchers to talk about how hormones influence these early events. This somewhat informal standard helps everyone communicate better, ultimately paving the way for more effective interventions and improved embryo viability (Zegers-Hochschild et al., 2017). We can't ignore genetics when it comes to cleavage and blastocyst formation either. Chromosomal abnormalities or even microdeletion events can disrupt the normal process of cell division, often resulting in embryos that struggle to reach the blastocyst stage. Some recent work has even suggested that manipulating specific genes may enhance the overall quality and number of cells within the blastocyst. For instance, studies on transcription factors such as Sox2, Nanog, and Oct4 consistently highlight their importance in maintaining pluripotency and self-renewal during early development (Chen et al., 2018). As our understanding of these genetic influences slowly evolves, it holds some real promise for not only refining assisted reproductive techniques but also for addressing broader fertility challenges in both clinical and research settings.

4.6.1. Environmental Influences (e.g., Temperature, Nutrients)

Cleavage and blastocyst formation initiate early on, and various environmental factors influence how cells behave during these initial stages. Temperature, for instance, is central – it's what drives key metabolic and enzyme activities that cells depend on to divide. When the temperature is just right, cells tend to hold together and function well. Still, even slight fluctuations can cause trouble, such as disrupting cell division or leading to abnormal developmental paths. Research in reproductive tech often highlights how keeping the culture environment thermally steady is key – in most cases, even minor deviations can hurt embryo quality and viability. Therefore, gaining a solid understanding of how temperature affects these processes is crucial for enhancing success in assisted reproductive methods. Nutrient availability jumps in as another big piece of the puzzle during the cleavage and blastocyst phases. The early embryo relies heavily on the resources it receives from its mother for energy and the basic building blocks necessary for growth. A lack of essential nutrients can slow down metabolism and stunt growth, which sometimes messes with gene expression and overall developmental outcomes. Recent advances, such as time-lapse imaging, have shed more light on how nutrient levels influence the timing and quality of cell division – offering a glimpse into these subtle changes as they occur. This blend of nutritional insights with modern imaging not only helps assess which embryos might be the most viable, but it also paves the way for better pregnancy outcomes, more often than not. Environmental cues like both temperature and nutrient gradients don't just affect cell metabolism – they also shape the whole embryonic setting. Take the endoplasmic reticulum (ER) as an example; it plays a crucial role in maintaining cellular balance, adapting quickly to stress or changes in available nutrients. If the ER becomes overloaded, it can trigger what's known as the unfolded protein response (UPR), and if homeostasis can't be restored, apoptosis might kick in, potentially reducing embryo viability. This dance between external stressors and what happens inside cells paints a complex picture of development. In most cases, understanding these interactions offers promising new routes for fine-tuning embryo culture conditions in the laboratory, thereby enhancing the effectiveness of fertility treatments and deepening our understanding of early embryonic development (Almanza et al., 2018; Apter et al., 2020).

4.6.2. Genetic Factors Impacting Development

Early on, genes set the stage. The very first divisions—what we call cleavage—and the eventual building of the blastocyst all lean heavily on these genetic cues. A fertilized egg splits repeatedly, and along the way, genes keep time and ensure even divisions. Complex players, such as transcription factors and various signaling messengers, jump into action, pushing the single zygote into a group of cells where each one begins to assume its role. Sometimes, if these genomic signals go off track, uneven splits happen, resulting in a weak blastocyst. This misstep can cause implantation issues or even an early glitch in development, underscoring once again the importance of maintaining good genetic direction. Things get trickier when we mix in epigenetic tweaks. Without altering the DNA code itself, these modifications can change how genes are read, especially during those early, rapid cell divisions. The embryo uses these flexible marks to adjust to signals coming from both inside and outside its little world. For example, the maternal environment can significantly alter the epigenetic landscape, subtly influencing which genes become active during the cleavage phase and later, as cells determine their paths. Therefore, managing these epigenetic factors is crucial for a smooth transition from initial cleavage to a stable blastocyst, ensuring that gene expression and cell differentiation occur precisely as intended. Understanding this delicate dance between genetic instructions and epigenetic adjustments is crucial—especially when it comes to challenges like infertility (Zegers-Hochschild et al., 2017). On another note, mixing deep genetic insights with reproductive medicine has spurred a push for a common language in discussing fertility and early embryonic growth. Scientists and healthcare providers often need to be on the same page to diagnose and treat infertility problems effectively. Recently, a consensus-based glossary of terms related to fertility and embryological processes was compiled to clarify any confusion (Zegers-Hochschild et al., 2017). This effort underscores the idea that while genes independently steer the course of development, having a shared vocabulary is equally essential. With a more standardized set of terms, researchers can tackle the genetic roots of developmental changes and help drive forward assisted reproductive techniques aimed at overcoming the hurdles of cleavage and blastocyst formation.

4.6.3. Implications of Abnormalities in Cleavage and Blastocyst Formation

Embryonic development's start is all about genetic make-up, and even minor missteps during the cleavage phase can set off a chain reaction. If the timing or smoothness of these early cell splits goes wrong, this results in aneuploidy—that is, having the wrong number of chromosomes. This kind of chromosomal mix-up can derail the shift from cleavage into the blastocyst stage, which, in turn, jeopardizes the embryo's overall viability. Some studies suggest that the transition between the second and third rounds of cell division is particularly susceptible to issues when oxidative stress from sperm is involved - a factor that can exacerbate developmental problems. It's interesting how these findings subtly point to paternal influences, suggesting that a broader view of reproductive health—and some tweaks in assisted reproduction practices—is usually in order (Barker et al., 2014). There's also the curious case of genetic normalization through the transition from cleavage to blastocyst. In many instances, embryos that initially show signs of aneuploidy appear to correct their course over the next stage; a fair number even display a diploid karyotype later on. This process demonstrates that the embryo's immediate environment can sometimes help nudge its genetic arrangement back into line, offering unexpected insights into potential corrective mechanisms that may one day be utilized therapeutically in reproductive medicine. Such observations tend to upend that old belief that early chromosomal errors are set in stone, and they remind us that there may be just the right moment for intervention during these critical stages (Barker et al., 2011). Looking at the bigger picture, issues in cleavage and blastocyst formation aren't just academic—they have real clinical implications. Aneuploidy, for example, might lead to problems like implantation failure or miscarriage, which can weigh heavily on the emotions and finances of hopeful parents. As preimplantation genetic screening (PGS) becomes more common, identifying these early chromosomal abnormalities takes on added urgency. By digging deeper into these early processes, we not only sharpen our scientific insights but also might open the door to innovative strategies that boost both embryo viability and overall reproductive outcomes (Barker et al., 2011, 2014).

SUMMARY

Oocyte maturation sets the stage for early embryo life – the whole process of cleavage and forming a blastocyst shows just how crucial it is. Recent studies, in most cases, point out that a bunch of factors can tip the scales one way or another. For example, when rapamycin is applied at just the right level, mature oocytes seem to stick around longer and even boost the rates of cleavage and blastocyst formation. It appears that tweaking pathways, such as the mTOR pathway, can lead to better developmental outcomes, hinting at new paths in both research and clinical work in reproductive technology (Yang et al., 2022). On the flip side, compounds such as butylparaben remind us that too much of a good thing can go wrong. High levels of butylparaben have been connected to lower fertilization rates and a spike in oxidative stress, which then messes with both cleavage and the formation of a proper blastocyst. These findings, in many cases, suggest that our environment can introduce some unwanted variables, with ROS and mitochondrial issues playing a role (Pil-Jeong et al., 2020). This balance (or lack thereof) underscores why we have to get a grip on both the helpful and harmful influences affecting oocyte quality. All in all, examining the factors that affect cleavage and blastocyst formation underscores the need for a comprehensive, holistic approach in reproductive biology. Leaning into beneficial tweaks, such as controlled rapamycin use, while keeping the negative effects of things like butylparaben in check, might just improve ART overall. When scientific insights blend with clinical practice, there's a real chance to nurture more successful embryonic development. This kind of wide-ranging understanding could lead to better protocols in fertility treatments – ultimately helping both human and animal reproduction to take a step forward. Early in embryonic life, the process of cell division and formation of a blastocyst reveals just how much a mother's condition can impact her developing baby. Research has started to point out that eggs from women who are overweight or obese end up being a noticeably different size when compared to those from women at a healthy weight, a size that seems to matter a lot. Smaller eggs, for instance, often don't have as good a chance of getting fertilized and then growing normally. And it's interesting, because even though these embryos might hit the morula stage faster, their metabolism looks off; they tend to use less sugar while sporting higher triglyceride levels. The clear-cut link between maternal BMI and early embryonic behavior suggests, in most cases, that a mother's health may have a lasting impact on her child's future (Leary et al., 2014). Physical pressures and gene signals appear to work together to shape how cells determine their roles during the blastocyst phase. Some studies into mammalian embryogenesis reveal that cells, lined up inside the zona pellucida, seem driven by basic physical ideas—almost like they're trying to reduce tension or elastic energy. At the same time, these same forces interact with genetic cues, helping to form structures such as the trophectoderm and even the beginnings of the endoderm. There are even two rival ideas floating around: one camp argues that a cell's position influences which genes fire up, while the other suggests it could be the other way around. Grasping this complex interplay of mechanical and genetic signals may significantly enhance our understanding of how multicellular organisms develop into distinct layers (Jedrusik et al., 2011). New findings in embryology make it clear that we still have much to learn about the mechanisms behind cleavage and blastocyst formation. When researchers combine ideas from both physical forces and gene behavior, they gain a deeper understanding of how cells interact, match, and fit together in those early moments. Some emerging ideas even suggest that directional forces may play a role in ensuring that cells adhere to one another in just the right way, creating a complex web of physical and biological influences.

CLOSER LOOK

PREIMPLANTATION GENETIC SCREENING (PGS)

PGS, now more commonly referred to as preimplantation genetic testing for aneuploidy (PGT-A), is a reproductive technology used during IVF to evaluate embryos for chromosomal abnormalities before implantation. The goal of PGS is to identify embryos with the correct number of chromosomes (euploid embryos) and avoid transferring those with abnormalities (aneuploid embryos), which are often associated with failed implantation, miscarriage, or genetic disorders such as Down syndrome. The process begins with the standard IVF protocol: eggs are retrieved from the ovaries, fertilized in the lab, and allowed to develop into embryos. On day five or six of development, when the embryos reach the blastocyst stage, a few cells are carefully biopsied from the trophectoderm—the part that will become the placenta—while leaving the ICM, which will form the fetus, untouched. These biopsied cells are then sent for genetic analysis using advanced techniques such as next-generation sequencing (NGS) or array comparative genomic hybridization (aCGH).

The information obtained from PGS allows fertility specialists to select the healthiest embryos for transfer, thereby increasing the chances of a successful pregnancy and reducing the risk of miscarriage. PGS is especially beneficial for women of advanced maternal age, as the risk of chromosomal abnormalities increases with age. It is also commonly used in cases of recurrent pregnancy loss, repeated IVF failure, or severe male factor infertility. Additionally, PGS may be used by couples who wish to avoid transferring embryos that carry chromosomal abnormalities, even if they are not known carriers of genetic diseases. By improving the accuracy of embryo selection, PGS can reduce the number of IVF cycles required to achieve a successful pregnancy, lowering emotional and financial burdens for patients.

Despite its benefits, PGS is not without limitations and controversies. One primary concern is the potential for mosaicism, where an embryo contains both normal and abnormal cells. In such cases, a biopsy might not represent the genetic status of the entire embryo, leading to potentially inaccurate results. Additionally, while PGS improves the chances of selecting viable embryos, it does not guarantee a successful pregnancy or a healthy baby, as other factors, such as uterine receptivity and overall embryo quality, also play crucial roles. Ethical considerations also arise, particularly around the selection or discarding of embryos based on genetic information. Moreover, PGS adds to the cost and complexity of IVF treatment, which may not be accessible or necessary for all patients.

Preimplantation genetic screening represents a powerful tool in assisted reproductive technology, enabling more informed and targeted embryo selection during IVF. By identifying chromosomally normal embryos, PGS can enhance pregnancy rates, reduce the risk of miscarriage, and increase the overall efficiency of fertility treatment. However, like all medical technologies, it requires careful consideration of its limitations, ethical implications, and appropriate use on a case-by-case basis. Ongoing advancements in genetic testing and embryo assessment continue to refine the accuracy and application of PGS, offering hope to many individuals and couples striving to build healthy families.

REFERENCES

1. Almanza, A., Carlesso, A., Chintha, C., Creedican, S., Doultsinos, D., Leuzzi, B., Luís, A., et al. (2018). Endoplasmic reticulum stress signaling–from basic mechanisms to clinical applications. *FEBS Journal, 286*(2), 241–278. https://doi.org/10.1111/febs.14608.
2. Apter, S., Ebner, T., Fréour, T., Guns, Y., Kovačič, B., Le Clef, N., Marques, M., et al. (2020). Good practice recommendations for the use of time-lapse technology. *Human Reproduction Open, 2020*(3), hoaa008. https://doi.org/10.1093/hropen/hoaa008.
3. Brezina, P., Barker, A., Benner, A., Ross, R., Nguyen, K., Anchan, R., Richter, K., Cutting, G., & Kearns, W. (2011). Genetic normalization of differentiating aneuploid human embryos. *Nature Precedings.* https://doi.org/10.1038/npre.2011.6045.1Barker, C. M., Burruel, V., Klooster, K., et al. (2014). Abnormal early cleavage events predict early embryo demise: sperm oxidative stress and early abnormal cleavage. https://core.ac.uk/download/323070233.pdf.
4. Bettegowda, A., Jurisicova, A., Crosier, A. E., Jakobsen, A. S., Robert, C., et al. (2011). Cell arrest and cell death in mammalian preimplantation development. https://core.ac.uk/download/12175482.pdf (accessed on 26 May 2025).
5. Blakeley, P., Fogarty, N. M. E., del Valle, I., Wamaitha, S. E., Hu, X., Elder, K., Snell, P., et al. (2015). Defining the three cell lineages of the human blastocyst by single-cell RNA-seq. *Development.* https://doi.org/10.1242/dev.123547.
6. Budrewicz, J., & Chavez, S. L. (2024). Insights into embryonic chromosomal instability: Mechanisms of DNA elimination during mammalian preimplantation development. *Frontiers in Cell and Developmental Biology, 12.* https://www.semanticscholar.org/paper/3c7a493377 3b4b4d56ca33b3ef8842775a8a91ee (accessed on 26 May 2025).
7. Cabral-Pacheco, G. A., Garza-Veloz, I., Castruita-De la Rosa, C., Ramirez-Acuña, J. M., Perez-Romero, B. A., Guerrero-Rodriguez, J. F., Martínez-Avila, N., et al. (2020). The roles of matrix metalloproteinases and their inhibitors in human diseases. *International Journal of Molecular Sciences, 21*(24), 9739. https://doi.org/10.3390/ijms21249739.
8. Capalbo, A., Rienzi, L., Cimadomo, D., Maggiulli, R., Elliott, T., Wright, G., Nagy, Z., et al. (2014). Correlation between standard blastocyst morphology, euploidy and implantation: An observational study in two centers involving 956 screened blastocysts. *Human Reproduction, 29*(6), 1173–1181. https://doi.org/10.1093/humrep/deu033.
9. Carlomagno, G., Minini, M., Tilotta, M., et al. (2018). From implantation to birth: insight into molecular melatonin functions. https://core.ac.uk/download/188824580.pdf (accessed on 26 May 2025).
10. Chen, X., Zhu, Z., Yu, F., Huang, J., Jia, R., & Pan, J. (2018). Effect of shRNA-mediated Xist knockdown on the quality of porcine parthenogenetic embryos. *Developmental Dynamics, 248*(2), 140–148. https://doi.org/10.1002/dvdy.24660.
11. Coticchio, G., Ezoe, K., Lagalla, C., Shimazaki, K., Ohata, K., Ninomiya, M., Wakabayashi, N., et al. (2021). Perturbations of morphogenesis at the compaction stage affect blastocyst implantation and live birth rates. *Human Reproduction, 36*(4), 918–928. https://doi.org/10.1093/humrep/deab011.
12. Davidson, A., Mantzouratou, A., Goldstein, A. H., Murdoch, A., Dale, B., Kea, B., Kovacic, B., et al. (2012). A novel isolator-based system promotes viability of human embryos during laboratory processing. https://core.ac.uk/download/9990449.pdf (accessed on 26 May 2025).

13. Dissanayake, K. (2022). Varastest embrüotest pärit ekstratsellulaarsed vesiikulid: Potentsiaal embrüokvaliteedi markeritena ja roll embrüo-emaka suhtluses [Extracellular vesicles from stored embryos: Potential markers of embryo quality and role in embryo-uterine communication]. https://core.ac.uk/download/491372072.pdf (accessed on 26 May 2025).

14. Ezoe, K., Miki, T., Akaike, H., Shimazaki, K., Takahashi, T., Tanimura, Y., Amagai, A., et al. (2023). Maternal age affects pronuclear and chromatin dynamics, morula compaction and cell polarity, and blastulation of human embryos. *Human Reproduction, 38*(3), 387–399. https://doi.org/10.1093/humrep/dead001.

15. Fragouli, E., Späth, K., Alfarawati, S., Kaper, F., Craig, A., Michel, C. E., Kokocinski, F., et al. (2015). Altered levels of mitochondrial DNA are associated with female age, aneuploidy, and provide an independent measure of embryonic implantation potential. *PLoS Genetics, 11*(6), e1005241. https://doi.org/10.1371/journal.pgen.1005241.

16. Giancani, A. (2020). Chromosomal and functional characterization of the early stages of human embryogenesis. https://core.ac.uk/download/286532767.pdf (accessed on 26 May 2025).

17. Gladyshev, V. N. (2020). The ground zero of organismal life and aging. *Trends in Molecular Medicine, 27*(1), 11–19. https://doi.org/10.1016/j.molmed.2020.08.012.

18. Jawad, A., Oh, D., Choi, H., Kim, M., Ham, J., Oh, B. C., Lee, J., et al. (2024). Myo-inositol improves developmental competence and reduces oxidative stress in porcine parthenogenetic embryos. *Frontiers in Veterinary Science, 11*. https://www.semanticscholar.org/paper/28f88c4f33af41d84b4bbb27521f909fdcf55f7d (accessed on 26 May 2025).

19. Jedrusik, A., Ralston, A., Plusa, B., Chazaud, C., Peterson, C., Thieffry, D., et al. (2011). Simulating the mammalian blastocyst: Molecular and mechanical interactions pattern the embryo. https://core.ac.uk/download/4889416.pdf.

20. Jeon, S. B., Jeong, P. S., Kang, H. G., Kim, M. J., Yun, J. H., Lim, K. S., Song, B. S., et al. (2024). NEK2 plays an essential role in porcine embryonic development by maintaining mitotic division and DNA damage response via the Wnt/β-catenin signaling pathway. *Cell Proliferation, 57*(1), e13626. https://doi.org/10.1111/cpr.13626.

21. Jeong, P. S., Lee, S., Park, S. H., Kim, M. J., Kang, H. G., Nanjidsuren, T., Son, H. C., et al. (2020). Butylparaben is toxic to porcine oocyte maturation and subsequent embryonic development following *in vitro* fertilization. *International Journal of Molecular Sciences, 21*(10), 3692. https://doi.org/10.3390/ijms21103692.

22. Jiang, Z., Kile, R. A., Krisher, R. L., et al. (2019). Dynamics of trophoblast differentiation in peri-implantation–stage human embryos. https://core.ac.uk/download/270056506.pdf (accessed on 26 May 2025).

23. Karamanos, N. K., Theocharis, A. D., Piperigkou, Z., Manou, D., Passi, A., Skandalis, S. S., Vynios, D. H., et al. (2021). A guide to the composition and functions of the extracellular matrix. *FEBS Journal, 288*(17), 6850–6912. https://doi.org/10.1111/febs.15776.

24. Kersten, K., de Visser, K. E., van Miltenburg, M. H., & Jonkers, J. (2016). Genetically engineered mouse models in oncology research and cancer medicine. *EMBO Molecular Medicine, 9*(2), 137–153. https://doi.org/10.15252/emmm.201606857.

25. Knöfler, M., Haider, S., Saleh, L., Pollheimer, J., Gamage, T. K. J. B., & James, J. L. (2019). Human placenta and trophoblast development: key molecular mechanisms and model systems. *Cellular and Molecular Life Sciences, 76*(17), 3479–3496. https://doi.org/10.1007/s00018-019-03104-6.

26. Komsky-Elbaz, A., Kalo, D., & Roth, Z. (2020). Effect of aflatoxin B1 on bovine spermatozoa's proteome and embryo's transcriptome. *Reproduction, 160*(6), 709–723. https://doi.org/10.1530/rep-20-0286.
27. Leary, C., & Leese, H. J. (2014). Human embryos from overweight and obese women display phenotypic and metabolic abnormalities. https://core.ac.uk/download/151160915.pdf (accessed on 26 May 2025).
28. Lenne, P. F., Munro, E., Heemskerk, I., Warmflash, A., Bocanegra-Moreno, L., Kishi, K., Kicheva, A., et al. (2020). Roadmap for the multiscale coupling of biochemical and mechanical signals during development. *Physical Biology, 18*(4), 041501. https://doi.org/10.1088/1478-3975/abd0db.
29. Lewis, N., & Sturmey, R. (2015). Embryo metabolism: what does it mean? https://core.ac.uk/download/151161377.pdf (accessed on 26 May 2025).
30. Li, C. M., Zhao, H., Song, J., Yi, M., Li, M., Hong, N., Liu, R., et al. (2010). Tracing blastomere fate choices of early embryos in single cell culture. https://core.ac.uk/download/pdf/289382.pdf (accessed on 26 May 2025).
31. Liebich, S., Testa, U., Castelli, G., Pelosi, E., Georges, F., Jin, J., Song, S., et al. (2020). [Title not provided]. *OBM Genetics, 4*(3). https://doi.org/10.21926/obm.genet.2003.
32. Łoboda, A., Damulewicz, M., Pyza, E., Józkowicz, A., & Dulak, J. (2016). Role of Nrf2/HO-1 system in development, oxidative stress response and diseases: An evolutionarily conserved mechanism. *Cellular and Molecular Life Sciences, 73*(16), 3221–3247. https://doi.org/10.1007/s00018-016-2223-0.
33. Ng, S. C., Daley, G. Q., & Cantley, L. C. (2013). Stem cell metabolism in tissue development and aging. *Development, 140*(13), 2535–2547. https://doi.org/10.1242/dev.091777.
34. Ono, Y., Shirasawa, H., Takahashi, K., Goto, M., Ono, T., Sakaguchi, T., Iwasawa, T., et al. (2024). O-069 The first mitotic spindle instability impacts nucleation, fragmentation, and development in human embryos. *Human Reproduction*. https://www.semanticscholar.org/paper/372c2f7043700a9a7dad502e6ec716dc5fd42498 (accessed on 26 May 2025).
35. Rienzi, L., Gracia, C. R., Maggiulli, R., LaBarbera, A. R., Kaser, D. J., Ubaldi, F. M., Vanderpoel, S., et al. (2016). Oocyte, embryo and blastocyst cryopreservation in ART: systematic review and meta-analysis comparing slow-freezing versus vitrification to produce evidence for the development of global guidance. *Human Reproduction Update.* https://doi.org/10.1093/humupd/dmw038.
36. Turner, S., Wong, H. P., Rai, J., & Hartshorne, G. M. (2010). Telomere lengths in human oocytes, cleavage stage embryos and blastocysts. https://core.ac.uk/download/46363.pdf (accessed on 26 May 2025).
37. Varshavsky, A., Gates, A. H., Kanzler, B., Colussi, C., Streffer, C., Li, C. B., Wong, C. C., et al. (2012). Nuclear reprogramming: Kinetics of cell cycle and metabolic progression as determinants of success. https://core.ac.uk/download/pdf/8712304.pdf.
38. Viotti, M. (2020). Preimplantation genetic testing for chromosomal abnormalities: Aneuploidy, mosaicism, and structural rearrangements. *Genes, 11*(6), 602. https://doi.org/10.3390/genes11060602.

39. Yang, Q., Xi, Q., Wang, M., Long, R., Hu, J., Li, Z., Ren, X., et al. (2022). Rapamycin improves the quality and developmental competence of mice oocytes by promoting DNA damage repair during *in vitro* maturation. *Reproductive Biology and Endocrinology, 20*, Article 109. https://doi.org/10.1186/s12958-022-00943-0.

40. Yoon, J. W., Lee, S. E., Park, Y. G., Kim, W. J., Park, H. J., Park, C. O., Kim, S. H., et al. (2020). The antioxidant icariin protects porcine oocytes from age-related damage *in vitro*. *Animal Bioscience, 34*(5), 546–557. https://doi.org/10.5713/ajas.20.0046.

41. Zegers-Hochschild, F., Adamson, G. D., Dyer, S., Racowsky, C., de Mouzon, J., Sokol, R. Z., Rienzi, L., et al. (2017). The International Glossary on Infertility and Fertility Care, 2017. *Fertility and Sterility, 108*(3), 393–406. https://doi.org/10.1016/j.fertnstert.2017.06.005.

42. Zegers-Hochschild, F., Adamson, G. D., Dyer, S., Racowsky, C., de Mouzon, J., Sokol, R. Z., Rienzi, L., et al. (2017). The International Glossary on Infertility and Fertility Care, 2017†‡§. *Human Reproduction, 32*(9), 1786–1801. https://doi.org/10.1093/humrep/dex234.

43. Zhang, J. Y., Dong, H. S., Oqani, R. K., Lin, T., Kang, J. W., & Jin, D. I. (2014). Distinct roles of ROCK1 and ROCK2 during development of porcine preimplantation embryos. *Reproduction, 148*(1), 99–107. https://doi.org/10.1530/rep-13-0556.

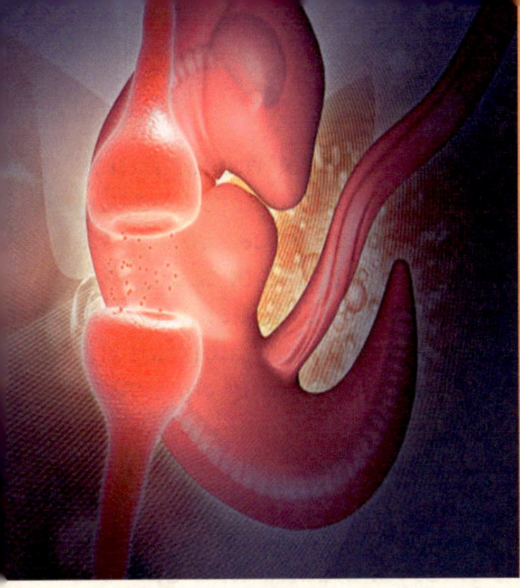

Chapter 5
GASTRULATION

Contents

Introduction

Transforming a totipotent zygote—a single cell with the potential to become anything—into a functioning, multicellular being is quite a wild ride, one that reveals some of biology's most captivating secrets. At its core, this journey relies on gastrulation, a pivotal moment when an embryo begins to differentiate into distinct layers. In many cases, this isn't just about shifting shapes; it's the stage that sets up later organ building and the overall body map. One can't help but recall the early work of individuals like Turing and Thompson, whose ideas on chemical cues and physical signals expanded our understanding of how cells and their mechanics interact. Generally speaking, these core ideas help us see how gastrulation manages a delicate mix of cell destinies and spatial setups, drawing together threads from developmental biology, physics, and evolution. Gastrulation depends significantly on the complex interplay of cell behaviors and the signals they exchange, which together rearrange embryonic tissue in unexpected ways. During this time, as cells acquire traits such as new shapes, altered adhesion to one another, and altered movement, the stage is suddenly set for the formation of the germ layers. Chemical messengers—often called morphogens—play a big hand here, nudging some cells to settle into specific roles and positions. At the same time, physical forces come into play, gently or sometimes rather abruptly pushing individual cells, and even groups of them, into coordinated movements. Recent studies on epithelial-mesenchymal transition (EMT) demonstrate that cells can, essentially, alter their characteristics in response to local signals, reinforcing the concept of a complex and dynamic interplay underlying gastrulation. There's a growing consensus among researchers; many feel that we need to agree on clear terms and methods. Yang et al. (2020) highlight just how essential standardized approaches are for advancing our understanding of EMT and gastrulation. Additionally, the way tissues behave—their rheology—has come into focus as another significant piece of the gastrulation puzzle. How tissues bend, twist, and respond to forces largely shapes the morphogenetic processes that form an embryo. Studies now suggest that the material properties of these tissues aren't fixed at all; instead, they can change suddenly, almost like a phase shift, which is critical for maintaining strong and adaptable development. In most cases, this connection implies that digging into the push-and-pull dynamics of tissue behavior could shine some light on the inner workings of embryonic construction, as Nicoletta et al. (2019) seem to suggest. With ongoing research and increasingly detailed models emerging, our understanding of tissue behavior during gastrulation is becoming even more nuanced. This broader perspective not only deepens our understanding of how embryos develop but also hints at practical applications for tackling related health issues, bridging the gaps between basic science and clinical insights (Figure 5.1).

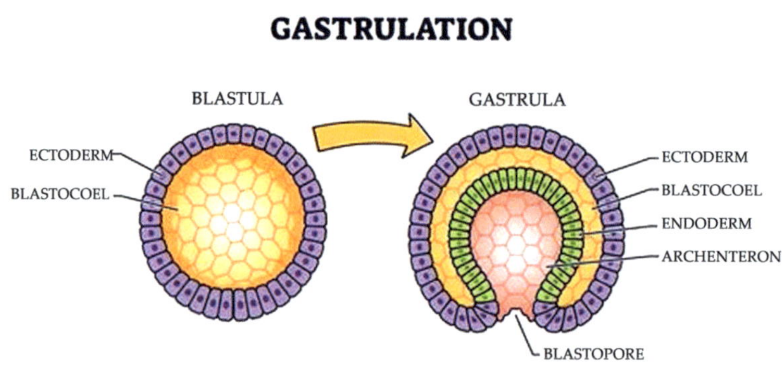

Figure 5.1. Gastrulation.

Source: https://www.shutterstock.com/image-vector/gastrulation-early-developmental-process-embryo-260nw-2306778309.jpg.

Definition of Gastrulation

A single-layer blastula suddenly twists into something more complex—a multi-layered structure we call gastrulation—and that shift is a real turning point in an embryo's life. During this phase, the embryo forms its basic structure by creating three primary layers—ectoderm, mesoderm, and endoderm—that later branch out into various tissues and organs. For instance, the ectoderm gives rise to the skin and nervous system, while the mesoderm contributes to the creation of muscles, bones, and the circulatory system. It's not just a quiet step leading into organ building; there's a wild cellular dance going on too. Cells fold inward, roll over, and spread out (processes named invagination, involution, and epiboly) to position themselves right, almost like nature's, slightly chaotic choreography, setting the stage for all that comes next. Digging a little deeper, gastrulation doesn't work in isolation; it's closely tied to the signals that guide each layer's destiny. In vertebrates, for example, signals from a small organizing region kickstart nerve development at just the right moment. Generally speaking, the process known as neural induction demonstrates how even a handful of molecules—such as TGFβ—can tip the scales, nudging ectodermal cells toward a neural fate rather than a non-neural one. Early embryologists (often tinkering with amphibian models) figured out that this trick was not just a fluke but a conserved mechanism across species (Ozair et al., 2013). Gaining insight into these molecular cues—especially the role of native neural inducers—highlights the complexity and importance of gastrulation in forming a functional organism. In addition to rearranging cells into place, the entire process sheds light on broader evolutionary patterns and even hints at why certain developmental disorders arise. Comparative studies tend to show that while the details of cell movements may vary from one species to another, the core principles remain largely consistent; even minor disruptions can sometimes lead to significant congenital issues. A closer examination of the multifaceted interactions during gastrulation is crucial to unlocking not only embryological puzzles but also understanding its pivotal role in the ongoing narrative of developmental biology (Tolera, 2023).

Importance in Embryonic Development

Gastrulation mother appears as a wild yet fundamental mother when life's blueprint begins to form. Cells start moving around in ways that might seem random at first—then, they end up creating three basic layers: ectoderm, mesoderm, and endoderm. These layers aren't just there for show; they become the raw materials for every organ and tissue that follows. It's not simply a matter of building structures, either—it's about laying down a rough plan for how the body will be arranged. Around this time, a phenomenon known as epithelial-mesenchymal transition (EMT) emerges. In a surprising twist, cells suddenly acquire new mobility, even exhibiting invasive behavior through a series of dynamic changes. These unexpected moves help steer how the layers form and, in turn, influence all that comes later in the embryo's development (Yang et al., 2020). Looking a bit closer, it turns out that behind the scenes of gastrulation, cell signaling, and molecular interactions are doing a lot more than one might expect. Consider epiboly—the process where the blastoderm spreads and thins over the yolk cell. This isn't just random stretching; it's a coordinated cell shuffle that gets all cells in line. Research generally shows that these events lean on some pretty intricate networks—take, for example, the syntenin-syndecan-PIP2-Arf6 complex. Networks like these are crucial for directing cells in just the right way early on. In most cases, these microscopic molecular "conversations" turn out to be the very factors that shape the physical framework of the embryo. Therefore, understanding these overlapping interactions is crucial for comprehending precisely how gastrulation shapes both the structure and function of the developing organism (Lambaerts et al., 2012). Gastrulation's impact isn't confined solely to developmental biology—it ripples out into the realm of medical research as well, especially when we look at congenital anomalies and the emerging field of regenerative medicine. When things go awry during this phase, profound developmental changes can arise, which only underscores the importance of studying. A solid handle on these complex signaling pathways and cellular behaviors can tip the balance in creating new strategies for regenerative therapies, be it through stem cell differentiation or tissue engineering. By untangling the complex details of early embryonic development, particularly the core processes of gastrulation, researchers gain a better understanding of how to modify these mechanisms for therapeutic purposes. Ultimately, the bedrock role of gastrulation in setting up the basic embryonic landscape shows just how central it is in both pure science and in efforts aimed at tackling medical challenges, marking it as a linchpin in our understanding of how life truly begins (Lambaerts et al., 2012; Yang et al., 2020) (Figure 5.2).

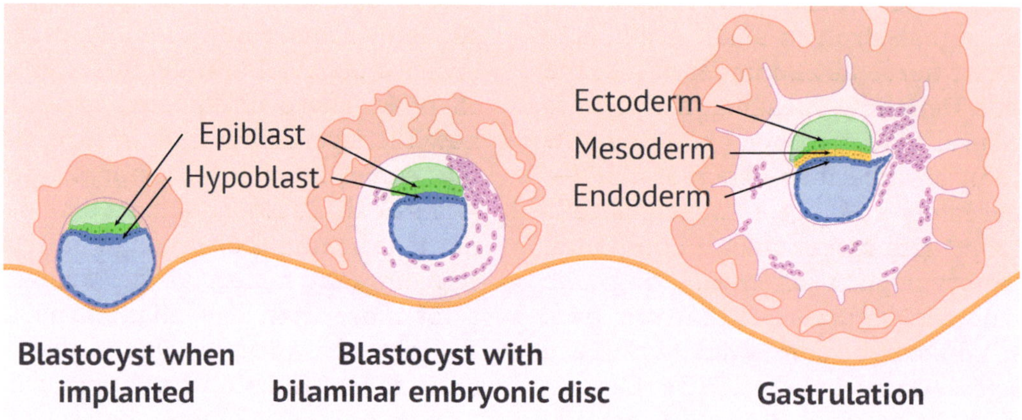

Figure 5.2. Gastrulation importance in embryonic development.

Source: https://www.invitra.com/en/wp-content/uploads/2019/04/how-gastrulation-works.png.

5.1. Historical Background

Gastrulation's complex process has reshaped our understanding of early development and sparked ethical debates about how we conduct research. The birth of Louise Brown in 1978 — a moment many still recall — kickstarted advances in IVF that transformed human reproduction. Soon after, the 14-day rule emerged as an offhand safeguard to ease concerns about intervening at life's very start; note that gastrulation itself begins around the 15th day, when key cell shifts occur. This guideline's impact ripples across many fields, marking a kind of consensus on where ethics should draw the line, even as we celebrate milestones like the formation of the primitive streak. Looking back, these evolving standards set the stage for today's tricky conversations on when and how to study embryos, always with a nudge toward balancing scientific curiosity and ethical care. If we rewind a bit further, the oversight of early embryo research - especially about the twists of gastrulation - has changed noticeably since the 1984 Warnock Report.

That detailed document not only shaped the UK's legal framework but also had a far-reaching influence on international guidelines. Researchers have persistently explored the intricate details of gastrulation, revealing how cells begin to differentiate and how germ layers form. In most cases, these explorations remind us why a deep understanding of developmental biology is crucial to medical progress, especially as new technologies enable us to culture embryos far beyond previous limits. As scientists continue to grapple with the tug-of-war between discovery and ethics, those early regulations still surface in debates over research timelines and the need to revisit outdated rules. Now, with breakthroughs like multi-omics analysis emerging, our historical backdrop in gastrulation highlights the need for rethinking ethical standards. New methods that enable us to examine cellular dynamics at the single-cell level have prompted a reevaluation of the strict rules of the past (Argelaguet et al., 2020). Since gastrulation lays down the blueprint for all future embryonic structures, discussions around it are loaded with implications for both science and bioethical oversight. Current chatter about extending the 14-day limit to 28 days echoes those earlier shifts, continually highlighting the push and pull between scientific potential and ethical reservations. In most cases, maintaining an awareness of our historical roots remains crucial when navigating the evolving ethical landscape of modern gastrulation research (Appleby et al., 2018).

5.1.1. Early Discoveries in Embryology

Early on, researchers uncovered clues about how embryos form by digging into gastrulation's messy beginnings. They tinkered with frogs, zebrafish, and other models—experiments that gave us unexpected snapshots into the dance of cells and how they sort themselves out. It quickly became apparent that signaling routes, with the Wnt pathway in the forefront, play a crucial role in helping cells move and form into tissues. As these studies in developmental genetics accumulated, each new finding built upon older ones in a somewhat patchy, conversational manner, slowly revealing the complex and intricate nature of embryonic morphogenesis (Katrin et al., 2018). This step-by-step, almost accidental journey into cell behavior laid the groundwork for all that we now understand about early development. New technological advances have nudged researchers even further into the secrets of embryology, uncovering a hidden knack among cells for self-organization. Models like embryoids, organoids, and even gastruloids have emerged unexpectedly, showcasing an almost artful mimicry of how real tissue forms. These three-dimensional constructs don't just display neat cellular interactions; they also subtly point to the microenvironment's influence in guiding development. In many cases, scientists have harnessed the cells' natural tendency to self-assemble, opening up entirely new avenues for understanding embryonic patterning and tissue design. It's a reminder that blending different scientific angles can lead to surprises in how we see developmental biology (Simunovic et al., 2017). Diving deeper into these embryological processes isn't just an academic exercise—it has real implications in clinics and regenerative medicine. Early insights now shape strategies for cell-based therapies and tissue engineering, even if the road isn't always smooth. By teasing apart the complex web of gastrulation and its signaling pathways, researchers are learning how to nudge cells into new roles and potentially enhance tissue repair in unexpected ways. The idea, as messy as it may seem, is that understanding how cells communicate and cluster early on could lead to breakthroughs in treating developmental disorders and diseases. In the end, those early discoveries in embryology have not only built a sturdy scientific base but also set the stage for innovations that might one day transform medical practice (Katrin et al., 2018) (Figure 5.3).

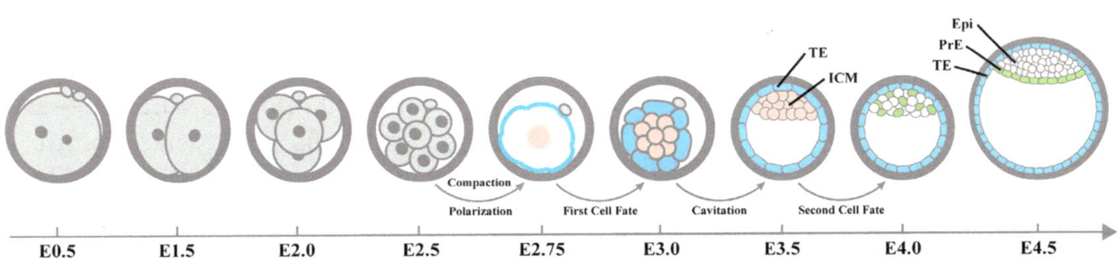

Figure 5.3. Early discoveries in embryology.

Source: https://ars.els-cdn.com/content/image/1-s2.0-S2667325822003521-gr2.jpg.

5.1.2. Key Figures in the Study of Gastrulation

Researchers have delved deeply into the genetic and molecular drivers behind gastrulation, providing a clearer understanding of this complex phase. Gene-regulatory network analysis, for instance, has changed how cell identity was seen at this stage; tools like Cell Oracle now let scientists simulate shifts in transcription factors, which in turn show how these proteins nudge cell differentiation. In one instance, zebrafish embryogenesis studies using *in silico* tests uncovered traits linked to loss-of-function scenarios—this not only points to the routes in notochord regulation but also stresses how transcription factors interact during gastrulation (Kamimoto et al., 2023). Another observation focuses on what happens immediately after fertilization, when the genome suddenly becomes active. Research shows that having a solid transcriptional ability is pretty crucial for switching from maternal cues to the embryo's control. Research on proteins such as Brd4 and P300 has revealed that they play a crucial role in controlling histone acetylation—essentially, the mechanism by which a silent genome is activated. The activation process unfolds gradually and, to be honest, somewhat unpredictably; this mirrors the complex system that governs gene expression during gastrulation. By breaking down these molecular talks, researchers generally argue that both inherited maternal mRNAs and active transcription factors jump-start the cell behaviors essential for early development (Chan et al., 2019). All in all, these efforts remind us that exploring gastrulation isn't a clean-cut task. Instead, it's a blend of computer-driven insights and classic lab work, often leaving us with a clearer yet still evolving picture of cellular signaling and gene networks. The findings—shedding light on both transcription factors and histone modifications—not only highlight crucial functions but also raise further questions in developmental biology. In most cases, this mix of approaches expands our overall grasp of how organisms develop and differentiate.

5.1.3. Evolution of Gastrulation Theories

Gastrulation has captured the attention of many developmental biologists due to its pivotal role in shaping the embryo's structure. Early research mostly zoomed in on how cells move and take on specific roles, but as time went on, the focus naturally shifted. Now it's more about spotting the echoes of evolution within these early steps. Scientists, in most cases, have observed that when comparing embryonic stages across different species, a recurring pattern emerges—gastrulation often marks a pivotal moments in developmental evolution (Irie et al., 2011). The idea that early cell patterns might signal broader evolutionary connections has prompted researchers to rethink traditional models. Network science and systems biology have also been up, revolutionizing research in gastrulation studies. In general, these fields are lending fresh perspectives to models of development, which in turn makes older, purely observational frameworks seem a bit too narrow. People are now discussing concepts like robustness and modularity, which help explain how cells appear almost predestined to particular fates and collaborate to form distinct tissues. Some evidence even hints that the initial groups of cells set the stage for what comes later, adding a layer of path-dependence to the story (Lenas et al., 2009). It appears that, in many cases, this combination of inherent cell behavior and signals from the surrounding environment creates a form of design logic behind gastrulation—even if the process still feels somewhat chaotic at times. The discussion around gastrulation is no longer static; blending traditional ideas with new data has become increasingly necessary. For instance, transcriptomic data keeps showing that gene expression remains surprisingly constant during the pharyngula stage, which reinforces the view of gastrulation as fundamental to setting up the vertebrate body plan (Irie et al., 2011). This convergence of hard data and fresh theories prompts us to view gastrulation not as an isolated process, but as a crossroads of evolution and development. Researchers are increasingly calling for interdisciplinary teamwork to unravel the complexities of embryonic development and shed light on how these processes have unfolded across different branches of life. Ultimately, the hope is that this collaborative future might finally bridge the long-standing gap between evolution and development in a way that feels, well, a bit more natural—even if there are still a few rough edges along the way (Figure 5.4).

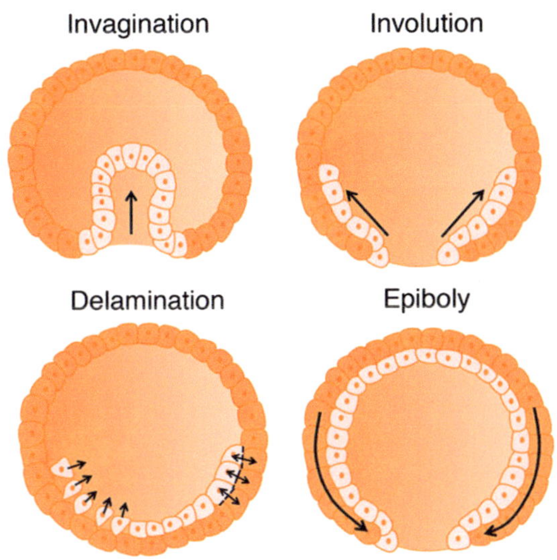

Figure 5.4. Evolution of gastrulation theories.

Source: https://ars.els-cdn.com/content/image/1-s2.0-S1084952121002056-gr1.jpg.

5.2. Stages of Gastrulation

Gastrulation kicks in early in development when a simple, one-layer blastula suddenly morphs into a layered structure called the gastrula. Cells start moving in unexpected ways—shuffling and differentiating until they form the ectoderm, mesoderm, and endoderm, which eventually lay out the plan for organs and tissues. Generally speaking, chemical messengers like fibroblast growth factor (FGF) fuel this transition; by regulating gene activity through helpers such as transcription factors, cells determine their future. Interestingly, some transcription factors act sequentially to steer each germ layer, weaving a complex network of signals that sets early development in motion (Claire et al., 2025). Understanding how these signals function during gastrulation greatly helps us comprehend later embryonic stages. When cells transition from an epithelial state to a more flexible mesenchymal form, they become more mobile—a crucial step in establishing the body plan. For example, the movement of the anterior visceral endoderm is vital for proper patterning; it initiates a chain reaction that leads directly to full gastrulation. If these busy processes go awry, developmental problems can follow, underscoring just how vital precise cell behavior is. Studies exploring how different signaling molecules influence cell identity have repeatedly highlighted the importance of specific genes and pathways in establishing an embryo's framework, thereby adding layers to our understanding of these complex events (Claire et al., 2024). Gastrulation isn't just about forming germ layers—it also lays down the groundwork for organ building and overall body balance. The combination of cell signals with behaviors such as growth, migration, and adhesion helps determine how those layers fine-tune into specialized tissues. When this balance is disrupted, a range of congenital issues can arise, underscoring the central role of gastrulation in normal development. Recent work even points to factors such as Etv4 and Etv5 as key players within FGF signaling, influencing both primitive endoderm formation and epiblast maturation. In most cases, this suggests that gastrulation is far more than a checklist of events—it's a carefully orchestrated process that ensures the embryo develops in harmony from the very beginning (Claire et al., 2025).

5.2.1. Formation of the Germ Layers

Gastrulation marks a turning point in early embryonic life. A simple two-layer disc suddenly reshuffles into three basic layers – ectoderm, mesoderm, and endoderm – that go on to build the body's essential framework. Each layer takes on its role, setting up tissues and organs in a way that feels almost spontaneous. Cells shift, move, and swap signals amid a flurry of activity, making this transformation possible. Lately, stem cell studies have shown that embryo-like models built from these cells can mimic these subtle early shifts, providing a new perspective on human embryogenesis (Oldak et al., 2023).

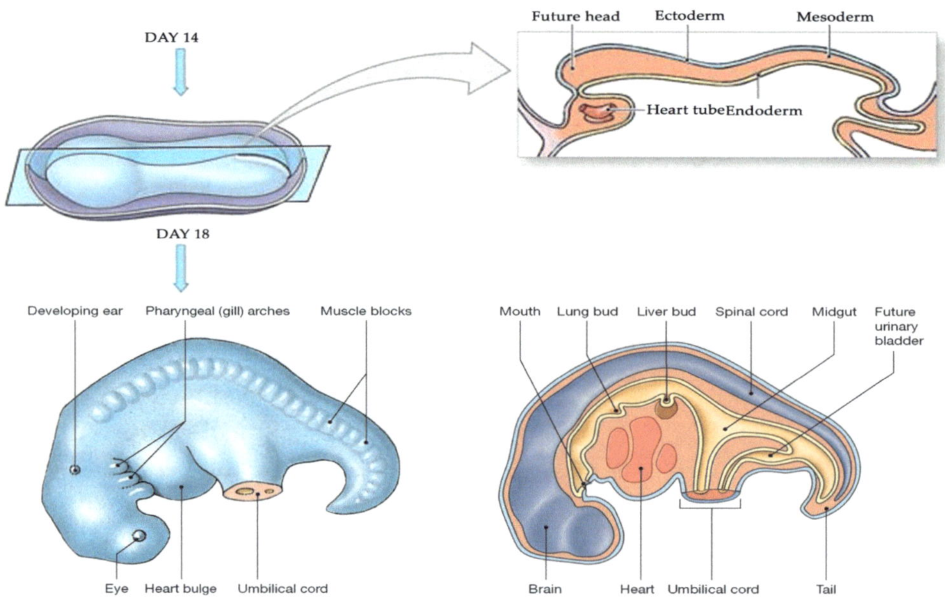

Figure 5.5. Formation of germ layers.

Source: https://lh3.googleusercontent.com/Ti-YXxU5xOn16Eq1ZW5-aMx_TyfZA_zbXWcsOQN653NJF6lDPSLOPDK2BW0R9GMaF4uC4Yth1XVON2DbDYYM2cJwof8TqtfG4gAgp3b2DquLr16xCZUhJWmT--4U0EA4APBwrN8Mu3d2l9kyVDjWszY.

Embryonic cells don't just multiply; they also wander and change shape, helping form these layers along the way. One key moment occurs when cells enter what is called the primitive streak – a pivotal point where they transition from the epiblast and begin to differentiate into mesoderm and endoderm. These movements are crucial. The endoderm, for instance, ultimately forms inner structures like the gut, while the mesoderm lays the groundwork for organs such as the heart, muscles, and even the skeleton. Recent work with mouse embryonic stem cell (ESC) models has yielded embryoids that exhibit features similar to those of neurulation-stage embryos, providing new insights into how these layers mix and interact (Peng-Xu et al., 2021). Having the power to tweak pluripotent stem cells upends biomedical research. When scientists coax these cells into forming organoids or embryo-like structures, they step into previously unreachable corners of development. This shift suggests a broader shift in how researchers approach not only human gastrulation but also related developmental disorders in the lab. As the field advances, more details emerge about the intricate signaling cues and unpredictable cell behaviors that shape these layers—insights that inform both our understanding of developmental biology and the future of regenerative medicine and therapies. Models like the new structured embryo-like systems may open up even more avenues to explore the early, sometimes messy, stages of life and what happens when things go right—or slightly off track (Oldak et al., 2023) (Figure 5.5).

5.2.2. Mechanisms of Cell Movement

Cells begin to move early in embryonic development, in a kind of organized chaos where physical forces and subtle chemical messages interact. In gastrulation, cells don't simply sit still; they shift, change shape, and reposition themselves—often thanks to the little reworkings inside their cytoskeletal systems. The actin-myosin setup, for instance, is key in allowing cells to contract and slide along, while sticky molecules like E-cadherin help them cling together in a loose formation. Even the way these adhesive spots are tweaked not only keeps cells stable but nudges them in specific directions.

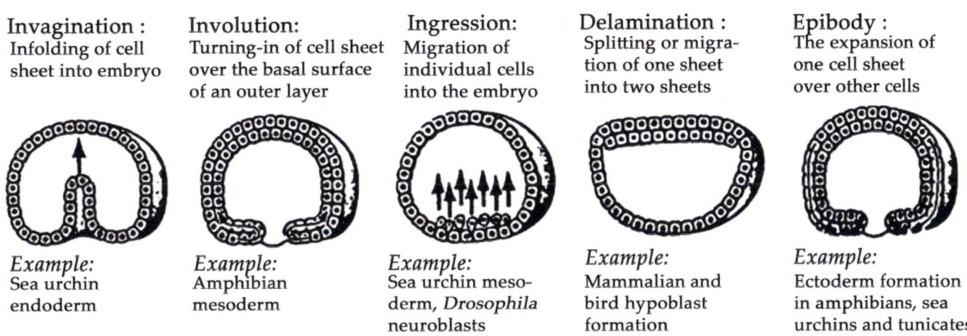

Figure 5.6. Mechanisms of cell movement in gastrulation.

Source: https://www.notesonzoology.com/wp-content/uploads/2016/07/clip_image002-103.jpg.

This balance plays a significant role in shaping the embryo's overall architecture, a feature observed in many species. At the same time, as cells glide past one another, the forces they generate start to tug on neighboring cells, which in turn reshapes the tissue landscape and sparks further cell-to-cell chatter. Different tissues, with some being softer than others, behave in varied ways; softer tissues bend quite easily, almost like they're shifting from a rigid solid to a more fluid state—much like a phase change in everyday life. In most cases, these mechanical feedback loops set the stage for what happens next in development, ensuring that the right moves are made during those critical transitions in gastrulation (Nicoletta et al., 2019). A further twist comes with the regulation of signals that guide these cells movements. Certain players—atypical Rho-GTPases such as Chp—show up to help localize E-cadherin at the right spots along the adherens junctions, which is essential for steering cells in the right direction. When this signaling goes slightly off track, epithelial movements tend to slow down, and cell adhesion falters, highlighting how even small disruptions can ripple through the entire process. Researchers have noted that proteins like PAK and PIX join this intricate network and further influence E-cadherin's behavior. In most cases, examining these molecular conversations provides a deeper understanding of how cell actions are coordinated during gastrulation and suggests why certain developmental disorders may arise when migration and adhesion aren't perfectly aligned (Tay et al., 2010) (Figure 5.6).

5.2.3. Timing of Gastrulation in Different Organisms

Embryonic development begins with a cascade of crucial events that prepare an organism for its future complexities. One standout phase is gastrulation—a moment when a clump of cells shifts into a more organized structure. The timing isn't uniform at all; generally speaking, different species handle this change in their way. For instance, mammals typically undergo gastrulation soon after the blastocyst forms, whereas amphibians usually wait until after a few early cell divisions have occurred. These differences, which reflect both evolutionary twists and the demands of distinct environments, underscore nature's knack for adapting its developmental blueprint—even though the end goal of establishing organized tissue layers remains a common thread. Another interesting turning point during this early period is what scientists refer to as the maternal-to-zygotic transition (MZT). Essentially, this occurs when control shifts from maternal factors to the embryo's genome. In many cases, as seen in species like zebrafish, this transition occurs pretty early, kick-starting rapid cell differentiation and helping trigger gastrulation. In contrast, mammals experience a slightly delayed MZT, leaving a longer window during which maternal influence still plays a significant role. This kind of variability reveals the subtle interplay between internal genetic instructions and external signals—a sort of tug-of-war that ultimately shapes how and when gastrulation unfolds, providing researchers with valuable clues about the regulatory mechanisms at work. At the core of gastrulation lie the active, almost dance-like movements of cells that eventually form distinct germ layers. In birds and reptiles, for example, the process is marked by the appearance of an elongated structure, commonly known as the primitive streak. This clever evolutionary adaptation helps tackle the unique challenges of egg-based reproduction. On the other hand, many fish species follow a different script, where gastrulation is defined by the involution of cells along the embryo's dorsal side. These varying strategies not only alter the timing of gastrulation but also reflect how each species has adapted to its unique environmental niche. As research continues to untangle the messy details of these processes, it's becoming clear that these differences aren't just biological quirks—they have significant implications for how we understand both developmental biology and the evolutionary relationships among species.

5.3. Cellular Mechanisms

Gastrulation begins when the firm epiblast layer starts breaking down into a mixture of germ layers—a change that's absolutely key. At the same time, a bunch of cell tricks get underway, with the EMT taking center stage. Basically, EMT nudges cells that usually stick together into adopting a more mobile, almost wanderlust-like behavior. Cells drop their usual polarity and let go of their tight-knit bonds, which sets them free to travel around; this change is pretty much what allows the three germ layers—ectoderm, mesoderm, and endoderm—to form. These cell tweaks carry enormous weight, laying down the blueprint for building organs later on. Investigating these processes reveals a convoluted but intriguing web of signals and cell conversations that ultimately form the intricate configurations our tissues require to function. At the heart of understanding gastrulation is how cells determine their identity and behavior, a process guided mainly by molecular factors. Examining the transcriptional profiles of over 400,000 cells from various post-conception weeks reveals that a rich molecular landscape underlies early gastrulation. This deep dive reveals that epiblast cells can switch gears, first transforming into neuroepithelial cells and later into radial glia, all under the influence of various signaling cues. Distinct groups of radial glial cells start to rise up along the neural tube; these clusters map out the paths that neurons will follow. Overall, these findings suggest that understanding the molecular shifts during gastrulation isn't just about early embryo development—it also provides a comparative playbook for how different species assemble themselves, highlighting the shared cellular blueprints between humans and common model organisms. It's hard to put a cap on how vital the actin cytoskeleton is during these shifts—it drives the shape changes and movements needed for tissues to form correctly. Researchers have been fortunate enough to capture these events live, in vivo, observing as the actin network directs processes such as invagination and migration, sometimes in real-time. Recent research shows that the kind of movements sparked by EMT isn't only vital for gastrulation in models like zebrafish and frog embryos but also offers clues about what happens when things go awry, such as in cancer metastasis. Seen from this perspective, the dance between actin dynamics and cell signaling during gastrulation provides a glimpse into how early development sets the stage for both normal body function and, potentially, disease later on. All in all, these insights underscore why getting into the nitty-gritty of cell mechanics is so essential to our broader understanding of developmental biology.

5.3.1. Role of Signaling Pathways

Gastrulation isn't a neat process—it involves various cell signals dancing together to pull off essential shape changes. TGF-β, for instance, stands out because it helps convert stationary epithelial cells into more fluid mesenchymal ones (a process known as EMT). In many cases, TGF-β works its magic even more effectively when teamed up with RAS-MAPK signals, so its impact isn't isolated. This complex mix of signals not only shapes cells but also guides processes such as cell specialization and the remodeling of the surrounding matrix. Researchers, by poking around these links, are beginning to show how TGF-β-driven EMTs mingle with early progenitor cell behavior during key moments like gastrulation, revealing core developmental cues (Lee et al., 2022). Immediately after implantation, the human embryo undergoes significant shape changes, laying the groundwork for everything that follows. FGF signaling plays a significant role here—it keeps both the embryo's main body and its extra-embryonic tissues growing, especially when switching from a pluripotent to a more settled state. Things become even more complicated when certain extra-embryonic hypoblast cells, oddly enough, position themselves asymmetrically and begin expressing inhibitors of signals like BMP, NODAL, and WNT.

These blockers are pretty important since they help map out the embryo's front-to-back, or anterior-posterior, layout. In most cases, observing how FGF interacts with these other signals provides insight into the complex dynamics that drive early human development, particularly during gastrulation, when proper axial patterning is crucial (Matteo et al., 2021). As gastrulation progresses, a complex network of signaling pathways not only shapes cell identities but also determines how tissues organize. TGF-β, FGF, and WNT signals get intertwined in a network that roughly coordinates the embryo's overall development. TGF-β, for one, does more than nudge cells along; it's a major force in moving cells from a pluripotent skim to more defined roles. Meanwhile, FGF steps in to boost cell growth and differentiation, setting up a kind of sturdy communication framework among cells. When these pathways converge, they help balance development and ensure that the embryo's front and back emerge correctly. Generally speaking, understanding this blend of signals is crucial for grasping the fundamentals of gastrulation—it lays the groundwork for later developmental stages and even sheds light on early-life anomalies (Matteo et al., 2021; Lee et al., 2022) (Figure 5.7).

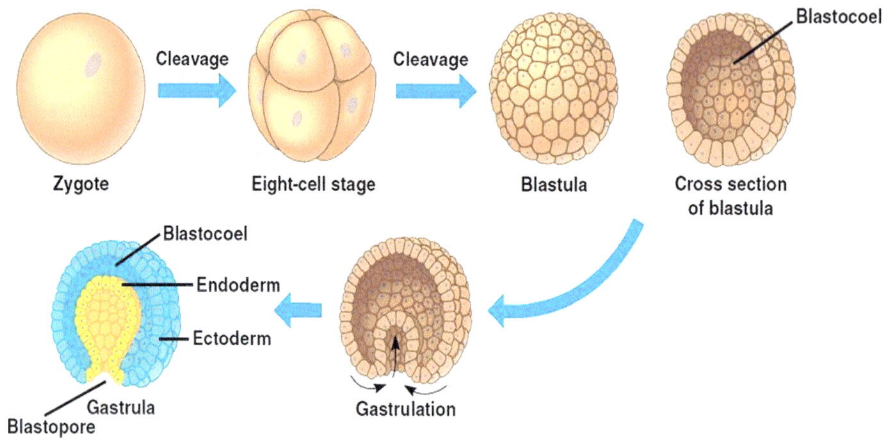

Figure 5.7. Role of signaling pathways.

Source: https://external-content.duckduckgo.com/iu/?u=http%3A%2F%2Fhannahleaanimalkingdom.weebly.com%2Fuploads%2F2%2F8%2F4%2F6%2F28462479%2F841039781.png&f=1&nofb=1&ipt=ae097e98b68dd07913c5a9edc30306b3270550646fa763fabe3f21f9f12db42d.

5.3.2. Cell Adhesion and Migration

Gastrulation kicks off a significant shift in an embryo's journey—cells stop sticking to one spot and start moving around in unexpected ways. At this point, cells essentially trade in their old, fixed roles for a more mobile lifestyle, allowing them to rearrange the embryo's layout. A process known as EMT is behind much of this switch; essentially, epithelial cells break apart their tight bonds and lose some order, acquiring traits that help them move. Studies, in most cases, point out that these changes not only shape tissues but also set the stage for later events in development. Cells, as they adjust and sometimes even repeat their fundamental tasks, bring adhesion molecules into the spotlight because these molecules are the driving forces behind cell migration during gastrulation (Jeffrey, 2021). At the heart of this movement is a reshuffling within the cell's framework, especially the actin fibers that let cells pull off shape changes and apply force. Signals emanating from the nearby extracellular matrix (ECM) and even some of the neighboring cells trigger this reorganization, resulting in the production of proteins that both promote adhesion and facilitate movement. There's a whole network of signals that gently dismantle old cell-cell bonds while beefing up connections with the extracellular surroundings. To understand what's happening, one must observe cells in action within living embryos—traditional methods fail to capture these rapid, dynamic shifts. Live imaging has become a go-to method for gaining insight into how cells behave during EMT, unveiling unexpected layers to the complex story of adhesion and migration (Yang et al., 2020). What's interesting is that cells getting better at moving isn't only a regular part of growing; it also ties into problems like cancer. As cells become more mobile, they can more easily invade nearby tissues, which often increases the risk of metastasis. This type of double-edged behavior is both an intriguing aspect of natural development and a significant concern in medical research circles. Generally speaking, understanding how EMT functions—and what maintains cell adhesion during gastrulation—is crucial because any misstep may lead to developmental abnormalities or even trigger malignant changes. By investigating the intricate web that regulates cell adhesion and migration, researchers are uncovering new insights into both developmental processes and potential cancer therapies (Jeffrey, 2021) (Figure 5.8).

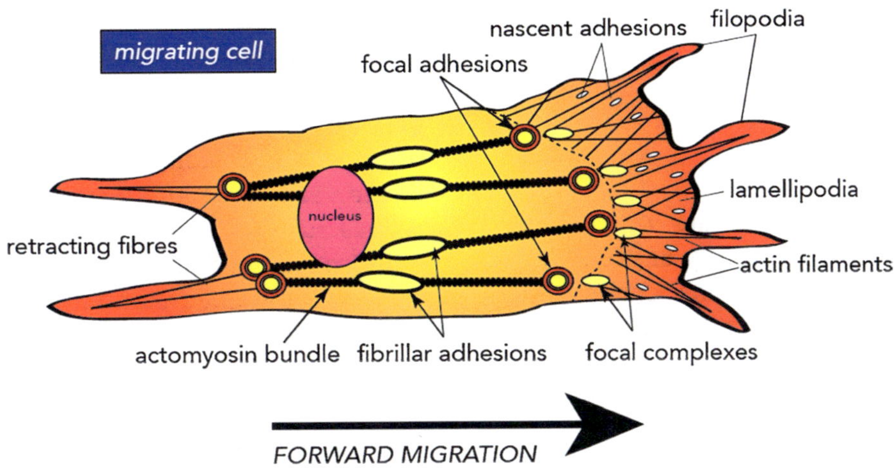

Figure 5.8. Cell adhesion and migration.

Source: https://external-content.duckduckgo.com/iu/?u=https%3A%2F%2Fwww.researchgate.net%2Fpublication%2F258168216%2Ffigure%2Ffig2%2FAS%3A297464360914952%401447932438493%2FOverview-of-structures-involved-in-cell-adhesion-and-migration-Schematic-of-the.png&f=1&nofb=1&ipt=ba0e3a3af1b8cb1b20cd36b8374796dadaa0c8568033881d822f67c0d5024bbf.

5.3.3. Cytoskeletal Dynamics During Gastrulation

Embryonic development is a wild mix of events where cells decide to change their roles. Take gastrulation, for instance – cells don't just remain epithelial with neat top and bottom sides; instead, they switch gears in a process known as the epithelial-mesenchymal transition (EMT). In most cases, this change allows cells to break free from their initial positions and participate in forming the germ layers. The actin cytoskeleton ultimately becomes intertwined with the process, driving those shape shifts and movements in ways that aren't immediately apparent. Live *in vivo* imaging, for example, has shown how these internal structures tweak adherens junctions (Jeffrey, 2021). Cytoskeletal dynamics aren't just about EMT either – they're part of a broader conversation in the cell, helping to steer decisions about fate and tissue organization. Generally speaking, actin filaments and even microtubules rally together to provide the forces needed for cell migration. It turns out that the way the actin network rearranges is closely tied to how adhesion molecules, such as cadherins, work to maintain tissue integrity, even while allowing cells some freedom to move about (Yang et al., 2020). Sometimes the links between these elements and various signals seem a bit unpredictable, suggesting that the exact timing and location of these changes are as crucial as they are fascinating. Taking a step back, understanding these early dynamics provides clues about phenomena like cancer metastasis, where cells once again act out a similar play. In many instances, reactivating a process reminiscent of EMT gives epithelial cells invasive traits that mirror those in embryonic development. It's almost as if the same strategies—those familiar cytoskeletal shifts and signaling cues—are being reused in different contexts. This crossover helps explain why studying gastrulation not only deepens our grasp of developmental biology but also lends insights into how things can go wrong in disease states (Jeffrey, 2021).

5.4. Comparative Gastrulation

Embryonic development bursts with activity, showcasing the unpredictability of gastrulation across vertebrate species. The driving force behind cell differentiation at this crucial juncture is the set of genes that guide the process. Take the Bmp gene family, for example—Bmp16, in particular, has taken a rather unexpected evolutionary detour compared to its peers. It appears that Bmp2, Bmp4, and Bmp16 all sprang from a single quartet kicked off by whole-genome duplications, leading to both similar functions being maintained and new adaptations cropping up in different species. Interestingly, while Bmp16 barely appears during development in the cloudy catshark, it plays a significantly larger role in species like the green anole lizard, underscoring how flexibly these genes can function during gastrulation (Feiner et al., 2019). Another twist comes from the transcriptional dynamics that steer cell fate. Recent studies using cutting-edge sequencing have revealed the diverse pathways that multiple zebrafish cell types follow during early somitogenesis. A cool development is the URD computational method, which helps piece together these routes and trace cells back to their original spots in the blastula. In most cases, research has identified Nodal signaling as a key player in guiding these pathways, also providing insight into how transcriptomes adapt under changing genetic conditions. All of this suggests that gastrulation isn't just a straightforward process—it's a careful balancing act between well-worn genetic routes and a surprising degree of changeability (Jeffrey et al., 2018). The reach of comparative gastrulation extends far beyond early development, encompassing our broader understanding of evolutionary biology and phylogenetics. By tracking differences in gene expression and the operation of regulatory systems across species, scientists can sketch out the evolutionary maps that shape vertebrate life. This approach not only taps into our shared genetic roots but also highlights how various lineages have adapted their developmental strategies to meet unique ecological challenges. As gastrulation research advances and gathers data from an ever-widening array of species, we gain a clearer understanding of the evolutionary forces and developmental limits that have woven the intricate tapestry of life on Earth. All in all, integrating insights from genetics, development, and evolution effectively highlights the importance of comparative studies in our quest to understand life's complexity (Feiner et al., 2019) (Figure 5.9).

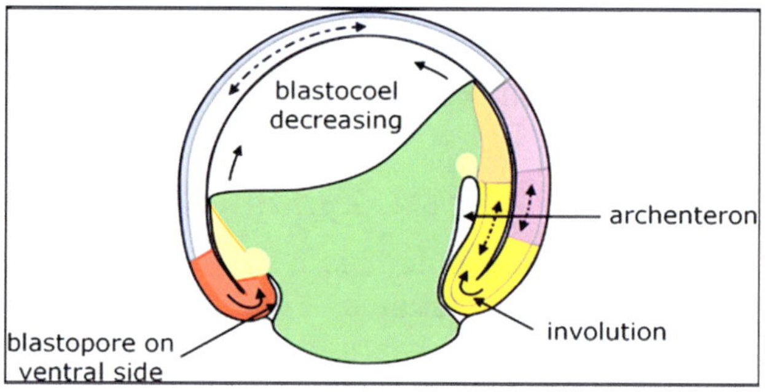

Figure 5.9. Comparison of gastrulation in vertebrates.

Source: https://evolutionunderthemicroscope.com/graphics/xenopus_gastrulation_2.jpg.

5.4.1. Differences in Gastrulation Among Species

Developmental biology reveals that gastrulation is a pivotal turning point in evolution—it initiates distinct developmental pathways in various species. Take cnidarians, for instance; these creatures sit at the very root of the animal family tree and give us clues about early gastrulation. They undergo unique changes that result in a two-layered (diploblastic) body plan, consisting of endoderm and ectoderm. Oddly enough, the way cnidarians handle gastrulation has some echoes in bilaterians, hinting that early methods have persisted. The sea anemone *Nematostella vectensis* grabs attention here, since studies on it have unraveled how cells and genes team up during gastrulation – and have pointed to key genes that help set up germ layers in bilaterian species (Technau, 2020). Differences in how gastrulation unfolds among organisms often stem from subtle variations in gene networks and cell movements. While cnidarians tend to stick with a simpler plan showing only two layers, bilaterians usually go a step further with a third, the mesoderm – a sign of more complicated signals at work. In most cases, even minor shifts in pathways like Wnt and FGF, as seen in *Nematostella*, can lead to significant changes in how an organism's body axis forms; this interplay makes one wonder how slight divergences can drive considerable results (Technau, 2020). Such nuances, repeated here in various contexts, open a window into comparing developmental strategies in a way that isn't always as neat as textbooks might suggest. It isn't all about just putting things in tidy categories, either. Learning about these variations gives us a glimpse into the inner workings of how cells determine their fate and how tissues ultimately develop. Techniques like single-cell RNA sequencing have started to lay bare the tangled hierarchies behind cell differentiation – showing that transcriptional diversity isn't just some academic fancy but a real clue into lineage choices. Researchers using tools like CytoTRACE have found that these details matter not only during early development but also in areas such as organ repair and even in weird cases of neoplastic transformation. In many ways, connecting these dots across species deepens our understanding of what gastrulation means in an evolutionary sense (Figure 5.10).

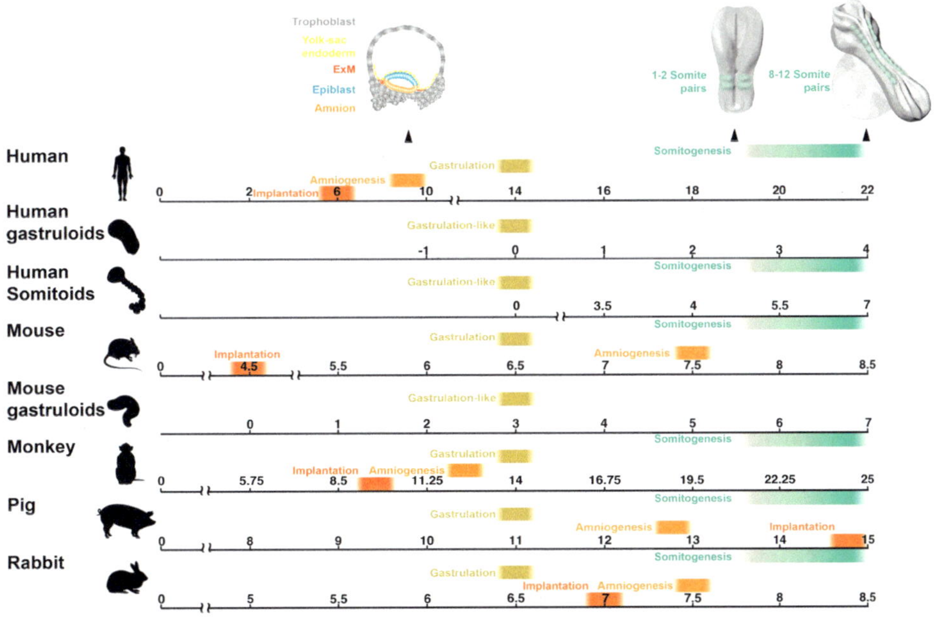

Figure 5.10. Comparing gastrulation across different species.

Source: https://www.researchgate.net/publication/375448536/figure/fig1/AS:11431281203792971@1699450434461/Comparing-gastrulation-across-different-species-in-vivo-and-in-vitro-There-are-clear.jpg.

5.4.2. Evolutionary Significance of Variations

Development is messy – differences start early on during gastrulation. Cells move around and shift roles, laying down a blueprint for tissues and organs in ways that aren't always neat. In most cases, gene activity changes thanks to both inherent quirks and outside influences, which ultimately shape an embryo's fate. Sometimes these shifts steer major pathways – think of the ones forming the mesoderm – and spark adaptive responses that prove vital in fluctuating environments. These natural differences not only allow species to settle into unique niches but also build up a kind of genetic reserve for future challenges. All in all, the messy details of early development drive the diversity we see across life. Evolution doesn't wait for perfection, and even slight variations during gastrulation can have a significant impact on an organism's fitness. Shifts in how cells communicate at this early phase might produce entirely new body shapes, boosting an organism's ability to thrive under harsh conditions. One can trace some of these finely tuned structures back to minor tweaks in gastrulation – generally speaking, it shows how internal genetic maps dance with outside cues. Studying these early differences provides researchers with insights not only into evolutionary biology but also into practical fields such as regenerative medicine and evo-devo. This mix of perspectives broadens our view of how life adapts in unpredictable ways. Variations at the gastrulation stage go far beyond keeping an embryo alive; they drive speciation and fuel biodiversity. Understanding how these quirks emerge can explain why distinct traits and forms come up, stitching together the patchwork of life on Earth. Comparative studies across different organisms reveal that, while the basic plan of gastrulation often remains consistent, the subtle variations tend to be fine-tuned for specific environmental challenges or evolutionary pathways. These differences can steer reproductive strategies and survival odds in directions that shape entire lineages. In breaking down these nuances, one sees clearly how evolution and development are tightly interwoven—even if the process is somewhat disorganized at times. There's still plenty to uncover here, as exploring these early shifts might offer fresh clues about the evolutionary past of today's life forms.

5.4.3. Implications for Developmental Biology

Gastrulation is a pivotal stage in early development that lays the groundwork for the formation of organs and the differentiation of tissues. During this hectic phase, cells shift and reorganize—displaying their natural flexibility, especially when they undergo the EMT. Researchers, examining these cell shifts, have found that such movements play a crucial role in determining how and where cells migrate to settle in the embryo. This kind of insight not only highlights the fundamental processes behind our development but also suggests how things can go awry—sometimes even sparking cancer—if the usual cell transitions are mismanaged. A shared, though sometimes evolving, understanding of what EMT truly involves is key to clarifying both embryonic development and disease research (Yang et al., 2020). Looking at gastrulation reveals how critical both EMT and the reverse process, mesenchymal-to-epithelial transition (MET), can be. A jumble of factors—transcription regulators, epigenetic tweaks, and even microRNA (miRNA) signals—work together to shepherd cells into their proper spots. These intricate yet surprisingly natural regulatory systems not only build up the cell layers necessary for proper organ formation but also indicate potential breakdowns that could cause severe developmental issues. In most cases, the ability of cells to transition into adulthood underscores their role in areas such as regenerative medicine and tissue repair. As our understanding of these transitions deepens, so too does the promise of harnessing EMT and MET for novel treatments in developmental disorders and cancer management (Ángela Nieto, 2013). The lessons from gastrulation extend far beyond early development, reaching into modern concepts of healing and therapy. By teasing out the drivers behind EMT and MET, scientists are beginning to craft interventions that may accelerate tissue repair or slow the spread of cancer. This crossover between understanding how life builds itself and how we might fix it has sparked a kind of collaborative energy, where experts trade ideas and sometimes even blur the lines between their specializations. Additionally, as guidelines for these processes become more refined—and our vocabulary around them becomes more consistent—it becomes easier for different fields to share insights seamlessly. Altogether, this spirit of cooperation is helping the scientific community untangle the many layers of gastrulation and its cell transitions, paving the way for advances in both fundamental biology and clinical practice (Ángela Nieto, 2013).

5.5. Gastrulation and Organogenesis

Gastrulation kick-starts the entire process of organ development by reshaping the embryo into a more complex structure. In this phase, the germ layers emerge, each type of layer assuming distinct roles that ultimately shape various tissues and organs. How these layers interact—setting up the body's blueprint, including where the axis lies and which cell types emerge—is pretty fascinating. Recent work, for instance, often highlights how certain molecular signals, such as R-spondin2, influence cell growth and even determine their fate, with this factor appearing in large amounts as gastrulation unfolds (Wang et al., 2018). In most cases, there's a subtle, yet crucial, exchange happening between the cells and these molecular cues that gets the whole organ-building act rolling. As gastrulation progresses, cells begin to assume more defined roles, laying the groundwork for later organ development. This shift is generally driven by a complex network of gene interactions that evolve and direct cells into their proper compartments over time. Single-cell RNA sequencing has significantly expanded our understanding of the diverse cell types emerging at this stage, each playing a distinct role in the development of organs (Ibarra-Soria et al., 2018). By charting the transcriptional profiles of over 20,000 cells during this critical moment, researchers have identified the key players and control switches that guide cell differentiation and organ formation. Such in-depth looks at early development not only clear up the cellular scene but also hint at ways we might tap into these processes for regenerative medicine later on. Our growing grasp of gastrulation sheds light on why congenital anomalies and developmental disorders occur when things don't go as planned. If the process gets disrupted, organs might not form correctly, leading to a range of health complications. By examining the molecular mechanics underlying both gastrulation and organ development, scientists can identify potential targets for therapeutic intervention. Take the role of R-spondin2 in muscle formation, for example—it shows pretty clearly how gene expression at this early phase can have lasting effects on tissue quality (Wang et al., 2018). Also, the way leukotriene pathways seem to impact the creation of blood progenitor cells suggests that certain factors could steer organ function, offering a sort of roadmap for future projects aimed at boosting developmental health and aiding recovery after birth (Ibarra-Soria et al., 2018).

5.5.1. Link Between Gastrulation and Organ Formation

Gastrulation emerges as a crucial event in early development—it marks the beginning of the process of organ formation. At this stage, cells begin to move and assume their roles, eventually forming three distinct layers: the ectoderm, the mesoderm, and the endoderm. Each of these layers goes on to create different organ systems, showing how this early shuffle ties into later body design. Even minor changes in this phase can lead to severe malformations later on, which tells us that getting the initial setup right is everything. In these early moments, cell movements and the jumble of signals begin to pave the way for organs to take shape, setting a rough blueprint for what's to come. As the process progresses, specific molecular cues begin to steer cells toward their final destinations. For instance, Pitx2 plays a significant role in distinguishing left from right when organs form. Within the gut, a pressure-sensitive pathway involving TGFβ regulates Pitx2 levels, allowing the intestine to twist just right. This feedback—not a neat, linear path but a mix of forces and chemical hints—shows how physical dynamics and molecular signals work together. Researchers have even found that any deviation from these pathways can trigger major issues, such as intestinal malrotation (Bhargav et al., 2022), underscoring the importance of every nuance during this phase. New techniques like single-cell RNA sequencing have opened our eyes to just how varied cells can be right after this critical period. By examining over 20,000 cells in the wake of gastrulation, scientists uncovered a surprising mix of cell types, each with its unique regulatory setup tied to specific organs. This level of detail reveals a complex web of signals that emerge during gastrulation, setting the stage for the eventual development of tissue and organ forms. For example, some studies suggest that the leukotriene pathway plays a key role in generating hematopoietic progenitor cells. This connection further links the narrative of early cell events to later organ development (Ibarra-Soria et al., 2018). All of this, even with its little imperfections and unexpected turns, reminds us just how pivotal those early, formative moments truly are (Figure 5.11).

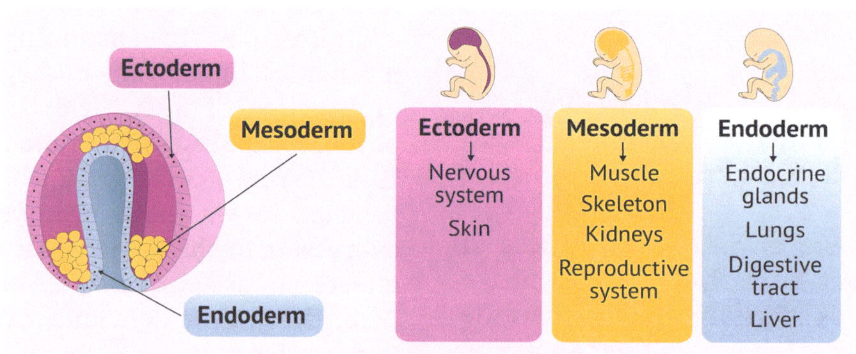

Figure 5.11. Gastrulation and development of organ systems.

Source: https://external-content.duckduckgo.com/iu/?u=https%3A%2F%2Fwww.invitra.com%2Fen%2Fwp-content%2Fuploads%2F2015%2F07%2Fembryonic-skin-development.png&f=1&nofb=1&ipt=89d9a31cc3259414ddf807e8188031fce15695901b88dca02cb5813147bb9dbb.

5.5.2. Role of Germ Layers in Organ Development

Gastrulation initiates embryonic development in a remarkably dynamic manner, laying the groundwork for the formation of the three germ layers. Cells start shifting around through moves like invagination and involution, and—surprisingly enough—it's these layers (ectoderm, mesoderm, and endoderm) that essentially build our organs. The ectoderm ends up making parts of the central nervous system and our skin, while the mesoderm handles muscles, bones, and even the circulatory system.

Then there's the endoderm, which takes charge of internal organs like the liver and lungs. When these layers mix their signals, they transform a simple cluster of cells into a complex, functioning organism—a process so crucial for healthy bodily operations. Sometimes things don't go as planned, though. If the germ layers aren't formed or organized correctly, significant developmental issues can arise. Researchers generally note that any deviation during germ layer differentiation can lead to congenital anomalies. For example, some studies have pointed out that exposure to chemicals such as TDCIPP may seriously disrupt gastrulation and proper germ-layer formation (Dasgupta et al., 2018). In most cases, understanding these subtle interactions provides insight into the molecular signals that direct cell fate. This insight isn't just academic—it's crucial for determining how to intervene when developmental disorders emerge. Meanwhile, there's considerable interest in utilizing these germ layer derivatives in regenerative medicine. Stem cells sourced from these layers offer a promising route, particularly for treating diseases associated with organ failure. Contemporary reviews even discuss how stem cell therapy can coax pluripotent cells into turning into distinct tissue types—whether they mimic ectodermal, mesodermal, or endodermal origins (Zakrzewski et al., 2019). This kind of control over cell destiny is nothing short of revolutionary and lays the groundwork for tissue engineering and organ replacement strategies. Recent progress in quality control and cell-assessment techniques suggests safer and more effective approaches. All in all, delving into the basics of how germ layers form is a crucial step for the future of regenerative treatments (Figure 5.12).

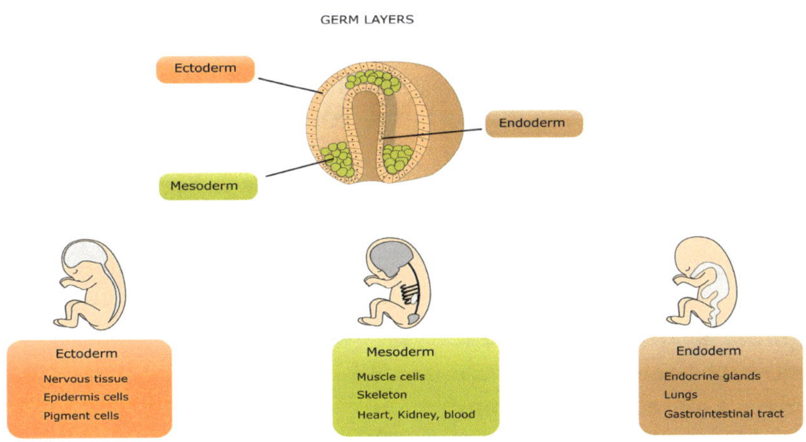

Figure 5.12. Role of germ layers in organ development.

Source: https://external-content.duckduckgo.com/iu/?u=https%3A%2F%2Fcdn.vmstudygroup.com%2Fwp-content%2Fuploads%2FGerm-layers-and-organs.jpg%3Fx99947&f=1&nofb=1&ipt=c79e0183c8e2f2a6aa62e91660bf6a59557e26dbf11d972db3773c5139b90ea8.

5.5.3. Consequences of Gastrulation Errors on Organogenesis

Gastrulation initiates organ formation and sets the stage for the development of tissues and structures. This early phase can be very fragile—minor errors here might mess up later processes. When cells stray from their typical paths or when patterns become slightly off, the tissue layers may form in the wrong order, which can slow or even derail the development of key features like the heart or brain. At its core, the process depends on carefully tuned cell movements and a cascade of signals that, in most cases, keep things roughly in line. Yet, even minor mix-ups can trigger a chain reaction of developmental issues, eventually manifesting as birth anomalies and functional problems later on. Even a slight deviation in this critical period can pose serious challenges for both organ formation and long-term health. Gastrulation also plays a significant role in the context of evolution. Generally speaking, mutations that disrupt this early stage often carry wide-ranging effects, putting tight limits on how species can adapt over time. Research shows that alterations in the regular order of early developmental events frequently lead to stiff, unchanging body plans and lower repair capacities, basically locking in an organism's design. These early errors, which affect individuals, sometimes ripple out to cause an evolutionary standstill within whole populations. The interplay between these mutations and their extensive effects underscores just how sensitive early development is—impacting not only personal health but also the evolutionary trajectory of species. Grasping these underlying mechanics becomes even trickier when tissue remodeling is examined on a global scale. Cutting-edge imaging studies reveal that the way forces are distributed in space plays a huge role in keeping the blueprint of life intact. These findings highlight that, aside from direct cell-to-cell contact, even distant mechanical cues play a role in shaping embryonic tissues. When these well-orchestrated forces falter, cells might end up too orderly or, conversely, too chaotic, which ultimately undermines proper organ building. As early errors accumulate through later stages, they trigger cascades that compromise organ function and lead to a range of physiological problems. Merging ideas from both mechanical and biological viewpoints thus offers a more rounded, if sometimes messy, picture of how mistakes in gastrulation impact the overall developmental process.

5.6. Experimental Approaches

New experimental methods have significantly advanced our understanding of gastrulation. Researchers now use motherlive-cell imaging to catch cells in action—watching as they move and decide their fates almost in real-time. Glowing markers enable us to observe precisely how cells behave during these early stages, providing key insights into how they establish their positions and begin forming tissues. Tracking individual cell dynamics shows us not only the traits of each cell but also how differences among them steer development. In many cases, these findings reveal that outside signals can influence cell fate during critical moments, which is why top-quality imaging tools are crucial in developmental biology research (Fiorentino et al., 2020). Mathematical modeling has also become a significant aid in interpreting gastrulation data. Researchers build computational models that mimic how cells interact and choose their destinies; such models can often predict what might happen under different developmental conditions. They combine ideas about what's happening inside the cell with signals from the cell's environment, providing a more nuanced—but richer—picture of cellular behavior. By blending hands-on experiments with computer simulations, scientists uncover potential regulatory networks that might otherwise be missed. As the field continues to evolve, refining these models alongside laboratory work is likely to deepen our understanding of the subtle dynamics of gastrulation (Fiorentino et al., 2020). There has also been exciting progress with systems like synthetic embryos and gastruloids, which provide scientists with solid alternatives for studying gastrulation in the lab. These setups more accurately imitate early embryonic development than traditional cell cultures, allowing researchers to more easily explore how cells communicate with one another and respond to their surroundings. Using these models, labs can dissect how cells react and determine the roles of specific signals as cells transition from a stem-like state to a more defined one. This line of research not only helps us understand normal developmental processes but also sheds light on what might go wrong in developmental disorders. As work in this area expands—and as methods gradually become more standardized—collaboration across different fields should only boost our overall understanding of developmental biology.

5.6.1. Techniques Used to Study Gastrulation

Gastrulation initiates the embryo's development by establishing the different germ layers, and scientists investigate this process using a combination of innovative techniques that reveal its molecular and cellular secrets. Live imaging, for example, allows researchers actually to see cells in action—tracking their movement, how they organize themselves, and even the subtle decisions they make as the embryo transitions from blastula to gastrula. Using fluorescent tags and high-tech microscopes, researchers follow the journey of mesoderm and endoderm precursors, uncovering their migration paths and interactions.

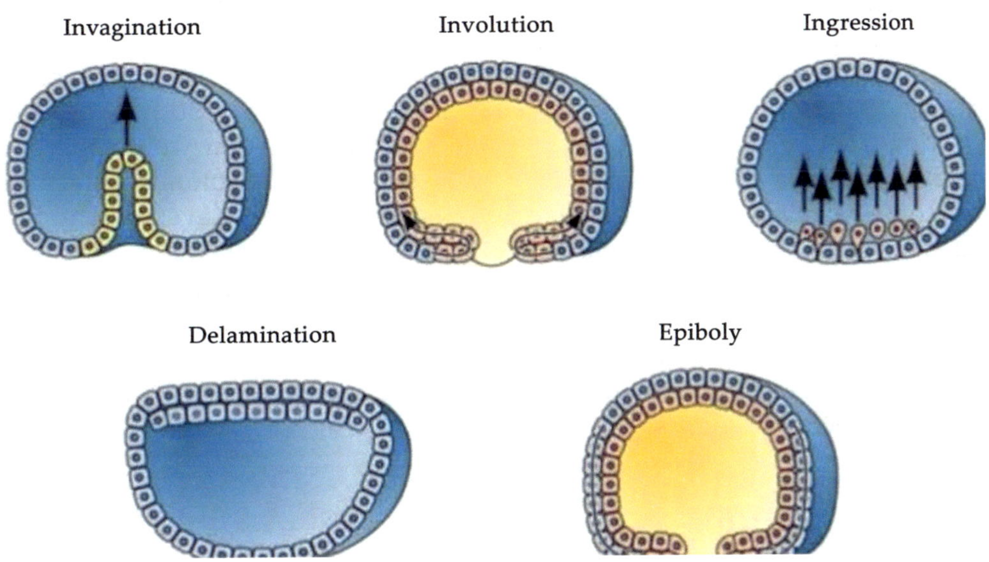

Figure 5.13. Techniques used to study gastrulation.

Source: https://external-content.duckduckgo.com/iu/?u=https%3A%2F%2Fimg.mudfooted.com%2F1663639291508.jpg&f=1&nofb=1&ipt=ca9be22d36b435e8572dd0078518af2052434b414cc42525c5fab5d974b22191.

In many instances, these live visuals are paired with computer models, which help predict cell behavior in real time. Altogether, this blend of methods deepens our understanding of how early embryonic development unfolds. Another popular way to study gastrulation focuses on the molecular aspects, examining gene expression and signaling networks that are crucial during this phase. Techniques such as quantitative PCR and *in situ* hybridization provide scientists with a means to measure mRNA levels for key genes involved in tissue differentiation and cell movement. These methods establish a kind of 'when-and-where' map for crucial regulatory genes—research has shown that pathways such as WNT, Notch, and BMP are active in distinct patterns during gastrulation, influencing cell fate decisions as the process progresses. High-throughput sequencing further expands this picture, providing a comprehensive view of the transcriptome and helping to unravel the complex genetic networks that drive embryonic patterning. Beyond traditional molecular and imaging approaches, newer technologies such as single-cell RNA sequencing (scRNA-seq) are revolutionizing our understanding of gastrulation. This innovative method enables researchers to examine gene expression in individual cells, revealing many hidden differences that bulk analyses previously overlooked. By combining scRNA-seq with spatial transcriptomics, scientists can begin to link specific gene expression patterns to precise locations within the embryo, thereby highlighting unique cell groups that play a significant role in forming the germ layers. Plus, catching those brief, transient cellular states provides fresh clues about developmental dynamics and lineage tracing. All in all, blending these advanced techniques gives us a more complete, and sometimes unexpectedly messy, picture of embryonic development during gastrulation (Figure 5.13).

5.6.2. Model Organisms in Gastrulation Research

Gastrulation research has long relied on a handful of go-to organisms to shed light on this complex phase. Take zebrafish and *Xenopus laevis*, for example. Zebrafish embryos are transparent, allowing scientists to observe live cell movements as they occur, while *Xenopus* has been a valuable workhorse in embryo experimentation and the growth of organoids. These species allow researchers to circumvent many of the ethical concerns associated with human studies while still providing numerous practical benefits. Generally speaking, the ease of tweaking their genes means it's simpler to draw ties between genetic signals and the cell shifts we see during gastrulation. Then there's another angle. Echinoderms—like sea urchins—add their twist by offering a cleaner view of early development. Their simple growth and distant evolutionary ties to vertebrates provide a unique kind of insight, one that highlights common threads in embryonic development. Recent work, as noted in some reviews, demonstrates that observing how sea urchins form gonads and sort out germ cell paths can further elucidate the controls operating at the onset of development (Li et al., 2025). Interestingly, social insects, often considered for aging research, also emerge as models to study how gastrulation may have evolved in more complex life forms. Examining these creatures reveals curious trade-offs—balancing long life with high reproduction—and networks like the TI-J-LiFe system appear to be at work in shaping both aging and embryonic development. When we compare different life histories within colonies, these patterns end up echoing across developmental processes. By piecing together evidence from fish, frogs, sea urchins, and even social insects, researchers are quietly sketching an evolutionary panorama that places gastrulation right at the heart of how diverse organisms adapt over time (Korb, 2024).

5.6.3. Recent Advancements in Gastrulation Studies

Fresh research into gastrulation reveals just how critical mechanical and chemical forces are in early development—it's pretty revealing. Scientists are now paying closer attention to the dynamic interplay between how cells move and the signals they send, which helps us understand how tissues gradually form during these crucial early moments. New imaging methods and computer models enable to observe these events in real time, revealing that physical pressures and chemical gradients interact to influence how cells behave. In some cases, these fresh insights have sparked the creation of models that hint at how complex tissue patterns form, subtly shedding light on why certain developmental disorders might arise. By studying in depth the mechanics of gastrulation, researchers hope to uncover treatment targets for congenital issues, suggesting that this line of inquiry isn't just theoretical—it's got tangible promise for medicine. Then there's the whole impact of organoid technology, which has switched up the way we study gastrulation. Using organoids grown from pluripotent stem cells, scientists are now able to recreate a tiny version of the embryonic environment in a dish. These mini models capture the same kind of signaling and physical traits observed in early development, offering a glimpse into the cell-to-cell communication that occurs during gastrulation. This clever method not only unpacks the details of how cells interact but also gives a testbed for exploring the effects of genetic mutations on early growth. Ethical considerations, such as ensuring proper informed consent and the potential future use of these organoids in transplants, have also been discussed in the community (Dide de Jongh et al., 2022). Balancing these ethical concerns with the rush of scientific progress is essential—even if it sometimes leads to a somewhat messy conversation. Mixing approaches from different disciplines has also opened new doors in gastrulation research. Recent work generally indicates that the interplay between mechanical forces and chemical signals influences how development unfolds across a range of organisms. Upgraded computational tools now enable scientists to mimic these complex interactions on the computer, sparking unexpected collaboration between biologists and mathematicians. Their joint efforts highlight that factors such as cellular flows and subtle tissue deformations play a crucial role even in these early stages, suggesting that mechanochemical influences are difficult to overlook. In many cases, these findings not only challenge our fundamental understanding of biology but also inform strategies in regenerative medicine aimed at repairing or replacing damaged tissues (Pierre-François Lenne et al., 2020).

SUMMARY

Gastrulation sits right at the heart of developmental biology. It's that process where a single cell slowly—almost imperceptibly at times—morphs into the design for an entire organism. Researchers have found that both these early transformations and what happens just after (think organ formation (Yuan et al., 2023) give us a sneak peek into how body parts are mapped out. In many cases, delving into these phases not only answers basic questions but also suggests ways to address developmental disorders and even opens doors to new regenerative medicine approaches. It's a curious mix of basic science and practical, clinical promise that ties all these ideas together in unexpected ways. Studying gastrulation in humans isn't always straightforward, primarily due to ethical limitations that prevent us from directly observing human embryogenesis. To work around this, scientists have developed creative models, such as gastruloids, made from pluripotent stem cells. These experimental setups yield essential insights into early development, and they even shed light on why early embryo loss or pregnancy issues can occur (Yuan et al., 2023). This trend toward using alternative models represents a significant step forward, allowing researchers to push the boundaries of what is known while sidestepping some of the ethical hurdles. There's also a genetic twist to consider. Specific genes, especially those linked to selenoproteins, seem to play a pivotal role in this drama. For instance, the SECIS-binding protein 2 (Secisbp2) is involved in controlling selenoprotein production, and if this system goes awry, early development can be disrupted even before gastrulation begins. Spotting these genetic influences—again, something researchers continually revisit—broadens our understanding of all the factors, both biological and ethical, that shape this stage. All in all, by weaving together findings from different lines of inquiry, we're gradually charting a course toward innovative therapies that might one day improve reproductive health outcomes. Gastrulation is a defining moment in embryonic development—it essentially sets the stage by forming the main layers that serve as a blueprint for the growing organism. Cell changes during this period aren't just a straight, simple path; a blend of internal cues and outside factors influences them. For example, the change from pluripotent stem cells to what we call definitive endoderm isn't just a neat, orderly shift. Instead, various signals—including factors such as low oxygen levels—tweak the process in unexpected ways. In most cases, these external conditions subtly steer the cells, opening up new questions about how nature fine-tunes each step. Lipid peroxidation, on the other hand, plays a more surprising role during the jumbled movements of gastrulation. Recent studies suggest that this process isn't solely about causing harmful damage; it also seems to help guide cell communication and even impact whether a cell survives or dies—consider, for instance, its role in ferroptosis. This controlled form of cell death may be an evolutionary adaptation, combining responses to oxidative stress with essential tissue remodeling. Across many species, including humans, the balance between enabling survival and triggering death through oxidative stress adds yet another layer of complexity to how we view embryogenesis. New methods, such as single-cell RNA sequencing, have, in a sense, revolutionized our approach to studying these early changes. By examining the RNA details of individual cells, researchers have identified key regulators that control the transition from mesendoderm to definitive endoderm. Take KLF8 as an example; this protein, acting as an unexpected modulator in the process, illustrates how targeted genetic tweaks can reveal deeply rooted developmental patterns. Generally speaking, as scientists continue to merge broader genetic data into their research, our overall picture of gastrulation becomes richer and more nuanced. This progress not only sharpens our fundamental understanding of embryo development but also hints at new potential targets for treating developmental disorders and advancing regenerative medicine.

CLOSER LOOK

EPIBLAST LAYER

The epiblast layer is a critical structure in early embryonic development, playing a foundational role in the formation of the entire embryo proper in amniotes, including humans. During the early stages of embryogenesis, following fertilization and the formation of the blastocyst, the inner cell mass (ICM) differentiates into two distinct layers: the epiblast and the hypoblast. The epiblast forms the upper layer and is composed of pluripotent columnar epithelial cells, meaning they have the potential to give rise to all three germ layers—ectoderm, mesoderm, and endoderm—through a process called gastrulation. This event marks the transition from a simple blastula to a complex, multilayered structure, laying the groundwork for organ and tissue formation.

Gastrulation begins with the formation of the primitive streak, a structure that appears on the surface of the epiblast. Cells of the epiblast migrate through the primitive streak, undergoing epithelial-to-mesenchymal transition (EMT), and then move inward and downward to form the mesoderm and endoderm layers. The remaining cells in the epiblast that do not migrate become the ectoderm. Thus, the epiblast is the sole source of all embryonic tissues, while the hypoblast primarily contributes to extra-embryonic structures such as the yolk sac. This pivotal role of the epiblast emphasizes its significance in developmental biology, as errors in epiblast differentiation or migration can lead to significant congenital anomalies or embryonic lethality.

In addition to giving rise to the body tissues, the epiblast also contributes to the formation of critical embryonic structures such as the amniotic cavity and the notochord. The amniotic cavity forms between the epiblast and the trophoblast, providing cushioning and protection for the developing embryo. The notochord, which arises from mesodermal cells originally part of the epiblast, serves as a key signaling center that patterns the surrounding tissues and helps establish the body axis. These events are tightly regulated by numerous signaling pathways, including those involving fibroblast growth factors (FGFs), bone morphogenetic proteins (BMPs), Wnt proteins, and Nodal signaling. These molecular cues orchestrate the spatial and temporal dynamics of cell movement and fate specification within the epiblast.

Furthermore, the study of the epiblast has become increasingly important in the field of stem cell research. Because epiblast cells are pluripotent, they share key characteristics with embryonic stem cells (ESCs), which are derived from the epiblast and can be cultured indefinitely *in vitro*. Understanding the behavior and regulation of epiblast cells has advanced regenerative medicine, including efforts to generate specific cell types for therapeutic use.

The epiblast layer is a central player in embryonic development, responsible for generating all the tissues and organs of the developing embryo. Through complex and highly regulated processes such as gastrulation and cell differentiation, the epiblast orchestrates the transformation from a simple cell mass into a structured organism. Its pivotal role in early development, disease modeling, and stem cell biology underscores its importance in both basic research and clinical applications.

REFERENCES

1. Amack, J. D. (2021). Cellular dynamics of EMT: Lessons from live *in vivo* imaging of embryonic development. *Cell Communication and Signaling, 19*. https://doi.org/10.1186/s12964-021-00761-8.

2. Appleby, J., & Bredenoord, A. L. (2018). Should the 14-day rule for embryo research become the 28-day rule? *EMBO Molecular Medicine, 10*(4), e9437. https://doi.org/10.15252/emmm.201809437.

3. Argelaguet, R., Arnol, D., Bredikhin, D., Deloro, Y., Velten, B., Marioni, J. C., & Stegle, O. (2020). MOFA+: a statistical framework for comprehensive integration of multi-modal single-cell data. *Genome Biology, 21*. https://doi.org/10.1186/s13059-020-02015-1.

4. Cai, Y., & Liu, A. (2024). Research on the evolution of ancient women's wedding attire. *International Journal of Social Sciences and Public Administration, 2*(3), 342–350. https://doi.org/10.62051/ijsspa.v2n3.48Chan, S. H., Tang, Y., Miao, L., Darwich-Codore, H., Vejnar, C. E., Beaudoin, J. D., Musaev, D., et al. (2019). Brd4 and P300 confer transcriptional competency during zygotic genome activation. *Developmental Cell, 49*(6), 867–881.e8. https://doi.org/10.1016/j.devcel.2019.05.037.

5. Chen, F., Wu, W., Li, M., Su, Y., Huang, M., Luo, X., You, W., et al. (2025). Cloning, characterization, and expression analysis of the DEAD-box family genes, Vasa and PL10, in Pacific abalone (*Haliotis discus hannai*). *Genes, 16*. https://www.semanticscholar.org/paper/a89b68c292c21edaabb0a6f9927333839fa7f5b4 (accessed on 26 May 2025).

6. Chu, L. F., Leng, N., Zhang, J., Hou, Z., Mamott, D., Vereide, D., Choi, J., et al. (2016). Single-cell RNA-seq reveals novel regulators of human embryonic stem cell differentiation to definitive endoderm. *Genome Biology, 17*. https://doi.org/10.1186/s13059-016-1033-x.

7. Conrad, M., Kagan, V. E., Bayır, H., Pagnussat, G. C., Head, B., Traber, M. G., & Stockwell, B. R. (2018). Regulation of lipid peroxidation and ferroptosis in diverse species. *Genes & Development, 32*, 602–619. https://doi.org/10.1101/gad.314674.118.

8. Dasgupta, S., Cheng, V., Vliet, S. M. F., Mitchell, C. A., & Volz, D. C. (2018). Tris(1,3-dichloro-2-propyl) phosphate exposure during the early-blastula stage alters the normal trajectory of zebrafish embryogenesis. *Environmental Science & Technology, 52*(19), 10820–10828. https://doi.org/10.1021/acs.est.8b03730.

9. de Jongh, D., Massey, E. K., Berishvili, E., Mar Fonseca, L., Lebreton, F., Bellofatto, K., Bignard, J., et al. (2022). Organoids: A systematic review of ethical issues. *Stem Cell Research & Therapy, 13*. https://doi.org/10.1186/s13287-022-02950-9.

10. Farrell, J. A., Wang, Y., Riesenfeld, S. J., Shekhar, K., Regev, A., & Schier, A. F. (2018). Single-cell reconstruction of developmental trajectories during zebrafish embryogenesis. *Science, 360*(6392). https://doi.org/10.1126/science.aar3131.

11. Feiner, N., Motone, F., Meyer, A., & Kuraku, S. (2019). Asymmetric paralog evolution between the "cryptic" gene *Bmp16* and its well-studied sister genes *Bmp2* and *Bmp4*. *Scientific Reports, 9*. https://doi.org/10.1038/s41598-019-40055-1.

12. Fiorentino, J., Torres-Padilla, M. E., & Scialdone, A. (2020). Measuring and modeling single-cell heterogeneity and fate decision in mouse embryos. *Annual Review of Genetics, 54*, 167–187. https://doi.org/10.1146/annurev-genet-021920-110200.

13. Galis, F., Metz, J. A. J., & van Alphen, J. J. M. (2018). Development and evolutionary constraints in animals. *Annual Review of Ecology, Evolution, and Systematics, 49*, 499–522. https://doi.org/10.1146/annurev-ecolsys-110617-062339.

14. Gladyshev, V. N. (2020). The ground zero of organismal life and aging. *Trends in Molecular Medicine, 27*(1), 11–19. https://doi.org/10.1016/j.molmed.2020.08.012.

15. Gulati, G. S., Sikandar, S. S., Wesche, D. J., Manjunath, A., Bharadwaj, A., Berger, M. J., Ilagan, F., et al. (2020). Single-cell transcriptional diversity is a hallmark of developmental potential. *Science, 367*(6476), 405–411. https://doi.org/10.1126/science.aax0249.

16. Ibarra-Soria, X., Jawaid, W., Pijuan-Sala, B., Ladopoulos, V., Scialdone, A., Jörg, D. J., Tyser, R. C. V., et al. (2018). Defining murine organogenesis at single cell resolution reveals a role for the leukotriene pathway in regulating blood progenitor formation. *Nature Cell Biology, 20*(2), 127–134. https://www.semanticscholar.org/paper/1a7c36c8750021f668ada9c30109be29e1372db4 (accessed on 26 May 2025).

17. Irie, N., & Kuratani, S. (2011). Comparative transcriptome analysis reveals vertebrate phylotypic period during organogenesis. *Nature Communications, 2*. https://doi.org/10.1038/ncomms1248.

18. Kamimoto, K., Stringa, B., Hoffmann, C. M., Jindal, K., Solnica-Krezel, L., & Morris, S. A. (2023). Dissecting cell identity via network inference and *in silico* gene perturbation. *Nature, 614*, 742–751. https://doi.org/10.1038/s41586-022-05688-9.

19. Korb, J. (2024). Termites and other social insects as emerging model organisms of ageing research: How to achieve a long lifespan and a high fecundity. *The Journal of Experimental Biology, 227*(22). https://www.semanticscholar.org/paper/4d383cab640762bb636bac1363ec6ecd75a59894 (accessed on 26 May 2025).

20. Lambaerts, K., Van Dyck, S., Mortier, E., Ivarsson, Y., Degeest, G., Luyten, A., Vermeiren, E., et al. (2012). Syntenic, a syndecan adaptor and an Arf6 phosphatidylinositol 4,5-bisphosphate effector, is essential for epiboly and gastrulation cell movements in zebrafish. *Journal of Cell Science, 125*, 1129–1140. https://doi.org/10.1242/jcs.089987.

21. Lee, J. H., & Massagué, J. (2022). TGF-β in developmental and fibro genic EMTs. *Seminars in Cancer Biology, 86*, 136–145. https://doi.org/10.1016/j.semcancer.2022.09.004.

22. Lee, M. T., Bonneau, A. R., & Giráldez, A. J. (2014). Zygotic genome activation during the maternal-to-zygotic transition. *Annual Review of Cell and Developmental Biology, 30*, 581–613. https://doi.org/10.1146/annurev-cellbio-100913-013027.

23. Lenas, P., Moos, M., & Luyten, F. P. (2009). Developmental engineering: A new paradigm for the design and manufacturing of cell-based products. Part I: From three-dimensional cell growth to biomimetics of *in vivo* development. *Tissue Engineering Part B: Reviews, 15*, 381–394. https://doi.org/10.1089/ten.teb.2008.0575.

24. Lenne, P. F., Munro, E., Heemskerk, I., Warmflash, A., Bocanegra-Moreno, L., Kishi, K., Kicheva, A., et al. (2020). Roadmap for the multiscale coupling of biochemical and mechanical signals during development. *Physical Biology, 18*, 041501. https://doi.org/10.1088/1478-3975/abd0db.

25. Li, Z., & Yang, Y. (2025). Reproductive physiology and molecular mechanisms underlying testicular development and spermatogenesis in echinoderms: A marine invertebrate

deuterostome. *Molecular Reproduction and Development, 92*(1), e70011. https://www.semanticscholar.org/paper/cee156f1f8e94fa11439031b90e64491c4a2363f (accessed on 26 May 2025).

26. Molè, M. A., Coorens, T. H. H., Shahbazi, M. N., Weberling, A., Weatherbee, B. A. T., Gantner, C. W., Sancho-Serra, C., et al. (2021). A single cell characterization of human embryogenesis identifies pluripotency transitions and putative anterior hypoblast center. *Nature Communications, 12*. https://doi.org/10.1038/s41467-021-23758-w.
27. Nieto, M. Á. (2013). Epithelial plasticity: A common theme in embryonic and cancer cells. *Science, 342*. https://doi.org/10.1126/science.1234850.
28. Oldak, B., Wildschutz, E., Bondarenko, V., Comar, M. Y., Zhao, C., Aguilera-Castrejon, A., Tarazi, S., et al. (2023). Complete human day 14 post-implantation embryo models from naive ES cells. *Nature*. https://doi.org/10.1038/s41586-023-06604-5.
29. Ozair, M. Z., Kintner, C., & Brivanlou, A. (2013). Neural induction and early patterning in vertebrates. *Wiley Interdisciplinary Reviews: Developmental Biology, 2*. https://www.semanticscholar.org/paper/09ec3c8494a9bfa4c7d309de0427ba66ad3ab9ea (accessed on 26 May 2025).
30. Petridou, N. I., & Heisenberg, C. P. (2019). Tissue rheology in embryonic organization. *The EMBO Journal, 38*. https://doi.org/10.15252/embj.2019102497.
31. Sanketi, B. D., Zuela-Sopilniak, N., Bundschuh, E., Gopal, S., Hu, S., Long, J. T., Lammerding, J., et al. (2022). Pitx2 patterns an accelerator-brake mechanical feedback through latent TGFβ to rotate the gut. *Science, 377*. https://www.semanticscholar.org/paper/ce3923fb386ce677039dd5ac5a03aaf972ef2990 (accessed on 26 May 2025).
32. Seeher, S., Atassi, T., Mahdi, Y., Carlson, B. A., Braun, D., Wirth, E. K., Klein, M., et al. (2013). Secisbp2 is essential for embryonic development and enhances selenoprotein expression. *Antioxidants and Redox Signaling, 21*, 835–849. https://doi.org/10.1089/ars.2013.5358.
33. Simon, C. S., Garg, V., Kuo, Y. Y., Niakan, K., & Hadjantonakis, A. (2024). ETV4 and ETV5 orchestrate FGF-mediated lineage specification and epiblast maturation during early mouse development. *bioRxiv*. https://www.semanticscholar.org/paper/2edcacd73663ed820e7c85195e3df956bba1921b (accessed on 26 May 2025).
34. Simon, C. S., Hur, W., Garg, V., Kuo, Y. Y., Niakan, K., & Hadjantonakis, A. (2025). ETV4 and ETV5 orchestrate FGF-mediated lineage specification and epiblast maturation during early mouse development. *Development*. https://www.semanticscholar.org/paper/cf38a014145e02ff73a47345a9895a8065b45482 (accessed on 26 May 2025).
35. Simunovic, M., & Brivanlou, A. H. (2017). Embryoids, organoids and gastruloids: new approaches to understanding embryogenesis. *Development, 144*, 976–985. https://doi.org/10.1242/dev.143529.
36. Strauß, L., Stegger, M., Akpaka, P., Alabi, A., Breurec, S., Coombs, G., Egyir, B., et al. (2017). Origin, evolution, and global transmission of community-acquired *Staphylococcus aureus* ST8. *Proceedings of the National Academy of Sciences of the United States of America, 114*, E10596–E10604. https://www.semanticscholar.org/paper/78581428d100108b069029ef0b77488d232f5a96 (accessed on 26 May 2025).

37. Streichan, S. J., Lefebvre, M. F., Noll, N., Wieschaus, E., & Shraiman, B. I. (2018). Global morphogenetic flow is accurately predicted by the spatial distribution of myosin motors. *eLife, 7*. https://doi.org/10.7554/elife.27454.

38. Tay, H. G., Ng, Y. W., & Manser, E. (2010). A vertebrate-specific Chp-PAK-PIX pathway maintains E-cadherin at adherens junctions during zebrafish epiboly. *PLoS ONE, 5*(8), e10125. https://doi.org/10.1371/journal.pone.0010125.

39. Technau, U. (2020). Gastrulation and germ layer formation in the sea anemone *Nematostella vectensis* and other cnidarians. *Mechanisms of Development, 163*, 103628. https://doi.org/10.1016/j.mod.2020.103628.

40. Tolera, M. (2023). The "Smart City" between urban narrative and empty signifier: Shaggar in focus. *World Journal of Education and Humanities*. https://www.semanticscholar.org/paper/25ed3db34ce39d30521eba05eecbd2b01cff1a4f (accessed on 26 May 2025).

41. Varnika, S., Arunasri, P. M., Keniit, J. J., & Pooja, P. S. (2025). Microgravity-induced alterations in embryonic development and stem cell differentiation. *International Research Journal on Advanced Engineering Hub (IRJAEH)*. https://www.semanticscholar.org/paper/1783a5fe5e8ee251aac4f2eb02a7983842895faa (accessed on 26 May 2025).

42. Wang, B., Yang, F., Li, R., Li, X., Wu, X., Sun, Z., Zhai, J., et al. (2018). Functional characterization of Cynoglossus semilaevis R-spondin2 and its role in muscle development during embryogenesis. *Genes & Genetic Systems, 93*(5), 181–190. https://www.semanticscholar.org/paper/7deda022c65cf8e549f8d043b6f580c411423f6b (accessed on 26 May 2025).

43. Wiese, K. E., Nusse, R., & van Amerongen, R. (2018). Wnt signaling: conquering complexity. *Development, 145*. https://doi.org/10.1242/dev.165902.

44. Xu, P. F., Moraes Borges, R., Fillâtre, J., de Oliveira Melo, M., Cheng, T., Thisse, B., & Thisse, C. (2021). Construction of a mammalian embryo model from stem cells organized by a morphogen signaling center. *Nature Communications, 12*. https://doi.org/10.1038/s41467-021-23653-4.

45. Yang, J., Antin, P. B., Berx, G., Blanpain, C., Brabletz, T., Bronner-Fraser, M., Campbell, K., et al. (2020). Guidelines and definitions for research on epithelial–mesenchymal transition. *Nature Reviews Molecular Cell Biology, 21*(7), 341–352. https://doi.org/10.1038/s41580-020-0237-9.

46. Yuan, G., Wang, J., Liu, Z., Chen, M., Zhu, P., Zhang, H., Hu, Z., et al. (2023). Establishment of a novel non-integrated human pluripotent stem cell-based gastruloid model. *bioRxiv* (Cold Spring Harbor Laboratory). https://doi.org/10.1101/2023.06.28.546720.

47. Zakrzewski, W., Dobrzyński, M., Szymonowicz, M., & Rybak, Z. (2019). Stem cells: Past, present, and future. *Stem Cell Research & Therapy, 10*, Article 68. https://doi.org/10.1186/s13287-019-1165-5.

48. Zeng, B., Liu, Z., Lu, Y., Zhong, S., Qin, S., Huang, L., Zeng, Y., et al. (2023). The single-cell and spatial transcriptional landscape of human gastrulation and early brain development. *Cell Stem Cell, 30*, 851–866.e7. https://doi.org/10.1016/j.stem.2023.04.016.

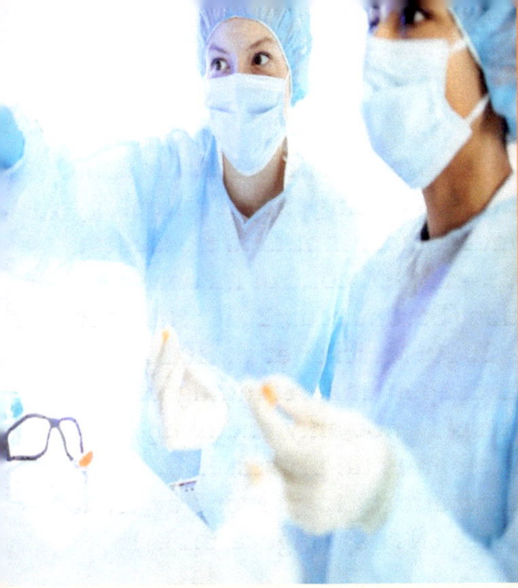

Chapter 6

NEURULATION

Contents

Introduction

Early on, the transition from a simple, totipotent zygote to a fully developed multicellular being remains a puzzle for researchers. Cellular and molecular tinkering drive the process in a complex yet fascinating way—neurulation, for instance, often stands out as a striking example. Alan Turing's "The Chemical Basis of Morphogenesis," among other classic works, helped establish our early ideas about how chemical signals interact with physical forces; it serves as a starting point for understanding how tissues shape themselves. Initially, a cell cluster is uniform, but then tiny imbalances begin to form due to both chemical nudges and mechanical forces (Blum et al., 2014; Zhang and Hiiragi, 2018). In most cases, if the neural tube isn't formed correctly, it can lead to serious birth defects, making the entire neurulation process important not only in developmental biology but also in clinical settings. When one looks closer at neurulation's inner workings, tissue rheology—the blend of stretchy (elastic) and slow, sticky (viscous) properties—has been grabbing more attention lately. How these tissues bend or resist pressure appears to influence processes such as tissue bending and ultimately neural tube closure. Researchers, by combining laboratory experiments with theory, have demonstrated that the material properties of tissues aren't merely background details; they facilitate cell shape changes during the critical transitions of development (Davidson, 2011; Lecuit et al., 2011).

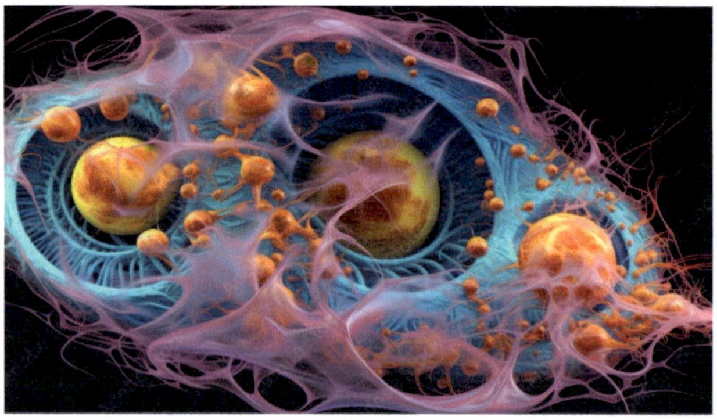

Figure 6.1. Overview of Neurulation.

Source: https://external-content.duckduckgo.com/iu/?u=https%3A%2F%2Fas2.ftcdn.net%2Fv2%2Fjpg%2F07%2F11%2F25%2F51%2F1000_F_711255126_UyUnKTM9yNqyle32KnFTo2KYjOZUbZMu.jpg&f=1&nofb=1&ipt=a56b9669824d793d16ada61d8f39bc8ace8cd610bfa1ea55d6a5ea1bc906fa94.

This type of investigation provides us with clues not only about cell behavior during neurulation but also about why similar developmental blueprints appear across so many species, suggesting an evolutionarily conserved design. Adding another layer, the growing realm of biomechanical studies offers some fresh insights into how cells and molecules work together to form the neural tube. Mechanosensitive pathways—even if they're a mouthful to say—turn mechanical pressures into chemical messages that can steer cell fate and behavior directly (Heisenberg and Bellaïche, 2013; Petridou et al., 2017). There even seems to be a feedback loop between these forces and signals, which underscores how intricate embryonic morphogenesis can be. Recent breakthroughs suggest that models mixing tissue rheology with other biomechanical inputs are essential for unraveling the tangled control mechanisms behind neurulation (Barone et al., 2017; Hannezo and Heisenberg, 2019; Mercker et al., 2016;). All in all, gaining a deeper understanding of this multifaceted interplay not only sheds light on fundamental developmental processes but may also inform future efforts to prevent or treat neural tube defects (NTDs) (Figure 6.1).

Definition of Neurulation

Neurulation kicks off early in embryonic growth and sets the stage for what later becomes the central nervous system. The ectoderm, that outer layer of the embryo, doesn't just sit there—it twists, folds, and stretches into a structure known as the neural plate, which then dips inward to form the neural tube. It's a process fueled by a complex interplay of genetic cues, cellular movements, and molecular signals, all interacting in unpredictable ways. Even slight changes here can lead to birth defects, so it's pretty crucial to understand how every little part works. Researchers continually revisit the roles of genetics and environmental influences, emphasizing that pinpointing these details is crucial to understanding successful neurulation—and what happens when things go awry. Much of our insight into this complex process comes from studying animals that mirror human development; consider mice and zebrafish, for example. These lab creatures allow scientists to manipulate genes and observe how these changes affect the course of neural tube formation. NTDs like spina bifida and anencephaly aren't just a human phenomenon—these conditions also appear in animal studies, indicating shared underlying causes (Zarzycki et al., 2020). Generally speaking, this kind of work not only unmasks the biology behind neural tube development, it also lights the way for interventions, especially in groups where genetic and environmental factors collide to up the risk. People are now taking an even broader view, combining ideas from genetics, epidemiology, and environmental science to unravel the complexities of neurulation. It turns out one can't fully grasp this developmental phase by sticking to just one field (Tolera, 2023). Instead, combining different angles gives us a more complete picture, even if it sometimes feels somewhat disjointed. This holistic take, with its occasional rough edges and unexpected turns, is paving the way for more innovative preventive healthcare efforts, all aimed at better outcomes for those facing congenital challenges.

Importance in Embryonic Development

Embryonic development isn't just one neat process. Cell death – or apoptosis, as it's often called – plays a big role in early growth by deciding which cells stick around and which don't.

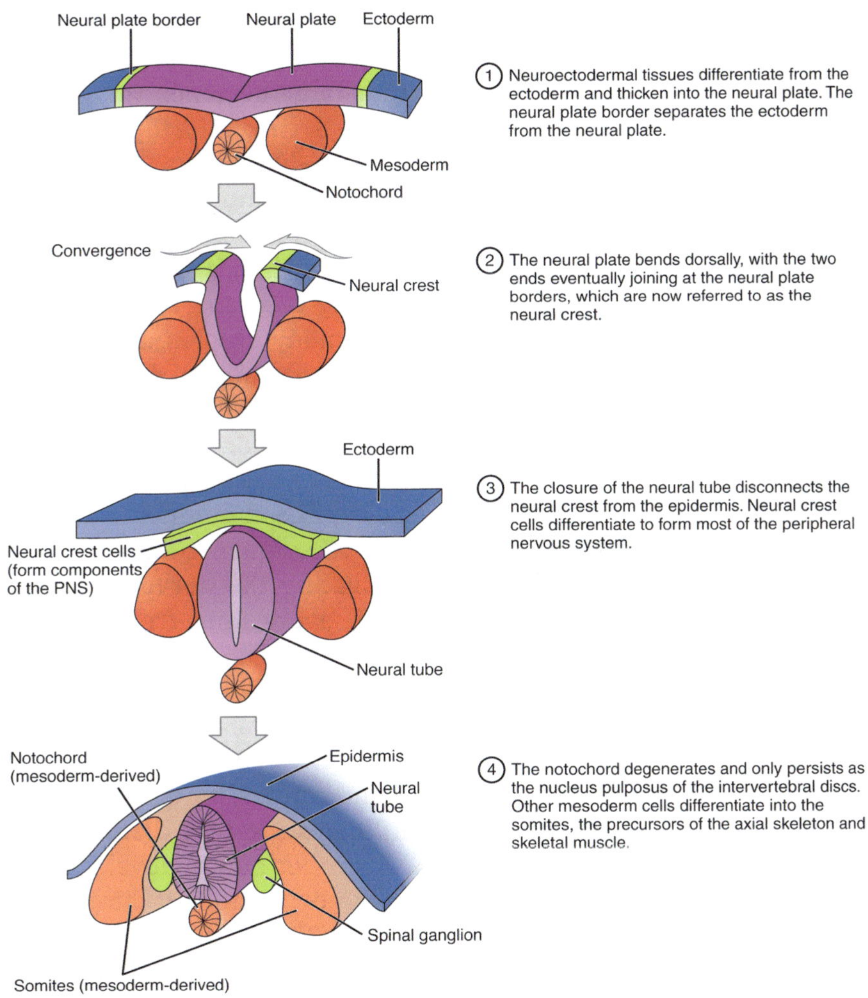

Figure 6.2. Neurulation importance in embryonic development.

Source: https://external-content.duckduckgo.com/iu/?u=https%3A%2F%2Fphilschatz.com%2Fanatomy-book%2Fresources%2F2912_Neurulation-02.jpg&f=1&nofb=1&ipt=67209e046c81f104c4caab22f678f1bbd1485ed4e7853c1ee41b5edce9ee758e.

Think about it: some cells need to survive while others are meant to vanish, and anti-apoptotic factors, notably those in the B-cell lymphoma-2 (BCL-2) clan, help keep this balance in check. They not only provide a helping hand to cells essential for building tissues but also ensure that extra or abnormal ones self-destruct, keeping things on track. Usually, congenital defects or other developmental glitches result when this balance breaks (Joseph et al., 2017). Therefore, understanding the function of these survival signals is crucial for a clear picture of early mammalian growth. It isn't just about cell survival, though. How cells get their polarity – or, put, how they know which way is up – is equally critical. The organization of tissues and the overall shape of the embryo depend on it. At the center of this process is the Wnt-Frizzled planar cell polarity (PCP) signaling pathway, which appears to guide cells into alignment without much effort. Various studies using organisms such as Drosophila, mice, and zebrafish have highlighted that genes like Vang/Vangl are key components in this arrangement, a role that's surprisingly conserved across species (Yang et al., 2015).

When cells fail to communicate or align correctly, the consequences can be severe, often leading to serious developmental defects. Both the fine-tuning of cell death and the setup of cellular orientation merge into what one might call the embryo's molecular dialogue. As tissues start to form and differentiate, especially during neurulation, the mix of survival signals and proper positioning becomes even more crucial. For instance, the creation of a proper neural tube doesn't rely solely on keeping neural precursor cells alive; those cells have to be in just the right spot, too. The interplay between the BCL-2 family and PCP signaling illustrates the profound interconnectedness of these systems (Yang et al., 2015; Joseph et al., 2017). Generally speaking, piecing together these molecular interactions may pave the way for new therapeutic approaches to developmental disorders, underscoring the crucial role these pathways play as a multicellular organism transitions from embryo to fully formed being (Figure 6.2).

6.1. The Process of Neurulation

Neurulation is one of those crucial early steps that sets the stage for a functioning nervous system. It starts when a flat ectoderm thickens into what we call the neural plate and then, almost as if by nature's whim, folds into a tube that later becomes the brain and spinal cord. Even a tiny misstep here can cause serious issues—like NTDs, which can be either open or closed and have a significant impact on a newborn's health. Genetics and the environment both play their roles in this delicate process, and getting the tube formation right is something that many studies have emphasized for years (Ricardo et al., 2024). Signals from various cells drive the whole process. One unexpected actor is the endocannabinoid signaling system (ECS). Research has shown that even at this early time point, ECS components are present, suggesting that they might have a foundational role in activating the nervous system. The ECS helps with everything from sparking neurogenesis and guiding neurons to their spots to tweaking the connections between them. Then, there are other factors, such as cannabis exposure, that can throw off this finely tuned mechanism. Some studies, for example, have noted that such influences might disturb the balance needed for proper neural development, adding another layer of complexity to neurulation (Ricardo et al., 2024). In a broader sense, the success of neurulation isn't dictated solely by our genes but also by how cells mingle with their surroundings. Many investigations generally indicate that factors such as a mother's nutrition and exposure to teratogens can significantly impact the integrity of the neural tube. Folic acid is often cited as a key factor that helps reduce the risk of NTDs, which underscores the need for good preventive care during pregnancy. It's also interesting to see how NTD rates differ from one region to another, offering valuable clues for public health strategies. All in all, ongoing research into neurulation—its mechanisms and risks alike—is gradually reshaping clinical practices, highlighting the interplay between our genetic blueprint and environmental cues in early development (Avagliano et al., 2018) (Figure 6.3).

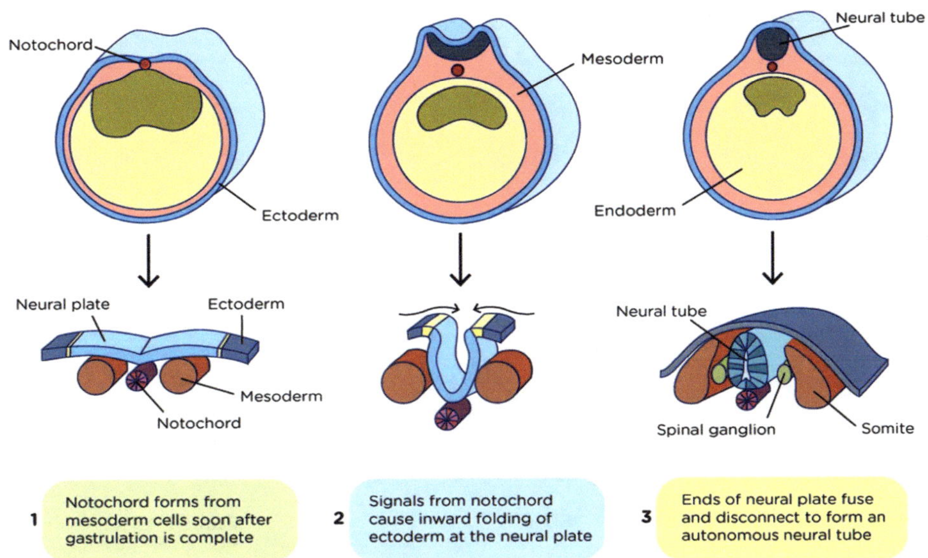

Figure 6.3. The process of neurulation.

Source: https://old-ib.bioninja.com.au/_Media/neurulation_med.jpeg.

6.1.1. Stages of Neurulation

Neurulation begins with a series of changes that eventually shape the neural tube—a process that lays down the foundation for the central nervous system. It all starts when cells along the embryo's back thicken up, forming what we call the neural plate (this clumping is primarily driven by signals coming from beneath, especially from the notochord). That initial thickening is like nature's green light for the whole transformation, hinting at the changes soon to come. Then, in a somewhat unexpected twist, the edges of the neural plate begin to rise into folds while the middle dips down—a subtle, yet critical, move toward fusion. This elaborate cell dance, full of motion and signaling, repeatedly demonstrates just how many small steps are required for early brain and spinal cord development. As the process continues, those neural folds slowly drift toward each other until they meet at the embryo's midline, starting the closure of the neural tube. Usually, this closure begins around the neck area and extends toward both the head and tail ends; in most cases, this coordinated action is vital because if the neural tube fails to close correctly, serious defects can occur. Cells then settle into distinct layers, a formation that helps set up the nervous system's symmetry. Key signals—BMP, Wnt, to name a couple—are busy regulating both how cells multiply and how they pick their future roles. Generally speaking, grasping these shifting interactions is crucial to our understanding of embryonic development and why even a minor disruption can lead to significant congenital issues. Once the neural tube is completely formed, the puzzle doesn't end there. The tube then begins to divide into distinct zones, each assigned to perform unique functions within the nervous system. The anterior part eventually morphs into the brain. At the same time, the back end develops into the spinal cord, driven by gradients of signaling molecules that gently guide the destiny of each neural progenitor cell. It's a delicate balancing act between genetic cues and environmental influences. Any misstep during this stage may trigger a range of neurological disorders, which is why many researchers closely monitor these early events. Ultimately, the interplay between cellular mechanics and external signals gives rise to our complex nervous system, making neurulation a truly awe-inspiring foundation of embryonic development (Figure 6.4).

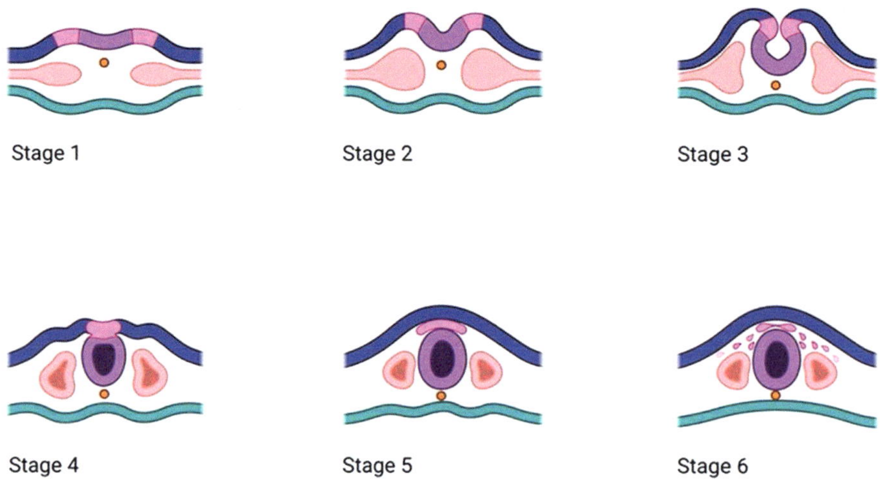

Figure 6.4. Main stages of the neurulation process.

Source: https://www.researchgate.net/publication/374272274/figure/fig1/AS:11431281194254906@1695991842010/Main-stages-of-the-neurulation-process-including-the-development-of-the-neural-tube.ppm.

6.1.2. Role of the Neural Plate

Neurulation begins when the neural plate takes center stage in establishing the central nervous system. Right along the embryo's back, this layer of ectoderm isn't just sitting there—it's shifting form in ways that mark key developmental milestones. As the process proceeds, the tissue gets firmer, hinting at its expanding role as it shapes into the neural tube. Generally speaking, recent imaging breakthroughs have shown that during neural tube closure (NTC), the stiffness of the neural plate steadily increases, aligning with events such as tissue thickening and bending, which, in most cases, are essential for proper tube formation (Handler et al., 2023). Building the neural plate goes hand in hand with a complex network of signaling pathways that steer cell fates in sometimes surprising ways. Just next door, the preplacodal region lays out a vivid example of how complex ectodermal interactions can be. Signals from fibroblast growth factors (FGFs), bone morphogenetic proteins (BMPs), and WNT pathways all get thrown into the mix, shaping this neighboring zone and reflecting the neural plate's deep involvement in kick-starting cranial placode formation. In a sense, the neural plate isn't only the forerunner to the neural tube, but it also plays an integral part in setting up the sensory organs (Singh et al., 2016).

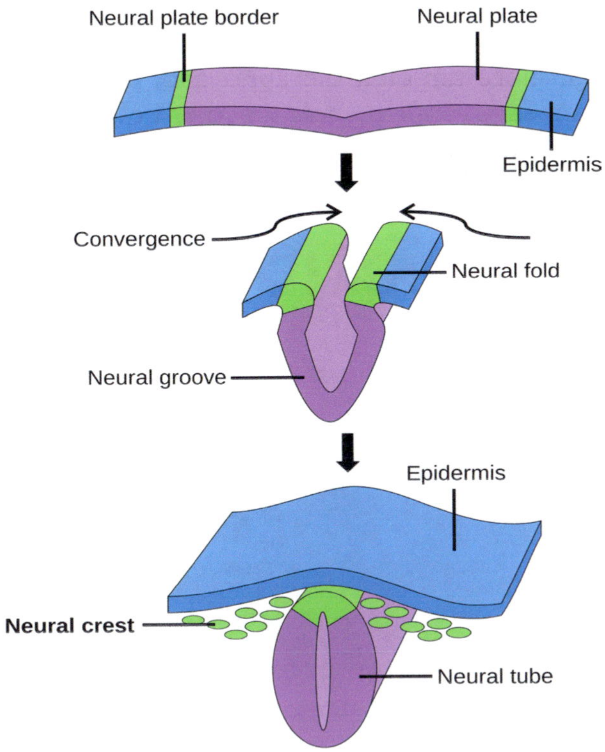

Figure 6.5. Neural plate.

Source: https://upload.wikimedia.org/wikipedia/commons/thumb/6/60/Neural_crest.svg/1200px-Neural_crest.svg.png.

In most cases, piecing together these signaling cues helps us glimpse the broader picture of vertebrate development. Transforming the neural plate into the neural tube is far more than a simple mechanical shift—it's a coordinated dance between cellular movements and molecular signals. As cells in the plate gradually lose their clear top-to-bottom order and morph in shape, they begin to move in concert, a necessary step for tube formation. At the same time, this change sparks cell differentiation, resulting in specific types that will ultimately contribute to the development of the nervous system and its associated structures. Both internal signals and external influences contribute, marking the neural plate as a hub of mechanical and biochemical activity. Ongoing research into these processes provides additional insights into developmental changes that may lead to serious health issues, underscoring the vital role of the neural plate during early embryogenesis (Handler et al., 2023) (Figure 6.5).

6.1.3. Formation of the Neural Tube

Embryonic development is a messy, fascinating process. A flat neural plate suddenly morphs into a three-dimensional neural tube—a stage most simply called neurulation, though it's way more than just a shape change. It all hinges on a mix of mechanical forces and genetics. For instance, understanding how stiff tissues are can help explain why the neural tube closes up (NTC). Recent research, in most cases, shows that when neuroepithelial tissues aren't stiff enough, NTC is thrown off balance. In models with NTDs, the local stiffness is oddly lower than in wild-type embryos (Yogeshwari et al., 2024). This highlights the need to investigate how these mechanical properties relate to overall embryonic growth, thereby putting mechanical biology squarely in the research spotlight. Recently, some innovative methods have emerged to examine the role of curvature and stiffness in neural tube formation. One interesting approach uses curved polydimethylsiloxane (PDMS) plates in cell cultures. This technique allows scientists to observe—in a controlled setting—how a simple bend in a plate affects cell behavior. Experiments with this setup have shown that human pluripotent stem cells tend to stretch out and even alter the angle of cell division when grown on concave surfaces (Ahn et al., 2023). Yet, the precise reason for the observed colony elongation remains somewhat unclear, suggesting that other biological pathways may be at work. In many ways, these novel techniques not only refine our grasp on tissue mechanics but also set the stage for further surprises on how physical properties influence neurulation. The broader implications here are far-reaching, especially when it comes to tackling NTDs. Neural tube closure is a crucial turning point in early development, so understanding what can go wrong may lead to more effective interventions. Recent experiments suggest that altering tissue stiffness with external supplements could offer a solution to developmental issues (Yogeshwari et al., 2024). Additionally, insights gained from studying mechanical biology enable us to design more targeted therapies and, potentially, improve clinical outcomes when NTC doesn't go as planned. Overall, piecing together both genetic influences and the quirks of biomechanics is essential if we genuinely want to understand neurulation and its many associated risks (Figure 6.6).

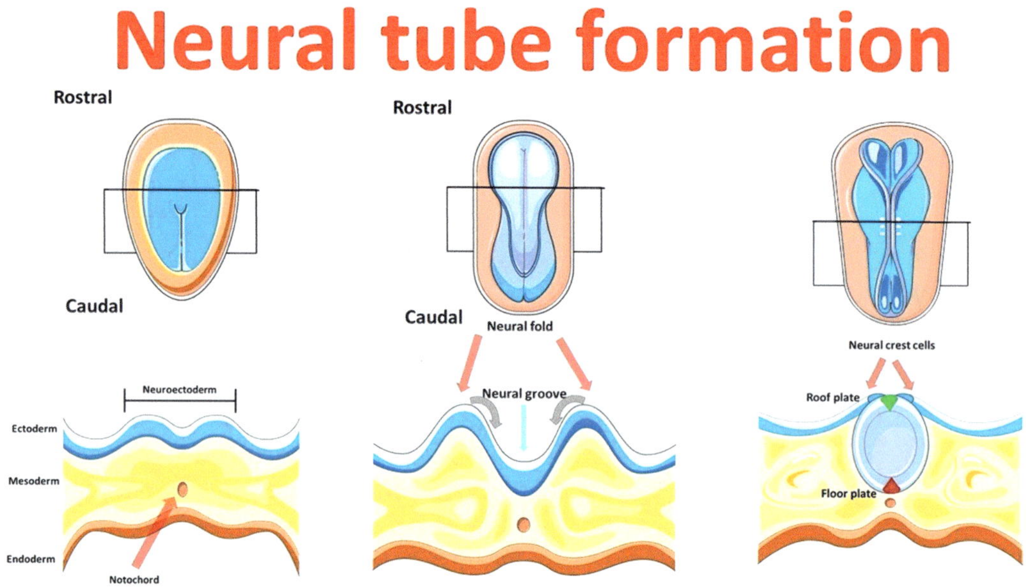

Figure 6.6. Neural tube formation.

Source: https://i.ytimg.com/vi/Fyiumno87H4/maxresdefault.jpg.

6.2. Molecular Mechanisms Involved

Neurulation is a complex process, driven by a combination of molecular signals that build our nervous system. It begins with a range of genes and pathways—each contributing its part—to form the neural tube properly. Take Hedgehog signaling, for example; its role is quite central, affecting everything from sparking neural induction to guiding how cells choose their fate. When the Hedgehog cues go off track, neurogenesis can get messed up, and that's tied to defects in the neural tube. MicroRNAs (miRNA) come into play, adding yet another twist by tweaking gene expression during key moments in embryo growth. Understanding these interactions, despite their complexities, is crucial for maintaining neurulation and preventing central brain and nerve issues. Signals don't act alone either. Beyond Hedgehog, pathways such as Wnt and Notch become involved, each contributing to the determination of cell roles and promoting differentiation. They're often all tangled together, working side-by-side to create an environment where neural development can flourish. For instance, Wnt helps expand the pool of neural progenitors while Notch kind of balances the mix between these cells and their cohort. Examining how these pathways interact reveals the complexity of the regulation underlying neurulation. It's a messy dance that not only deepens our grasp of normal development but also offers clues on where we might step in when things go sideways. Looking ahead, future research in this area needs to fill in the gaps about how these molecular signals interact. Scientists are poking around to see how both outside factors and what's happening inside the embryo nudge these signaling routes, hoping this will explain why NTDs crop up. Think about it: the blend of genetic predispositions and environmental exposures might just be the missing piece in our puzzle. And while we're at it, exploring miRNAs a bit more to see how they fine-tune gene activity could open up new perspectives on early development. Recent reviews—generally speaking—suggest that a deeper examination of Hedgehog and its interactions with other pathways may lead to new approaches for treating or even preventing these issues (Casale et al., 2024; Farhadi et al., 2024). By slowly bridging these knowledge gaps, researchers may well spark innovative treatments that improve outcomes for folks with neural developmental disorders.

6.2.1. Key Signaling Pathways

Neurulation is a messy, twisting process steered by a range of signaling cues that set the stage for making a proper neural tube.

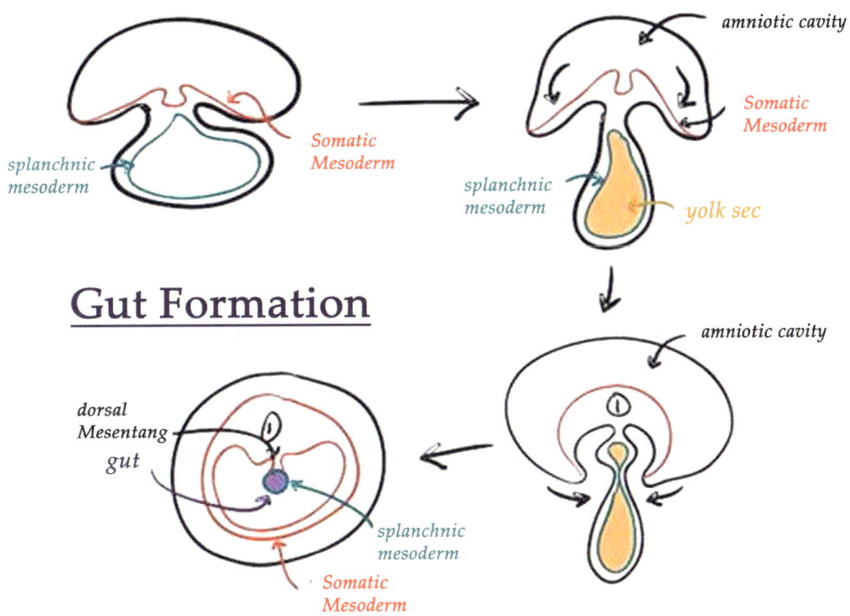

Figure 6.7. Signaling pathways.

Source: https://external-content.duckduckgo.com/iu/?u=https%3A%2F%2Ftse2.mm.bing.net%2Fth%3Fid%3DOIP.ABMKKtXhEvu3 dkQB0jFLAgHaFY%26cb%3Diwc1%26pid%3DApi&f=1&ipt=fa2c4966ef3e6df7ef0354872287e744855b26f2ddfc572c958652958d0fe7a3.

The PCP pathway, for instance, acts somewhat like a behind-the-scenes organizer—getting cells to move in sync during these dramatic changes. When this pathway is disrupted, notable developmental defects occur, highlighting just how crucial the embryo's reliance on it is. Then there are miRNAs, which jump in to fine-tune gene activity in a way that shifts with the situation. In most cases, this jumble of signals and subtle controls reveals the complexity of neurulation (Mukhopadhyay et al., 2020). EMT—short for epithelial-to-mesenchymal transition—brings another twist, influencing how cells behave and how tissues remodel to wrap up neural tube closure. It usually kicks off when cells swap out E-cadherin for N-cadherin, a change that ramps up their ability to move. A network of signals manages this switch and transcription factors chattering away to adjust cell traits. Sometimes, though, when those signals lose their rhythm, EMT suffers, and the neural tube only partially closes, leading to further changes in development. Therefore, understanding how these various cues overlap is crucial to determining why things sometimes go off track (Loh et al., 2019). It's not just an academic exercise; these signaling pathways help us understand some nerve-related disorders that stem from neurulation mistakes. Early missteps can result in serious conditions like spina bifida or even anencephaly. As research continues to progress, there's a growing sense that tweaks in pathways such as PCP and EMT have significant implications for future therapies. Discovering miRNA targets associated with these pathways might open up new avenues to correct—or at least mitigate—the impact of these developmental errors. All in all, delving into these intertwined signaling networks not only deepens our understanding of routine neural development but also suggests promising biomarkers and treatment targets for neurulation-related disorders (Mukhopadhyay et al., 2020) (Figure 6.7).

6.2.2. Role of Transcription Factors

Neurulation isn't just a neat, linear event; it's a messy, fascinating sequence of events where special transcription factors step in to guide gene expression during early development. The neural tube forms when the neural ectoderm begins to fold, and these factors essentially determine which genes are activated to shape cell types and tissue structure. Think about the mammalian grainy head-like gene group—Grhl2 in particular seems to be a star here, helping to build the essential epithelial traits needed for smooth neurulation. In most cases, if these regulators lose their grip, things can go awry, leading to serious defects (Marina et al., 2020). By peeling back the layers of how these factors operate, we gain a clearer understanding of the molecular mechanisms behind neural tube formation and the anomalies that sometimes arise. Besides playing a structural role, transcription factors are involved in a complex network of regulatory pathways that balance the epithelial and mesenchymal states throughout neurulation. It turns out that Grhl2, interacting with others like Ovol1 and Ovol2, is vital for preserving epithelial integrity. When Grhl2 function drops, there's a noticeable spike in mesenchymal markers—this tilt can nudge cells toward undergoing an epithelial-mesenchymal transition (EMT). Too many mesenchymal traits, as observed in Grhl2-null mice (Marina et al., 2020), can tip the balance toward problems such as cleft palate and other neural defects. Essentially, these proteins wear many hats, and their interactions highlight the delicate balance that normal embryogenesis relies on. Zooming out a bit, the influence of transcription factors in neurogenesis stretches well beyond fiddling with individual genes. Research generally suggests that these molecules help set the stage for early neural progenitors while also playing a hand in forming a range of neural subtypes. For example, transcription factors associated with Delta/Notch signaling have been shown to affect both the differentiation and spatial organization of neural tissues, suggesting a broader and more intricate regulatory network. These observations, woven together, reveal that the specialized structure and function of neurons during neurulation are tightly bound up in hierarchies crafted by these factors. All in all, understanding this tangled web of interactions is key to unraveling the evolutionary and developmental complexity of neural systems in vertebrates—and, likely, even further afield (Figure 6.8).

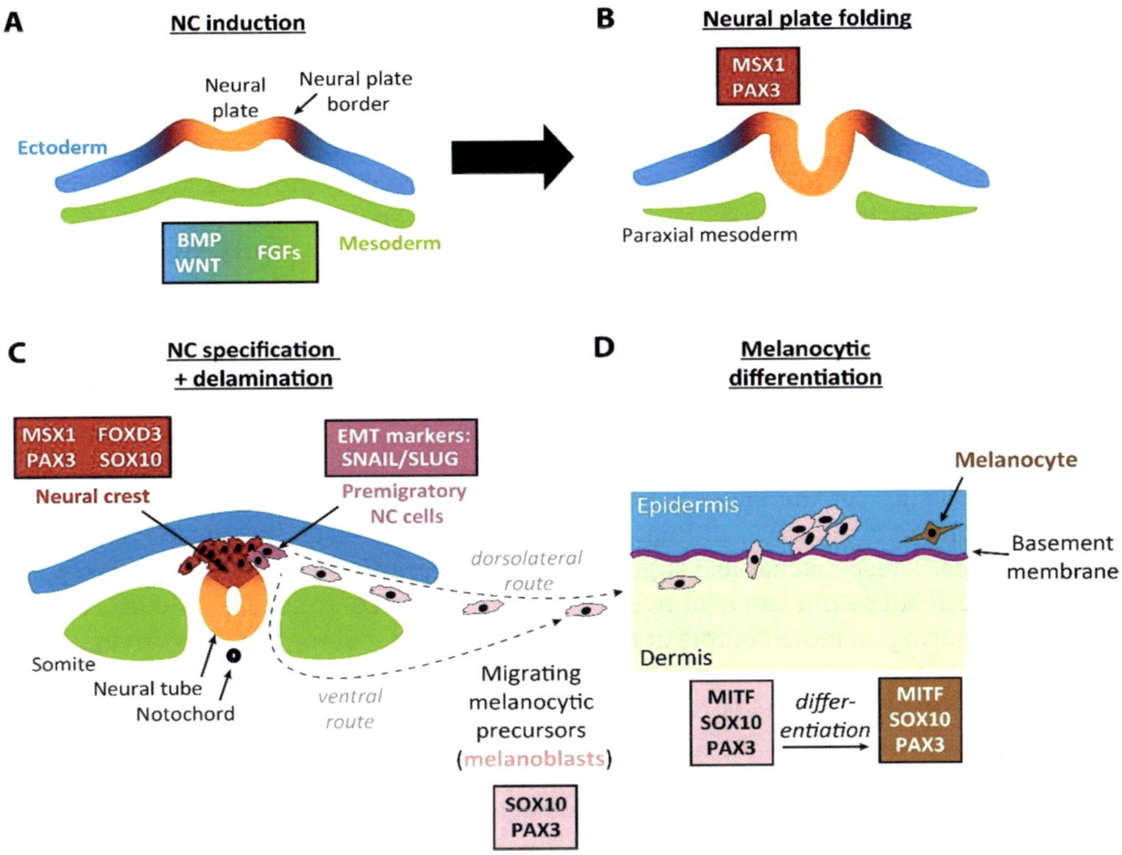

Figure 6.8. Neurulation role of transcription factors.

Source: https://www.mdpi.com/ijms/ijms-22-05761/article_deploy/html/images/ijms-22-05761-g001-550.jpg.

6.2.3. Influence of Extracellular Matrix (ECM)

Neural tube formation kicks off with lively cellular and molecular interactions, and the extracellular matrix (ECM) jumps right in as a kind of unsung hero. Cells begin to organize into place as the neural tube forms, and the ECM acts like a flexible framework, nudging cells in ways that are sometimes difficult to predict. Processes such as convergent extension and even the tightening of cells at their tops (apical constriction) ultimately become closely tied to the composition of the ECM. Sometimes, if the ECM changes even a little, it can mess with the balance of forces needed to close the neural tube just right—leading, in most cases, to serious birth issues known as neural tube defects. In this delicate dance, the back-and-forth between the ECM and cell signals reminds us just how crucial it is to get these dynamics right (David et al., 2017). The ECM isn't just a static support—it also laces into the signaling cues that steer neurulation. In most instances, pathways like the non-canonical Wnt/planar cell polarity and the Shh/BMP signals wind their influence together with the ECM to trigger the essential reactions for neural tube buildup. Researchers have noted that the ECM can alter the availability or activity of these signals, subtly changing the fate and behavior of nearby cells. At the same time, the matrix helps establish the layout of signaling centers, ensuring that important growth factors are directed to the correct locations. This entire web of interactions demonstrates how minor adjustments in the ECM can have a profound impact on the signaling networks that govern embryonic shape formation, underscoring its pivotal role (David et al., 2017). Not to be overlooked, the biomechanical properties of the ECM also come into play during neurulation. Its stiffness and elasticity can directly influence how cells migrate, divide, and re-shape in response to both internal cues and outside nudges. Recent studies even suggest that a tougher, stiffer ECM may set the stage for the amount of tissue folding required to ultimately form the neural tube. These mechanical signals not only mold the cell shape but can also tweak gene expression, layering on more complexity to the whole process. All told, this view underlines a broader picture—where the ECM is far more than a passive bystander, instead being an active partner in shaping development (Nikolopoulou et al., 2017).

6.3. Types of Neurulation

Neural development in embryos hits a crucial turning point when the neural plate shifts into a neural tube—a key step often referred to as neurulation. Generally speaking, this process can be divided into two broad categories: primary and secondary forms. Primary neurulation, which many vertebrates follow, involves the dorsal ectoderm thickening and then folding in on itself. As the tissue gradually fuses, it forms a hollow tube that later gives rise to different parts of the nervous system. This stage is delicate; even small missteps can lead to serious congenital issues. Researchers have noted that factors like UBE3D play a significant role in regulating genes during this phase, a point underscored in recent studies (Mi et al., 2025). Secondary neurulation, on the other hand, pops up mostly in some amphibians and reptiles. Instead of the ectoderm doing the folding, cells from early mesoderm come together—the cells aggregate and condense to form a solid neural cord, which then eventually hollows out. In most cases, this method is crucial for proper spinal cord formation, illustrating the remarkable diversity of evolution in building nervous systems. Some comparative studies have provided a detailed picture of these different routes, highlighting the distinct mechanisms that operate across species (Kim et al., 2024). In a broader sense, examining both types of neurulation provides essential insights into normal developmental patterns as well as the origins of NTDs that can arise when these processes go awry. Advances such as three-dimensional culture techniques now allow scientists to peer into early developmental stages with surprising clarity. These breakthroughs not only deepen our grasp of embryonic blueprints but also pave the way for new strategies in regenerative medicine. By exploring both primary and secondary pathways, researchers can gain a deeper understanding of why and how congenital anomalies occur (Kim et al., 2024).

6.3.1. Primary Neurulation

Neurulation initiates vertebrate development by forming the neural tube, which ultimately gives rise to the central nervous system. In its earliest phase—what we call primary neurulation—the neural plate twists and folds into a tube, a process so sensitive that even minor disturbances might trigger NTDs. These defects typically fall into two categories: one where the tube fails to close completely (resulting in conditions such as anencephaly or myelomeningocele), and another, less obvious type. In most cases, breaking down this process helps us understand why approximately 1 in every 1,000 pregnancies (Boschen et al., 2020) may face these serious anomalies. Genetics and the environment both leave their mark here, reminding us that primary neurulation isn't a one-track affair. Recent work, for example, suggests that during key moments of gestation, alcohol exposure—especially near the rostroventral neural tube (RVNT) region—can throw the system off balance. To put it mildly, alcohol appears to interfere with gene expression, disrupting the normal process of cell division and organ formation. In one study, over 2300 genes showed changes after alcohol exposure, a clear sign of the tangled network at work. These shifts don't just stop at improper closure; they can have a lasting impact on brain structure and function (Boschen et al., 2020). Upon closer examination, it becomes apparent that a complex interplay of signals directs neurulation. Take the BMP and Sonic hedgehog pathways—they work together to help bend the neural plate into shape. This balance generally ensures that the tube stays on track, separating correctly from the surrounding tissue. Still, challenges remain, especially when it comes to untangling genetic contributions to NTDs. While maternal folic acid supplementation has been a solid line of defense against many NTDs, there are cases where this measure falls short, hinting at other, not fully understood factors. Further research into these complex mechanisms is necessary to develop more effective preventive strategies (Copp et al., 2013) (Figure 6.9).

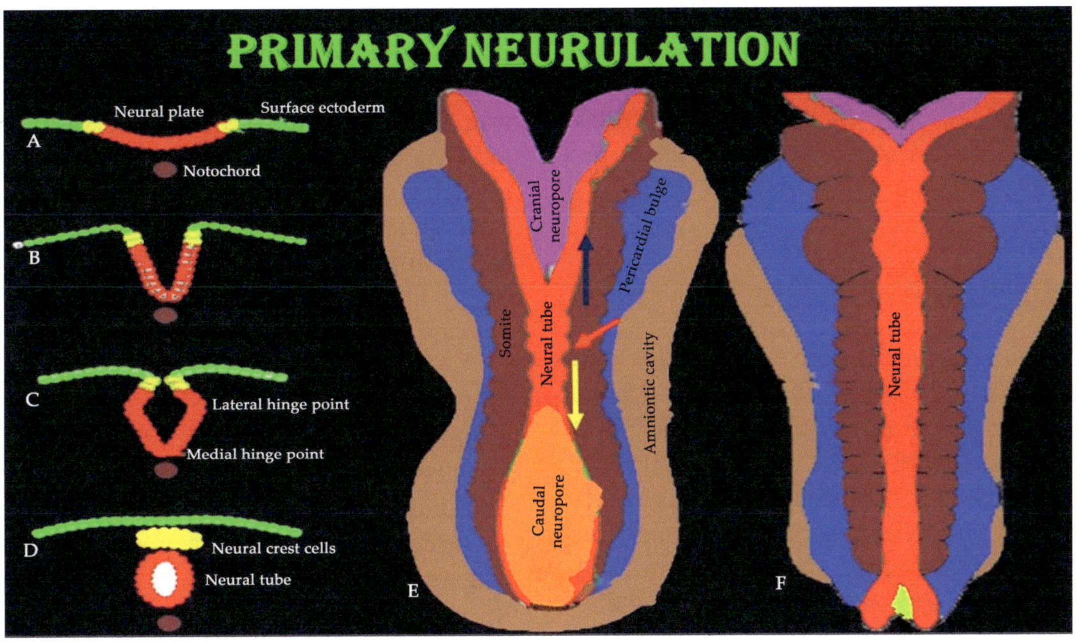

Figure 6.9. Primary neurulation.

Source: https://epos.myesr.org/posterimage/esr/ecr2019/146842/media/791032.

6.3.2. Secondary Neurulation

Neurulation shapes our central nervous system — a process that's messy, fascinating, and a bit unpredictable. Primary neurulation lays down the neural tube, and then, sort of in its shadow, secondary neurulation steps in. Here, a solid rod of mesodermal tissue unexpectedly reshapes into a hollow structure that ends up helping form the tailbud and parts of the spinal cord. In most cases, models like *Xenopus laevis* prove remarkably helpful by illustrating how cells move and signal during these stages. The tailbud, blending awkwardly with trunk tissues, reveals some complex interactions that extend beyond simply maintaining connections (Beck, 2015).

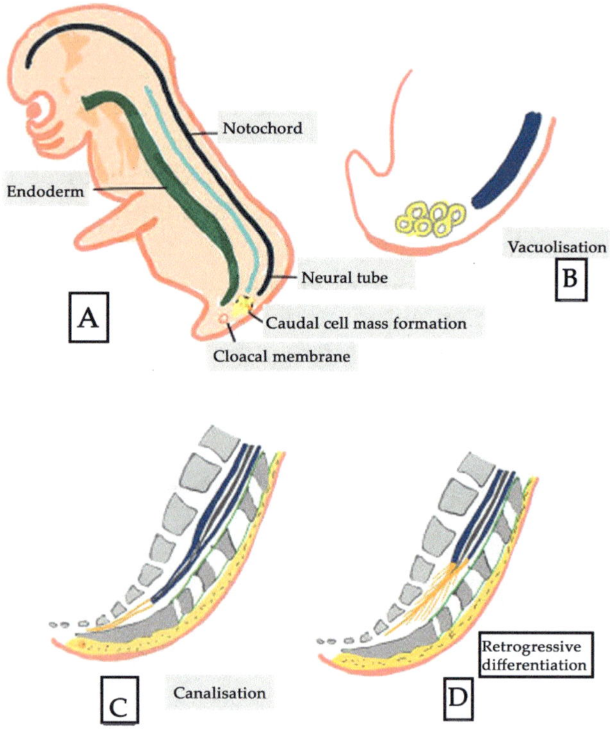

Figure 6.10. Secondary neurulation.

Source: https://external-content.duckduckgo.com/iu/?u=https%3A%2F%2Fwww.researchgate.net%2Fpublication%2F357775820%2Ffigure%2Ffig8%2FAS%3A1121968568963076%401644509560915%2FStages-of-secondary-neurulation-beginning-just-as-the-posterior-neuropore-closes-A.jpg&f=1&nofb=1&ipt=eff3b9a9fe4c2abe44b9efea55e2403c0b9c567283901e20874f92809ee84e4f.

Understanding secondary neurulation involves noticing a few unusual details. Tailbud cells house multipotent progenitors—cells that, generally speaking, can birth tissues from several germ layers. This ability, which sometimes seems almost like an accidental talent for regeneration, challenges older ideas about fixed cell lineages in vertebrate development. One might even suggest that ancient genetic tools were combined in this process. Comparative research across different vertebrates even hints at a shared genetic beat behind it all (Beck, 2015). These insights not only push our understanding of developmental biology forward, but they also shed light on congenital issues linked to neurulation, like NTDs. Neural tube defects, or NTDs, arise as clear signals when neurulation goes a bit off track—often with secondary neurulation playing its quirky role. Open defects, such as myelomeningocele, tend to be connected to problems in primary neurulation, whereas closed types frequently trace back to irregularities in the secondary phase. The whole picture of NTDs is messy: it involves a jumble of genetic predispositions and environmental quirks. Recent studies, for example, have linked pathways such as the planar cell polarity pathway to these defects, underscoring the nuanced regulation of neurulation. Understanding these mechanisms isn't merely academic; it's a crucial step towards crafting effective prevention and intervention strategies for disorders linked to neural tube formation (Figure 6.10).

6.3.3. Differences Between the Two Types

Examining how neurulation unfolds provides insight into some key developmental processes—especially when comparing primary and secondary types. During primary neurulation, the neural plate folds in on itself and forms a hollow tube that eventually cradles the central nervous system; this step is crucial. On the other hand, secondary neurulation begins when mesenchymal cells cluster together to form a solid neural cord, which later develops into a hollow tube. It's worth noting that these methods aren't just different evolutionary tweaks—they spring from distinct embryonic origins and feature varying cell behaviors, all of which shape the neural layout. Additionally, the makeup and sturdiness of tissues are crucial; properties like stiffness can significantly impact developmental outcomes, as NTDs demonstrate

(Yogeshwari et al., 2024). Digging a little deeper into the cellular side of things, apparent differences emerge in how these two neurulation types are orchestrated—particularly when it comes to signaling and genetic regulation. For primary neurulation, there's a pretty intricate dance involving a mix of growth factors and morphogens that's needed to fold and fuse the neural plate properly. In contrast, secondary neurulation relies more on cells gathering and migrating together, all under a different set of genetic cues. Interestingly, research suggests that genes critical for the primary process might not be as crucial for the secondary one, hinting at an evolutionary split in how these pathways work. Generally speaking, any disruption in these finely tuned pathways can lead to various NTDs, adding yet another layer of complexity to our understanding of the genetic underpinnings (Yogeshwari et al., 2024). Examining the results of these neurulation processes reveals clear distinctions in both the structures formed and the functions they perform. Primary neurulation usually produces a well-defined neural tube that eventually gives rise to the brain and spinal cord—essentially setting up the central nervous system's framework. Meanwhile, secondary neurulation tends to result in a more ambiguous and loosely organized neural cord, which may affect overall neural function. The physical stability here is key; primary neurulation, for example, depends heavily on solid mechanical support provided by the ECM and the inherent stiffness of cells. In most cases, when that stiffness isn't quite right, the neural tube fails to close properly—underscoring just how vital the mechanical environment is for proper differentiation and function (Yogeshwari et al., 2024).

6.4. Evolutionary Perspectives

Embryonic development isn't a neat, straightforward process—especially when one looks at that unclear phase known as neurulation. At this stage, the neural tube, which eventually forms the brain and spinal cord, emerges in a manner that may seem similar among many animals at first glance. However, upon closer examination, the genetic and molecular blueprints are remarkably diverse. Even though vertebrates tend to have a similar appearance during the early phylotypic stage, the actual path each one takes to get there is surprisingly different. Researchers often emphasize that evolution doesn't just come from random mutations; in most cases, there's a lot more going on. This realization prompts us to consider alternative development models that more accurately capture the diverse range of stages observed in embryonic development. Figuring out the role of neurulation in evolution is a bit like watching different species end up looking remarkably similar despite taking their unique paths. One might notice visual similarities during these critical stages. A straightforward, universal conception of lineage is called into question by the complexities of genetic expression and environmental factors, which reveal an entirely different side of the tale. Environmental pressures and natural shifts appear to nudge each species into developing its unique version of a neural design, which undermines the notion of a strict, shared origin. Researchers have even begun to tweak our evolutionary frameworks to accommodate these deviations, suggesting that the way species adapt during neurulation can lead to distinct functional outcomes among vertebrates (Liu et al., 2024). Examining neurulation from an evolutionary perspective also sheds light on developmental disorders. Slight differences in how neurulation unfolds can reveal clues about why certain congenital conditions, such as spina bifida or anencephaly, develop. When scientists draw connections between these evolutionary tweaks and the appearance of such conditions, it reinforces how deeply intertwined evolutionary biology and medical research are.

As our understanding of developmental biology continues to evolve, there's a growing call to view these early processes within their broader evolutionary context—even if it means accepting a few rough edges along the way (Liu et al., 2024).

6.4.1. Neurulation in Different Species

Evolution doesn't follow a strict script when it comes to building the nervous system. In many vertebrates, the early twist of the neural plate into what becomes the neural tube marks a crucial moment – one that, surprisingly, isn't uniform across all species. Different creatures can switch up the details entirely.

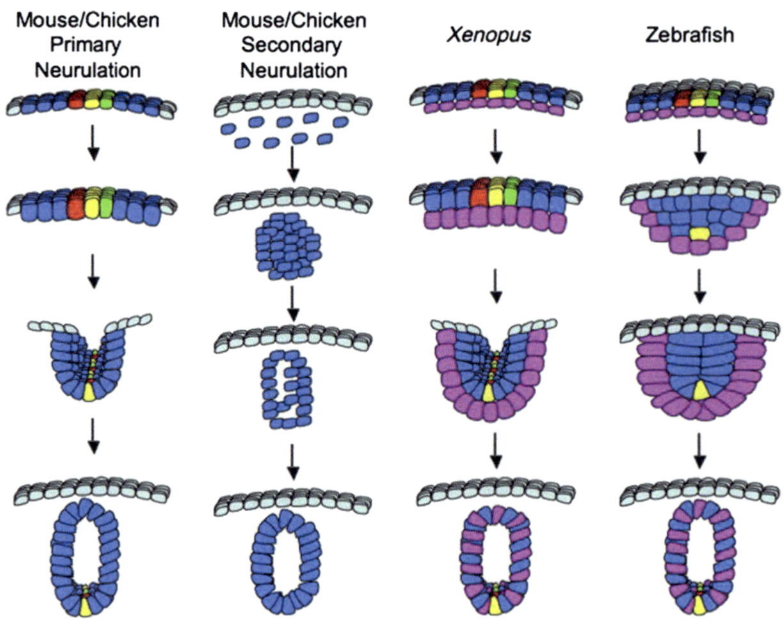

Figure 6.11. Neurulation in different species.

Source: https://ars.els-cdn.com/content/image/3-s2.0-B9780124059450000375-f37-03-9780124059450.jpg.

Take amphibians like *Rana ridibunda*, for example; they develop some unusual shapes during their transition from water-bound larvae to life on land, hinting that genes and the environment might be co-writing the developmental script. One can see how varied the neurulation process is, and that variety tells its story about evolution's knack for mixing things up. Neurulation's diversity isn't just about adapting to different habitats – it also opens a window into how tangled genetic regulation can be. Research generally indicates that even a phenomenon as fundamental as osmotic tolerance during cell development, particularly in erythrocytes, can exhibit significant variation among vertebrates (Gerda et al., 2024). Then there's the fact that distinct embryonic methods often end up crafting noticeably different nervous systems. Birds, for instance, form their neural tube through a pathway that appears more refined compared to what is seen in many mammals, a reminder that evolution sometimes takes surprisingly unique routes. These differences hint at a complex interaction, where genetic components and environmental pressures blend in ways that are anything but predictable. A closer examination of these trends raises several interesting questions about the genetic mechanisms underlying neural development. Some species appear to possess a built-in flexibility that enables their neural structures to adapt when circumstances change, whereas in others, rigid genetic pathways may lock in a more fixed design. In most cases, the interplay between nature and nurture provides us with fresh perspectives on evolution, prompting researchers to reassess what we know about early development. As more studies emerge, it becomes clear that every unique developmental strategy not only broadens our grasp of neural formation but also paves the way for exciting future research in comparative embryology and evolutionary neuroscience - a field that, despite its complexity, never fails to fascinate (Figure 6.11).

6.4.2. Comparative Embryology

Embryonic development in different species provides a window into how neurulation may influence evolution. A closer look at various early life blueprints reveals that vertebrates adjust their neural designs almost on the fly to fit unpredictable surroundings. Take the killifish, for example—they follow a quirky, practically annual cycle that seems built for toughness. Their eggs, which are strangely resistant to drying out, let them hang on in temporary water patches—a neat mix of survival tactics and early growth. In many cases, these natural tweaks remind us that comparing how embryos develop can help explain the shifting shapes and roles of neural systems during neurulation (Andrew, 2015). Neurulation's defining quirks start showing up during the embryonic phases in vertebrates, where those important neural crest cells step in like unsung heroes. Unique to vertebrate embryos, these cells not only help form sensory ganglia and bits of facial cartilage but also seem to switch roles in ways that keep scientists guessing. A closer look at their development reveals that the complex gene networks operating behind the scenes are crucial for understanding how these cells move and transform. It's interesting, —evolutionary forces have, generally speaking, molded the neural crest into a sort of template for studying cell variability and identity.

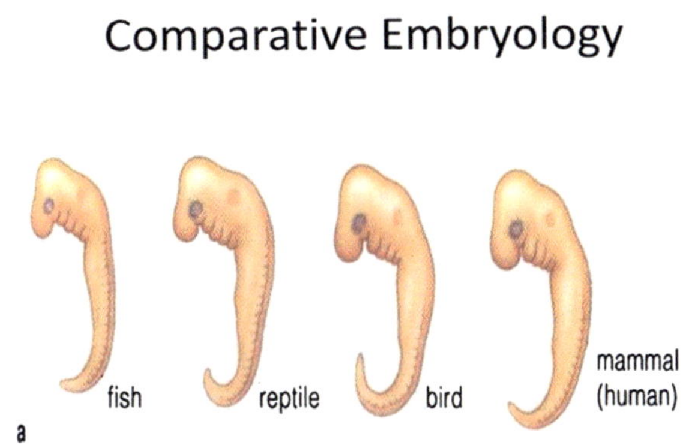

Figure 6.12. Comparative embryology.

Source: https://external-content.duckduckgo.com/iu/?u=https%3A%2F%2Fimage1.slideserve.com%2F2461880%2Fcomparative-embryology-n.jpg&f=1&nofb=1&ipt=c547a7a3518a7faae8af228845a54ba551e153cede665780aae2ae5f1423dca9.

Mapping out the transcriptional and epigenetic signals involved further highlights subtle differences across species, showing how each twist becomes crucial during neurulation (Sim Mões-Costa et al., 2015). Comparative embryology isn't just about one species—it opens up a broader narrative about how neural structures evolve. Different embryonic journeys, such as the unique life cycles seen in killifish, suggest that even minor reproductive changes can have a profound impact on neural development. Such observations often prompt researchers to speculate about ancestral traits and the processes that ultimately led to the diverse array of anatomical features in vertebrates. When exploring these winding evolutionary paths through comparative embryology, it becomes clearer how environmental hurdles and biological adaptations are closely linked, underscoring the significant role of neurulation in shaping nervous system architecture and function across diverse ecological niches (Andrew, 2015) (Figure 6.12).

6.4.3. Evolutionary Significance of Neurulation

Neurulation is a game-changer in the evolution of vertebrates, where basic forms suddenly shift toward more intricate designs. The process builds the neural tube—a structure that essentially lays down the groundwork for the central nervous system—and, in doing so, it enhances neural complexity. In most cases, this increase in complexity is precisely what enables vertebrates to exhibit their adaptive, even clever, behaviors. When viewed through an Evo-Devo lens, this change isn't just a slow, step-by-step tweak; instead, it hints that development might be doing a lot more heavy lifting in evolution than we once thought. Alberch's findings, for instance, indicate that peeling back the layers on neurulation can expose those sudden breaks in morphology, neatly tying early development with broader evolutionary trends (Manuel, 2024). Neurulation also tends to steal the spotlight when scientists explore larger evolutionary puzzles, such as atavism—where old traits reappear in modern species. Researchers, by examining these throwback features, sometimes unravel the messy interplay of gene expression and the subtleties of epigenetic control that are at work. This mix often makes us wonder just how differentiated developmental processes can be, mainly when they cater to our evolutionary past. Recent studies have implied that during neurulation, subtle changes can indeed trigger these ancestral throwbacks, showcasing evolution's knack for adaptability; in a way, this process underlines that the formation of the neural tube isn't merely an early developmental event but a real evolutionary strategy that helps organisms handle their environments, bumping up their survival and reproductive odds (Sun, 2024). Looking beyond individual species, the impact of neurulation ripples out to explain evolutionary relationships among vertebrates. Comparing how different creatures form their neural tubes allows scientists to trace the origins of those complex traits that define neural development. This side-by-side comparison often reveals a shared blueprint among vertebrates, lending weight to the idea that common developmental mechanisms are at play. Thus, the study of neurulation extends beyond its immediate role in early growth, opening a window onto evolutionary biology by connecting body shape, function, and even genetic regulation. In many ways, neurulation acts as a crossroads, a point where embryonic development intersects with broader evolutionary changes. It reveals that subtle adjustments in early life can trigger significant shifts across a wide range of forms (Manuel, 2024).

6.5. Disorders Related to Neurulation

Neurulation isn't just a fancy word—it's the process that builds our central nervous system. When this stage goes off track, a variety of issues can emerge, with NTDs being one of the most striking examples. These defects are a real health worry, ranking as the second most common congenital problem affecting brain and spinal development. They show up in different ways, be it anencephaly or spina bifida, and a lot depends on what kind of lesion is present and exactly where it's located. It seems that both genetic and environmental factors come into play, suggesting that there is still much to be understood about how these issues originate. Studies over the years have pointed out that some populations seem to be hit harder by NTDs, which puts a spotlight on the need for more innovative public health measures. The numbers suggest that both inherited traits and a mother's health—especially if she's low in folate—combine to drive these defects. Early on in pregnancy, what a mother eats turns out to be critically important; even chat before conception about folic acid can make a difference. There's a substantial body of research supporting this claim, with reports of notably fewer NTD cases in communities that implemented folic acid fortification programs (Avagliano et al., 2018). NTDs, however, aren't just about immediate physical hurdles—they also ripple out into social and emotional challenges. Children and adults facing these conditions often encounter difficulties with mobility and learning, which can impact their overall quality of life. Handling these issues effectively means assembling a team of doctors, therapists, educators, and other professionals. With prenatal tests continually improving, more families are receiving early, well-rounded advice on what the future may hold. These insights not only inform medical choices but also help parents and caregivers navigate the complex reality of these developmental difficulties (María Jiménez-Sánchez et al., 2016) (Figure 6.13).

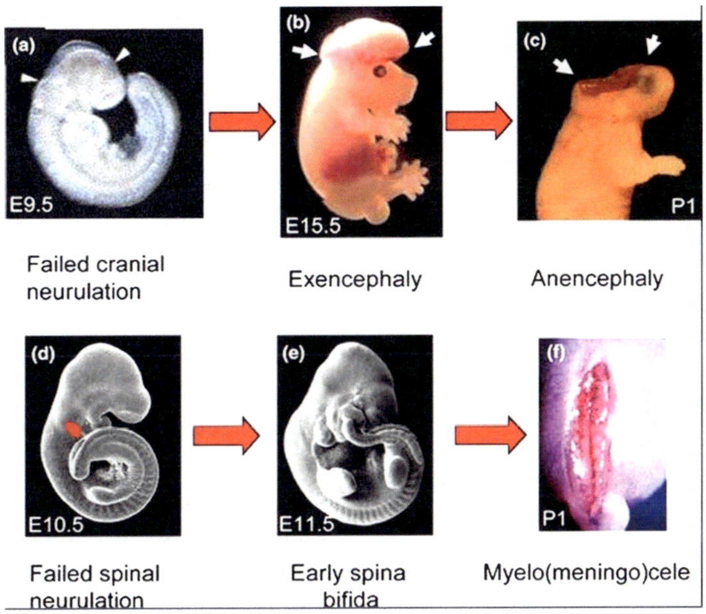

Figure 6.13. Disorders related to neurulation.

Source: https://wires.onlinelibrary.wiley.com/cms/asset/0ae6f483-c9d9-46de-8bea-3b880300c6ad/mfig001.jpg.

6.5.1. Neural Tube Defects (NTD)

Embryonic development isn't as straightforward —issues can crop up when the neural tube doesn't close at just the right moment during early growth. NTDs, such as spina bifida and even anencephaly, vividly illustrate how things can go awry in the central nervous system. It appears that a complex interplay of genes and environmental factors is behind these issues, although the exact genetic blueprint remains unclear. Researchers have, for instance, identified over 200 genes in animal studies, suggesting that the situation in humans may be equally complex. In most cases, grasping this cause-and-effect puzzle is crucial not only for understanding neurulation itself but also for developing more effective treatment and prevention methods in clinical practice (Nicholas et al., 2014). Despite the challenges in identifying NTD triggers, steady progress has been made in pinpointing risk factors. One important factor turns out to be maternal nutrition—with folate levels playing a surprisingly significant role.

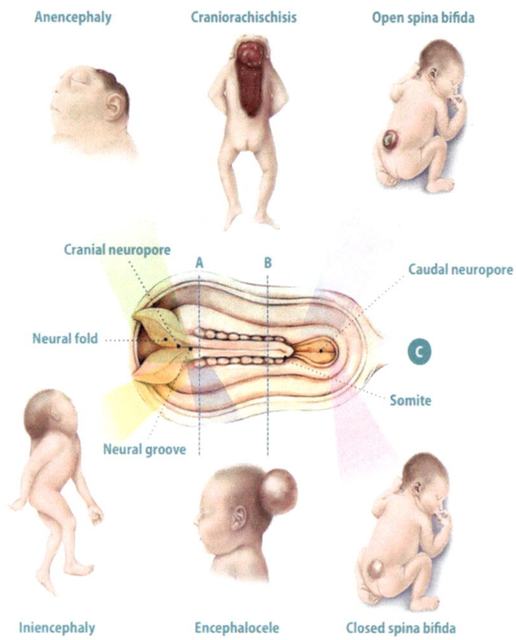

Figure 6.14. Neural tube defects (NTDs).

Source: https://archive.cdc.gov/www_cdc_gov/ncbddd/birthdefects/surveillancemanual/quick-reference-handbook/neuralTubeDefects_html_files/fig1-pt2.jpg.

Many studies suggest that taking folic acid before conception and during early pregnancy can lower the chances of these defects significantly in populations that follow this practice. That said, folic acid isn't a magic bullet; its benefits, though clear, don't cover every single case. Given the messy nature of NTD causes, it seems likely that additional nutritional or genetic tweaks might be needed, too. Early work on other supplements, such as inositol—which has shown promise in animal studies—offers hope that our preventive toolkit for human NTDs may soon expand (Andrew et al., 2009). Getting the neural tube to close properly is a critical early event in development, and any disruption along the way can result in NTDs. A host of cell-level processes come into play here, from how the cell's inner framework is organized to the way it sends signals and keeps itself alive. Key signaling routes—such as those involving sonic hedgehog and planar cell polarity—are considered central to ensuring everything fits together just right. There's a fascinating yet intricate interaction between these pathways and their gene regulators, which highlights the complexity of cellular communication during embryonic growth. Ongoing investigations into how these proteins function are essential, as they could pave the way for targeted interventions aimed at reducing NTD risk in vulnerable groups (Nicholas et al., 2014) (Figure 6.14).

6.5.2. Causes and Risk Factors

Neurulation doesn't unfold in a neat, step-by-step fashion; rather, both genetic quirks and everyday environmental factors mix to shake up how NTDs might occur. Generally speaking, some mutations mess with the molecular signals that help the neural tube seal properly. One might find, for example, that oddities in genes tied to the non-canonical Wnt pathway or in parts of the BMP signaling pathway can disrupt things, and this can gently nudge the risk upward. It's not just about the genes, though—when a mother doesn't get enough folate during pregnancy, that nutritional gap adds to the mix. And in many cases, health issues like diabetes or obesity in the mother make matters more complex, highlighting why attentive, all-around prenatal care is so critical. In addition to these inner workings, broader life contexts—such as socioeconomic background—also play a significant role. Women who struggle to access healthcare services often miss out on key nutritional advice or the timely boost of folate, and that delay can compound the already present genetic risks. In most cases, individuals from lower socioeconomic groups are more likely to face instances of neural tube problems, indicating a clear interaction between internal bodily processes and external social factors.

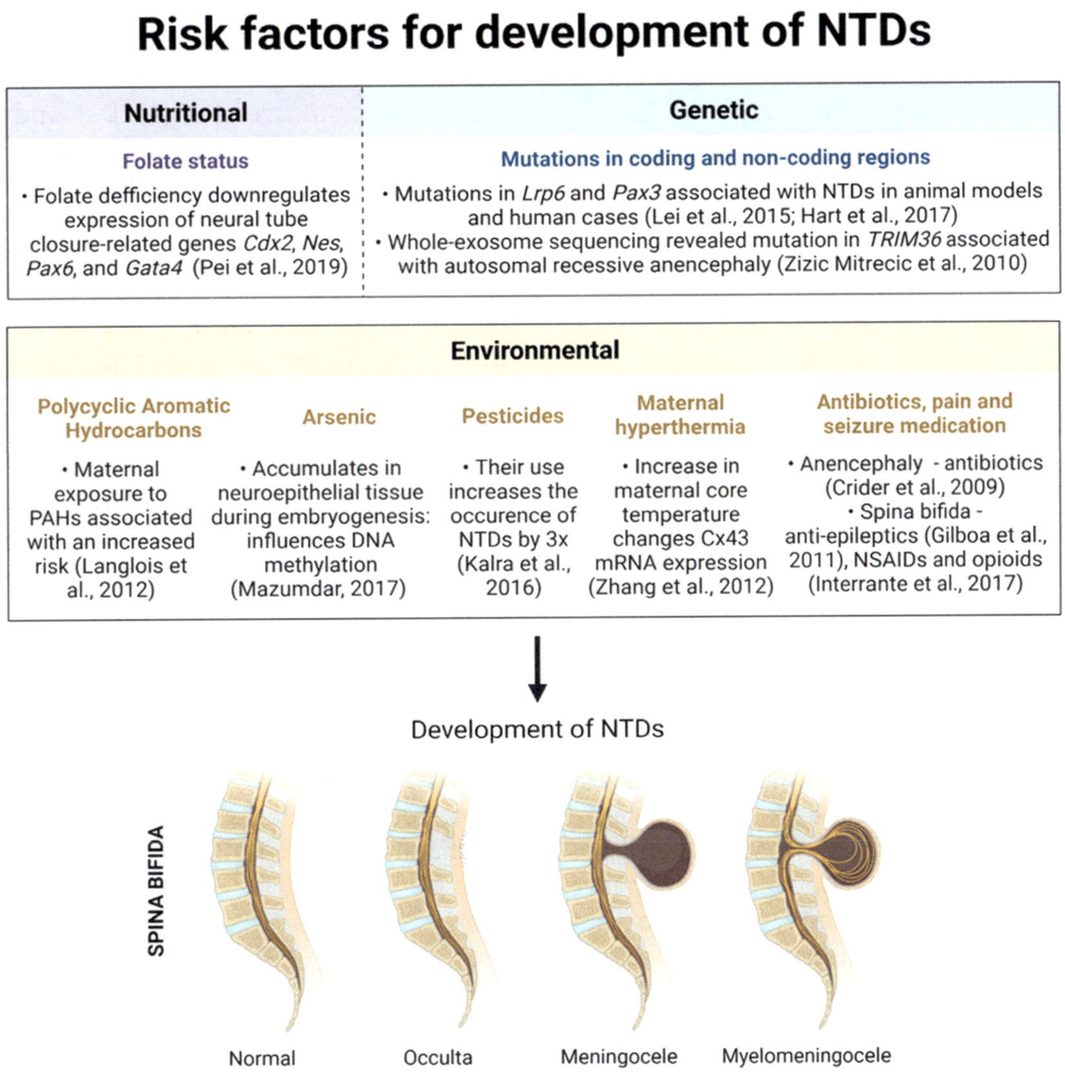

Figure 6.15. Causes and risk factors of NTDs.

Source: https://www.researchgate.net/publication/360137166/figure/fig2/AS:11431281210445581@1702045289780/of-risk-factors-leading-to-development-of-NTDs-Created-with-wwwBioRendercom-accessed.tif.

Ethnic and regional differences also emerge, suggesting that the interplay of genes, environment, and local access to quality care significantly influences how these defects manifest. Public health efforts that promote awareness about maternal nutrition and wellness are, therefore, not only helpful but also necessary. Recent breakthroughs in understanding the physical mechanics of neurulation add yet another layer to the picture. Researchers now tell us that processes like apical constriction and convergent extension—cellular actions that may sound technical but are crucial—help drive the tube's closure. These cellular movements, which are influenced by genetic signals and the embryo's mechanical forces, can also be disrupted by external toxins, making the entire process even more vulnerable. Exposure to such harmful substances during pregnancy has been linked to broader neurodevelopmental issues, further muddying the waters of risk. In a way, examining both biology and biomechanics brings us closer to understanding how a combination of factors can ultimately lead to congenital malformations (Nikolopoulou et al., 2017; Avagliano et al., 2018) (Figure 6.15).

6.5.3. Prevention and Treatment Options

Neurulation might seem like a complicated process, but it's key to building a healthy nervous system. In many cases, understanding how the neural tube forms provides clues to preventing and treating issues associated with its faulty development. For instance, one standard method involves expectant mothers taking folic acid—this supplement is known to lower the risk of NTDs during early growth. Sufficient folate often helps the neural tube develop properly, reducing the chances of problems like spina bifida and anencephaly. Public health efforts, which boost both awareness and easy access to folic acid, also play a big part here; such initiatives typically call for close teamwork between healthcare professionals and community groups so that pregnant women get the nutritional advice and support they need, ultimately leading to better neural outcomes. Beyond these preventive steps, new surgical and pharmaceutical treatments are also recognized as vital for addressing these conditions that arise from abnormal neurulation. Take hydrocephalus, for example—a condition sometimes linked to NTDs that is treated by diverting cerebrospinal fluid to reduce brain pressure. However, recent studies note that these surgeries can often fall short, which means there's a pressing need to explore improved drug therapies. Although earlier pharmacological efforts haven't always hit the mark, current research probing the molecular underpinnings of hydrocephalus might, generally speaking, pave the way for more effective treatments. Increased investment in research—bridging both public and private sectors—is crucial to deepening our understanding of neurulation and its impact on therapy, ultimately aiming for better outcomes for patients. The overall treatment picture for NTDs and similar neurological conditions could become even richer if we adopt a multidisciplinary approach. Instead of relying solely on surgery, it may be time to consider alternative therapies targeting the ECM, which plays a central role in neural development. Interestingly, cellular fibronectin has been linked to tumor progression and may, in some cases, shed light on how ECM components influence both normal and pathological neurulation. Understanding how the ECM and neural tissues interact could lead to innovative methods that enhance the natural regenerative capacity of nerve tissues or even improve responses to traditional treatments. Ultimately, innovative therapeutic frameworks based on this knowledge may not only broaden our prevention and treatment strategies but also reshape clinical management in neurology, ultimately promoting improved health outcomes for affected populations (Efthymiou et al., 2020; Hochstetler et al., 2022).

6.6. Research and Advances in Neurulation

Neurulation has turned heads lately—it's that process where the neural tube comes from what starts off as the neural plate. People are increasingly curious because it touches on how the neural systems develop and sometimes go off-track. Scientists have noticed that when things slip up at this stage, conditions like spina bifida or even anencephaly can crop up. digging. They have been looking into gene activity and cell signaling—yes, those muddled, intertwined details—to figure out exactly how everything works. For example, observing cases like pediatric hydrocephalus, which often hint at a common cellular misstep, has led many to wonder if a better understanding of these pathways might open doors for treatments that would significantly improve patient outcomes, underscoring the need for broader research in the field (Hochstetler et al., 2022). Recently, technological advancements have introduced a new dimension to the study of neurulation. Taking advantage of induced pluripotent stem cells (iPSCs) has revolutionized the field. These cells now serve as a kind of hands-on laboratory model for human neural development, allowing researchers to observe this process in a dish. By nudging iPSCs to become neurons or glial cells, scientists can break down neurulation dynamics in ways that weren't possible before. Interestingly, these moves have even helped mimic neurodegenerative diseases like Alzheimer's, paving the way for fresh drug discovery and testing ventures (Bar Mák et al., 2022). In many cases, being able to craft specific cell types sharpens our understanding of what normal neurulation should be, while also highlighting the genetic and environmental factors that might disrupt the course of developmental disorders—bridging the gap between lab bench insights and real-world clinical needs. Research into neurulation doesn't stop at understanding development—it's spilling over into the world of treatments and prevention, too. With discoveries emerging, scientists are generally homing in on common molecular pathways thought to trigger various neurodevelopmental disorders, such as hydrocephalus. Given the high failure rates we see with surgeries, the push for solid non-surgical treatments is more urgent than ever. Investing in studies that zoom in on those shared cellular changes could, in most cases, reshape our therapeutic strategies. And let's face it, getting patient groups, government, and even the private sector to hash things out together seems like a no-brainer for sparking innovative solutions and boosting outcomes for folks affected by disorders that stem from abnormal neurulation (Hochstetler et al., 2022) (Figure 6.16).

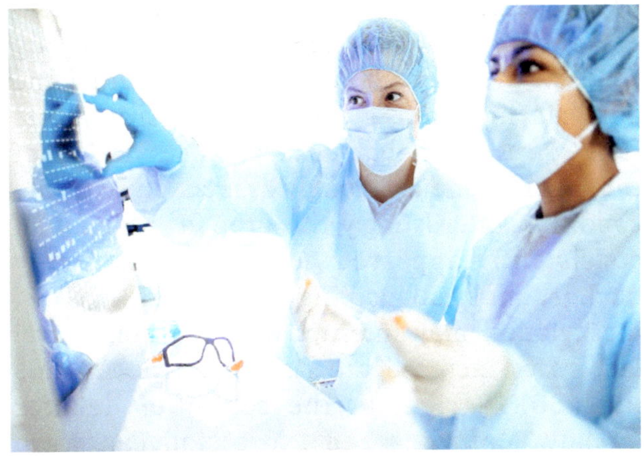

Figure 6.16. Neurulation Research.

Source: https://external-content.duckduckgo.com/iu/?u=https%3A%2F%2Fbepartofresearch.nihr.ac.uk%2FdA%2F732d5bab53%2FHealth%2520breakthroughs.jpg&f=1&nofb=1&ipt=fde2b6331995f159f71c262e834ba1bc849542d04266e38d6432939e4e9eab64.

6.6.1. Current Studies and Findings

Neurulation kicks off early in an embryo's life and turns out to be a lot more twisty than one might assume. New research continues to suggest that, although forming the embryo's neural structures is essential, the process is accompanied by its set of complex processes. One clinical study, for example, zeroed in on the mix of hormonal cues and reproductive outcomes in women with diminished ovarian reserve (DOR). In this study, efforts like ovarian biopsy and auto transplantation didn't immediately bump up the number of follicles suitable for IVF/ICSI; still, about 60% of the participants managed to secure clinical pregnancies within a year. This odd interplay between surgical moves and hormone shifts points to a deeper, if unexpected, connection to early development processes—underscoring the importance of examining the biological underpinnings of neurulation (Lunding et al., 2019). Meanwhile, other researchers are peeling back layers on the molecular side of things, focusing on NTDs. It now appears that factors beyond the raw DNA—epigenetics, in plain terms—might cast long shadows over neurulation. A detailed methylome analysis in patients with myelomeningocele (MMC) revealed that reduced methylation of the SOX18 gene is strongly associated with the condition. Interestingly, this drop in methylation consistently appeared across various family backgrounds, suggesting that shifts in DNA methylation may interact with environmental factors to increase the risk of NTDs. All this puts SOX18 right at the center of debates on how shifts in gene expression can warp developmental paths, adding yet another twist to the neural tube formation story (Rochtus et al., 2016). All in all, these findings paint a picture that's both evolving and layered. On one side, delving into hormonal dynamics could spell new hope for women grappling with reproductive hurdles; on the other, a sharper focus on genetic and epigenetic changes might pave the way for more innovative prevention strategies against defects like NTDs. There's a real need for studies that blur the borders between basic biology and clinical outcomes—even if the results are a bit messy at first glance. By bridging these fields, researchers may unlock fresh insights into neurulation that could ripple out to improve our broader understanding of human health (Rochtus et al., 2016; Lunding et al., 2019).

6.6.2. Technological Advancements in Research

Recent technological advancements have significantly altered our understanding of neurulation. High-throughput sequencing now plays a central role in untangling the molecular dance behind neural tube formation—it's quite the game-changer. Single-cell RNA sequencing (scRNA-seq) enables researchers to examine cell states at an individual level during early embryonic stages, revealing a spectrum of cellular diversity and gene expression differences that bulk methods might easily overlook. Still, scRNA-seq doesn't retain spatial details, which makes comprehending the whole-cell interplay a bit tricky (Desta et al., 2025). Lately, spatial transcriptomics has begun to step in, promising a more nuanced look at where RNA is located inside tissues, even if the transition isn't entirely smooth yet. Big data has begun to play a significant role in biomedical research, combining everyday analytical power with cutting-edge ideas. Massive, layered datasets offer fresh insight into both normal and off-track processes that shape neural development. Advanced computer techniques, such as deep learning and enrichment analysis, help sort through vast amounts of information to pinpoint functional patterns. In embryology, these approaches go beyond number crunching; they spot critical molecular pathways that guide neurulation. Additionally, biomedical ontologies help bridge the differences among diverse data sources, making it easier to integrate information (Fu et al., 2025). Sure, there's a bit of redundancy here and there, but these methods are proving essential for a richer, more detailed picture of development. All of these advances are doing more than just upgrading our lab tools—they're sparking unexpected teamwork across fields like neurology and developmental biology. Genomics, bioinformatics, and even computational modeling are converging to provide a broader, more natural perspective on the complex process of neurulation. Researchers are now better able to ask pointed questions and even craft targeted interventions for issues such as NTDs. In most cases, as our research landscape continues to shift and technology blends with biology, we're opening new doors to understand how genes and environmental cues interact during development, promising improvements in human health overall.

6.6.3. Future Directions in Neurulation Research

Mechanical forces appear to drive early brain development more than previously thought. Researchers have been noticing that these forces might steer how the embryonic brain develops. Generally speaking, studies point out that feedback from these forces is crucial in shaping the young brain. The neuroepithelium doesn't respond the same everywhere—stiffer patches tend to show stretched, unusual nuclear shapes while softer spots keep things more round. This fresh view on tissue flexibility and mechanical loads opens the door to asking how stress signals might influence cell shape and, in a roundabout way, the overall brain layout. It creates a foundation for understanding both normal growth and, potentially, how errors in these forces could trigger NTDs, prompting us to explore potential solutions further (Filas et al., 2012). Cells chatting with each other also seem to play a surprising role during neurulation, especially when one considers the surface ectoderm's biomechanics. Transcription factors like Grhl-2 and Grhl-3, for instance, have been identified as essential messengers in the process of neural tube closure. In most cases, functional tests reveal that when mutations interfere with these factors, cell shape and their mechanical balance are disrupted—sometimes leading to severe NTDs. Additionally, there's the issue of cells sticking together; consider E-cadherin, for example, which illustrates the critical role adhesion plays in the process. It is possible that future work, by teasing apart how desmosome dynamics and other adhesive molecules function in various genetic contexts, could guide us toward targeted treatments for defects arising from these mechanical missteps (Marshall et al., 2021). Mixing computer models with lab experiments is another route that's starting to interest researchers. Recent findings indicate that bumping up contractility in the embryonic chicken brain can produce shapes reminiscent of those seen in more primitive vertebrates—an observation that, in most cases, invites a closer look at evolution's role in brain development. Using digital simulations to map how local cell contractions vary may help decode the flexible nature of brain formation and explain why species differ significantly in brain design. This kind of cross-disciplinary approach not only deepens our understanding of evolutionary developmental biology but also suggests how to build experimental systems that mimic developmental quirks. Over time, merging these methods could significantly enhance our understanding of neurulation and its broader effects across a range of organisms (Filas et al., 2012).

SUMMARY

Neurulation kicks in as a critical moment during early growth—it's not only about forming the central nervous system, but also about how the whole shape of the little organism comes together. Neural tubes, for instance, seem to spring from a messy mix of genes, cell shifts, and even mechanical pushes; it's almost as if they're wedded to randomness and order at the same time. New research continues to highlight that, in many cases, the contractile networks within cells serve as the backbone for movement during this stage. One can also see how mathematical models and good old quantitative checks (a nod to ideas proposed initially by D'Arcy Thompson) help us grasp the concept of morphogenesis. This mash-up of methods, although not neatly laid out, demonstrates that tracking everything from cell motion to tissue buildup can significantly enhance our understanding of neurulation's role at the beginning of life (Natalie et al., 2017). Understanding neurulation doesn't stop at the lab bench. It spills over into real-world challenges, such as congenital conditions like holoprosencephaly (HPE). A glitch in this developmental flip can throw off both anatomy and function—kind of a double whammy that stresses why it matters to get neurulation right. Studies on HPE have, in most cases, shed light on how a combination of genetic predispositions and environmental influences can shape forebrain development. This layered, sometimes confusing view not only maps out the routes leading to nerve system quirks but also suggests ways to address them. Ongoing investigations into HPE and its relatives suggest that expanding our understanding in this area may significantly impact how we approach a range of malformation syndromes (Roessler et al., 2010). In essence, neurulation ties form and function together in ways that are anything but simple. As more research incorporates numbers and cell checks into the mix, we begin to unravel the tangled threads of this key stage. Our growing insight into how neurulation works adds both to scholarly debates and to practical strategies for addressing congenital issues—it's, well, a significant development in both theory and practice. So, looking into neurulation isn't merely an exploration of early development; it's a peek into the broader laws that govern life, affirming that sometimes a little interdisciplinary chaos is precisely what we need to solve nature's puzzles (Roessler et al., 2010; Natalie et al., 2017). Neurulation kicks off one of the most critical stages in early development—the very moment when the outer cell layer, the ectoderm, starts to reshape into what we call the neural plate, which then folds into the neural tube. This phase is not just about forming one structure; it's central to setting up the whole body plan. In most cases, digging into these molecular details helps us understand issues like spina bifida and anencephaly. Researchers, for example, have shown that various signaling routes, with cadherins (those sticky molecules) playing a key role, are crucial in ensuring that cells clump together properly. Since cadherins help cells switch from an epithelial state to a more mobile one, they're pretty essential for keeping tissues stable—even when things go a bit off track during tube formation (Noronha et al., 2021). Examining cadherin expression during this period can also shed light on the genetic origins of neural development. There's a mix of external signals and internal messaging that influences how these proteins appear, which then affects how cells move and determine their fate. This kind of back-and-forth is critical in the central nervous system, where solid cell adhesion is crucial in wiring up the correct neural networks. Some studies even suggest that changes in cadherin patterns may be linked to tumors, such as gliomas, underscoring once again the crucial role these proteins play in smooth development (Noronha et al., 2021). When one sees that link between everyday cell functions and potential tumor growth, it's a reminder that a slight misstep in cadherin signaling can have consequences both during early development and later on. On another note, the twist of evolution in gene regulation—especially in things like the Wnt signaling pathway—adds even more layers to our picture of neurulation.

CLOSER LOOK

NEURAL TUBE CLOSURE (NTC)

NTC is a vital process during early embryonic development in vertebrates, leading to the formation of the neural tube, which ultimately gives rise to the central nervous system, including the brain and spinal cord. This event occurs during the third to fourth week of human gestation, shortly after gastrulation, when the three germ layers—ectoderm, mesoderm, and endoderm—are established. NTC begins when a specialized region of the ectoderm, called the neural plate, thickens along the dorsal midline of the embryo in response to inductive signals from the underlying notochord and mesoderm. The lateral edges of the neural plate then elevate to form neural folds, which curve toward the midline and eventually fuse to form the neural tube. The process initiates at multiple closure points along the anterior-posterior axis and proceeds bidirectionally, sealing the tube in a zipper-like fashion.

Successful neural tube closure is crucial for the proper development of the brain and spinal cord. Failure of this process results in serious congenital disorders known as neural tube defects (NTDs). The most common NTDs include spina bifida, where the lower portion of the neural tube fails to close, leading to incomplete development of the spinal cord and vertebrae, and anencephaly, where the upper part of the neural tube remains open, resulting in the absence of a significant portion of the brain and skull. These conditions can lead to lifelong disability or even death, emphasizing the importance of precise regulation of NTC. Genetic and environmental factors both play significant roles in NTC. Genes involved in cell adhesion, cytoskeletal dynamics, and signaling pathways, such as Wnt, BMP, and Shh (Sonic Hedgehog), are essential for proper closure. Environmental influences include maternal nutritional status, with folate (vitamin B9) being particularly important. Folic acid supplementation before and during early pregnancy has been shown to significantly reduce the risk of NTDs, which is why it is recommended for women of reproductive age.

Cellular mechanisms underlying NTC are highly coordinated. Neural plate cells undergo changes in shape, such as apical constriction, driven by actomyosin contraction, which helps to bend the neural plate. Cell proliferation, migration, and intercalation also contribute to the dynamic remodeling of tissues necessary for closure. The surrounding non-neural ectoderm and mesoderm play supporting roles, providing mechanical and signaling inputs that guide the elevation and fusion of the neural folds. The fusion of the neural folds involves precise molecular interactions, including the expression of specific cell adhesion molecules, such as N-cadherin and E-cadherin, as well as the roles of filopodia and lamellipodia that extend across the midline to bring opposing cells together.

Neural tube closure is a complex and tightly regulated morphogenetic process essential for the development of the central nervous system. Disruptions in any part of this process—whether genetic, molecular, or environmental—can result in severe developmental disorders. Continued research into the mechanisms of NTC is not only vital for understanding basic developmental biology but also for improving strategies to prevent and manage NTDs through genetic counseling, nutritional guidance, and early diagnosis.

REFERENCES

1. Ahn, H., & Sun, W. (2023). Plate-curving cell culture as a model for assessing curvature-induced cellular responses during neural tube morphogenesis. *Animal Cells and Systems, 27*(1), 413–424. https://doi.org/10.1080/19768354.2023.2287085Ambekar, Y. S., Caiaffa, C. D., Wlodarczyk, B. J., Singh, M., Schill, A. W., Steele, J., Zhang, J., et al. (2024). Optical coherence tomography-guided Brillouin microscopy highlights regional tissue stiffness differences during anterior neural tube closure in the *Mthfd1l* murine mutant. *Development.* https://www.semanticscholar.org/paper/cd23d10dbb7425dd0d058f6b02b8eb83c0806b7a (accessed on 26 May 2025).
2. Amjad, A., Qaiser, S., Błaszczyszyn, M., & Szczęsna, A. (2024). The evolution of frailty assessment using inertial measurement sensor-based gait parameter measurements: A detailed analysis. *WIREs Data Mining and Knowledge Discovery, 14.* https://www.semanticscholar.org/paper/26c76f2155fa2996e9836ba837fee34c91ea95b4 (accessed on 26 May 2025).
3. Avagliano, L., Massa, V., George, T. M., Qureshy, S., Bulfamante, G., & Finnell, R. H. (2018). Overview on neural tube defects: From development to physical characteristics. *Birth Defects Research, 111*, 1455–1467. https://doi.org/10.1002/bdr2.1380.
4. Barák, M., Fedorová, V., Pospíšilová, V., Raška, J., Vochyánová, S., Sedmík, J., Hříbková, H., et al. (2022). Human iPSC-derived neural models for studying Alzheimer's disease: From neural stem cells to cerebral organoids. *Stem Cell Reviews and Reports, 18*, 792–820. https://doi.org/10.1007/s12015-021-10254-3.
5. Beck, C. (2015). Development of the vertebrate tailbud. *Wiley Interdisciplinary Reviews: Developmental Biology, 4.* https://www.semanticscholar.org/paper/bcc04770e807f0481375d2767aa78c6948506274 (accessed on 26 May 2025).
6. Boschen, K., Ptacek, T. S., Simon, J. M., & Parnell, S. (2020). Transcriptome-wide regulation of key developmental pathways in the mouse neural tube by prenatal alcohol exposure. *Alcoholism: Clinical and Experimental Research.* https://www.semanticscholar.org/paper/482a458069624f5a2f7b4b0e36b2ff6f9181ddf7 (accessed on 26 May 2025).
7. Carpinelli, M. R., de Vries, M. E., Auden, A., Butt, N. H., Deng, Z., Partridge, D., Miles, L. B., et al. (2020). Inactivation of *Zeb1* in GRHL2-deficient mouse embryos rescues mid-gestation viability and secondary palate closure. *Disease Models & Mechanisms, 13*, dmm042218. https://doi.org/10.1242/dmm.042218.
8. Copp, A. J., & Greene, N. D. E. (2009). Genetics and development of neural tube defects. *The Journal of Pathology, 220*, 217–230. https://doi.org/10.1002/path.2643.
9. Copp, A., & Greene, N. (2013). Neural tube defects—disorders of neurulation and related embryonic processes. *Wiley Interdisciplinary Reviews: Developmental Biology, 2.* https://www.semanticscholar.org/paper/e31e1dfe03119ef82377c86e4d05b8c454efb4bc (accessed on 26 May 2025).
10. Del Casale, A., Modesti, M. N., Gentile, G., Guariglia, C., Ferracuti, S., Simmaco, M., & Borro, M. (2024). Is the Hedgehog pathway involved in the pathophysiology of schizophrenia? A systematic review of current evidence of neural molecular correlates and perspectives on drug development. *Current Issues in Molecular Biology, 46*, 5322–5336. https://www.semanticscholar.org/paper/e8dc9c920da4640cb5702593f780945ed5e1d5ce (accessed on 26 May 2025).

11. Desta, G. M., & Birhanu, A. (2025). Advancements in single-cell RNA sequencing and spatial transcriptomics: Transforming biomedical research. *Acta Biochimica Polonica, 72*. https://www.semanticscholar.org/paper/8242b8eb0f45c6f5b5cf16b8ec7b8ce82d36e19b (accessed on 26 May 2025).

12. Efthymiou, G., Saint, A., Ruff, M. W., Rekad, Z., Ciais, D., & Van Obberghen-Schilling, E. (2020). Shaping up the tumor microenvironment with cellular fibronectin. *Frontiers in Oncology, 10*, Article 641. https://doi.org/10.3389/fonc.2020.00641.

13. Farhadi, A., Zhao, Q., & Tan, K. (2024). The molecular mechanism of embryonic development in decapod crustaceans. *Reviews in Aquaculture*. https://www.semanticscholar.org/paper/347da0b2e1ac0690443825cbd15693f3a44fd725 (accessed on 26 May 2025).

14. Filas, B. (2012). *Mechanisms of Early Brain Morphogenesis* [Doctoral dissertation, University of Iowa]. CORE. https://core.ac.uk/download/233205484.pdf (accessed on 26 May 2025).

15. Fu, H., Liu, Y., Zhang, M. Y., & Yang, H. (2025). Enrichment analysis and deep learning in biomedical ontology: Applications and advancements. *Chinese Medical Sciences Journal*. https://www.semanticscholar.org/paper/def9fa239d3d16401a3f0a82a1e34ee85f1b5d4c (accessed on 26 May 2025).

16. Furness, A. I. (2015). The evolution of an annual life cycle in killifish: Adaptation to ephemeral aquatic environments through embryonic diapause. *Biological Reviews, 91*, 796–812. https://doi.org/10.1111/brv.12194.

17. Gerda, B. A., Skverchinskaya, E. A., Andreeva, A. Y., Volkova, A., Gambaryan, S., & Mindukshev, I. (2024). Comparative analysis of the osmotic fragility of erythrocytes across various taxa of vertebrates. *Žurnal evolutional biohimii i fiziologii*. https://www.semanticscholar.org/paper/10fe5db95986e30c063a1444da2f5a3089d8fd5f (accessed on 26 May 2025).

18. Greene, N. D. E., & Copp, A. J. (2014). Neural tube defects. *Annual Review of Neuroscience, 37*, 221–242. https://doi.org/10.1146/annurev-neuro-062012-170354.

19. Handler, C., Scarcelli, G., & Zhang, J. (2023). Time-lapse mechanical imaging of neural tube closure in live embryo using Brillouin microscopy. *Scientific Reports, 13*. https://doi.org/10.1038/s41598-023-27456-z.

20. Heer, N. C., & Martin, A. C. (2017). Tension, contraction and tissue morphogenesis. *Development, 144*, 4249–4260. https://doi.org/10.1242/dev.151282.

21. Hinman, V. F., & Burke, R. D. (2018). Embryonic neurogenesis in echinoderms. *Wiley Interdisciplinary Reviews: Developmental Biology, 7*(3), e316. https://doi.org/10.1002/wdev.316.

22. Hochstetler, A., Raskin, J. S., & Blazer-Yost, B. L. (2022). Hydrocephalus: Historical analysis and considerations for treatment. *European Journal of Medical Research, 27*. https://doi.org/10.1186/s40001-022-00798-6.

23. Jiménez-Sánchez, M., Licitra, F., Underwood, B. R., & Rubinsztein, D. C. (2016). Huntington's disease: Mechanisms of pathogenesis and therapeutic strategies. *Cold Spring Harbor Perspectives in Medicine, 7*, a024240. https://doi.org/10.1101/cshperspect.a024240.

24. Kim, H., & Kim, E. (2024). Current status of synthetic mammalian embryo models. *International Journal of Molecular Sciences, 25*. https://www.semanticscholar.org/paper/99a63c237aec64c43d31b97f7d05cb141c8d211b (accessed on 26 May 2025).

25. Liu, X., Ning, X., Wu, C., & Zhang, Y. (2024). Evolutionary trends in carbon market risk research. *Energies*. https://www.semanticscholar.org/paper/8c754e5ed5aa2fee20e709117ba92c4a7ff815de (accessed on 26 May 2025).

26. Loh, C. Y., Chai, J., Tang, T., Wong, W. F., Sethi, G., Shanmugam, M. K., Chong, P. P., et al. (2019). The E-Cadherin and N-Cadherin switch in epithelial-to-mesenchymal transition: Signaling, therapeutic implications, and challenges. *Cells, 8*, Article 1118. https://doi.org/10.3390/cells8101118.

27. Lunding, S. A., Pors, S., Kristensen, S., Landersoe, S. K., Jeppesen, J. V., Flachs, E., Pinborg, A., et al. (2019). Biopsying, fragmentation and auto transplantation of fresh ovarian cortical tissue in infertile women with diminished ovarian reserve. *Human Reproduction*. https://www.semanticscholar.org/paper/05f085e3e5faaf855c408ae602674bf7ef3e3783 (accessed on 26 May 2025).

28. Marshall, A. R. (2021). *Biomechanical and Genetic Analysis of Neural Tube Closure in The Mouse Embryo* [Doctoral dissertation, University of Cambridge]. CORE. https://core.ac.uk/download/477685991.pdf (accessed on 26 May 2025).

29. Mi, Y., Yan, L., Wu, Y., & Zheng, Y. (2025). Deficiency of UBE3D in mice leads to severe embryonic abnormalities and disrupts the mRNA of homeobox genes via CPSF3. *Cell Death Discovery, 11*. https://www.semanticscholar.org/paper/9d4a11192d2b19703cee863977bcba44d550fb93 (accessed on 26 May 2025).

30. Mukhopadhyay, P., Greene, R. M., & Pisano, M. (2020). MicroRNA targeting of the non-canonical planar cell polarity pathway in the developing neural tube. *Cell Biochemistry and Function, 38*(7), 905–920. https://doi.org/10.1002/cbf.3512.

31. Nikolopoulou, E., Galea, G. L., Rolo, A., Greene, N. D. E., & Copp, A. J. (2017). Neural tube closure: Cellular, molecular and biomechanical mechanisms. *Development, 144*, 552–566. https://doi.org/10.1242/dev.145904.

32. Noronha, C., Ribeiro, A. S., Taipa, R., Castro, D. S., Reis, J., Faria, C. C., & Paredes, J. (2021). Cadherin expression and EMT: A focus on gliomas. *Biomedicines, 9*, Article 1328. https://doi.org/10.3390/biomedicines9101328.

33. Nurifah, C., Rosida, D., & Munarko, H. (2025). Differences in nutritional value of rice crackers with the addition of three types of leaves (Moringa, Torbangun, and Katuk). *AJARCDE (Asian Journal of Applied Research for Community Development and Empowerment)*. https://www.semanticscholar.org/paper/df36b26704f56d941e95c5d2a52dbbea3ef37a2a (accessed on 26 May 2025).

34. Opferman, J. T., & Kothari, A. (2017). Anti-apoptotic BCL-2 family members in development. *Cell Death and Differentiation, 25*, 37–45. https://doi.org/10.1038/cdd.2017.170.

35. Petridou, N. I., & Heisenberg, C. P. (2019). Tissue rheology in embryonic organization. *The EMBO Journal, 38*, e102497. https://doi.org/10.15252/embj.2019102497.

36. Price, D. J., Jarman, A. P., Mason, J. O., & Kind, P. C. (2017). *Building Brains: An Introduction to Neural Development*.

37. Rochtus, A., Winand, R., Laenen, G., Vangeel, E., Izzi, B., Wittevrongel, C., Moreau, Y., et al. (2016). Methylome analysis for spina bifida shows SOX18 hypomethylation as a risk factor with evidence for a complex (epi)genetic interplay to affect neural tube development. *Clinical*

Epigenetics, 8. https://www.semanticscholar.org/paper/1875fda0b7de4b1e4ab354e697bb7e9ee28ef322 (accessed on 26 May 2025).

38. Rodrigues, R. J., Marques, J. M., & Köfalvi, A. (2024). Cannabis, endocannabinoids and brain development: From embryogenesis to adolescence. *Cells, 13*(22), 1875. https://doi.org/10.3390/cells13221875.
39. Roessler, E., & Muenke, M. (2010). The molecular genetics of holoprosencephaly. *American Journal of Medical Genetics Part C: Seminars in Medical Genetics, 154C*, 52–61. https://doi.org/10.1002/ajmg.c.30236.
40. Sánchez Arteaga, J. M. (2024). "The logic of monsters:" Pere Alberch and the evolutionary significance of experimental teratology. *Journal of the History of Biology, 57*, 379–401. https://www.semanticscholar.org/paper/e6cd50579cd94c5ed0d77f85c2010cebb744d29b (accessed on 26 May 2025).
41. Simões-Costa, M., & Bronner-Fraser, M. (2015). Establishing neural crest identity: A gene regulatory recipe. *Development, 142*, 242–257. https://doi.org/10.1242/dev.105445.
42. Singh, S., & Groves, A. K. (2016). The molecular basis of craniofacial placode development. *Wiley Interdisciplinary Reviews: Developmental Biology, 5*(3), 363–376. https://doi.org/10.1002/wdev.226.
43. Somorjai, I., Martí-Solans, J., Diaz-Gracia, M., Nishida, H., Imai, K. S., Escrivà, H., Cañestro, C., et al. (2018). Wnt evolution and function shuffling in liberal and conservative chordate genomes. *Genome Biology, 19*, Article 92. https://doi.org/10.1186/s13059-018-1468-3.
44. Sun, J. (2024). Unveiling the evolutionary significance: Atavisms transition from ancestral traits to a fundamental biological phenomenon. *Theoretical and Natural Science*. https://www.semanticscholar.org/paper/48f0929ac6bdbc1744c9a4ff080a984948d0c39d (accessed on 26 May 2025).
45. Swift, D. (2022). The diverse early embryonic development of vertebrates and implications regarding their ancestry. *BIO-Complexity*. https://www.semanticscholar.org/paper/7bc7a46a6fcfd94b7f275fb9057c3f239956dca7 (accessed on 26 May 2025).
46. Thornton, M., Eder, G., Amman, F., Pantielieieva, A., Vierheilig, J., & Bergthaler, A. (2025). Comparative wastewater virome analysis with different enrichment methods. *bioRxiv*. https://www.semanticscholar.org/paper/7b1c4afd6671365c34519abee38687b90fdd1a2a (accessed on 26 May 2025).
47. Tolera, M. (2023). The "smart city" between urban narrative and empty signifier: Shaggar in focus. *World Journal of Education and Humanities*. https://www.semanticscholar.org/paper/25ed3db34ce39d30521eba05eecbd2b01cff1a4f (accessed on 26 May 2025).
48. Yang, Y., & Mlodzik, M. (2015). Wnt-Frizzled/planar cell polarity signaling: Cellular orientation by facing the wind (Wnt). *Annual Review of Cell and Developmental Biology, 31*, 623–646. https://doi.org/10.1146/annurev-cellbio-100814-125315.
49. Yu, H., Zhong, T., Xu, Y., Zhang, Z., Ma, J., Yuan, J., Wang, M., et al. (2025). Molecular profiling of skin cells identifies distinct cellular signatures in radiation-induced skin injury across various stages in the murine dataset. *Experimental Hematology & Oncology, 14*. https://www.semanticscholar.org/paper/77637e1bbb3f686235eb0539c52ccaa5035493bf (accessed on 26 May 2025).

50. Zarzycki, A., Thomas, Z. M., & Mazrier, H. (2020). Comparison of inherited neural tube defects in companion animals and livestock. *Birth Defects Research, 113*, 319–348. https://www.semanticscholar.org/paper/3e071a7c1410c6089cc4937775ca20871293bb5a (accessed on 26 May 2025).

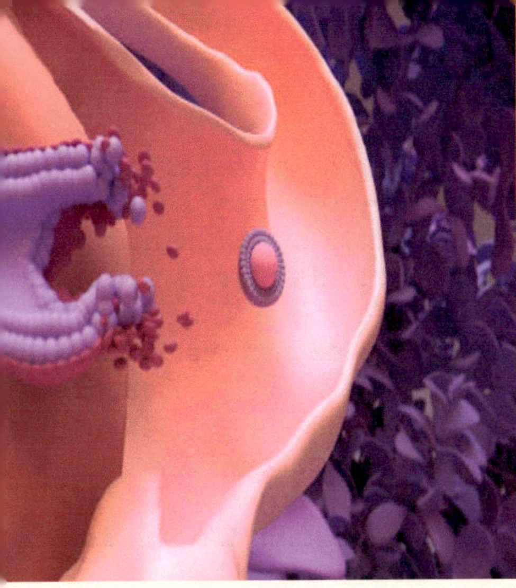

Chapter 7

EXTRAEMBRYONIC MEMBRANES AND PLACENTA

Contents

Introduction

Early on, mammalian development begins with cells and molecules interacting in unpredictable ways that set the stage for a functioning organism. Extraembryonic membranes and the placenta, though different, work together to support the fetus—one provides protection and structure while the other. At the same time, the other takes on tasks like shuffling nutrients and clearing out waste, and understanding how these parts form and function is crucial to unraveling the mysteries of embryonic growth. In most cases, understanding how these membranes and the placenta behave sheds light on the delicate dance between mother and fetus. At the same time, even minor deviations might throw a wrench into pregnancy or a child's later development. There's more to these extraembryonic players than just physical support. They pack a biochemical punch that influences both mother and baby. Take the extracellular matrix (ECM) for example—it isn't just a background scaffold, but a lively environment where cells stick, move, and even change roles. Research has generally shown that the

ECM pulls together the signals that guide these cellular responses, helping keep tissues intact during gestation. Additionally, components such as collagens and glycoproteins play a crucial role in ensuring that membranes and the placenta remain both firm and adaptable as the body's needs change (Nikos et al., 2021). Among all of this, the placenta stands out as the narrow border between mother and fetus, crucial for managing nutrient exchange and waste removal. Trophoblast cells, which drive the placenta's development, have a unique knack—they invade maternal tissues and tweak the uterine blood vessels to create a nurturing setting for the growing baby (Maltepe et al., 2015). People have taken a keen interest in the intricate biology of the placenta, and it has become clear that its health is deeply intertwined with the overall well-being of both the fetus and the mother. Ongoing exploration of this vital interface will undoubtedly reveal new treatment ideas and reaffirm the significance of the extraembryonic membranes and the placenta in the broader context of health (Figure 7.1).

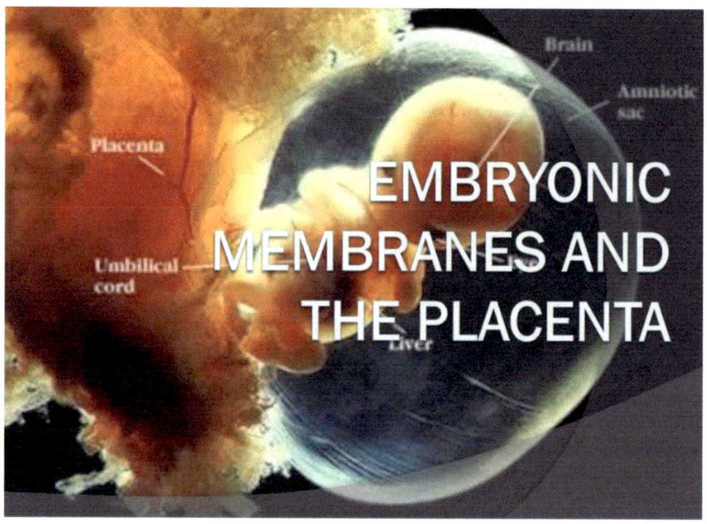

Figure 7.1. Embryonic membranes and the placenta.

Source: https://external-content.duckduckgo.com/iu/?u=https%3A%2F%2Fimage1.slideserve.com%2F2271625%2Fembryonic-membranes-and-the-placenta-l.jpg&f=1&nofb=1&ipt=1befe765a5e9cb042f41788552bf0529460f6658241b11e4b6939e18ddb1c536.

Definition of Extraembryonic Membranes

Early on, an embryo's development kicks off with a tangle of interactions that spark the emergence of key structures. Extraembryonic membranes show up—not as part of the embryo proper, but as essential byproducts of the zygote—that help keep the little one growing inside the womb. The yolk sac, chorion, amnion, and allantois are among the components that contribute to life support. In many cases, the fact that these membranes appear in so many vertebrates suggests a deep, shared reproductive strategy and a role in forming placentas. Take the amnion, for instance, probably the most well-known among them; it builds a protective, fluid-filled sac that cushions the developing embryo. The amniotic fluid not only creates a steady environment but also smooths out movements, serving as a sort of shield against external disturbances. The chorion, on the other hand, handles nutrient and gas exchange between the mother and the embryo, laying the groundwork for what later becomes part of the placenta. Their mutual reliance reveals a surprisingly complex system that's vital for survival—and it's worth noting that these membranes don't just offer physical support. They also send out signals, subtly guiding the whole process of development. Lately, studies employing cutting-edge methods, such as single-cell transcriptomics, have begun to reveal just how diverse the cells in these extraembryonic tissues can be. New findings reveal a complex yet fascinating network of cell interactions in the early placenta and decidua, underscoring that this phase is far from straightforward. The ECM plays its part too, acting as both a supportive scaffold and a messenger that nudges cells in different directions. As our understanding grows, it becomes increasingly apparent that these membranes aren't passive bystanders—they're active players in managing pregnancy and fetal growth. In most cases, this evolving view underscores the vital role extraembryonic membranes play not only in nourishing the embryo but also in shaping overall maternal-fetal health (Suryawanshi et al., 2018; Nikos et al., 2021) (Figure 7.2).

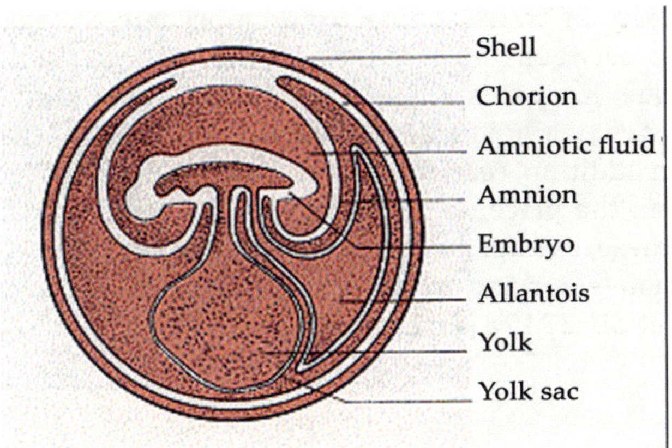

Figure 7.2. Extraembryonic membranes.

Source: https://files.mtstatic.com/site_4463/7219/0?Expires=1746698417&Signature=ctvs6nlEX~krrrYJGd5XJJdwPWfEHm7V2clXd7mz6qhJhqB-51PlCUmoZxj6A0GEC2yQ-eeR--MWJIjGzkzEReDkNE~OU6nzVje0VogkPo8eNRSxtLKZx4gzx61TkLGcCwmr99N~HhKA6zSmfutw6MpAnkUJhb1ZalRRTSa6MoY_&Key-Pair-Id=APKAJ5Y6AV4GI7A555NA.

Importance of the Placenta in Mammalian Development

The placenta does a lot more than act as a structural support. It's busy regulating the tricky balance of nutrients and gases necessary for the baby's growth, almost like a live wire connecting the mother's and fetus's bloodstreams. It handles oxygen and essential nourishment while taking care of waste removal. The trophoblast cells—even though they come from the baby—adapt in surprising ways that keep the mother's immune system from overreacting. This type of immune tolerance is crucial, allowing the placenta to settle into the uterus without triggering alarm bells in the mother's defenses. Research continues to uncover new layers of these complexities, revealing how the placenta supports both fetal development and long-term maternal health (Maltepe et al., 2015). The placenta also plays a vital role in guiding how the baby's organs take shape and how its metabolism runs. It even mimics the work usually done by organs like the lungs, liver, and kidneys, ensuring that the supply of food and oxygen is just right. Its design is clever—a broad surface area speeds up the exchange of gases and nutrients while keeping the wall between maternal and fetal blood as thin as possible. In fact, by remodeling the mother's uterine arteries, it tweaks blood flow to meet changing needs. And since the fetal brain is extremely energy-demanding, its needs get extra attention, underscoring, in most cases, the placenta's central role in mammalian development (Graham et al., 2015). Hormones from the placenta mix into the mother's body and have a pretty significant impact. Early on, these hormones help build up the mother's energy reserves, which later get mobilized to support the growing baby. This hormonal chatter kind of syncs the metabolic needs of both, setting up a nurturing environment inside the womb, to some extent. The placenta's ability to adapt—even to challenges like bipedalism—demonstrates its evolutionary knack for handling the unique blood flow dynamics of humans. Of course, these same adaptations sometimes contribute to complications like pre-eclampsia, an issue that appears more frequently in human pregnancies. All in all, the placenta isn't just about keeping the baby alive; it takes an active part in a complex biological symphony that affects immediate fetal growth and influences longer-term changes in the mother (Graham et al., 2015).

7.1. Types of Extraembryonic Membranes

Gestation can be a real juggling act that needs some exceptional support along the way. Extraembryonic membranes—like the yolk sac, amnion, chorion, and allantois—come up unexpectedly to help the embryo get through its early stages. These parts don't just hang around; they each do different jobs that, when mixed, keep development on track. For example, the yolk sac jumps in early to supply nutrients and even kick-starts blood formation, a key step in the embryo's early life. Then the amnion forms a soft, protective cushion that guards against sudden bumps and helps with hydration. At the same time, the chorion and allantois handle the movement of nutrients, waste clearance, and gas exchange—roughly speaking, they work as a loose team to ensure everything goes smoothly. In mammals, the yolk sac gets extra attention during those early days when the mother's nutrient channels aren't fully set up. It's interesting because, in reptiles and birds, the yolk sac is like a bulky storage unit complete of yolk reserves, whereas in mammals it's much more modest. This change hints at a gradual shift toward a more efficient placental system. In most cases, as development progresses, the yolk sac recedes into the background, allowing newer structures to assume the roles of nutrient and gas exchange between the mother and the baby. Meanwhile, the allantois appears later, playing a crucial part in handling waste and even aiding in the formation of the umbilical cord. Such gradual role changes not only move and demonstrate the adaptability of these membranes but also highlight the complexity of transitioning from embryonic to fetal life. The chorion stands out as a significant bridge between the mother and the embryo. Built from trophoblast cells that invade the maternal tissue, it creates a network of blood vessels that smooths the exchange of nutrients and gases. This delicate dance of signals and immune checks helps ensure the embryo is both fed and protected. In addition, recent research has highlighted that various mesenchymal stem cells (MSCs) derived from the placenta may offer promising potential for regenerative medicine applications. All in all, these extraembryonic membranes combine in a way that's a bit unpredictable and uniquely human—working together to secure a successful pregnancy outcome (Hass et al., 2011; Zakrzewski et al., 2019) (Figure 7.3).

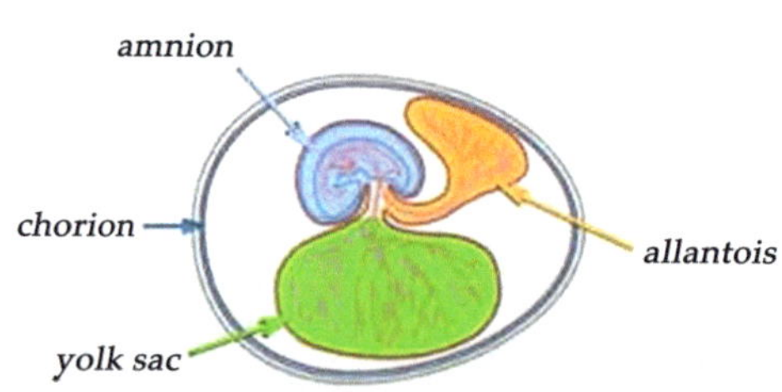

Figure 7.3. Types of extraembryonic membranes.

Source: https://study.com/cimages/multimages/16/Extraembryonic-Membranes-In-Egg-Laying-Vertebrates.jpg.

7.1.1. Amnion and Its Protective Role

The amnion takes center stage in setting up a safe, nurturing environment for the growing embryo. It creates a fluid-filled sac that cradles the embryo and absorbs sudden mechanical impacts that might disrupt development. In those early stages of gestation, when the embryo is extra delicate, this cushioning matters. The amniotic fluid inside not only maintains a steady temperature but also supplies the hydration needed to keep things running smoothly. All of these little jobs help create conditions that are just right for growth, stressing how vital the amnion is in mammalian reproduction. Beyond simply acting as a basic protective barrier, the amnion becomes involved in the biochemical environment surrounding the embryo.

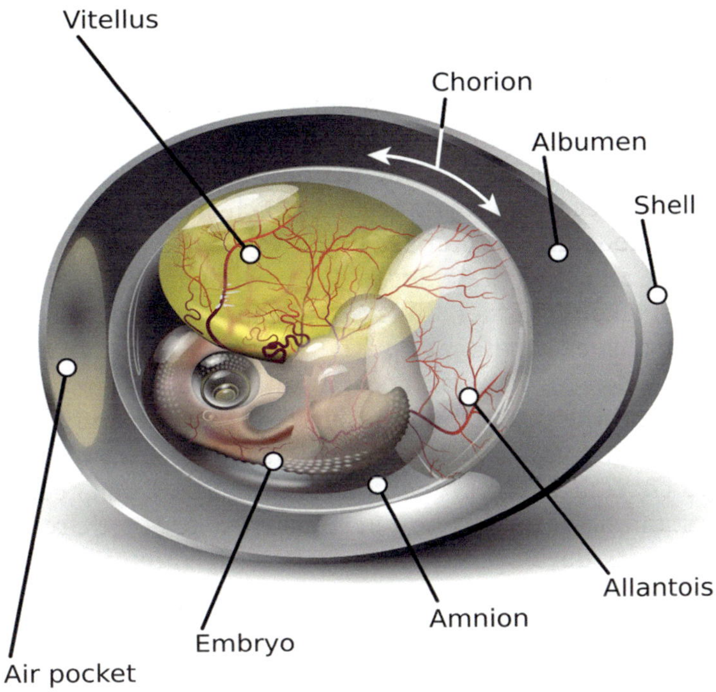

Figure 7.4. Amnion.

Source: https://upload.wikimedia.org/wikipedia/commons/2/20/Chicken_egg_diagram.svg.

It generates various factors—and yes, this occurs repeatedly—to help establish the molecular environment crucial for development. For instance, recent studies generally speaking show that it supplies growth factors and cytokines which aid tissue repair and boost cell multiplication. Its role has even expanded beyond simple protection during embryogenesis; now, in clinical settings, the amnion is being integrated into regenerative medicine, showing promise in wound healing and tissue engineering applications (Elkhenany et al., 2022). By offering a kind of natural, biocompatible scaffold, it stitches together developmental biology with therapeutic possibilities. Recent advances in embryology and regenerative medicine have further highlighted the amnion's protective functions. Comparative research across different mammalian models has helped unravel the secrets of human embryonic growth; these studies suggest that the amnion's method of shielding the embryo may be a common strategy in nature. In most cases, these fundamental processes appear to function similarly across species, suggesting some basic biological principles. This broader investigative framework not only reiterates the amnion's essential role but also sparks ideas for potential treatments that tap into its unique properties in clinical practice. Thus, exploring extraembryonic membranes, such as the amnion, deepens the conversation on their vital contributions to both developmental biology and regenerative therapies (Gerri et al., 2020) (Figure 7.4).

7.1.2. Chorion and Its Function in Nutrient Exchange

In early embryonic life, a smooth nutrient transfer is a must, and the chorion – that extra layer outside the embryo – steps up to make it happen. It starts working relatively early, around implantation, when it penetrates the mother's tissues to form a crucial link with the placenta. As the pregnancy rolls on, the chorion acts like a selective barrier, managing which essential metabolites and gases move from the mother's bloodstream to the growing embryo. This process, although complex, helps the embryo obtain sufficient fuel for its rapid growth, setting the stage nicely for proper embryogenesis. The chorion isn't just sitting there; it's actively involved in making some crucial biomolecules. It churns out proteins and hormones that help create a cozy environment for the developing baby. Sometimes, it secretes growth factors which encourage new blood vessel formation in the placenta – a bit like boosting the nutrient highway. It also plays a role in modulating the mother's immune response, allowing the embryo to grow even when conditions aren't perfectly favorable. All these actions, taken together, underscore a kind of dynamic back-and-forth between the chorion and maternal tissues, highlighting its significant role in healthy gestation. Studies have generally shown that when the chorion doesn't function at its best, complications can arise, affecting both the embryo and the mother. Conditions like intrauterine growth restriction (IUGR) often occur due to issues in the chorion or placenta, resulting in a lack of vital nutrients. This marks how essential the chorion is for proper placentation and balanced nutrient exchange on both sides. As our understanding of the chorion deepens, recent genetic research has revealed that more genes are involved in its development than previously thought (Woods et al., 2018). This growing insight into chorionic mechanisms might just open up new ways to address pregnancy complications and improve reproductive outcomes (Figure 7.5).

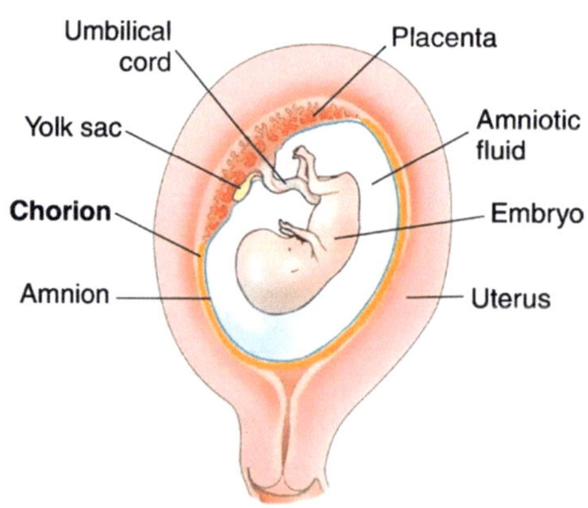

Figure 7.5. Chorion.

Source: https://cdn-ildfibj.nitrocdn.com/qaWeLntkRcyxNUcEoWbLpZLQkcgLFsiJ/assets/images/optimized/www.biologyonline.com/wp-content/uploads/2021/09/Structure-of-Chorion.png.

7.1.3. Yolk Sac and Its Role in Early Blood Cell Formation

Early on, embryo growth depends on a mix of parts and functions—and the yolk sac quickly emerges as the standout in making blood cells. This extraembryonic membrane appears early and becomes the primary site for blood cell formation before more complex blood-making organs are even established. In most cases, without this early boost, the embryo wouldn't have the right cells to carry oxygen or shuttle nutrients when it needs them. It's interesting to note that the yolk sac also teems with unique MSCs, which help form blood vessels, ensuring the little one can continue until the placenta takes over (Mançanares et al., 2019).

One cannot overlook that the yolk sac's blood cell-making knack is tied to its two different inner layers—the parietal and visceral endoderms. These layers not only hold things together but also gently guide the embryo along by providing the necessary support and facilitating the transition to placental function. In most cases, research suggests that the visceral layer, in particular, is rich in factors such as SOX17, a key protein that helps maintain cell identity during those early, fragile moments. All in all, the yolk sac ends up wearing two hats—both feeding the embryo and jump-starting the blood-making process (Igarashi et al., 2018). As gestation moves on, the placenta gradually takes over, and the yolk sac starts to fade from the spotlight. Still, its early work in generating blood cells is hard to ignore since it lays the groundwork for everything that follows. The overall health of the embryo often hinges on how well these early blood cells function, which is why the yolk sac remains crucial in those initial stages. Generally speaking, understanding these processes not only sheds some light on congenital issues but also opens up new avenues for therapies that target those early developmental paths. The yolk sac continues to be a key focus in studying extraembryonic membranes and placental development (Mançanares et al., 2019) (Figure 7.6).

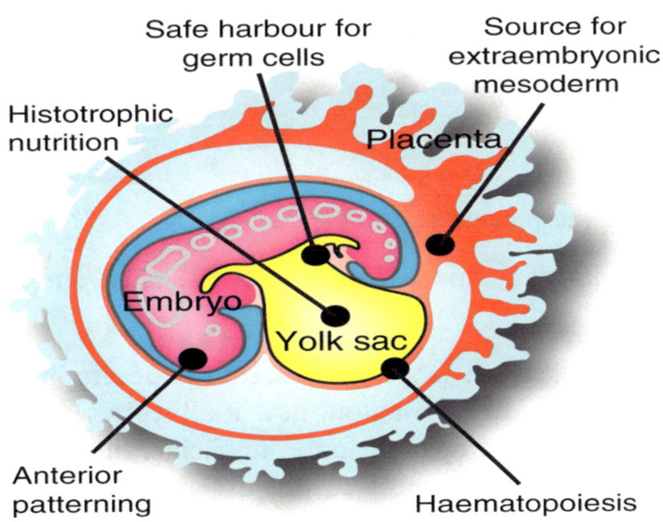

Figure 7.6. Yolk sac.

Source: https://media.springernature.com/lw1200/springer-static/image/art%3A10.1038%2Fs41467-020-17575-w/MediaObjects/41467_2020_17575_Fig6_HTML.png.

7.2. Development of the Placenta

Placenta formation is essential for an embryo's early growth—it makes sure the fetus gets the nutrients, oxygen, and even handles waste removal. A lot of this comes down to how the mother and fetus tissues mix; this interaction builds a kind of barrier, often called the feto-maternal interface, that selectively passes molecules. This filtering process is seen in many mammals, which strongly suggests that evolution has highly valued this system.

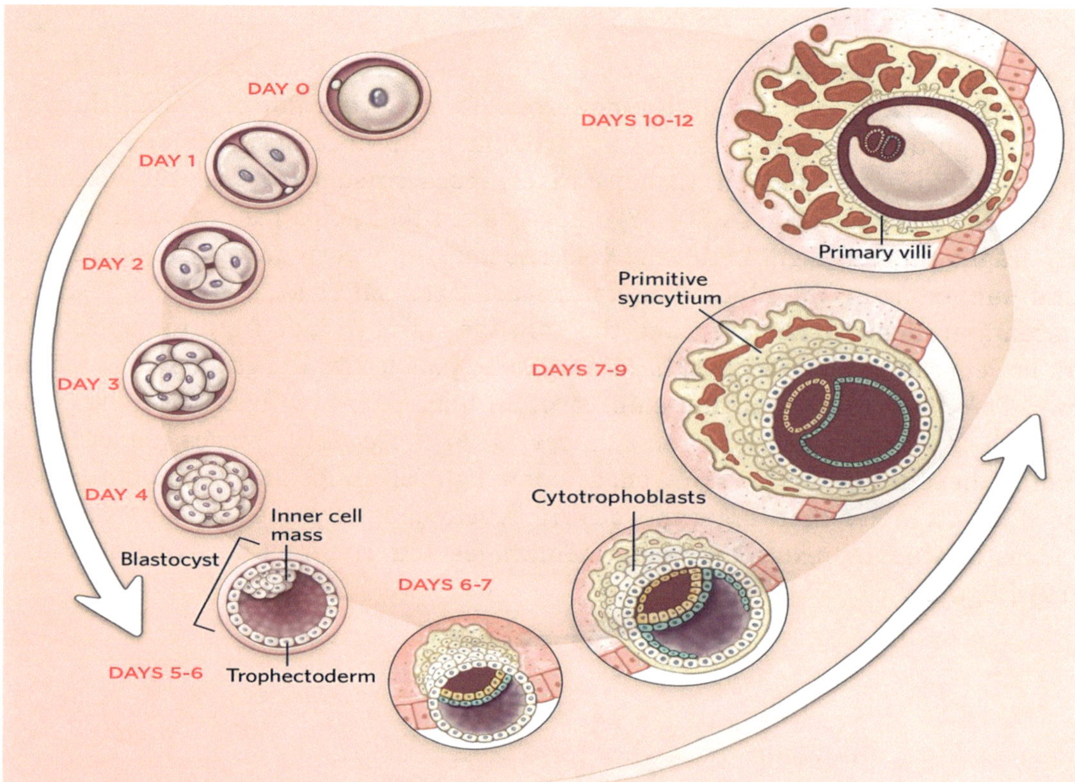

Figure 7.7. Development of the placenta.

Source: https://cdn.the-scientist.com/assets/articleNo/71518/iImg/51622/12-23-placenta-infographic-online-l.jpg.

Suppose something goes off track while the placenta is developing. In that case, it can lead to severe developmental setbacks, so figuring out how it all works is key not just for embryology but also for better handling placental dysfunction in medicine. Understanding the signaling trails that steer placental development is, in most cases, just as crucial—especially when one looks at protease activity and how cells chat with one another in these tissues. Recent studies have highlighted that specific serine proteases, such as matriptase and prostasin, play a crucial role in establishing the feto-maternal barrier. These proteins trigger signals that stimulate blood vessel growth, essential for nutrient exchange and ultimately, embryo survival. Research in mice even suggests that the physical interactions alongside these intricate signaling networks are indispensable for the placenta to work correctly, hinting at a complex biochemical dance behind its development.

At the same time, the overall effectiveness of the placental barrier also hinges on how well tight junction proteins, such as claudin-1, are expressed. Generally speaking, these proteins are crucial for maintaining the integrity of epithelial layers; even a slight deficiency can compromise the barrier and have severe consequences for the developing embryo. Moreover, since some signaling routes overlap, any disruption in proteins like matriptase or in receptors such as PAR-2 tends to cause notable problems, leading to both placental and embryonic complications (Zakrzewski et al., 2019). Examining these pathways not only broadens our understanding of reproductive biology but also reveals new avenues for therapeutic interventions in placental disorders, underscoring the ongoing need for advanced research in this area (Zakrzewski et al., 2019) (Figure 7.7).

7.2.1. Formation of the Placenta from Trophoblast Cells

Human embryonic development is a marvel of cell transitions and specialization—almost like an unpredictable dance. Right after fertilization, a blastocyst appears that holds two core groups of cells: the inner cell mass (ICM) (destined to form the embryo) and the trophoblast, which later builds the placenta. Trophoblast cells rapidly adapt and morph into various subtypes to establish their position within the maternal uterus.

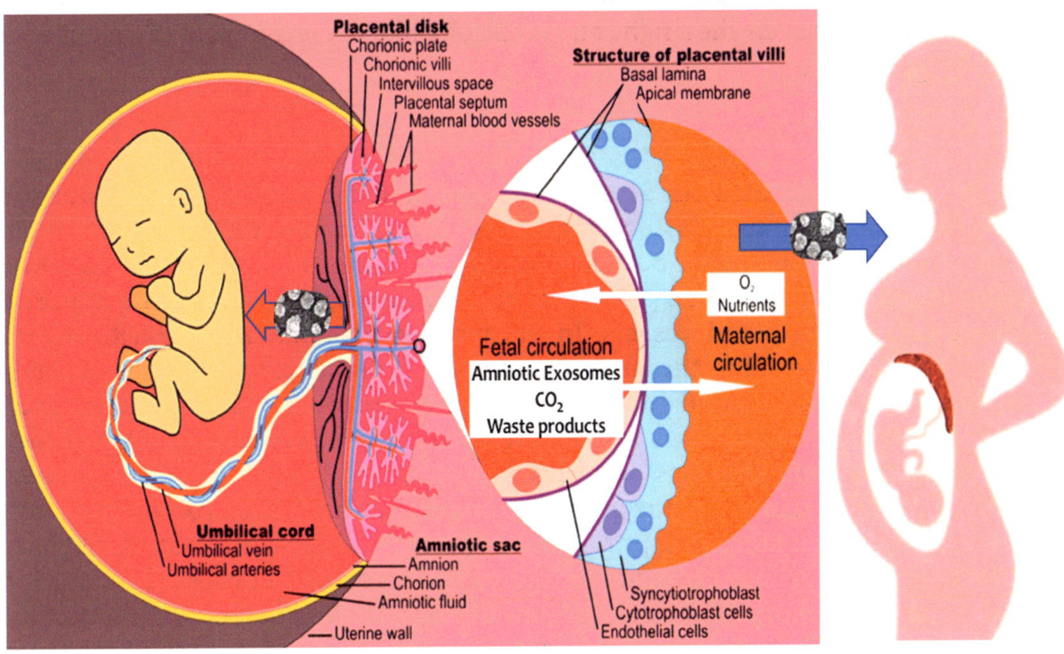

Figure 7.8. Formation of the placenta from trophoblast cells.

Source: https://stemcellthailand.org/wp-content/uploads/2014/01/placenta-development-human.jpg.webp.

This change is vital because these cells burrow into the uterine lining and create tight connections with the mother's blood vessels, allowing for the exchange of nutrients and oxygen necessary for the developing fetus. In many cases, the lively interactions between these cells and the surrounding maternal tissues set the stage just right for fetal growth. Specific signaling routes play a bigger role than one might initially expect in steering how trophoblasts develop. Research generally indicates that inhibiting Activin/Nodal signaling prompts human embryonic stem cells (hESCs) to adopt the trophoblast pathway. Often, these cells respond to subtle cues by gradually shifting their fate until they start showing markers typical of placental tissue. Notably, BMP signaling comes into action just as the Activin/Nodal cues are held back, highlighting a mix of signals that keeps the entire process balanced.

This interplay is crucial for ensuring that trophoblasts mature properly, and such carefully graded signals are key for forming placental structures responsible for nutrient delivery and waste removal during pregnancy. Ultimately, shaping the placenta from trophoblast cells involves assembling several distinct layers and features that facilitate smooth maternal–fetal communication. Current research highlights that the placenta's design is optimized to maximize oxygen and nutrient transfer, thanks to its vast surface area in conjunction with a fragile interhemal membrane. As time goes on, the trophoblast layer matures into syncytiotrophoblast—a barrier that delicately manages maternal immune responses while still letting essential substances pass through. Additionally, these cells produce hormones that play a critical role in sustaining pregnancy and helping the mother adapt, for example, by boosting nutrient storage and metabolism. Given the placenta's intricate build and varied functions, understanding how trophoblasts evolve offers essential insights into reproductive health and may even shed light on conditions like pre-eclampsia (Graham et al., 2015; Wu et al., 2008) (Figure 7.8).

7.2.2. Stages of Placental Development During Pregnancy

The placenta's formation kicks off with a series of steps that matter for a successful pregnancy. Early on, trophoblast cells from the blastocyst split into two groups—the syncytiotrophoblast and the cytotrophoblast—which then reach out to the mother's lining. This initial interaction isn't just a simple meeting; it sparks a short-lived phase where the cells begin to invade the maternal tissue, setting up a basic network of blood vessels. In most cases, proteins such as TRIML2 appear to play a beneficial role by fine-tuning the inflammatory response during this early bonding stage, which in turn helps establish a solid foundation for both placental development and smooth maternal-fetal connections (Emily et al., 2025). All in all, this phase lays the groundwork for a more elaborate vascular system as things progress. After implantation, things take a dramatic turn. Around the end of the first trimester, the placenta undergoes a kind of robust remodeling. The internal blood vessel network starts adapting, and a strong umbilical circulation begins to form, which is key for the baby's growth. It's interesting to observe how, during this period, both the secondary yolk sac and the chorioallantoic placenta develop their blood supply networks, linking up with the maternal flow (Burton et al., 2018). At the same time, placental villi show up—these structures are crucial because they help nutrients and gases get exchanged. The entire process is highly dynamic; the placenta must adjust to changing nutritional and hormonal signals from the mother while meeting the increasing needs of the developing fetus. As the pregnancy moves further along, the placenta reaches a point where it's mature and finely tuned to the fetus's needs. Around 12 to 14 weeks, there's a noticeable boost in placental blood flow that lowers resistance in its circulation—an adjustment that's pretty much essential for the baby's heart and overall development (Burton et al., 2018). At this stage, the vascular architecture becomes even more intricate, with an extensive web of capillaries that boost both gas exchange and nutrient delivery. Meanwhile, proteins like TRIML1 and TRIML2 continue to play a vital role, helping the placenta manage stress from oxidation and ensuring it functions smoothly to support both maternal and fetal health throughout the remainder of the pregnancy (Emily et al., 2025) (Figure 7.9).

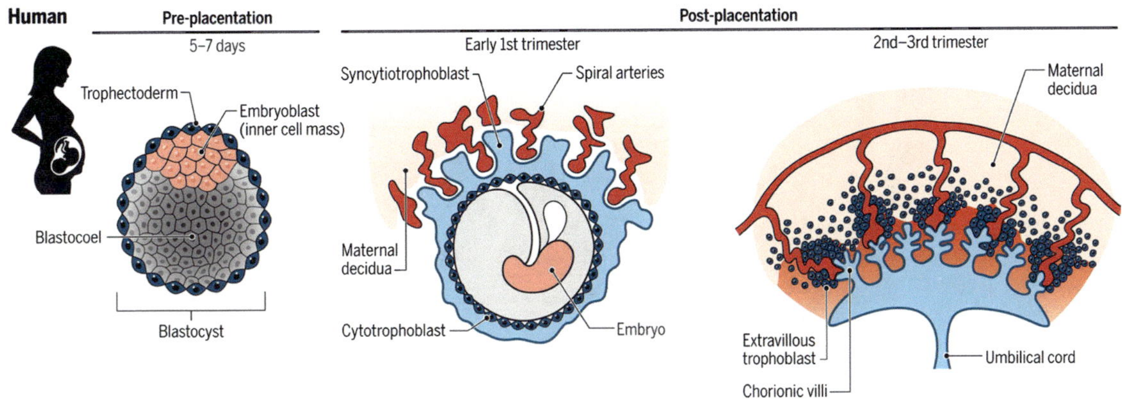

Figure 7.9. Stages of placental development during pregnancy.

Source: https://www.researchgate.net/publication/368680745/figure/fig1/AS:11431281258752692@1720128085374/Stages-pre-and-post-placentation-of-placenta-development-12.tif.

7.2.3. Role of Maternal Tissues in Placental Formation

Maternal tissues and the growing placenta mix in a way that's both complex and crucial for a healthy pregnancy. The endometrium, for instance, suddenly shifts its structure to help the placenta form. At the same time, the syncytiotrophoblast—the outer layer—pushes into the uterine lining, setting up those key maternal–fetal links. This push not only secures the placenta but also kick-starts changes in the mother's blood vessels so that the fetus gets enough oxygen and nutrients. A variety of cytokines and growth factors, coming from both the mother and the embryo, generally keep this process in check, which in many cases underlines nature's clever tweaks for supporting a growing baby. The way these maternal tissues change is at the heart of meeting the unique demands of fetal growth. Uterine arteries, for example, often undergo dilation and structural changes as the placenta develops, increasing blood flow. This adjustment isn't just a reaction to the physical pressures of a growing fetus; it also mirrors a subtle interplay of hormonal signals. Placental hormones encourage the mother's metabolism to shift to balance nutrient availability. The tissues' ability to adapt not only fuels the pregnancy but also plays a significant role in overall placental development, ultimately affecting fetal health in a somewhat interconnected fashion. On a related note, the maternal immune system exhibits surprising flexibility during placental formation, managing to protect while still accommodating fetal growth. The unique immune setting during pregnancy allows both maternal and fetal elements to coexist; trophoblast cells, for example, have evolved ways to modulate the mother's immune response—preventing the fetus from being rejected. Immune players, such as regulatory T cells, help sustain a tolerant environment, even when the genetic makeup of the placenta is distinctly different. This delicate balancing act is key, particularly when the maternal and fetal tissues sometimes clash. In most cases, examining these intertwined relationships provides valuable insight into complications such as pre-eclampsia, which can emerge when these careful processes go awry (Graham et al., 2015; Bangs et al., 2016) (Figure 7.10).

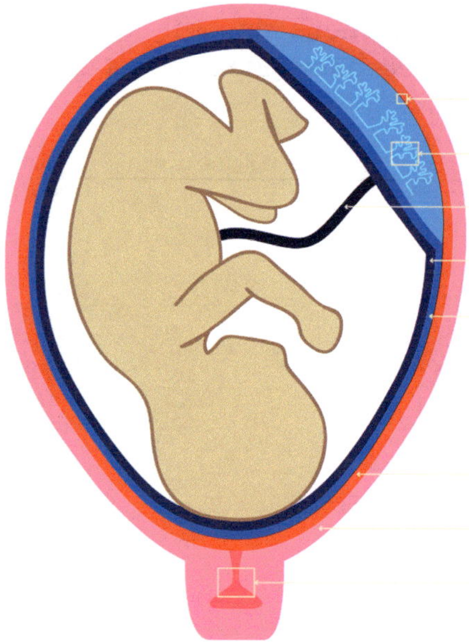

Figure 7.10. Role of maternal tissues in placental formation.

Source: https://www.researchgate.net/publication/277801598/figure/fig4/AS:267659585519674@1440826426894/The-tissues-of-pregnancy-Our-systematic-literature-review-surveyed-a-total-of-9-distinct.png.

7.3. Functions of the Placenta

The placenta stands out as one of those fascinating organs that does more than one might expect. It isn't just a bridge between a mother and her baby; rather, it juggles several key jobs. For instance, it carries oxygen and essential nutrients from the mother's blood to the growing fetus while at the same time clearing away wastes and even creating hormones. In many cases, moving these vital elements around ensures steady growth throughout gestation. It also works like a barrier, filtering out some harmful pathogens and softening certain specific maternal immune responses, so that the environment remains as safe as possible for the developing child. All this shows that the placenta isn't merely a passive link but, indeed, an active actor that has evolved to suit live-bearing species. But there's more to the story. Besides shielding and nourishing the fetus, the placenta turns out to be a crucial hormone factory. Hormones such as human chorionic gonadotropin (hCG) and progesterone are produced here; these chemicals generally help prevent additional ovulation and maintain the uterus's stability. They also adjust the mother's metabolism—reconfiguring her body to meet the ever-growing demands of her baby—and even fine-tune her cardiovascular system to allow for ample blood flow to the uterus. Altogether, this intricate hormonal interplay establishes a sort of conversation between mother and fetus, underscoring that the placenta plays an active role in orchestrating the numerous complex processes essential for a healthy pregnancy. In early development, the placenta also dives into another set of critical duties. It helps shape several extraembryonic structures that support growth along the way. Take the yolk sac, for example; even though it is only temporary in some species, it remains crucial during the embryonic period by absorbing nutrients and initiating early blood formation. Then there's the allantois—which, in its various forms across species, seems to influence gene expression and blood vessel development. As researchers continue to investigate these differences, it becomes increasingly clear that the placenta does far more than sustain life—it actively shapes the developmental pathway of organisms (Hassan et al., 2017; Shibata et al., 2023) (Figure 7.11).

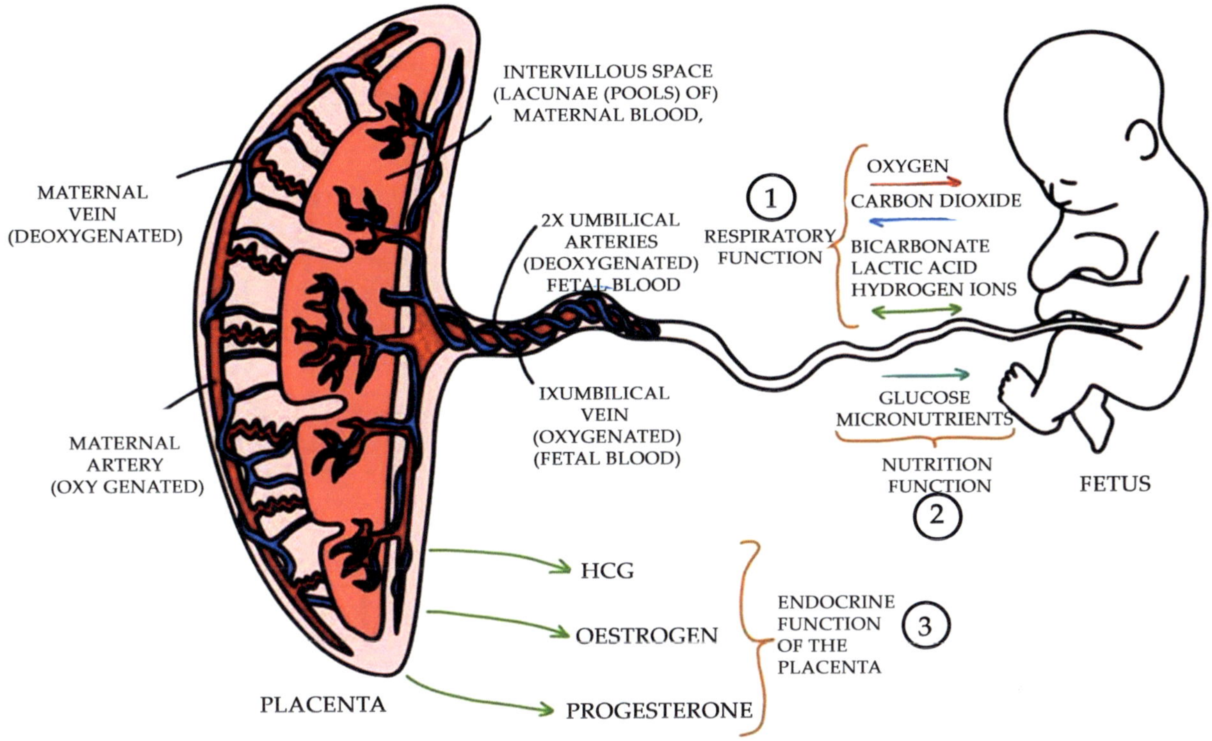

Figure 7.11. Function of the placenta.

Source: https://zerotofinals.com/wp-content/uploads/Placenta-1024x576.jpg.

7.3.1. Nutrient Transfer from Mother to Fetus

The placenta plays a wild role during pregnancy – it's not just a barrier but the very bridge that shuttles life's essentials between mother and baby. It sits at the center of the maternal and fetal bloodstreams, passing on key nutrients such as oxygen, glucose, and amino acids. Even a minor glitch in this handoff can sometimes lead to issues like IUGR. Lately, it turns out that a whole mix of genes is up to the task, weaving a pretty complex web behind nutrient transfer. In brief, a sound placental function lays the groundwork for a healthy pregnancy, while a lagging one can hurt both the baby and the mother (Woods et al., 2018). Take a closer look at those placental cells – the trophoblasts – which seem to be running the show. These cells infiltrate the maternal blood vessels and carve out a specialized niche that even quiets the mother's immune response, helping the genetically distinct fetus to thrive. They handle nutrient uptake and waste disposal in a highly selective and controlled manner. New insights into their differentiation and function suggest deep connections with fetal metabolism and overall health. It's almost as if these cells are orchestrating an intricate balance, rather than simply acting as a barrier (Maltepe et al., 2015). But the placenta's influence goes way beyond immediate nutrient transfer. Its efficiency—or lack thereof—can significantly impact the baby's long-term health by influencing metabolic programming and affecting broader developmental outcomes. When placental function falters due to defects, nutrient delivery suffers, which in most cases links to an increased risk of cardiovascular and metabolic issues later on. Recent research is slowly mapping out the critical pathways that underlie this effect, showing just how much placental physiology lays the groundwork for a healthier postnatal life. As studies shift from animal models to human implications, it becomes increasingly clear that maintaining the placenta in good working order is crucial for managing pregnancy complications (Maltepe et al., 2015; Woods et al., 2018) (Figure 7.12).

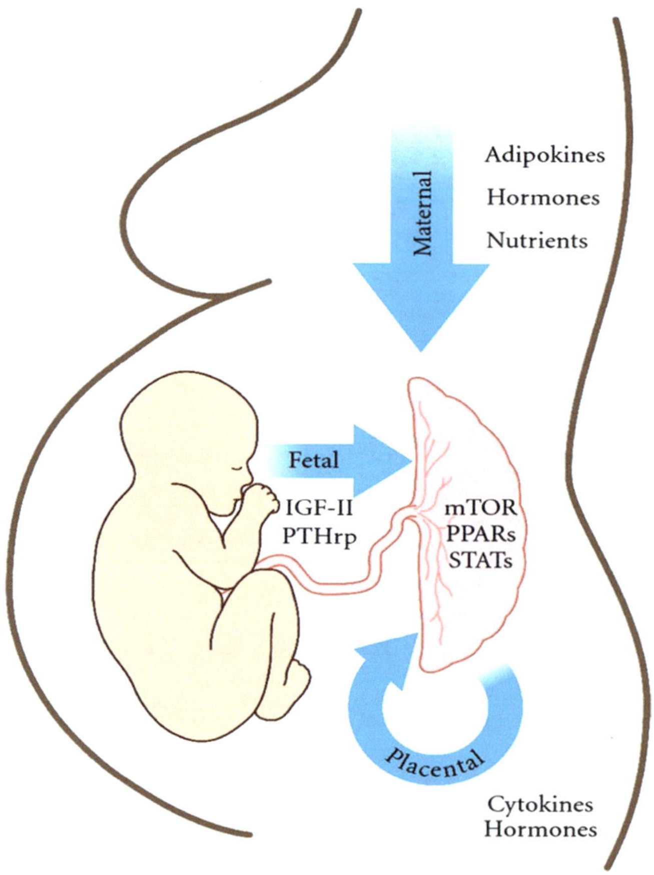

Figure 7.12. Nutrient transfer from mother to fetus.

Source: https://onlinelibrary.wiley.com/cms/asset/5626a96d-41d2-41cd-8d5f-251dfd8d8872/jp179827-fig-0002-m.jpg.

7.3.2. Gas Exchange and Waste Removal

Gas exchange and waste removal in early development happen through some pretty unique structures. The embryo grows in an environment where, generally speaking, the placenta serves as a crucial intermediary—supplying oxygen and nutrients while also removing unwanted byproducts. There are these tiny, branching surfaces—placental villi—that boost the area available for diffusion, and the placenta's rich blood supply from the mother makes sure that conditions stay just right for the baby. In a clever evolutionary move, this system balances both intake and clean-up, keeping the developing embryo safe in a controlled setting. Trophoblasts, those key cells in the placental mix, add another layer to the story. They not only help absorb the nutrients needed for growth but also remodel maternal blood vessels to handle the increased flow demanded by the embryo. Remarkably, these cells seem to dodge the mother's immune responses—a subtle trick that ensures the exchange process is left undisturbed. This tolerance, which is essential given that the genetics come from both parents, means oxygen, nutrients, and waste removal continue smoothly, underscoring the delicate balance during gestation. Recent research has shed even more light on the mystery behind these processes. Studies now highlight unexpected interactions between the mother's tissues and those of the fetus, offering fresh insights into how the placenta manages both gas exchange and waste elimination. In most cases, these findings not only deepen our understanding of placental function but also point to potential ways to address complications such as preeclampsia and intrauterine growth restriction. The placenta isn't just a passive structure—it actively shapes long-term health for both mother and child, a role that modern discoveries increasingly confirm (Maltepe et al., 2015; Camilla et al., 2020).

7.3.3. Hormonal Functions and Their Impact on Pregnancy

Pregnancy triggers a whirlwind of hormones that help both the mother and her embryo adjust and grow. Immediately after the embryo settles in, a key hormone called human chorionic gonadotropin (hCG) begins to flow from the trophoblastic cells. In most cases, hCG doesn't just keep the corpus luteum busy—it also cranks up progesterone production, which in turn helps hold the uterine lining in place and stops menstruation. This mix of hormones sets up a friendly environment for the baby and nudges changes in the mother's body, easing nutrient sharing and tweaking metabolism. There's a kind of back-and-forth chat between the extraembryonic membranes and the maternal endocrine system that quietly lays the groundwork for what comes next. As the pregnancy progresses, other hormones take center stage unexpectedly. Take estriol, for instance—a steroid produced by the placenta that plays a pretty crucial role in smoothing out uteroplacental circulation and keeping the uterus relaxed. This connection between the placenta and hormone control is further illustrated when hormones like progesterone and relaxin join the process, preparing the mother's body for labor and regulating uterine contractions. Generally speaking, these hormones balance out to signal how well the pregnancy is holding together, all thanks to a system of natural feedback loops running between the placenta and the extraembryonic membranes. Recent studies have shown that the placenta isn't just a passive bridge for exchanging nutrients; it's an active hormone hub with a diverse mix of cells. New research using single-cell transcriptomics has revealed distinct cell types within the human placenta, each contributing its unique contribution to hormonal secretion and immune function (Suryawanshi et al., 2018; Ross et al., 2020). This cellular variety suggests that if the delicate hormone balance gets thrown off, complications such as preeclampsia or gestational diabetes might occur. In most cases, understanding these hormonal interactions in the placental microenvironment proves key to grasping how extraembryonic membranes, including even the yolk sac, contribute to keeping the gestational journey on track—even if the picture isn't always perfectly tidy (Figure 7.13).

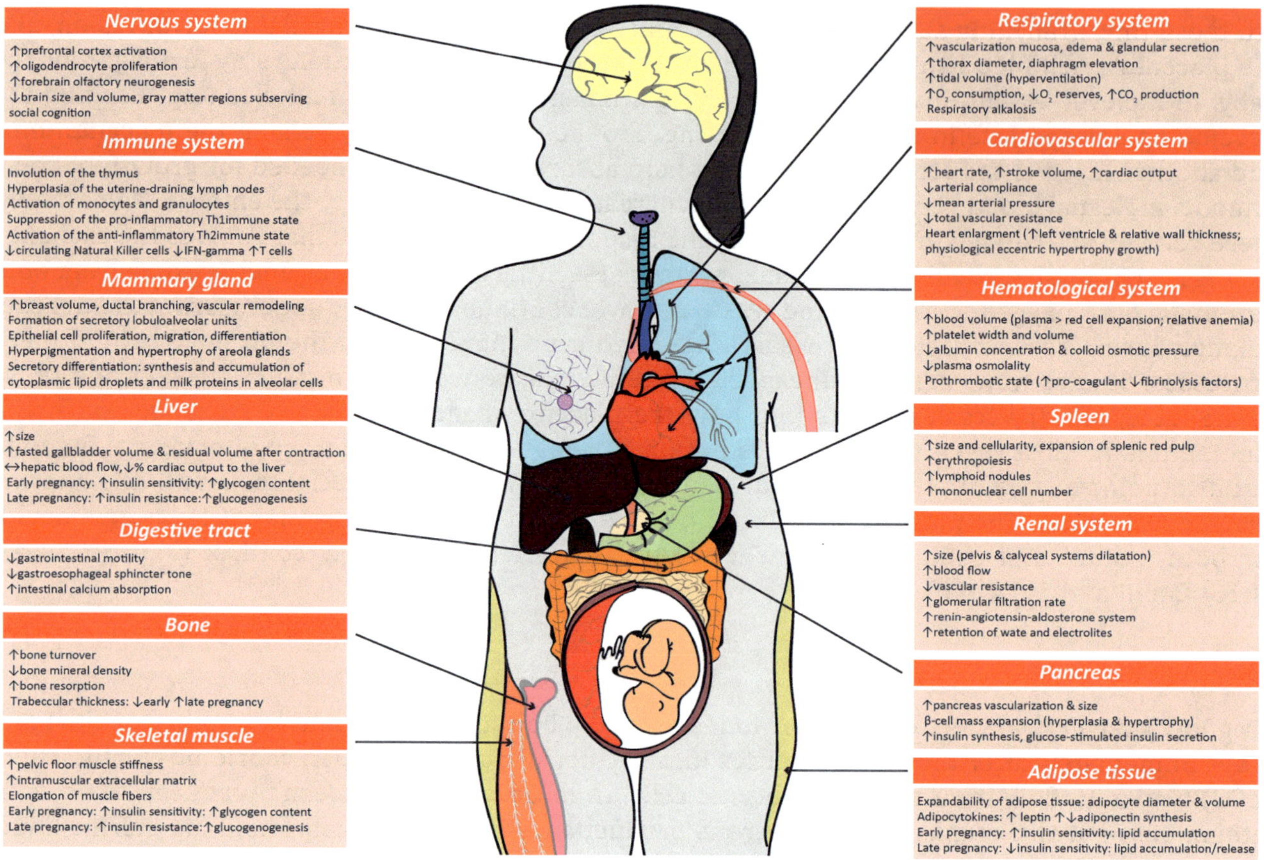

Figure 7.13. Hormonal functions and their impact on pregnancy.

Source: https://www.frontiersin.org/files/Articles/387601/fphys-09-01091-HTML/image_m/fphys-09-01091-g001.jpg.

7.4. Placental Structure

Embryonic development depends on the placenta—it acts as a bridge between mother and baby. It isn't just sitting there passively; it helps manage nutrient exchange, gas transport, and even facilitates waste removal. It's made up of mostly trophoblast cells that mingle with the mother's tissues, keeping the placenta firmly attached to the uterine wall. Then there are the villous structures, which increase the available surface area for rapid transfers and highlight how this intricate design supports both maternal systems and the baby's growth. In most cases, understanding this structure is crucial, as it establishes vital roles such as hormone signaling, which generally influence the mother's health and the overall pregnancy outcome. Looking closer under a microscope, the placenta reveals a fascinating mix of tissues that seem to come together in a natural, yet unpredictable, way to sustain life. The chorionic villi, with tiny fetal capillaries hidden inside, extend into pools of maternal blood—creating a kind of circulation that thankfully avoids direct blood-to-blood contact. This design usually helps lower the chance of the mother's immune system turning against the baby while still ensuring oxygen and nutrients are passed along. Plus, that special syncytiotrophoblast layer doesn't just stand guard; it also gets involved in hormonal actions that adjust how the mother's metabolism works. Every layer has its specific functions and processes, highlighting how the placenta adapts to meet the developing fetus's needs, and overall, it's essential for a successful, healthy pregnancy. When things go awry, placental issues highlight why its detailed structure matters so much. Abnormal development or function of the placenta can cause serious problems for both mother and child—from limited growth to neurological deficits, among other concerns. Studies generally indicate that when the placenta's integrity is compromised, the transfer of necessary nutrients suffers, which highlights its role as more than just a basic support system. Researchers are now investigating the robustness of placental tissues and their associated stem cells, potentially opening up new avenues for treating these complications. As the scientific community continues to unravel the many layers of placental biology, it is clear that understanding these details is crucial for improving maternal-fetal health outcomes (Bangs et al., 2016; Zakrzewski et al., 2019) (Figure 7.14).

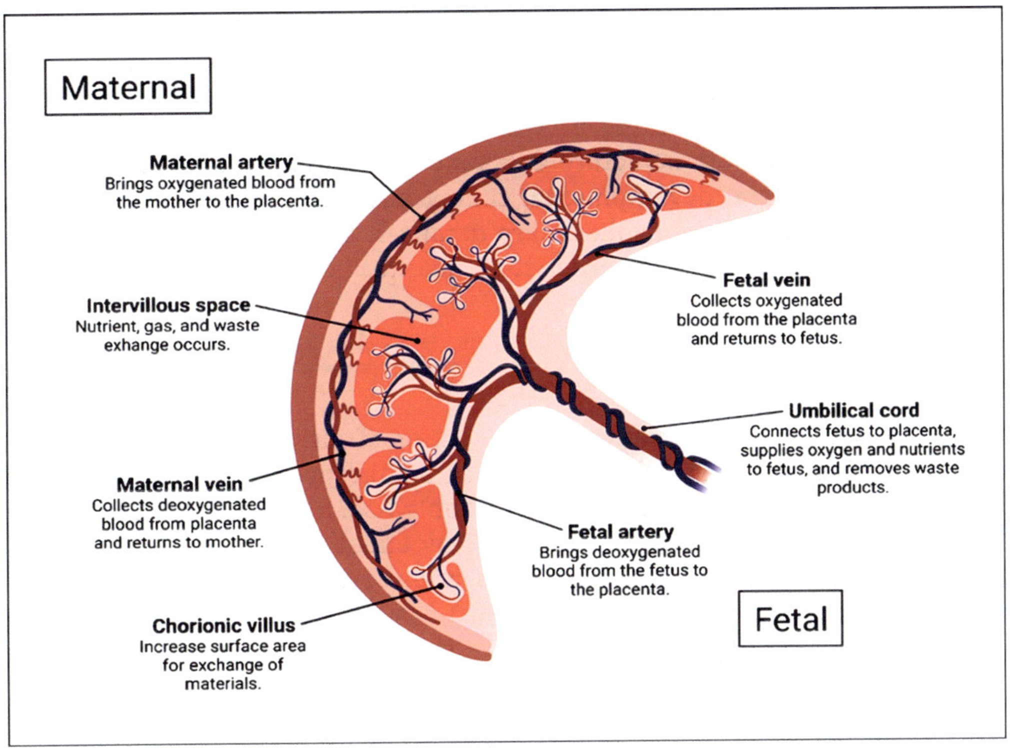

Figure 7.14. Human placental structure.

Source: https://www.researchgate.net/publication/366017486/figure/fig2/AS:114312811156827 52@1675052186865/Human-placental-structure-and-function.png.

7.4.1. Layers of the Placenta and Their Significance

The placenta's design is fascinating—a busy bridge linking a mother with her developing embryo. It isn't just a simple wall; instead, its layered setup quietly manages vital exchanges, such as passing on nutrients and eliminating waste. Right on the outer edge sits the chorion, which not only helps form the placenta but also chats, in a manner of speaking, with the mother's immune cells. At the same time, the allantois becomes involved in forming new blood vessels and eliminating waste, eventually developing into the structure that anchors the umbilical cord. Interestingly, differences in allantoic development across species seem to hint at evolutionary adaptations that affect nutrient sharing and the arrangement of blood vessels (Hassan et al., 2017). Understanding this layered arrangement can, generally speaking, offer us clues about the placenta's remarkable roles across various mammals—and its impact on both fetal development and maternal health. The layers don't just handle nutrients and waste; they also help steer the immune environment during pregnancy. The decidua, which originates from the maternal side, creates a space where immune cells—such as natural killer cells and macrophages—take up positions to support the pregnancy. These cells aren't merely hanging around; they often interact dynamically with both the mother and the embryo, playing a crucial role in embryo implantation and maintaining a delicate immune balance. In most cases, a slip in this careful balance might lead to complications like preeclampsia or even spontaneous abortion. Research into how immune cells function at the maternal-fetal boundary has revealed that they can sometimes be both protective and problematic (Erlebacher, 2013). Across different mammals, the varied nature of placental layers tells its evolutionary story. Consider the allantois, which differs noticeably between species; its size and shape often reflect the distinct reproductive strategies and environmental demands of each species. This diversity doesn't just broaden our understanding of what the placenta does; it also underscores how evolutionary pressures shape both structure and function. Differences in placentation can affect not only nutrient allocation and developmental timing but also the overall viability of offspring. As studies continue to dig into these evolutionary details, it becomes clear that the placenta, with all its layers, offers key insights into reproductive health and evolutionary biology (Erlebacher, 2013; Hassan et al., 2017).

7.4.2. Vascularization and Blood Supply

Vascularization and blood supply shape the very foundation of early life. Extraembryonic membranes like the chorion, yolk sac, amnion, and allantois kick off the process by building a network that moves nutrients and gases around—a setup that not only boosts the embryo's growth but also lets the maternal and fetal circulatory systems mingle. Tiny endothelial cells lining these vessels help control what seeps through, effectively acting as a barrier between mother and baby. All in all, this patchwork of blood vessels shows, in most cases, just how finely tuned placental design is during early gestation. As the embryo grows, the placenta gradually morphs into a highly vascularized organ that reliably delivers oxygen and nutrients to the fetus. New blood vessels form through angiogenesis, a process generally guided by different elements in the ECM. The ECM isn't just a block of structure; it quietly steers cell signals that drive angiogenesis. Key proteins—such as collagens, laminins, and others—sculpt a microenvironment that nudges endothelial cells to differentiate and multiply, thereby laying down the paths for a complex vascular network. This blend of blood vessel formation and ECM action, in most cases, opens up potential therapeutic routes for placental insufficiency (Nikos et al., 2021). Stem cells add another fascinating layer to the picture of vascular development in extraembryonic tissues, particularly when forming placental structures. The way these cells branch out into endothelial and vascular smooth muscle cells is crucial for establishing the intricate blood supply a healthy placenta depends on. Recent advances in stem cell therapy and the engineering of biomaterials—including, surprisingly, graphene scaffolds—offer promising new routes to enhance vascular maturity. Researchers are harnessing extracellular vesicle-based approaches to optimize stem cell behavior, aiming to create networks that mimic natural placental development. This line of work, promising for tackling issues of poor vascularization that can affect both maternal and fetal health, points the way toward breakthroughs in reproductive medicine and therapies for placental dysfunction (Zakrzewski et al., 2019) (Figure 7.15).

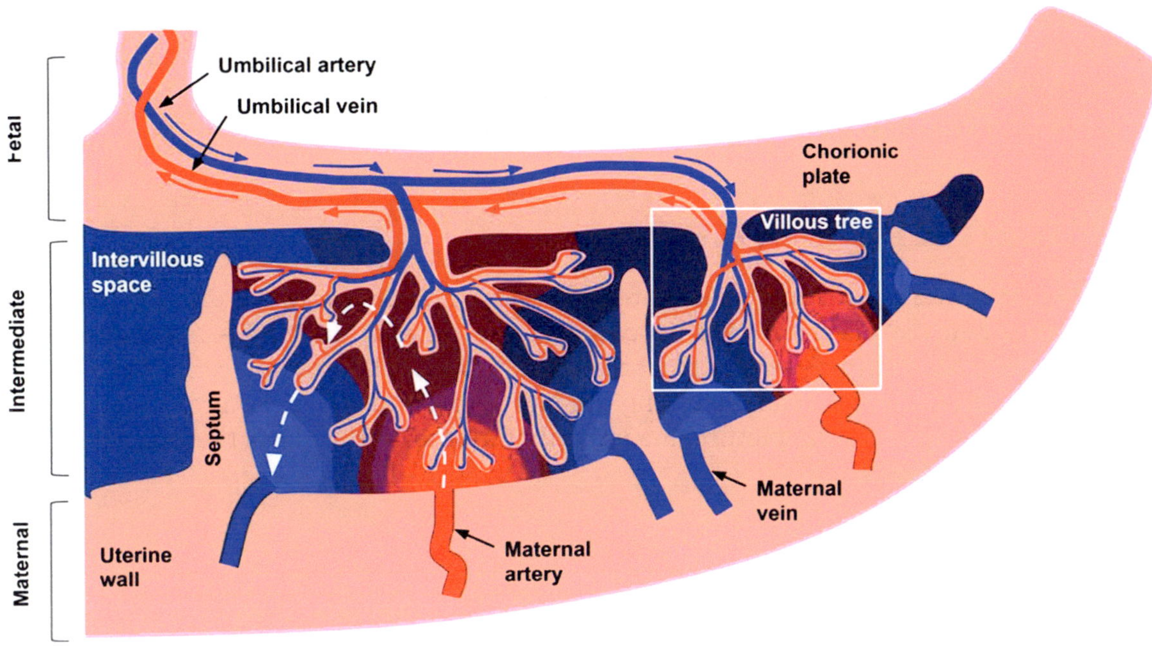

Figure 7.15. Vascularization and blood supply.

Source: https://www.researchgate.net/profile/Paddy-Slator/publication/321751342/figure/fig3/AS:667820589330435@1536232244486/Schematic-representation-of-blood-flow-through-the-placenta-and-surrounding-tissue-Blue.png.

7.4.3. Interface Between Maternal and Fetal Blood Systems

Pregnancy success hinges a lot on how the mother's and baby's blood work together. When the placenta forms, it builds a vital barrier that lets nutrients and gases pass to the fetus while also keeping out potentially harmful substances. Tiny projections called placental villi help shuttle oxygen, carbon dioxide, glucose, amino acids, and more across this filter. The barrier's permeability matters—if even a small part falters, it can lead to complications like restricted fetal growth or preeclampsia. In essence, this delicate balance of nourishment and protection is crucial, and any disruption could have serious consequences. Examining the details of these exchange processes reveals a surprisingly complex picture. Maternal blood flows into the intervillous space and surrounds the chorionic villi—this close contact lets diffusion work its magic between the baby's capillaries and the mother's blood. New lab models, which are *in vitro* setups that mimic the human placental barrier, are providing us with fresh insights. For example, co-cultures of trophoblasts and endothelial cells are showing unexpected details about how nutrients and even drugs get transferred. It turns out that where specific proteins like LAT1 and P-glycoprotein end up makes a huge difference in moving amino acids and medications back and forth (Fuenzalida et al., 2024). These findings underscore the critical importance of the physical setup of the placenta to fetal health. Beyond simply exchanging nutrients and gases, this interface signals and shapes development and immune responses in distinct ways. It not only handles the vital exchange but also sends hormonal cues that may tweak the mother's body—a process that, in most cases, seems to require a fair bit of adaptation. Research shows that the maternal immune system adjusts to accept the semi-allogeneic fetus, supported in part by the placenta's special structures. Still, breaking into the mysteries of early placental development is no easy feat because of ethical and technological hurdles. New methods, such as microfluidic models and advanced computer simulations, are gradually peeling back these layers (Masserdotti et al., 2024). All in all, these advances could pave the way for improved prenatal care and healthier outcomes for both mothers and their babies.

7.5. Placental Disorders

A healthy pregnancy starts with how well a mother's body and her placenta work together. Placenta previa happens when the placenta ends up covering the cervical opening – a situation that can create serious issues at delivery—while placental abruption is when the placenta pulls away from the uterine wall a bit too soon, often stressing the baby. Age, unusual structural traits, and even a past cesarean can all mix into the picture, meaning that mothers who show these factors generally need closer prenatal checks.

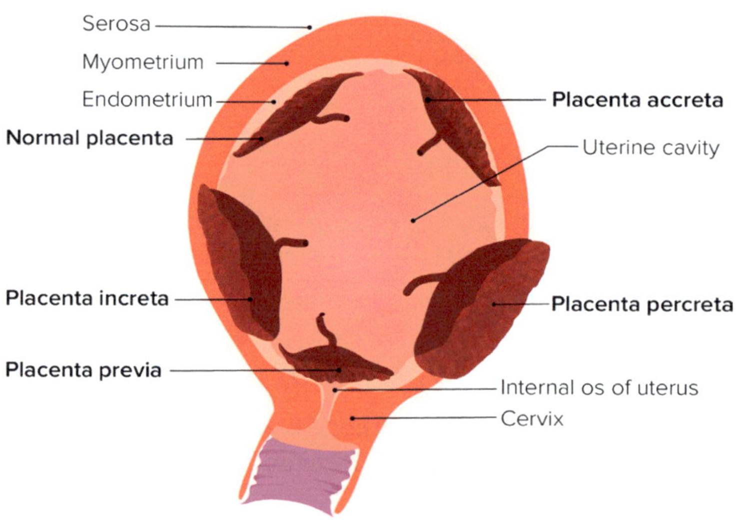

Figure 7.16. Placental abnormalities.

Source: https://cdn.lecturio.com/assets/Types-of-placental-invasion.png.

Another concern is gestational trophoblastic disease, a type of disorder that occurs when the trophoblastic cells of the placenta grow in abnormal ways, sometimes forming tumors such as hydatidiform moles or even choriocarcinoma. In most cases, a combination of genetic quirks and environmental influences disrupts normal placental development. This set of issues often necessitates surgery and underscores the importance of early detection—measured by serum hCG levels—is essential. Understanding these underlying biological processes, in most cases, can help steer us toward better treatments and boost outcomes for both mother and baby. Leptin, a hormone made by both body fat and the placenta, has also grabbed a lot of attention lately. It helps control energy balance and sends signals throughout the placental system. When leptin levels go a bit off, especially in mothers struggling with obesity (and perhaps even gestational diabetes), things can get messy for placental function. Keeping an eye on metabolic health during pregnancy isn't just crucial for the here and now; it might have lasting effects on the offspring's health. Recent studies generally underscore that a mother's overall condition plays a role in how well the placenta develops (Carter, 2020; Pic Có et al., 2021) (Figure 7.16).

7.5.1. Placenta Previa and Its Implications

The link between how the placenta forms and fetal growth gets pretty tangled when placenta previa comes into play. Sometimes the placenta ends up covering part or even all of the cervix, which not only makes a vaginal delivery way trickier but also hikes up the risk for severe bleeding. Mothers can end up dealing with preterm labor, placental abruption, or find themselves needing a cesarean more often. It turns out that getting what's happening at the heart of placentation is crucial – and recent studies show that the way the placenta mingles with the uterine environment plays a significant role. Any glitch in this delicate interaction may set the stage for complications, such as placenta previa (Vornic et al., 2024). There has also been some interesting work lately on identifying biomarkers and unraveling the molecular details behind placental issues. Researchers have been poking at the regulatory RNA network, which oddly enough sheds light on why there might be extra blood loss during cesareans. In cases of placenta previa, it appears that disruptions in the growth of blood vessels and the function of trophoblasts can compromise placental attachment and growth. By following these signaling pathways – and, in most cases, understanding these subtle molecular quirks – clinicians can gain a competitive advantage in predicting and managing delivery risks. This kind of molecular insight proves essential not only for understanding placenta previa but also for advancing maternal-fetal care (Yang et al., 2020). Managing placenta previa isn't a one-person show; it requires a whole team, blending obstetric expertise, surgical tactics, and constant monitoring. Doctors often have to keep a watchful eye with ultrasounds and other tests to map out exactly how the placenta is positioned, and as things move along, picking the correct delivery method becomes a careful balancing act. It's about weighing the threat of hemorrhage against keeping both mother and baby as safe as possible. Even discussing placenta previa with expectant mothers becomes critical. Combining knowledge about the relationship between extraembryonic membranes and placental health in general allows for a more adaptable strategy that, even under trying circumstances, can help reduce difficulties and improve outcomes for both mother and child. (Vornic et al., 2024) (Figure 7.17).

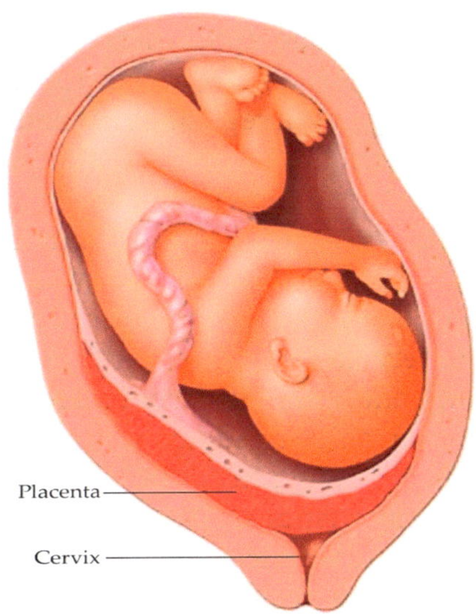

Figure 7.17. Placenta previa.

Source: https://assets.mayoclinic.org/content/dam/media/en/images/2023/02/03/Placenta%20previa.jpg.

7.5.2. Gestational Trophoblastic Disease

The placenta's role in various pregnancy complications makes it worth examining conditions like gestational trophoblastic disease (GTD) in the context of extraembryonic tissues. GTD isn't just a straightforward disorder—it springs from issues with trophoblastic cells that typically help form the placenta but, instead, start multiplying in odd ways. This is frequently observed as hydatidiform moles, which can be partial or full and are characterized by the atypical development of chorionic villi. These abnormal growths not only throw off placental function but also bring real health risks to the mother, ranging from lingering GTD to a shift toward gestational trophoblastic neoplasia. When the delicate early development of the placenta goes awry due to GTD, the need for early detection and management becomes crystal clear, especially during those critical weeks of placental formation (Graham et al., 2018). To understand GTD, one must dig into its underlying workings—a picture that remains only partially clear. The offbeat proliferation of trophoblastic tissue appears to be linked to chromosomal abnormalities, and factors such as the mother's age or irregular fertilization can sometimes contribute to the issue. Usually, the placenta adjusts its blood flow and remakes its vessels to support both baby and mother, but GTD disrupts that natural rhythm. In most cases, such disturbances lead to problems like heavy bleeding, severe morning sickness (*hyperemesis gravidarum*), and spikes in serum markers such as human chorionic gonadotropin (hCG). Since the placenta has a significant influence on how a mother's body adapts, GTD's impact goes well beyond a mere anatomical glitch—it rattles the whole system. No wonder treatment can be challenging, ranging from surgical interventions to simply monitoring hCG levels, depending on the specifics of the case (Ghi et al., 2016). Improved imaging techniques and biomarkers have, in recent years, made it easier to catch and tackle GTD sooner. Ultrasound, for instance, has become a key tool—it can reveal unusual patterns in placental growth and help clinicians decide the best course of action. Organizations like the International Society of Ultrasound in Obstetrics and Gynecology (ISUOG) emphasize the importance of precise imaging protocols when addressing these complex issues. Meanwhile, blood tests measuring markers such as hCG are now indispensable for checking if treatments are working and for keeping tabs on any potential relapse. As research continues (and our understanding deepens), it seems clear that solving the puzzles of GTD requires a team effort—drawing on expertise from obstetrics, gynecology, and oncology—to get the best outcomes. A better grasp of how GTD interferes with placental development gives us clues for interventions aimed at setting pregnancies back on a healthier track, reducing complications, and boosting well-being for both mother and baby (Graham et al., 2018) (Figure 7.18).

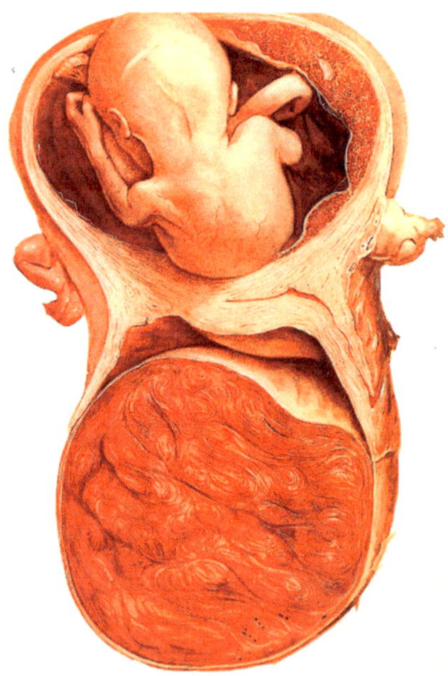

Figure 7.18. Gestational trophoblastic disease.

Source: https://cdn.storymd.com/optimized/8ojyGxcLA7/original.jpg.

7.5.3. Pre-Eclampsia and Its Effects on Placental Function

Pre-eclampsia shakes up how the placenta works during pregnancy—it isn't just the mother's health that gets hit, but the baby suffers too. Often, the trouble starts when the maternal spiral arteries don't remodel quite right, so the placenta ends up with less blood than it should have. This shortage can push the placenta into a state of ischemia, and subsequently, a series of problems, including oxidative stress and inflammation, can ensue. These issues then wear down the placental barrier, meaning it can't deliver all the nutrients and oxygen needed for the baby's growth. In most cases, this chain reaction results in consequences such as intrauterine growth restriction (IUGR) or even preterm birth, making it clear that early action is crucial for maintaining the maternal vascular system and placental function in proper balance. In the midst of this, melatonin emerges as a potential lifesaver. Research, generally speaking, shows that this molecule acts as a robust antioxidant right inside the placenta, countering the oxidative stress that often worsens pre-eclampsia. Interestingly, the placenta even manages to synthesize some of its melatonin, which helps it maintain a stable environment. By scavenging free radicals, melatonin helps bolster placental integrity, fostering a healthier connection between mother and child. Its further role in tweaking immune responses adds another layer of steadiness during gestation, opening up hopeful therapeutic avenues for cases of pre-eclampsia. The interplay between immune cells and the uterine environment is another big piece of the pre-eclampsia puzzle. Uterine natural killer (uNK) cells, for example, have been getting a lot of attention since they're key to helping remodel the maternal spiral arteries—a process vital for ensuring proper blood flow to the placenta. When pre-eclampsia rears its head, these uNK cells can go off track, failing to help the arteries adapt the way they need to; this can eventually lead to placental insufficiency. As the balance of immune activity shifts, both the functions of the placenta and the overall course of the pregnancy are disrupted. In most cases, examining these immune dynamics could be crucial for finding better ways to manage the complications associated with pre-eclampsia (Figure 7.19).

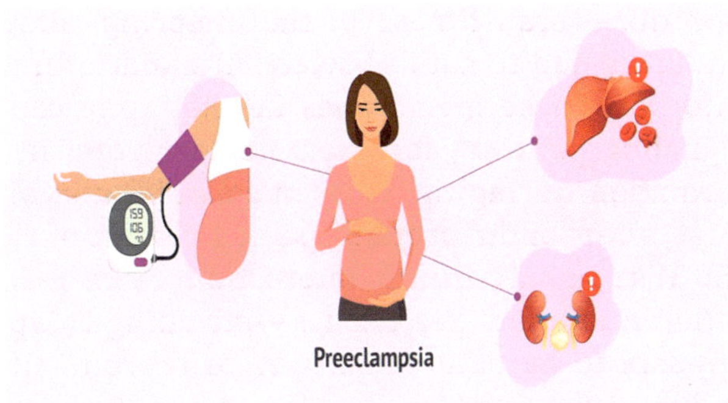

Figure 7.19. Preeclampsia.

Source: https://maxlab.co.in/categoryimage/1667973920.jpg.

7.6. Evolutionary Aspects of Extraembryonic Membranes

Extraembryonic membranes have evolved significantly in mammalian history, and they play a crucial role as creatures transitioned onto land. Early on, when embryos left the water, they suddenly needed better ways to protect themselves and obtain nutrients. The amnion, for example, is a fluid-filled sac that not only softens impacts but also helps keep the embryo from drying out. Then there's the chorion, which evolved to handle gas exchange and remove waste in environments that varied a lot. In many respects, the entire setup of these membranes demonstrates how nature, bit by bit, crafted systems that enhance reproductive success, allowing more advanced life forms to flourish in various terrestrial settings. Shifting gears a bit, it appears that the combination of genetic signals and environmental pressures has also played a significant role in shaping the development of these membranes across species. Several studies have highlighted that molecular pathways—such as those involving B-cell lymphoma-2 (BCL-2), for instance—are crucial in maintaining cell activity balance during embryogenesis. These pathways, which balance cell growth and cell death, repeat themselves as a central theme in the formation of extraembryonic structures. Early survival strategies have been refined over time, enabling mammals and other vertebrates to adapt. The protective function of these membranes naturally ups the overall fitness of the offspring, allowing them to thrive even in harsh conditions—an enduring nod to natural selection's knack for fine-tuning life (Joseph et al., 2017). Looking further into how these membranes develop, one can't ignore the role of cell-to-cell signaling. The Wnt signaling pathway, for example, is pivotal in regulating stem cell behavior and directing tissue formation during the early stages of embryogenesis. Molecules such as Lgr5, its receptor, and a host of R-spondin proteins paint a picture of a complex yet elegant regulatory network. By boosting the Wnt signal through interactions with R-spondin, stem cells receive the support they need to differentiate into key tissues—including components of the placenta. This fine-tuning in signaling appears to be nature's answer to reproduction on land, demonstrating just how essential those cellular conversations are for maintaining extraembryonic membranes and ultimately ensuring species survival (Wim de Lau et al., 2014) (Figure 7.20).

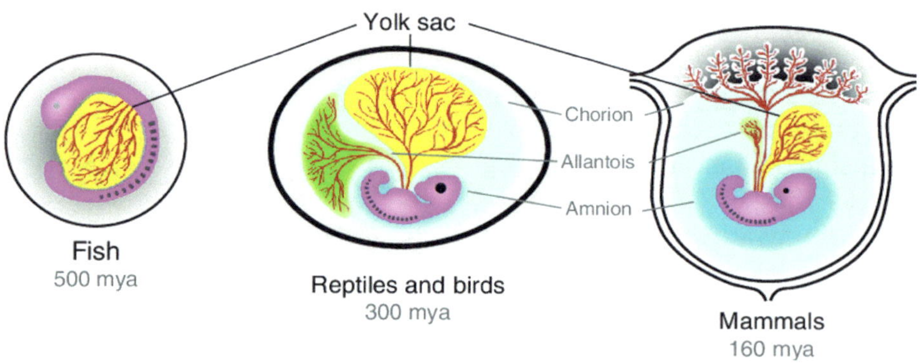

Figure 7.20. Evolutionary aspects of extraembryonic membranes.

Source: https://www.researchgate.net/publication/343261694/figure/fig1/AS:922991223373824@1597069664368/Extraembryonic-membranes-in-fish-birds-and-mammals-The-yolk-sac-dates-back-to-our.png.

7.6.1. Comparison of Extraembryonic Membranes Across Species

Extraembryonic membranes have evolved in surprising ways that are key to an embryo's survival and growth. Different vertebrates can tweak these membranes so that mothers and offspring swap nutrients and toss out waste more effectively—an adaptation that shows off nature's ingenuity. Take amniotes, for example; reptiles, birds, and mammals each have specialized layers, such as the chorion and allantois, which, in most cases, aid in breathing and waste control during development. Their shapes and designs aren't random either—they reveal how nature's tinkering meets local environmental and reproductive needs. All these variations in membrane structure—repeatedly observed across groups—highlight the importance of maternal support in vertebrate evolution and hint at a complex interplay between developmental processes and evolutionary forces. This point is pivotal to our understanding of placental evolution (Roberts et al., 2016). Beyond vertebrates, extraembryonic structures also appear in invertebrates, offering a curious parallel in reproductive development. Many invertebrate groups—such as Platyhelminthes and Arthropods—supply nutrients directly to their young via specialized membranes or even through maternal tissues, demonstrating that evolution in these lineages sometimes experiments with similar ideas. This nutrient handoff varies from cases of histotrophy to placentotrophy; such differences demonstrate an adaptive radiation of reproductive strategies across an impressive range of organisms. In this way, comparing extraembryonic membranes highlights the idea that these adaptations aren't isolated oddities, but somewhat convergent solutions to common reproductive challenges (Andrew et al., 2015). Mammals, however, take things a step further; the evolution of extraembryonic membranes there culminates in the formation of intricate placentae—a true milestone in reproductive biology. Generally speaking, the placenta becomes the keystone of nutrient transfer, while also serving as an immunological barrier between the mother and the embryo. Different types of placentae—whether choriovitelline or chorioallantoic—reflect a variety of evolutionary journeys, each one shaped by differing levels of maternal investment and environmental quirks. The link between increasingly complex placental structures and rapid fetal development suggests a strong evolutionary drive to optimize reproductive success. This deep specialization seen in mammalian membranes weaves together a rich narrative, emphasizing how our evolutionary past influences reproductive strategies and overall survival in vertebrates (Roberts et al., 2016).

7.6.2. Evolutionary Advantages of Complex Placentation

Complex placentation has set an evolutionary course that comes with numerous benefits for mammalian reproduction. Animals inhabiting different environments suddenly found that better fetal support was essential. Complex placentation improves nutrient sharing and gas exchange while tying the growing embryo way closer to its mother; this close connection often means that survival chances go up when resources are unpredictable. Instead of acting like a mere pipeline, the placenta shows up as an active helper in nurturing embryonic growth and overall health. It ultimately reshapes reproductive approaches across mammals, with the mother's investment supporting offspring viability. In short, by channeling more maternal energy into fewer, stronger babies, these placental innovations offer a clear advantage, especially on land. Curiously, digging into these effects raises the idea of convergent evolution. Across many vertebrate groups, complex placentas have evolved independently - each with its unique twists in shape and function that mirror distinct ecological pressures. Generally speaking, this adaptive convergence suggests that the benefits of advanced placentation are substantial enough to drive parallel evolutionary adaptations. The close interplay between maternal tissues and fetal membranes isn't just about nutrient transfer; it also throws in some immune protection, easing the usual conflicts between the two. In this way, the placenta appears to have evolved not only to support growth but also to create a stable environment for fetal development, enabling young ones to thrive in increasingly complex ecosystems. These evolutionary tweaks underscore the importance of placentation in maintaining species diversity and adaptability. Beyond the physical benefits, complex placentation also steers broader ecological and evolutionary moves. It can shape everything from mating behaviors and parenting investments to overall population trends. Species sporting this kind of placentation often pump more resources into each pregnancy, resulting in fewer—but tougher—offspring. This trade-off points to a shift toward quality over quantity, linking reproductive efforts closely with nature's fluctuations. In environments where success depends on an organism's ability to grow and handle challenges, such adjustments become especially key. All the layers of benefit wrapped up in complex placentation clearly show that this organ plays a central role in shaping the evolutionary paths and life histories of mammals.

7.6.3. Adaptations in Response to Environmental Factors

Species must quickly adjust to the pressures of their surroundings if they're to keep on thriving, especially when it comes to reproduction. Take mammals, for example: over time, extraembryonic membranes, such as the placenta, evolved as a clever workaround to deal with shifts in nutrient supplies and oxygen levels. The placenta isn't just a delivery route for nourishment; it also works as a sort of gatekeeper, keeping unintended intruders like pathogens and toxins at bay. This type of selective filtering plays a crucial role in creating the optimal conditions for a baby's development—a close and often complex connection between a mother's health, her surroundings, and the future success of her offspring. In most cases, recent studies even suggest that the mix of bacteria a mother carries may influence these adaptive moves, potentially affecting reproductive outcomes and overall maternal-fetal health (Al Nasiry et al., 2020). Additionally, a mother's body must adapt to a constant back-and-forth with environmental cues throughout pregnancy. For instance, when oxygen dips—what we call hypoxia—it can spark notable shifts in energy management for both her and the developing embryo. The placenta appears to handle low-oxygen scenarios by responding to cues from factors such as hypoxia-inducible factor 1 (HIF-1), which prompts its metabolism to shift from one mode to another, transitioning from oxidative processes to more glycolytic pathways. This kind of metabolic agility is crucial for ensuring that, come what may, the embryo still receives enough fuel. The entire process highlights the importance of a mother and her baby synchronizing well, with the surrounding environment influencing those vital energy pathways (Radka Čerychová et al., 2018). Looking even farther down the road, these adjustments don't just affect the here and now—they can influence long-term health for both mother and child. A slip in the balance of the mother's usual microbial crew, for example, might lead to problems like preterm births or gestational diabetes, clearly showing just how powerfully the environment can impact reproductive health. And when things go awry, say through conditions like maternal diabetes, crucial messengers such as HIF-1 can get thrown off, potentially interfering with the baby's heart development and bumping up the risk of birth defects. This all goes to show why digging into these fine-tuned and sometimes quirky processes—within the mix of a mother's overall health and her environmental exposures—is so essential for understanding the long-run prospects of offspring (Radka Čerychová et al., 2018; Al Nasiry et al., 2020).

SUMMARY

Extraembryonic membranes and the placenta share a profound, yet understated, bond that is crucial for maintaining an embryo's viability and ensuring proper development. A successful pregnancy depends on these structures being built correctly, with the appropriate specialization and integration. Modern techniques, such as single-cell RNA sequencing, have begun to unravel the complex web of gene networks involved in trophoblast differentiation, providing a fresh perspective on how placentation works. In bovine studies, even slight disruptions in gene expression have shown that minor alterations can lead to significant fertility issues in cattle populations (Kimberly et al., 2025). Maternal health, of course, adds another twist to the story. Conditions such as preeclampsia, anemia, and chorioamnionitis tend to disrupt the balance by altering the architecture of the placenta and the expression of collagen.

Generally speaking, research has found that these inflammatory states—especially in chorioamnionitis—result in noticeable decreases in important collagen types, creating a domino effect that heightens the risk of complications (Zats et al., 2024). This connection highlights the importance of maintaining maternal health to support a robust placenta and promote healthy fetal growth. In summary, the dynamic dance between extraembryonic membranes and the placenta lies at the heart of successful reproduction. Ongoing studies into the cellular and molecular details provide important clues about both normal pregnancies and those that deviate from the norm. By deepening our understanding of these systems, not only can we better tackle infertility, but we can also craft interventions aimed at easing complications linked to maternal pathologies. As our research steadily advances, the crucial role of the placenta and its related membranes is likely to continue opening new paths in improving reproductive health for both mothers and their babies (Zats et al., 2024; Kimberly et al., 2025).

Extraembryonic membranes and the placenta share a connection that's not only complex but also key to how embryos grow. These structures don't just shuttle nutrients and clear out waste—they also play a bunch of other roles that keep an embryo viable. Right in the mix, the ECM acts as more than just a framework; it nudges various cell behaviors along the way. Recent studies, in general, have shown that the ECM is involved in wakeful tasks such as cell signaling and migration, which in turn shape and influence the function of trophoblastic cells. Even small changes in the ECM can tip the balance, potentially leading to developmental issues such as placental insufficiency or other fetal complications (Nikos et al., 2021). In short, examining these membranes extends far beyond basic reproductive biology and is beginning to hint at some promising therapeutic possibilities. At the same time, genetic integrity within embryos remains a significant concern. Chromosomal quirks or abnormalities aren't just minor changes; they can seriously disrupt an embryo's chance at success, whether in natural conception or assisted reproduction.

Some recent reviews have pointed out that methods like preimplantation genetic testing for aneuploidy (PGT-A) and tests for structural rearrangements (SR) help flag embryos with genetic issues before they're even implanted. These advances not only make it easier to pick out healthy embryos, but they also shed light on why miscarriages and congenital disorders crop up so frequently when chromosomal errors are in the mix (Viotti, 2020). By letting clinicians cut out the embryos that carry these issues, our overall outcomes get a meaningful boost—and that's a win for the field of reproductive medicine. Taking a step back, the way extraembryonic membranes, the placenta, and genetic integrity all interact forms a sort of tangled web, one that's vital for a thriving gestation. Determining which ECM elements perform specific functions provides insight into the structural framework that supports embryonic growth, while advanced genetic screening methods continue to refine our practices in clinical settings. The blend of these two areas not only deepens our grasp of early development but also opens up new avenues for potential therapies. Ongoing research into how these parts work together remains crucial in facing infertility and pregnancy complications—efforts that will likely benefit the generations to come.

CLOSER LOOK

TROPHOBLAST CELLS

Trophoblast cells are specialized cells that form the outer layer of the blastocyst during early embryonic development, playing a critical role in the establishment and maintenance of pregnancy. These cells are the first to differentiate from the fertilized egg. They are essential for implantation of the embryo into the uterine wall, as well as for the formation of the placenta. This organ facilitates the exchange of nutrients and gases between the mother and fetus. Trophoblasts originate from the trophectoderm, the outermost layer of the blastocyst, and undergo further differentiation into various subtypes with distinct functions. The two main lineages of trophoblast cells are cytotrophoblasts and syncytiotrophoblast. Cytotrophoblasts are mononuclear, proliferative cells that serve as progenitors for other trophoblast subtypes. They can fuse to form syncytiotrophoblast, which are multinucleated, terminally differentiated cells that cover the surface of the placental villi and are directly involved in nutrient and gas exchange, hormone production (such as hCG, human chorionic gonadotropin), and immune modulation to prevent maternal rejection of the fetus.

A third type of trophoblast, known as extravillous trophoblasts, invades the maternal decidua and remodels the spiral arteries to ensure an adequate blood supply to the growing fetus. This invasive capability is a hallmark of early placental development and is tightly regulated; abnormal trophoblast invasion is associated with pregnancy complications such as preeclampsia, intrauterine growth restriction (IUGR), and miscarriage. The ability of trophoblasts to modulate immune responses is also crucial, as the maternal immune system must tolerate the semi-allogeneic fetus. Trophoblasts achieve this by expressing unique surface molecules, such as HLA-G, which help mediate immune tolerance at the maternal-fetal interface.

Trophoblast biology is also of interest in cancer research due to similarities between trophoblast invasion and tumor metastasis. Both processes involve cell proliferation, migration, invasion through extracellular matrices, and angiogenesis; however, trophoblast activity is tightly controlled, whereas cancer is characterized by deregulation. Furthermore, abnormalities in trophoblast development or function can lead to gestational trophoblastic diseases, a group of rare disorders that include hydatidiform mole and choriocarcinoma, in which trophoblast cells grow abnormally and may become malignant.

Understanding the molecular and cellular mechanisms that regulate trophoblast differentiation, function, and interaction with maternal tissues is crucial for improving pregnancy outcomes and developing treatments for related complications. Trophoblast cell lines and placental organoids are commonly used in research to study these processes in vitro. In addition, advances in single-cell RNA sequencing and imaging techniques have allowed researchers to explore the heterogeneity and dynamics of trophoblast populations with unprecedented resolution. Overall, trophoblast cells are not only central to the success of pregnancy but also provide a valuable model for studying cell invasion, immune regulation, and cellular differentiation in both physiological and pathological contexts. Their unique role at the interface between maternal and fetal tissues underscores their importance in reproductive biology and maternal-fetal medicine.

REFERENCES

1. Al-Nasiry, S., Ambrosino, E., Schlaepfer, M., Morré, S. A., Wieten, L., Voncken, J. W., Spinelli, M., et al. (2020). The interplay between reproductive tract microbiota and immunological system in human reproduction. *Frontiers in Immunology, 11*, 378. https://doi.org/10.3389/fimmu.2020.00378.
2. Bangs, F., & Anderson, K. V. (2016). Primary cilia and mammalian Hedgehog signaling. *Cold Spring Harbor Perspectives in Biology, 9*, a028175. https://doi.org/10.1101/cshperspect.a028175.
3. Burton, G. J., & Fowden, A. L. (2015). The placenta: A multifaceted, transient organ. *Philosophical Transactions of the Royal Society B: Biological Sciences, 370*, 20140066. https://doi.org/10.1098/rstb.2014.0066.
4. Burton, G. J., & Jauniaux, E. (2018). Development of the human placenta and fetal heart: Synergic or independent? *Frontiers in Physiology, 9*, 373. https://doi.org/10.3389/fphys.2018.00373.
5. Carter, A. M. (2020). Animal models of human pregnancy and placentation: Alternatives to the mouse. *Reproduction, 160*(6), R129–R143. https://doi.org/10.1530/rep-20-0354.
6. Čerychová, R., & Pavlínková, G. (2018). HIF-1, metabolism, and diabetes in the embryonic and adult heart. *Frontiers in Endocrinology, 9*, 460. https://doi.org/10.3389/fendo.2018.00460.
7. Davenport, K. M., Lowke, M. T., Ortega, M. S., Kelleher, A. M., Warren, W. C., & Spencer, T. E. (2025). Single cell multiome analysis of the bovine placenta identifies gene regulatory networks in trophoblast differentiation. *Biology of Reproduction*. https://doi.org/10.1093/biolre/ioaf036de Lau, W., Peng, W. C., Gros, P., & Clevers, H. (2014). The R-spondin/Lgr5/Rnf43 module: Regulator of Wnt signal strength. *Genes & Development, 28*, 305–316. https://doi.org/10.1101/gad.235473.113.
8. Eitel, E. K., Sponchiado, M., Sullivan, R. M., Lucas, C. G., Redel, B., Chen, P. R., Wells, K. D., et al. (2025). Expression of tripartite motif family-like protein 1 and 2 in early conceptus development and placentation in the pig. *Reproduction & Fertility, 6*. https://www.semanticscholar.org/paper/05cbd88e064afb842b122659d2b7a9cfe06adc25 (accessed on 26 May 2025).
9. Elkhenany, H., El-Derby, A. M., Abd Elkodous, M., Salah, R. A., Lotfy, A., & El-Badri, N. (2022). Applications of the amniotic membrane in tissue engineering and regeneration: The hundred-year challenge. *Stem Cell Research & Therapy, 13*, Article 84. https://doi.org/10.1186/s13287-021-02684-0.
10. Erlebacher, A. (2013). Immunology of the maternal-fetal interface. *Annual Review of Immunology, 31*, 387–411. https://doi.org/10.1146/annurev-immunol-032712-100003.
11. Fuenzalida, B., Basler, V., Koechli, N., Yi, N., Staud, F., & Albrecht, C. (2024). Modelling the maternal-fetal interface: An *in vitro* approach to investigate nutrient and drug transport across the human placenta. *Journal of Cellular and Molecular Medicine, 28*. https://www.semanticscholar.org/paper/892c259525dfc820bf0ac86635c081fb92f027cc (accessed on 26 May 2025).
12. Gerri, C., Menchero, S., Mahadevaiah, S. K., Turner, J. M. A., & Niakan, K. K. (2020). Human embryogenesis: A comparative perspective. *Annual Review of Cell and Developmental Biology, 36*, 411–440. https://doi.org/10.1146/annurev-cellbio-022020-024900.

13. Ghi, T., Sotiriadis, A., Calda, P., da Silva Costa, F., Raine-Fenning, N., Alfirević, Ž., & McGillivray, G. (2016). ISUOG practice guidelines: Invasive procedures for prenatal diagnosis. *Ultrasound in Obstetrics and Gynecology, 48*, 256–268. https://doi.org/10.1002/uog.15945.

14. Hass, R., Kasper, C., Böhm, S., & Jacobs, R. (2011). Different populations and sources of human mesenchymal stem cells (MSC): A comparison of adult and neonatal tissue-derived MSC. *Cell Communication and Signaling, 9*, 12. https://doi.org/10.1186/1478-811x-9-12.

15. Hassan, W., & Viebahn, C. (2017). A correlative study of the allantois in pig and rabbit highlighting the diversity of extraembryonic tissues in four mammalian species, including mouse and man. *Journal of Morphology, 278*, 600–620. https://doi.org/10.1002/jmor.20657.

16. Igarashi, H., Uemura, M., Hiramatsu, R., Hiramatsu, R., Segami, S., Pattarapanawan, M., Hirate, Y., et al. (2018). Sox17 is essential for proper formation of the marginal zone of extraembryonic endoderm adjacent to a developing mouse placental disk. *Biology of Reproduction, 99*, 578–589. https://www.semanticscholar.org/paper/3500b7f763b3a409706124cfc718bf6df653df8f (accessed on 26 May 2025).

17. Joseph, T. T., Schuch, V., Hossack, D. J., Chakraborty, R., & Johnson, E. L. (2024). Melatonin: The placental antioxidant and anti-inflammatory. *Frontiers in Immunology, 15*, 1339304. https://doi.org/10.3389/fimmu.2024.1339304.

18. Karamanos, N. K., Theocharis, A. D., Piperigkou, Z., Manou, D., Passi, A., Skandalis, S. S., Vynios, D. H., et al. (2021). A guide to the composition and functions of the extracellular matrix. *FEBS Journal, 288*, 6850–6912. https://doi.org/10.1111/febs.15776.

19. Maltepe, E., & Fisher, S. J. (2015). Placenta: The forgotten organ. *Annual Review of Cell and Developmental Biology, 31*, 523–552. https://doi.org/10.1146/annurev-cellbio-100814-125620.

20. Mançanares, C. A., de Oliveira, V. C., Oliveira, L. J., Miglino, M., Meirelles, F., & Ambrósio, C. (2019). Morphological and molecular analysis of *in vitro* tubular structures from bovine yolk sac-derived MSCs. *Stem Cells International, 2019*. https://www.semanticscholar.org/paper/00cc9b1fc7e7dd2306160087471cc07ea25f05f6 (accessed on 26 May 2025).

21. Masserdotti, A., Gasik, M., Grillari-Voglauer, R., Grillari, J., Cargnoni, A., Chiodelli, P., Papait, A., et al. (2024). Unveiling the human fetal-maternal interface during the first trimester: Biophysical knowledge and gaps. *Frontiers in Cell and Developmental Biology, 12*. https://www.semanticscholar.org/paper/b89becfad2c19ab4b866462103cd81a9952400f5 (accessed on 26 May 2025).

22. Opferman, J. T., & Kothari, A. (2017). Anti-apoptotic BCL-2 family members in development. *Cell Death and Differentiation, 25*, 37–45. https://doi.org/10.1038/cdd.2017.170.

23. Ostrovsky, A. N., Lidgard, S., Gordon, D. P., Schwaha, T., Genikhovich, G., & Ereskovsky, A. (2015). Matrotrophy and placentation in invertebrates: A new paradigm. *Biological Reviews, 91*(3), 673–711. https://doi.org/10.1111/brv.12189.

24. Picó, C., Palou, M., Pomar, C. A., Rodríguez, A. M., & Palou, A. (2021). Leptin as a key regulator of the adipose organ. *Reviews in Endocrine and Metabolic Disorders, 23*, 13–30. https://doi.org/10.1007/s11154-021-09687-5.

25. Roberts, R. M., Green, J. A., & Schulz, L. C. (2016). The evolution of the placenta. *Reproduction, 152*, R179–R189. https://doi.org/10.1530/rep-16-0325.

26. Ross, C., & Boroviak, T. (2020). Origin and function of the yolk sac in primate embryogenesis. *Nature Communications, 11*, Article 3061. https://doi.org/10.1038/s41467-020-17575-w.

27. Shibata, M., Makihara, N., & Iwasawa, A. (2023). The yolk sac's essential role in embryonic development. *Reviews in Agricultural Science, 11*, 243–258. https://doi.org/10.7831/ras.11.0_243.

28. Suryawanshi, H., Morozov, P., Straus, A., Sahasrabudhe, N., Max, K. E. A., Garzia, A., Kustagi, M., et al. (2018). A single-cell survey of the human first-trimester placenta and decidua. *Science Advances, 4*, eaau4788. https://doi.org/10.1126/sciadv.aau4788.

29. Szabo, R., Peters, D. E., Kósa, P., Camerer, E., & Bugge, T. H. (2014). Regulation of feto-maternal barrier by Matriptase- and PAR-2-mediated signaling is required for placental morphogenesis and mouse embryonic survival. *PLoS Genetics, 10*, e1004470. https://doi.org/10.1371/journal.pgen.1004470.

30. Viotti, M. (2020). Preimplantation genetic testing for chromosomal abnormalities: Aneuploidy, mosaicism, and structural rearrangements. *Genes, 11*, 602. https://doi.org/10.3390/genes11060602.

31. Vornic, I., Buciu, V., Furău, C., Baderca, F., Novacescu, D., Barb, A. C., Cumpănaş, A. A., et al. (2024). The interplay of molecular factors and morphology in human placental development and implantation. *Biomedicines, 12*, 2908. https://doi.org/10.3390/biomedicines12122908.

32. Wang, F., Qualls, A., Marques-Fernandez, L., & Colucci, F. (2021). Biology and pathology of the uterine microenvironment and its natural killer cells. *Cellular and Molecular Immunology, 18*, 2101–2113. https://doi.org/10.1038/s41423-021-00739-z.

33. Whittington, C. M., & Friesen, C. R. (2020). The evolution and physiology of male pregnancy in syngnathid fishes. *Biological Reviews, 95*(5), 1252–1272. https://doi.org/10.1111/brv.12607.

34. Woods, L., Pérez-García, V., & Hemberger, M. (2018). Regulation of placental development and its impact on fetal growth—New insights from mouse models. *Frontiers in Endocrinology, 9*, 570. https://doi.org/10.3389/fendo.2018.00570.

35. Wu, Z., Zhang, W., Chen, G., Cheng, L., Liao, J., Jia, N., Gao, Y., et al. (2008). Combinatorial signals of Activin/Nodal and bone morphogenic protein regulate the early lineage segregation of human embryonic stem cells. *Journal of Biological Chemistry, 283*, 24991–25002. https://doi.org/10.1074/jbc.M803893200.

36. Yang, T., Li, N., Hou, R., Qiao, C., & Liu, C. (2020). Development and validation of a four-microRNA signature for placenta accreta spectrum: An integrated competing endogenous RNA network analysis. *Annals of Translational Medicine, 8*, 919. https://doi.org/10.21037/atm-20-1150.

37. Zakrzewski, W., Dobrzyński, M., Szymonowicz, M., & Rybak, Z. (2019). Stem cells: Past, present, and future. *Stem Cell Research & Therapy, 10*, Article 68. https://doi.org/10.1186/s13287-019-1165-5.

38. Zats, O. S., Sherstiuk, S., & Panov, S. (2024). Expression of interstitial collagens in fetal membranes and placenta against the background of maternal pathology. *Karazin Journal of Immunology.* https://www.semanticscholar.org/paper/fe3123fcfc8111cd33763ae0233f7f4d459c1cac (accessed on 26 May 2025).

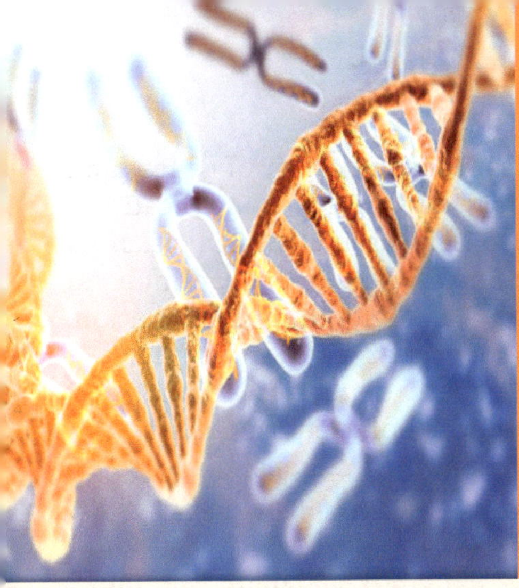

Chapter 8
GENETICS

Contents

Introduction

Living organisms exhibit certain basic traits that scientists investigate from various angles. Genetics, for example, isn't just another field—it digs into how traits pass from one generation to the next and why we end up so varied. At its core, it's about understanding how those instructions, tucked away in the spiral of DNA (that twisty, life-making ladder), are passed along, shaping all the little features we notice. Over time, as our understanding of these processes deepened, their effects spread to areas such as medicine, farming, and even our concepts of evolution. No wonder genetics now stands as a real cornerstone in biology, linking tiny molecular details with the big picture of health and disease. Digging a bit deeper, it all comes down to the gene—the basic unit of heredity. A gene is just a stretch of DNA holding the orders for making proteins, the workhorses in our cells that drive growth and function. Back in the mid-20th century, when Watson and Crick uncovered the famous double helix, a whole new way of looking at mutations and variations opened up. These variations manifest themselves in visible ways, such as eye color, or in more complex characteristics where a variety of genes (and perhaps the environment) interact.. This research often finds its way into practical applications, such as genetic counseling, where tracing inheritance patterns can help predict health risks. As scientists continue to unravel how genes interact with the environment, the subject continues to offer surprises for everything from individual health to our overall understanding of evolution. Recent breakthroughs in genetics have significantly impacted many areas of the life sciences. With tools like CRISPR-Cas9 now available, researchers can tweak genetic material with a level of precision that was once unimaginable. This sort of targeted gene editing holds enormous promise for treating genetic disorders. Still, such power isn't without its debates; ethical questions crop up when we consider the potential for modifying genes in humans and other organisms. Meanwhile, large-scale genomic studies are uncovering markers linked to diseases, deepening our insight into complex conditions like Alzheimer's disease and various cancers. Generally speaking, the move toward understanding diseases at a molecular level has refined how we diagnose and treat many conditions. All in all, ongoing work in genetics not only expands our knowledge of how life works but also paves the way for personalized medicine and fresh perspectives on evolution—even if some details get a bit messy along the way (Figure 8.1).

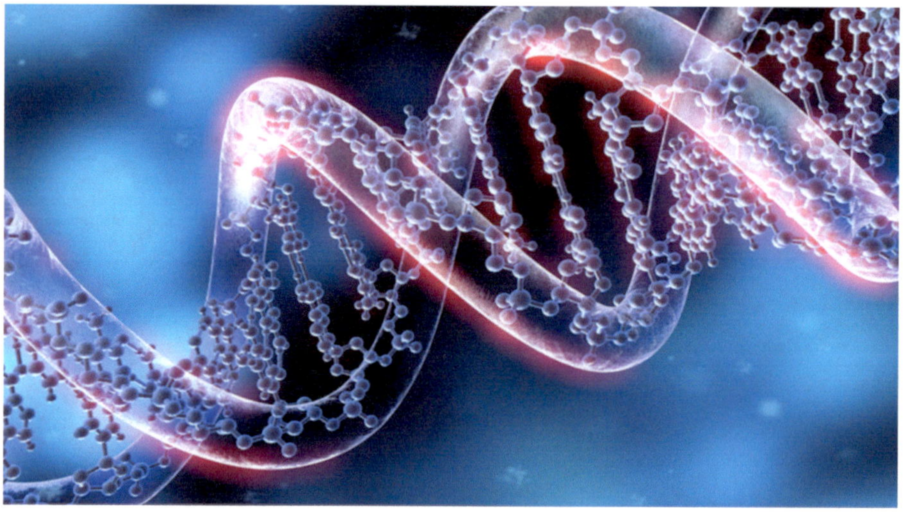

Figure 8.1. Genetics.

Source: https://study.com/cimages/course-image/genetics-101-intro-to-genetics_175592_large.jpg.

Explanation of Genetics as a Branch of Biology

Life's rich variety boils down to how traits get passed along—a mix of heredity and variation kicking off everything. Genetics, that branch of biology that delves into the nitty-gritty of genes at a microscopic level, examines how features are passed from parent to child. It covers a bunch of stuff—DNA's twisting structure, how genes fire up, even the odd little mutations that sneak in—so we can see how our genetic info is stored, copied, and tweaked over time. This kind of work isn't just about understanding life's inner mechanics; it also helps tackle real-world issues, such as controlling diseases or spurring breakthroughs in farming. Overall, genetics pulls back the curtain on both the basic blueprint of life and the curveballs that lead to new adaptations, driving evolution along the way. Research tools aren't standing still either. New computational methods—such as Molecular Evolutionary Genetics Analysis (MEGA) software—are enabling scientists to delve deeper into genetic relationships and map out evolutionary patterns. There are rapid relaxed-clock methods on the scene, which, in most cases, help trace family lines and pinpoint when splits occurred; this demonstrates a neat blend of technological innovation and genetic inquiry (Tamura et al., 2021). Moreover, these tools enable researchers to tag gene sequences with hints about when and where they emerged, adding a rich layer of context to our understanding of species differences. In many ways, this evolving toolkit is reshuffling the genetic landscape, uncovering old links between organisms and hinting at trends that could guide future studies. These days, genetics isn't just an academic thing—it's a real-world player in global health.

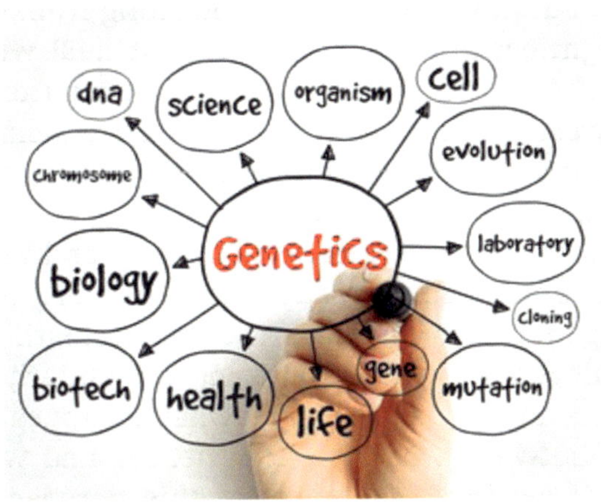

Figure 8.2. Genetics as a branch of biology.

Source: https://www.shutterstock.com/image-photo/genetics-mind-map-medical-concept-260nw-2445256651.jpg.

The COVID-19 outbreak, for example, highlighted how tracking genetic clues can pinpoint the origin of a pathogen and its mode of transmission. The case of SARS-CoV-2—identified as a new coronavirus—serves as a clear example of how genetics informs our understanding of zoonotic diseases and their connections to human health. By mapping out the family trees of viruses, scientists can spot how these bugs might jump hosts, which then helps shape public health strategies (Alexander et al., 2020). This mix of genetics with epidemiology not only deciphers our genetic codes but also sets the stage for tackling emerging global threats. Overall, genetics remains a cornerstone of our scientific approach, influencing our grasp of life, health, and the world around us (Figure 8.2).

Historical Context and Development of Genetic Science

Heredity and change have been part of our understanding for ages, although it was only around the mid-1800s that science began to delve into genetics. Gregor Mendel—many refer to him as the father of genetics—conducted these meticulous, yet seemingly casual, pea plant experiments, which, in most cases, revealed how dominant and recessive traits function. His findings, which initially didn't get the attention they deserved, eventually turned heads in the early 1900s. As more researchers got involved, it became clear that traits were passed along in little, specific packets we now call genes—a pretty significant shift from the old idea of blending traits. Between 1900 and 1910, the rediscovery of Mendel's work not only revived interest but also laid the groundwork for genetics to emerge as a distinct branch of biology, paving the way for deeper discussions on how heredity functions. Around the early 20th century, things started to mix up in interesting ways, with Mendelian genetics merging with the study of cells—cytology. Scientists like Thomas Hunt Morgan, among others, were busy exploring how genes are placed on chromosomes and just how they move around during cell division. With new techniques, such as various staining methods, researchers could suddenly see genetic material in ways that were, frankly, almost unimaginable before. This unexpected pairing of cell study and genetics led to significant leaps, such as identifying mutations and exploring their roles in various biological processes. Gradually, as experts began to appreciate the complex interplay of gene interactions, they took on a broader view of how an organism's genetic code is actually connected to its observable traits, effectively stretching the boundaries of gene science. Then in the latter half of the 20th century, a real turning point arrived when James Watson and Francis Crick revealed DNA's structure in 1953. Generally speaking, this discovery not only cleared up how genetic information is stored and passed on, it also triggered a burst of research in molecular genetics, firmly placing DNA at the heart of heredity. Soon after, breakthroughs such as recombinant DNA techniques and the polymerase chain reaction (PCR) emerged, providing scientists with the means to manipulate genes with ever-greater accuracy. These advances have significantly advanced our understanding of genetic disorders, the intricate role of the microbiome, and their various implications for human health and medicine. As the understanding of the genetic roots of diseases evolved, so too did opportunities for new therapies—underlining, in most cases, why genetic research is key to tackling today's health challenges. This progress even paved the way for fresh insights into complex ideas, such as the microbiota-gut-brain axis and its influence on neurological disorders (John et al., 2019), as well as for understanding sport-related concussions (McCrory et al., 2017).

Importance of Genetics in Understanding Heredity

Genetics and heredity significantly influence our understanding of biological inheritance. Scientists dig into the messy, intertwined details of genes to figure out how traits are passed along from one generation to another in ways that aren't always straightforward. It matters a great deal when it comes to health—after all, knowing about genetic predispositions can shed light on patterns within families, such as those associated with cystic fibrosis or sickle cell anemia, where a single gene mutation can lead to significant problems. Doctors have begun using this genetic information in clinics to guide diagnoses and treatments, providing them with a kind of predictive power that once seemed out of reach. In most cases, this demonstrates just how crucial genetics is (Vendramin et al., 2021). Genetics isn't just about single traits; it encompasses a broader picture where gene interactions intersect with environmental influences. Epigenetics, for instance, is quite fascinating—it demonstrates how external factors can influence gene activity without altering the underlying DNA, resulting in changes that can be inherited. Indeed, it may appear somewhat complicated, but this shows that heredity is an intricate interaction between what one experiences and what one inherits rather than a straightforward relay race of genes. In many cases, this perspective opens new doors for understanding complex diseases where multiple genes intersect with life's curveballs, an insight that's especially vital in fields like psychology and pharmacology, where responses to treatment can vary significantly based on genetic makeup and personal history (John et al., 2019). When various strands of gene research are considered, the importance of genetics in decoding heredity becomes even more apparent. Cracking the human genome didn't just give us a blueprint for our bodies—it also unraveled some of the winding evolutionary paths that drive genetic diversity. While the basics of heredity were laid out by Mendelian genetics, modern discoveries add layers that point to a far more intricate picture of variation across populations. Generally speaking, as research advances, it's becoming increasingly clear that understanding the fundamentals of genetics is crucial to addressing today's challenges in health, agriculture, and conservation. In many ways, this genetic insight forms the backbone of new ideas and practical solutions, keeping the study of heredity as relevant as ever (Vendramin et al., 2021) (Figure 8.3).

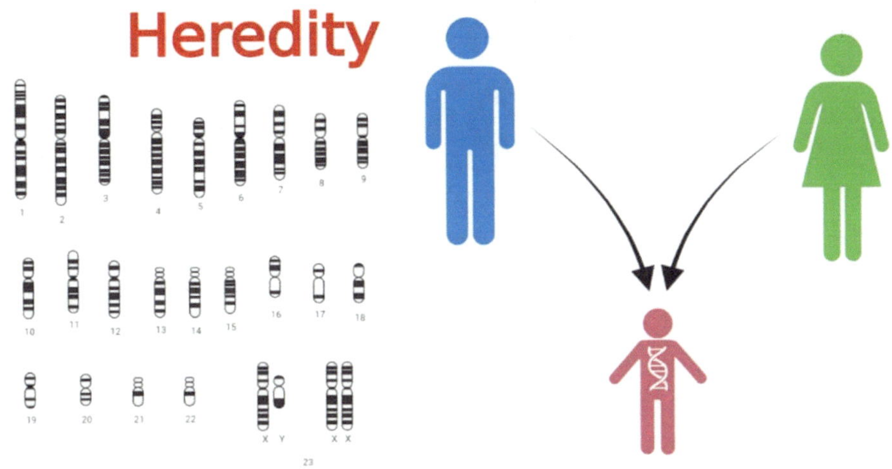

Figure 8.3. Importance of genetics in understanding heredity.

Source: https://microbenotes.com/wp-content/uploads/2022/10/Heredity.jpg.

8.1. Basic Concepts of Genetics

Traits are passed down generation after generation, and this simple truth lies at the heart of genetics. Genes—those little blueprints nestled in chromosomes— call the shots when it comes to everything humans look like and how they function. DNA (short for deoxyribonucleic acid) is the instruction manual for building and operating a living being. In most cases, when gametes form, different versions of a gene—called alleles—separate, a process that Gregor Mendel first highlighted. This is seen in classic monohybrid and dihybrid crosses, which give us a rough idea of how often certain traits are likely to appear. Concepts like dominant versus recessive, along with whether an organism is homozygous or heterozygous, recur frequently and help piece together the picture of diversity found in everything from crops to humans. Building on Mendel's early ideas, researchers have developed more complex models that capture the nuances of genetic inheritance. Traits governed by several genes—think height or skin color—don't always fit neatly into a dominant-recessive box but instead vary continuously. There's also epistasis, where one gene can mask or modify the effect of another, making predictions more challenging. And it isn't just about the genes themselves; the environment plays a significant role too, nudging how traits appear. Lately, scientists have shifted some focus toward epigenetics—a field that looks at heritable changes that occur without altering the DNA sequence itself. Generally speaking, these layered interactions show that genetics is neither a rigid roadmap nor a one-trick pony, but a dynamic dialogue between what's inherited and what's experienced. Understanding these basic genetic principles matters far beyond textbooks—it impacts our health, disease management, and even advances in biotechnology. Genetic predispositions to certain conditions underscore the importance of genetic counseling and personalized medicine, which are becoming increasingly important every day. Understanding how inheritance works can help patients identify potential risks, leading to more active and informed health choices. Then there's CRISPR, a tool making gene editing a real possibility for treating disorders once thought untouchable. As society enters this brave new world of modifying genetic material, ethical questions naturally arise, prompting scientists and the public alike to weigh in.

When we weave genetics into our overall health strategies, it isn't just about the science; it's about grappling with ethical responsibilities and making decisions that affect us all (Figure 8.4).

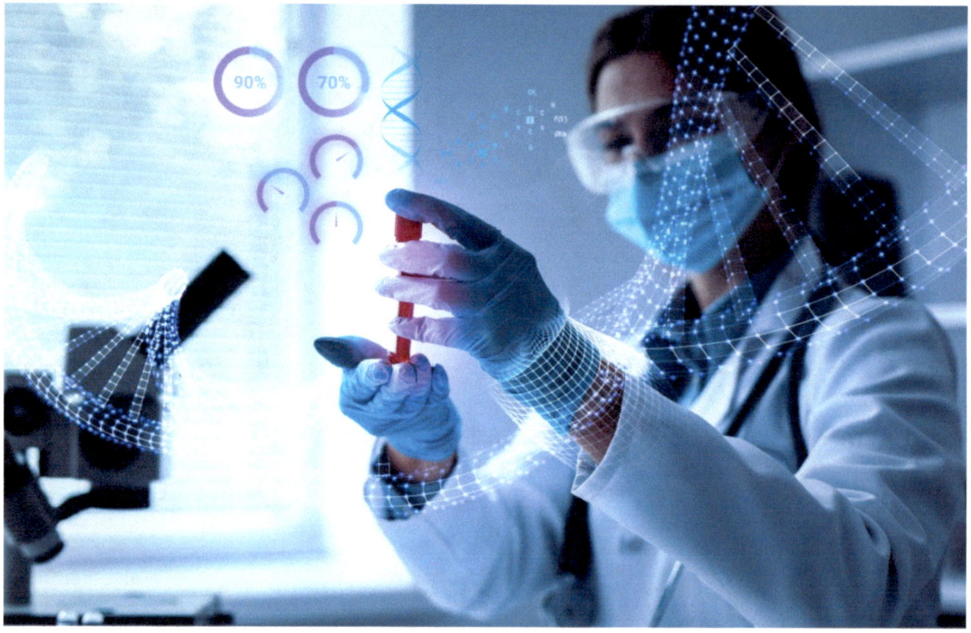

Figure 8.4. Concepts of Genetics.

Source: https://media.licdn.com/dms/image/D4D12AQEOYfRp2EuGag/article-cover_image-shrink_720_1280/0/1708013719263?e=2147483647&v=beta&t=zttr-awD3bQuC3Az8RarOSNlDcrnHytPCUI5DMUTGOc.

8.1.1. Genes and Alleles: Definitions and Differences

When studying genetics, genes and alleles become the basic building blocks. Genes are simply segments of DNA that code for proteins and are placed at specific spots on a chromosome. They can change a little here or there – those minor tweaks are what we call alleles, and they're pretty important for creating the diverse traits we notice in a population. In most cases, understanding the difference between a gene and its alternative forms helps us determine how traits are passed from one generation to the next. This idea, repeated over and over, establishes a more natural approach to studying genetic inheritance without getting too caught up in overly formal details. If one studies deeper, alleles begin to tell an even more interesting story. Each gene can come with several alleles that may differ by only a few nucleotide bases, which sometimes results in a significant difference in how an organism expresses its traits. Take flower color, for instance – a plant could have a gene for color that comes in variations, such as red or white. In many cases, a dominant red allele masks a recessive white one, so a red blossom is the result even when both versions are present. This back-and-forth between dominant and recessive types, while straightforward, underpins the classic ideas of Mendelian genetics and lays a foundation for exploring more complicated patterns in trait expression and even disease spread. Beyond just academic interest, this entire genes-versus-alleles picture has practical implications in fields such as medicine and agriculture. Geneticists often use what we understand about alleles to develop targeted therapies for specific disorders – here, pinpointing causal gene variants becomes central. Tools such as Combined Annotation-Dependent Depletion (CADD) help scientists assess the potential harm of a variant, which in turn determines which alleles are further studied in clinical settings (Rentzsch et al., 2018). Meanwhile, in agriculture, tweaking alleles leads to crops that reliably resist disease or produce better yields. All in all, figuring out the differences between genes and alleles isn't just a textbook exercise; it's a key part of applying genetic knowledge to real-world challenges (Figure 8.5).

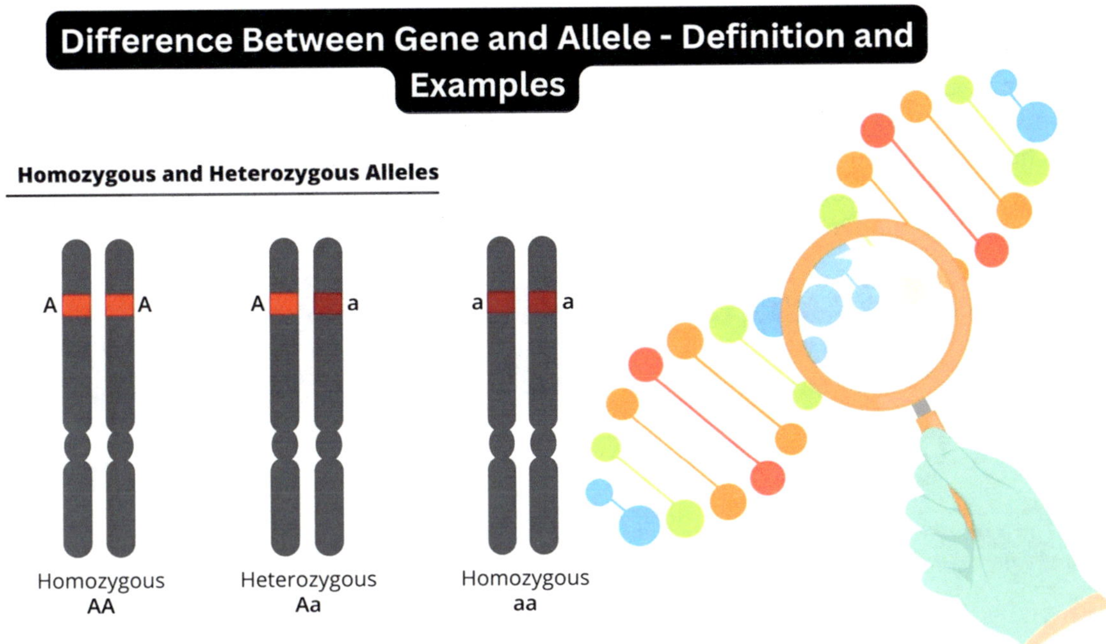

Figure 8.5. Genes and alleles: Definitions and differences.

Source: https://biologynotesonline.com/wp-content/uploads/2024/09/Difference-Between-Gene-and-Allele-Definition-and-Examples.jpg.

8.1.2. Chromosomes and Their Role in Inheritance

Chromosomes play a crucial role in the overall puzzle of genetic inheritance. At their core, these bundles of DNA and proteins are like nature's way to store handy blueprints—arranged into little units that help keep things in order as cells split. In a way, each chromosome carries a load of instructions that guide everything from growth to everyday function. It's interesting to note that when examining how traits are passed from one generation to another, the layout and quirks of chromosomes play a key role. Back in the day, Mendelian genetics shone a light on these basics, and that kick-started much of what we understand about genetic variation, eventually guiding modern genetics as we know it. Exploring the intricacies of inheritance, researchers are uncovering new insights into chromosome behavior during meiosis. This isn't just about splitting up the genetic material into gametes—it also involves processes like crossing-over and independent assortment, which, in most cases, boost genetic diversity. In simpler terms, the way chromosomes mix and match during sexual reproduction shows that passing on traits is far from a straightforward hand-me-down of DNA. Studies on organisms like *Trypanosoma brucei* even suggest that traditional Mendelian ideas hold true even in species that receive less attention. All these pieces together hint that chromosomes aren't solely responsible for inheritance; they also shed light on the broader evolutionary impact of genetic exchange (MacLeod et al., 2007). When examining chromosomal dynamics, the influence extends to broader scientific debates, encompassing genetics-related diseases and evolutionary biology. Researchers now examine how even minor glitches in chromosome setup can give rise to a range of disorders, stressing—sometimes repeatedly—the need for precise chromosomal operation to protect genetic stability. By bridging classic genetic theories with the latest genomic methods, scientists have created a more comprehensive understanding of how traits and diseases emerge, impacting both human health and biodiversity. They combine time-honored studies with new technology to develop innovative tools for examining genetic variations and their impact on how organisms appear and behave. In the end, chromosomes do more than define individual traits—they help mold entire species and populations over time, opening up exciting roads for future research in genomics (Novick et al., 2017) (Figure 8.6).

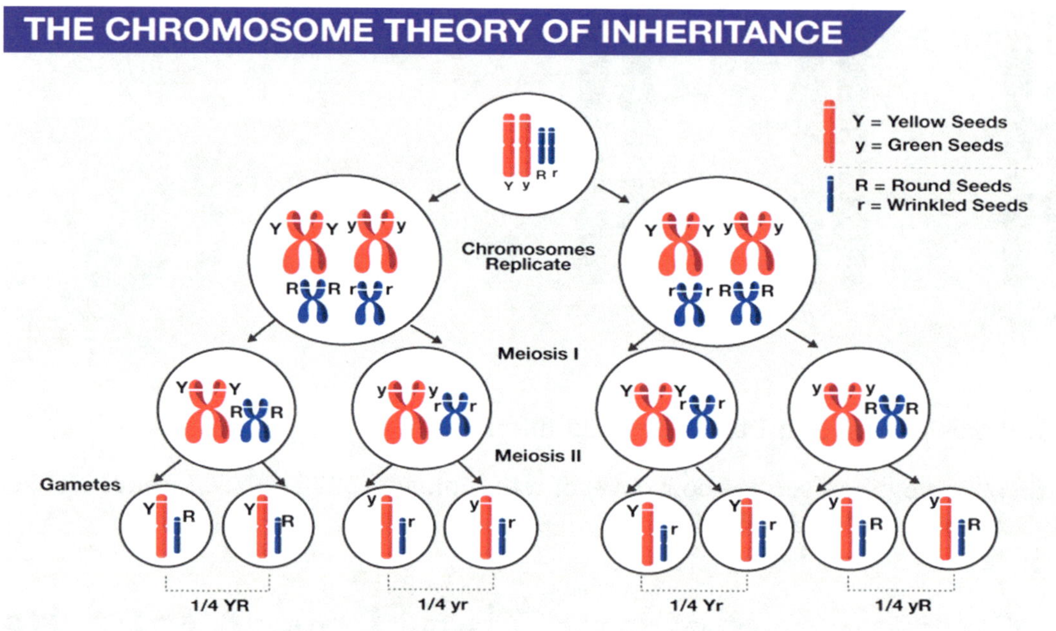

Figure 8.6. Chromosomal theory of inheritance.

Source: https://cdn1.byjus.com/wp-content/uploads/2017/11/THE-CHROMOSOME-THEORY-OF-INHERITANCE.png.

8.1.3. Genotype Versus Phenotype: Understanding Expression of Traits

Genotype and phenotype are tightly intertwined in genetics—even if it sounds all very theoretical, it's the way our genetic code morphs into what we see. Think of the genotype as the basic genetic recipe passed down from our parents —a mix of alleles. The resulting traits, the phenotype, aren't just about those inherited instructions. Environmental factors, such as diet, weather, and even the people we interact with, also play a role. In most cases, this mix of genes and surroundings is what leads to differences, even among organisms that share nearly identical blueprints. Studies with model organisms demonstrate that genetic interactions play a significant role in determining the traits we observe. Research generally suggests that the way traits add up depends on how often specific alleles appear at interacting spots—meaning individual genes can have more or less impact depending on their neighbors. Some investigations even suggest that networks of gene interplay, known as epistatic interactions, can enhance our predictions about phenotype outcomes. When scientists take the time to map these tangled webs, they gain a clearer picture of the genetic makeup behind trait diversity, which is crucial for anticipating how these traits might shift in response to new environmental stresses and selection pressures (Bloom et al., 2016).

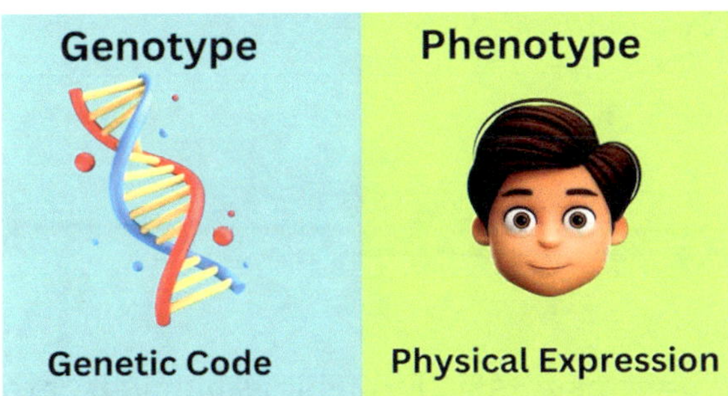

Figure 8.7. Genotype versus phenotype.

Source: https://i.ytimg.com/vi/4eK2JBctUa0/hq720.jpg?sqp=-oaymwEhCK4FEIIDSFryq4qpAxMIARUAAAAAGAElAADIQj0AgKJD&rs=AOn4CLB59Vv1gs690UvxPehvexa-WLhfbA.

Environmental tolerance further complicates and enriches our understanding of how genes and their surroundings work together over time. Reaction norms—basically explanations for how a gene's success varies with different conditions—shed light on both how a trait tends to appear and how widely it can vary. The ability of a genotype to adjust to changes in its environment can widen the range of traits it produces, suggesting that natural selection might favor creatures for reasons that blend both genetic predispositions and local conditions. Contemporary research, in most cases, demonstrates that these tolerance curves provide a valuable framework for predicting how populations adapt in response to ecological challenges. All in all, examining how broadly organisms can adapt provides us with essential clues about the ongoing interplay between genetics and the environment, and enriches our overall understanding of phenotype expression (Gabriel et al., 1992) (Figure 8.7).

8.2. Mendelian Genetics

Gregor Mendel sparked a whole new way of thinking about heredity when he started tinkering with pea plants—back then, the idea of traits passing down wasn't nearly as clear. His experiments, conducted with meticulous care and a hint of unexpected insight, revealed that traits don't simply blend; instead, they emerge in distinct ways, with some traits standing out and others receding into the background. Mendel's detailed notes, often repeated and refined over time, laid the groundwork for what we now call the laws of segregation and independent assortment. This isn't just an old theory tucked away in textbooks—it shapes our entire approach to modern genetics. It influences research on everything from simple traits to much more complicated genetic conditions. One can see his mark in gene mapping and studies of genetic disorders, a testament to his lasting influence and a reminder of how systematic, though sometimes unexpectedly informal, observation led to major scientific breakthroughs. Victor A. McKusick then applied those Mendelian ideas in a practical context within the field of medical genetics. He wasn't one to stick to abstract theories; instead, he wedded careful, everyday clinical observations with genetic analysis, showing off a knack for blending abstract concepts with real-life health issues. His work—especially mapping hereditary disorders in groups like the Amish—

helped bring Mendel's theories out of the lab and into everyday medical practice. By setting up courses and producing key resources such as "Mendelian Inheritance in Man," McKusick paved the way for holistic approaches in clinical care and research. In most cases, his teachings, laced with careful yet conversational insights, act as a bridge between theory and practice in medical genetics (Rasmussen et al., 2021). Around the same time, the field of genetics received a significant boost from new techniques—tissue culture, for instance, changed the game completely. Emerging in the mid-20th century, along with the widespread use of antibiotics, these techniques enabled researchers to delve into cytogenetics, gene localization, and even mutagenesis in ways that earlier methods couldn't accommodate. There's a kind of natural synergy here, a blending of Mendel's early insights with modern, sometimes unpredictable, approaches that dig deep into the fabric of genetic interactions and the roots of various diseases. As scientists continue to push the envelope, building on the legacy of those first observations with fresh, if occasionally rough-edged methods, the hope for breakthroughs in understanding complex genetic disorders remains as strong as ever (Nichols, 2009) (Figure 8.8).

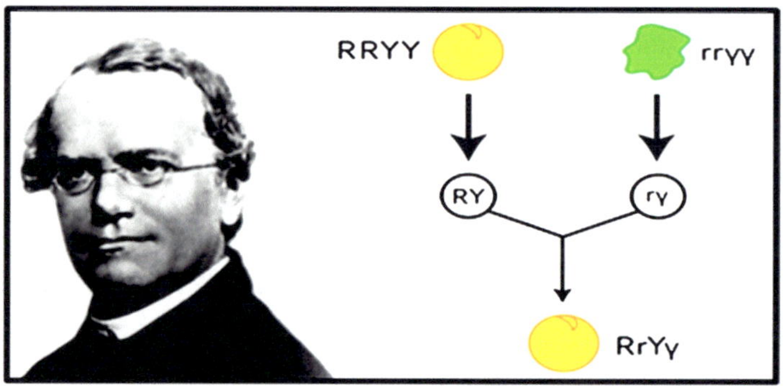

Figure 8.8. Mendel genetics.

Source: https://external-content.duckduckgo.com/iu/?u=https%3A%2F%2Fblogs.biomedcentral.com%2Fbmcseriesblog%2Fwp-content%2Fuploads%2Fsites%2F9%2F2015%2F03%2FMendel.png&f=1&nofb=1&ipt=dd3db0ff364ba519b138daecbcf48b7b3b1595af94ef9278d130f55dbf1c29f4.

8.2.1. Gregor Mendel's Experiments with Pea Plants

Gregor Mendel's work with pea plants in the mid-1800s set off a chain reaction in how we view inheritance. He casually mixed different pea varieties—tweaking flower color and seed shape—to see what might happen, and his careful yet sometimes uneven observations laid the groundwork for what we now call modern genetics. He wasn't just busy in a lab for the sake of it; his experiments matched the everyday needs of farmers and plant enthusiasts. Oddly enough, his studies even stepped outside the quiet walls of his monastery to engage with local communities curious about plant hybrids, showing that his discoveries mattered far beyond pure theory (Gliboff et al., 2013). Mendel's findings were published in 1866, and although his work didn't receive much attention during his lifetime, it eventually had a profound impact on biology. His idea that traits could be dominant or recessive—what we now label as Mendelian inheritance—provided a statistical foundation for predicting how traits might appear in future generations. Yet, later on, Ronald Fisher in 1936 pointed out that Mendel's data might have been biased too neatly toward his expectations, and this sparked debates that, to be honest, still persist in scientific circles (Branco et al., 2011).

It appears that even the earliest research can be viewed from many perspectives. We can't ignore how far Mendel's trials extend; his experiments overflowed well beyond botany into areas such as evolutionary biology and medicine, linking genetics with broader life processes. Today, scientists revisit his work—admiring his breakthrough while also wrestling with the ethical and methodological quirks that marked his early studies. Generally speaking, this ongoing discussion advocates for a more open and transparent scientific process, serving as a reminder of the importance of examining research from multiple angles. Ultimately, his legacy continues to challenge and shape our modern understanding of heredity and the science of genetics (Gliboff et al., 2013).

8.2.2. Laws of Inheritance: Segregation and Independent Assortment

Genetic inheritance isn't just a dry set of rules—it's the pulse behind how traits show up in every living thing. Think of it like this: each individual carries a couple of alleles for every trait, and when gametes form, these alleles split apart, so that each gamete gets its copy. That's what the law of segregation is all about, and it keeps things diverse.

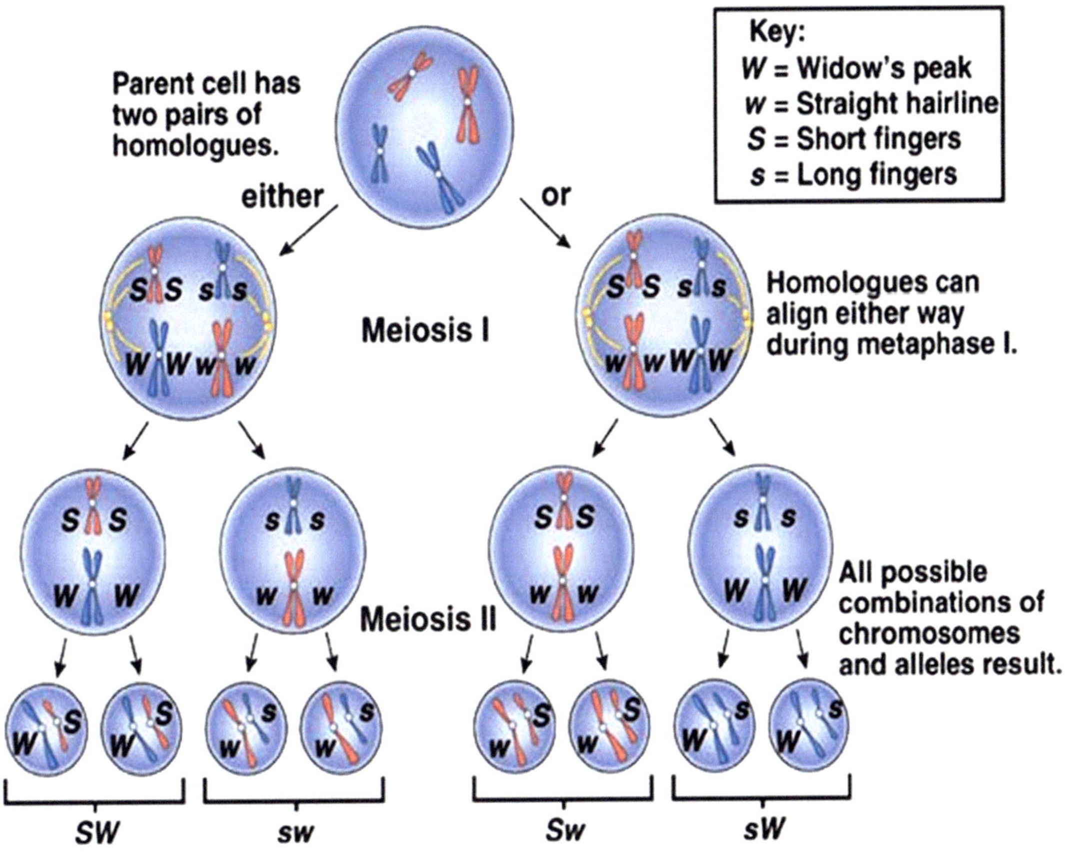

Figure 8.9. Segregation and independent assortment.

Source: https://external-content.duckduckgo.com/iu/?u=https%3A%2F%2Fimage.slideserve.com%2F281608%2Fsegregation-and-independent-assortment-l.jpg&f=1&nofb=1&ipt=320e8345b283346d65ead7a53ed78e878fdbe6cad942ed17f7bdc394b1d47f21.

Then there's independent assortment, which means that alleles from different genes mix it up on their own, not following a strict order. This spontaneous shuffling lays the groundwork for new combinations in offspring, and, generally speaking, it's a big reason why species can adapt to new challenges over time. Scientists have explored these ideas to gain a deeper understanding of more complex traits and diseases. When one realize that many traits arise from the interplay of multiple alleles, it opens up a whole puzzle about predictability and variation. Sure, simple traits—those governed by one gene—fit neatly into these ideas, but traits influenced by several genes (polygenic inheritance) make the picture much fuzzier. In most cases, this layered genetic blueprint helps researchers grasp just how intricate and interconnected our inherited traits can be, even if there's occasional overlap or redundancy in how they express themselves. Beyond just theory, these genetic principles extend into practical realms such as genetic engineering and genome editing. Researchers in agriculture and medicine, for example, rely on the idea that understanding how alleles segregate and mix can help them predict inheritance patterns with a fair degree of accuracy. This predictive power is crucial when attempting to develop more resilient crops or novel treatments for genetic diseases. In essence, by understanding and playing with these fundamental laws, scientists can better navigate the messy, beautiful landscape of life—and that's what makes studying genetics so endlessly fascinating (Figure 8.9).

8.2.3. Applications of Mendelian Principles in Modern Genetics

Gregor Mendel's ideas continue to shape modern genetics in ways that aren't always presented in a straightforward, step-by-step manner. His fundamental insights about how traits get passed down now underpin studies that dig into the links between our DNA and a range of characteristics. Researchers, for example, sift through countless genetic markers – sometimes hundreds of thousands – to identify differences that hint at why certain diseases or traits occur. In most cases, this hands-on approach, built on Mendel's early work, even allows scientists to gauge how much of a trait is due to genetics; it's a technique that plays a significant role in designing new medicines and public health strategies. These time-tested ideas extend far beyond academic theory, influencing everyday medical decisions and sparking new research innovations (Uffelmann et al., 2021).

The push to integrate genetics into everyday medical training is also catching on. Schools are mixing things up by introducing active learning modules that don't simply rehash textbook material. Medical students, for instance, now dive right into resources like the Online Mendelian Inheritance in Man (OMIM) database, using it to analyze real patient cases where inheritance isn't always straightforward. Generally speaking, these hands-on sessions help build confidence – and sometimes involve a little trial and error – when it comes to spotting genetic clues in complex conditions. This shift indicates that, in most settings, healthcare educators feel the need to equip future professionals with practical genetic knowledge, preparing them for an era when hereditary issues are at the forefront of patient care (Anderson et al., 2021). Genetic counseling stands out as another area where old ideas meet new technology in unexpectedly fluid ways. Counselors now rely on the very frameworks Mendel established, using them to sort through genetic test results and offer families a clearer picture of their health risks. That said, things become more complicated when multiple genes – and even environmental factors – complicate the picture. In such cases, merging those classic Mendelian ideas with the latest genomic tools can sharpen a counselor's insight, leading to care that's more tailored to individual needs. All in all, blending tradition with innovation shows that Mendel's early work remains a reliable guide, even as the methods and models of genetics continue to evolve (Uffelmann et al., 2021) (Figure 8.10).

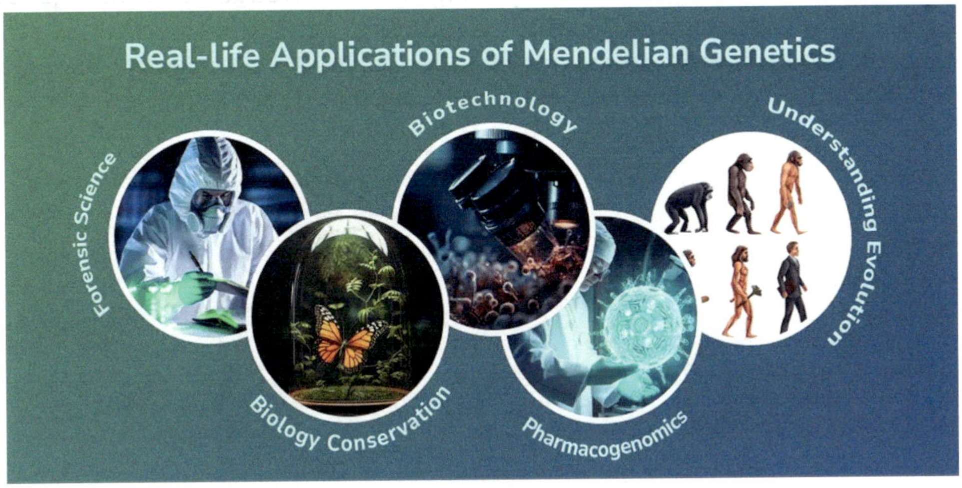

Figure 8.10. Applications of Mendelian principles in modern genetics.

Source: https://media.geeksforgeeks.org/wp-content/uploads/20240404144816/Real-life-Applications-of-Mendelian-Genetics.webp.

8.3. Molecular Genetics

Life at the molecular scale uncovers secrets about heredity and genetic changes. Early biophysics initiated a journey that combined ideas from various fields, and now molecular genetics is all about integrating those insights. Erwin Schrödinger, for instance, set a new course with his well-known book—he envisioned the genetic code long before many of us did. He pictured genetic material as a kind of solid, an aperiodic crystal, which, in turn, laid the groundwork for the later discovery of DNA's double helix. His thoughts on "negative entropy" suggested that life, constructed from tiny parts, could resist chaos. In most cases, that early spark led researchers to explore genes in greater detail and connect them to broader biological functions (Danylova, 2020). In medicine, the impact of molecular genetics is clear, especially when examining diseases like glioblastoma multiforme (GBM). This grade IV tumor shows how digging into gene details can unravel the messy process of tumor formation—specific mutations seem to create very varied genetic profiles even within similar tumors. Interestingly, the story of gliomas dates back to early notes from over two centuries ago, which eventually blended with work by researchers like Bailey and Cushing, painting a narrative that becomes richer with each new genetic insight. With molecular testing now in the mix, the link between genotype and what is observed in patients (the phenotype) becomes clearer, and treatment can be more tailored. Generally speaking, understanding GBM's genetic roots has altered clinical practices, demonstrating how genetics can inspire new ideas in oncology and potentially enhance patient outcomes (Stoyanov et al., 2018). Molecular genetics also shifts our view on evolution, not constantly in textbook-style order. Studying nucleotide sequences and gene expression reveals how species adapt over time to small changes in their environment. By examining gene differences in populations, researchers can piece together evolutionary relationships and even the details of speciation and genetic drift. This hands-on method provides us with a deeper, albeit sometimes messy, understanding of biodiversity and life's many layers. Cutting-edge tools like CRISPR gene editing are further revolutionizing the field, opening up new avenues to tackle genetic disorders and enhance agriculture. As molecular genetics continues to integrate into various scientific fields, its implications continue to broaden our understanding of both fundamental biological processes and the complex systems that sustain life (Danylova, 2020) (Figure 8.11).

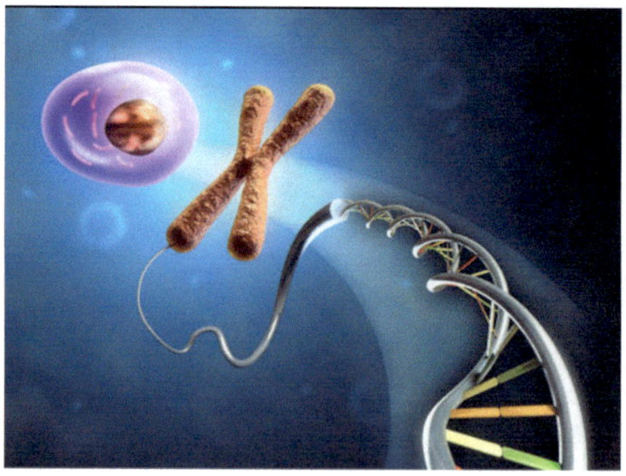

Figure 8.11. Molecular genetics.

Source: https://www.simply.science/images/content/biology/genetics/molecular_genetics/conceptmap/image1.gif.

8.3.1. Structure and Function of DNA

At its core, genetic information is stored in DNA. This molecule, made of two strands running in opposite directions that twist into a double helix, doesn't just keep our genetic material safe—it also makes replication and transcription possible. The helix holds itself together through specific base pairing (adenine joins up with thymine, and cytosine with guanine), which means that every time a cell divides, it's generally able to make a nearly perfect copy of its genetic code. And then there are the grooves—both broad and narrow—that serve as docking sites for proteins like transcription factors. In many cases, these small details in DNA's design directly shape how it works within the cell, showcasing a neat link between its structure and function. But there's more to DNA than just a sturdy, predictable structure. It's surprisingly flexible when it comes to modifications that can tweak how genes are expressed and how the genome stays stable. Chemical changes, such as methylation occurring at specific cytosine sites, can either silence or enhance gene activity depending on the cell's immediate needs. These epigenetic tweaks add an extra, sometimes redundant, layer of complexity to genetic expression—helpful for processes such as development, differentiation, and responding to environmental cues. At times, DNA can twist into loops or supercoil in unexpected ways, which might change how accessible its instructions are. This adaptability highlights DNA's versatile nature, providing organisms with a dynamic means to fine-tune gene expression. Researchers generally see great promise in harnessing these modifications for applications in gene therapy and biotechnology. DNA's role isn't limited to simply encoding genetic instructions, either—it also plays a hand in extensive repair work. A host of proteins is assigned the task of spotting and repairing errors or damage in the DNA, which is critical for maintaining the genomic blueprint intact. Think about the replication process: enzymes like DNA polymerases add nucleotides with such precision it's almost remarkable, yet when there's damage from environmental stress or replication slip-ups, repair systems jump in. Mechanisms like base excision repair and nucleotide excision repair provide backup, mending the flaws as they occur. This repair work underscores DNA's essential function not only in heredity but also in protecting the genetic framework of life across generations. In this way, the interwoven nature of structure, modification, and repair paints a pretty complete picture of the many roles DNA has in our biology (Figure 8.12).

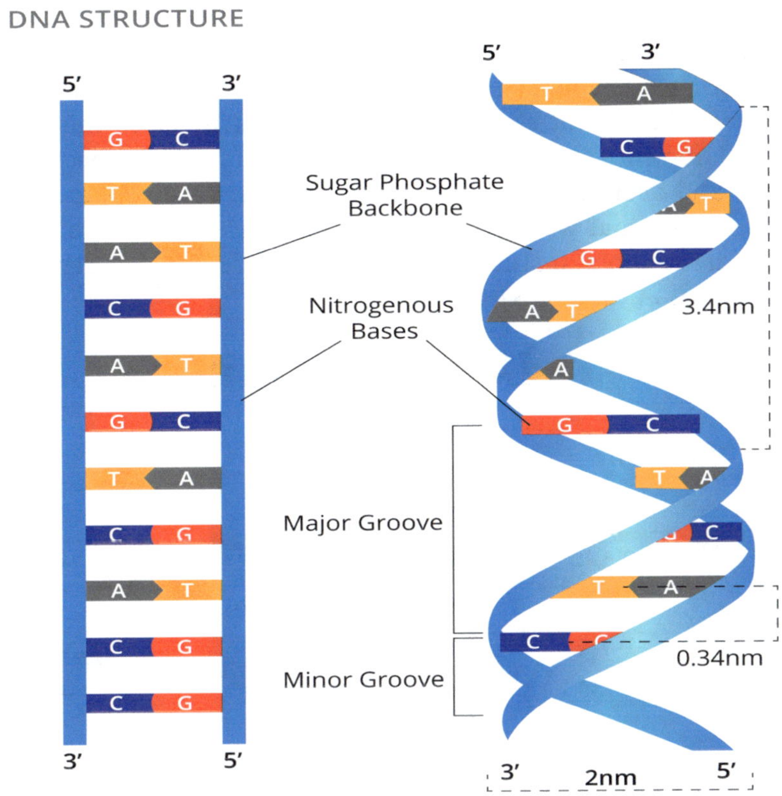

Figure 8.12. DNA structure and function.

Source: https://www.earthslab.com/wp-content/uploads/2017/07/DNA_structure.jpg.

8.3.2. The Process of DNA Replication

Genetic info getting passed on correctly in every cell division isn't something that just happens by chance. DNA replication—the process of unwinding our double-stranded blueprint so new, matching strands can be put together—kicks things off. Instead of following a neat, step-by-step plan, the cell gets started at several points simultaneously. At these replication forks, helicase enzymes unwind the twist of the DNA, leaving behind two single strands that then serve as guides for the next round of building, primarily facilitated by DNA polymerases. These polymerases not only add the new bits but also check their work as they go, fixing errors on the fly; without this built-in proofreading, mistakes would pile up and could even trigger significant changes over time—so , accurate replication is key to keeping things running smoothly in the cell. As the process progresses, unexpected snags can arise, especially in complex areas like centromeres. These regions are a headache because their repetitive sequences tend to fold into unusual shapes, which can significantly disrupt the usual unwinding routine. In many cases, specialized proteins—such as DNA2, for example—jump in to clear the mess. DNA2 isn't just busy removing obstacles; it also helps tidy up Okazaki fragments on the lagging strand. This mix of unwinding and cleanup illustrates the complexity of the entire protein effort, as these molecular workers collaborate in unpredictable ways to ensure that even the most intricate parts of the genome are copied accurately, a crucial step for proper chromosome segregation during cell division (Li et al., 2018). Generally speaking, accurately wrapping up DNA replication is absolutely vital for cell survival and maintaining genome stability. When the process encounters a snag—whether due to genetic mutations or environmental disturbances—replication forks can stall and trigger checkpoint responses. Pathways involved in the DNA damage response, often mediated by ATR, step in to handle these issues; if things can't be set right, the cell might end up halting its cycle and even undergo apoptosis. Ongoing research continues to shed light on these replication details, and what we learn not only deepens our grasp of basic genetics but also paves the way for new treatments against diseases like cancer, where errors in replication are a common challenge (Galluzzi et al., 2018) (Figure 8.13).

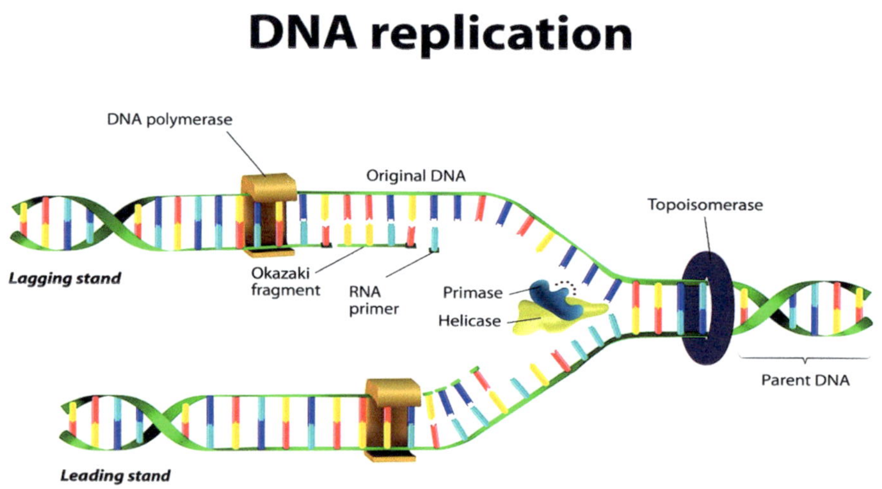

Figure 8.13. The process of DNA replication.

Source: https://d2jx2rerrg6sh3.cloudfront.net/image-handler/picture/2018/7/shutterstock_201778373.jpg.

8.3.3. Role of RNA in Protein Synthesis

Cells buzz with activity, and a lot of it comes down to tiny molecules that "talk" between genes and proteins. RNA sits right in the middle of this buzz—acting as both messenger and translator in a process that unfolds in unexpected steps. mRNA, which is a copied blueprint from DNA, carries instructions straight from the nucleus to the cell's bustling inner space. Once out there, it buddies up with ribosomes, which read its code and piece together an amino acid chain that eventually shapes a protein. This shift from simple nucleic acid info to a complex protein is kept in check by various natural regulators (Philip et al., 2020). Then there's more to the story than just mRNA. Take tRNA, for example—it's a little helper that hitches specific amino acids and matches them up with the corresponding bits on the mRNA through its anticodon. It's almost like each tRNA is on a mission to deliver just the right piece of the puzzle. Meanwhile, rRNA joins forces with proteins to form ribosomes: those busy, built-to-work factories churning out proteins. In many cases, the collaboration among these different RNA types keeps the process on track, even if it can seem a bit unpredictable at times (Wang et al., 2019). Diving a bit deeper, RNA's role isn't limited to everyday cell chatter—it also shows up when things go wrong. Generally speaking, if RNA is disrupted due to mutations or regulatory issues, the resulting protein assembly line can be thrown off, potentially leading to a range of genetic problems. In most cases, however, this very knowledge has opened doors to clever fixes, such as RNA-based vaccines and cutting-edge gene-editing tools. As researchers continue to unravel the mechanisms of RNA function—both in healthy conditions and in disease—the insights they gather continually expand our understanding of genetics and cellular behavior in new and unexpected ways (Philip et al., 2020) (Figure 8.14).

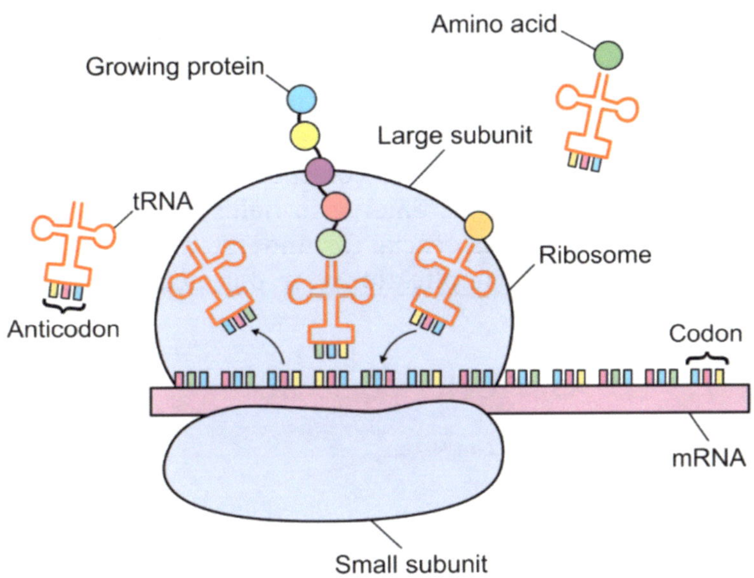

Figure 8.14. A new role for transfer RNA in protein synthesis.

Source: https://www.pnas.org/cms/asset/9a303b9d-0bc7-495d-932b-a72e1106c9b9/sciencesourceimages_2479214_mediumres_croptranslation.jpg.

8.4. Genetic Variation

Genetic variation is the engine behind natural selection—it's hard to overemphasize its role. Without a mix of different genes, populations would not be able to adjust when their surroundings change or when threats like diseases emerge unexpectedly. This variety manifests in several ways: through mutations, gene flow, and even a bit of randomness that we call genetic drift. Mutations introduce new alleles into a group, laying the groundwork for evolution. And then there's gene flow; when individuals move between groups, they pass along their genetic bits, which adds to the overall mix. In small populations, chance can play a considerable role—genetic drift can suddenly change allele frequencies, sometimes in ways that seem almost random. In many cases, these processes merge, weaving a pretty complex tapestry of genes that's crucial for both evolution and everyday adaptation. In addition to that big picture, genetic variation impacts individual health and disease risk. Variations in genes can lead to different traits, not just in how we look, but also in how our bodies respond to medications or fight off illnesses. For instance, studies on Drosophila melanogaster have revealed some interesting insights into how even minor genetic differences can have a profound impact on a whole population. These patterns spill over to human genetics too, where specific sets of alleles seem linked to conditions like diabetes or even some cancers. This kind of information, generally speaking, is vital for personalized medicine—helping tailor treatment plans to match an individual's unique genetic makeup. As we delve deeper into the intricacies of genetic variation, its role in health and disease continues to garner increasing attention in both research and clinical circles. And it's not just about the little letter-by-letter differences in DNA; there's also a whole realm of change that comes from big structural tweaks. Think chromosomal inversions, transposable elements, or other genome rearrangements that can mess with how genes are expressed—sometimes causing rapid changes in how an organism appears or functions. Thanks to recent advances in genomic techniques, scientists have been able to examine these larger alterations with greater detail than ever before, uncovering just how much they contribute to evolution. These findings, in most cases, underscore that genetic variation is much more than just single-nucleotide differences. As researchers continue to explore these structural shifts, we can expect to see fresh and innovative ideas emerge in fields ranging from evolutionary biology to medicine. All in all, this broader view is crucial for understanding the complex and fascinating nature of genetics and its far-reaching implications for our health, evolution, and biodiversity (Figure 8.15).

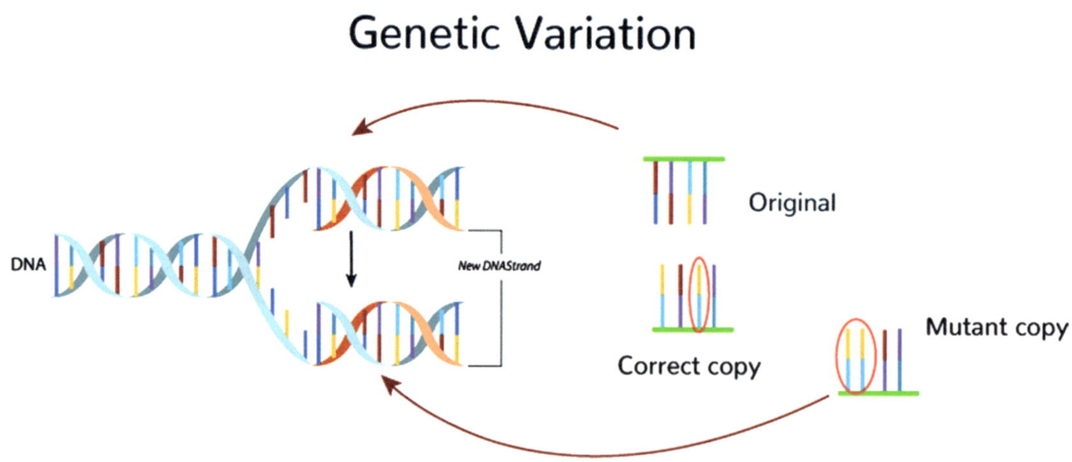

Figure 8.15. Genetic variation.

Source: https://external-content.duckduckgo.com/iu/?u=https%3A%2F%2Fmedia.geeksforgeeks.org%2Fwp-content%2Fuploads%2F20240119101553%2FGenetic-Variation-660.png&f=1&nofb=1&ipt=6ee961b1b66adc2b8117def4760d475116323079f259dcd9cba5ccf5ec78407c.

8.4.1. Sources of Genetic Variation: Mutations and Recombination

Genetic variation kicks off with unexpected shifts that lie at the heart of evolution. Mutations, in a lot of cases, are the sparks that light up new genetic possibilities—they show up when DNA slips during replication or when the environment pushes it off course. Take, for instance, bacteria; they've been known to have mutation rates between 1.4×10^{-6} and 4.5×10^{-6} changes per nucleotide each year, which steadily builds up genetic diversity over time. This spontaneous variability helps organisms adapt, yet if these changes stack up too often without correction they can also cause trouble, showing mutations to be both creative and sometimes, honestly, a bit problematic (Gelman et al., 2010). Recombination also plays its part by mixing the genetic material in ways that are anything but routine. During sexual reproduction, genetic material gets reshuffled almost like dealing a new hand in a card game—with alleles swapping between chromosomes in a process that feels more like natural mischief than mere chance. In most cases, this isn't just a random scrambling; a quirk known as GC-biased gene conversion (gBGC) tends to favor G/C pairs over A/T pairs, adding a subtle twist that not only adjusts the nucleotide balance but can also spur speedy evolution in specific regions (Auton et al., 2013). It's almost as if nature enjoys mixing things up with a dash of unpredictability. When viewed as a whole, mutations and recombination work together in a delicate dance that shapes life's genetic story. New genetic variations are introduced through mutations, and then recombination picks up these variations, remixing them over generations to enhance a population's adaptability. Natural selection usually steps in too—filtering out the harmful missteps while keeping the beneficial ones around. Studies on bacteria and model organisms generally show that these rates can vary significantly, meaning the entire evolutionary outcome isn't set in stone. In many cases, these insights deepen our understanding of genetic diversity and reveal how organisms manage to navigate a constantly changing world (Gelman et al., 2010; Auton et al., 2013) (Figure 8.16).

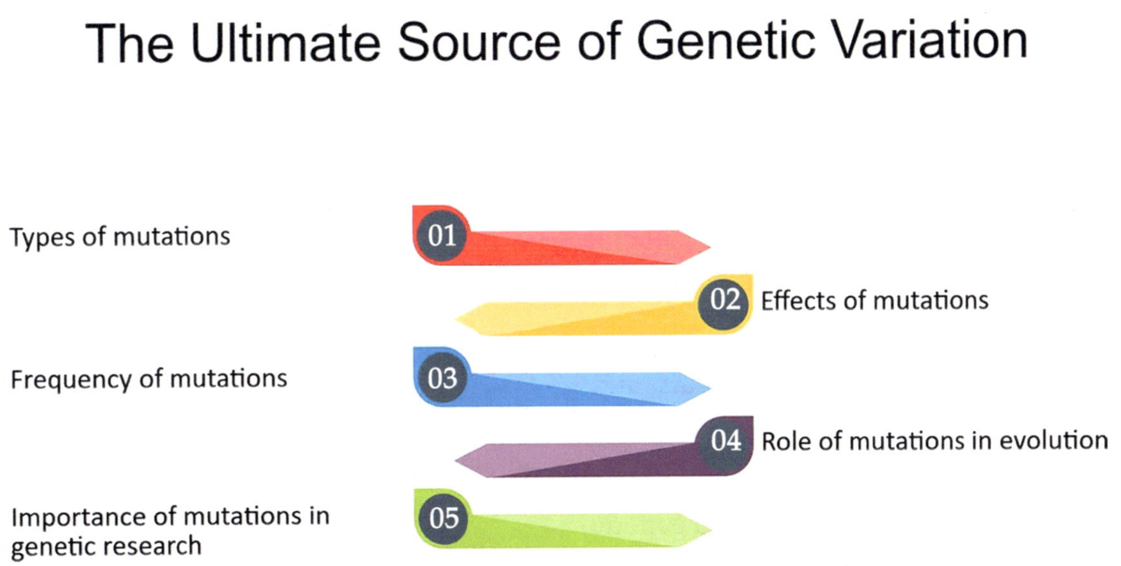

Figure 8.16. The ultimate source of genetic variation.

Source: https://fastercapital.co/i/Genetic-Variation--The-Fuel-behind-Natural-Selection--The-Ultimate-Source-of-Genetic-Variation.webp.

8.4.2. Importance of Genetic Diversity in Populations

Genetic variety truly matters. Different genes mixed together help species adapt to sudden changes in the environment—whether it's shifts in climate, unexpected diseases, or other stress factors. Some studies on population differences have shown that certain genetic traits can be advantageous under specific conditions, thereby increasing the odds of survival and reproduction. Forests, for example, appear to benefit from a cocktail of genes that enables them to withstand human-caused pressures and climate fluctuations. In many cases, research on Mediterranean forests has suggested that managing these gene mixes is crucial when preparing for future challenges, such as changing weather patterns or invasive species (Fady et al., 2022). Essentially, monitoring areas with high genetic diversity helps maintain nature's balance. More than just an environmental safety net, a diverse mix of genes plays a significant role in maintaining population health. When genetic diversity drops too low, inbreeding can occur, making groups more susceptible to diseases and less capable of adapting to new threats. Consider the recent COVID-19 outbreak—when coronaviruses jumped to humans—which clearly shows how our genetic set-up may affect our vulnerability to infections. Examining the genetic makeup of populations enables researchers to identify weaknesses, allowing public health plans to be more effectively tailored. With viruses like SARS-CoV-2 reminding us of the stakes, it has become clear that examining genetic differences in both individuals and groups is crucial (Alexander et al., 2020). In most cases, diving into genetic studies now means we can be better prepared when the next outbreak occurs. Efforts to expand genetic variety are fundamental for how we approach conservation and manage natural resources over the long haul. Projects aimed at reviving and protecting species appear to have a significant impact on the way ecosystems function. For instance, effective forest management often begins with identifying and protecting areas rich in diverse genetic resources, especially in regions renowned for their biodiversity. Recent work reveals that understanding the genetic structure of these populations can inform actions such as assisted migration and restoration—with some studies even showing that collaboration between researchers and land managers pays off when it comes to enhancing a forest's ability to adapt (Fady et al., 2022). By keeping our focus on sustaining genetic diversity, we not only help ensure that species continue to thrive, but we also make ecosystems more resilient when faced with the unexpected in our ever-changing world.

8.4.3. Impact of Genetic Variation on Evolution

Genetic variation lies at the core of evolution. Populations host a jumble of genes that natural selection works on—almost like raw clay waiting to be molded. Mutations, gene flow, and recombination all contribute to creating a constantly shifting mix, and this ever-changing blend fuels evolutionary change in species over time. For example, studies on *Daphnia galeata* populations across Europe; researchers noted surprisingly high clonal variety and marked differences among groups. Local conditions, it turns out, and that same genetic mix help shape a species' ability to adjust when the environment shifts, which drives home how intertwined genes and surroundings are (Dove et al., 2005). In agriculture, things aren't much different—genetic variation spills over into our farms too. Weeds, for instance, develop an almost uncanny resilience as they evolve under the pressure of crop cultivation and the use of herbicides. This rapid adaptation (which, in many cases, leads to resistance) shows a direct tie between a species' gene pool and its survival tactics. A closer look at the genetic frameworks within these weeds can help craft strategies to slow down adaptation and curb their spread, highlighting how evolution-informed practices are key to handling adaptation, persistence, and overall management challenges on our fields (Ainsworth et al., 2009). Conservation also relies heavily on the genetic diversity available within a species. For endangered populations, a diverse genetic pool is essential for survival and enhancing resilience when abrupt changes—such as climate shifts or new outbreaks of disease—occur. In most cases, maintaining this diversity enables species to better cope with and adapt to new challenges. Genetic insights, when integrated into conservation strategies, enable us to identify crucial gene reservoirs and refine breeding techniques for population restoration. Ultimately, the interplay between genetic diversity and evolution not only deepens our theoretical understanding but also underscores the practical steps necessary for effective ecological management (Dove et al., 2005).

8.5. Genetic Disorders

Genetic disorders captivate us with a curious mix of scientific allure and ethical puzzles—especially as the field of genetics continues to evolve. Sometimes, a tiny gene slip-up triggers a problem, and other times it's a whole chromosomal mess or even a combination of factors, such as one's daily habits and the environment. Generally speaking, these complications don't just touch one person; they ripple out into communities. Nowadays, identifying these issues early is crucial, and clinical genetics has taken center stage in achieving this goal. Oddly enough, even art—think Velázquez's Las Meninas—hints at old-school observation techniques that once helped identify unusual traits and overlooked syndromes, nudging modern evaluations along (Peralta et al., 2025). Clinical genetics has steadily become the go-to approach for managing these conditions, opening the door to early action and treatments tailored to individual needs. Take, for example, cystic fibrosis or Duchenne muscular dystrophy: breakthroughs in genetic testing have flipped the script, letting families weigh their options when it comes to treatment and even future planning. As we delve deeper into the human genome, gene therapy emerges as a promising, albeit sometimes complex, solution. Of course, these advances aren't free of ethical questions—issues like who gets access and the real effects of tinkering with our genes. Even in fields like andrology, where the focus shifts to how genetics might influence male infertility, the debate broadens, merging hands-on clinical care with cutting-edge genetic technology (Akbari et al., 2025).

Then there's the bigger picture. Genetic disorders push their influence well past the lab, impacting public health policies, genetic counseling, and community outreach. Tackling the lingering stigmas is key to building acceptance and support for those affected. In many cases, public health efforts now aim to raise awareness about genetic risks and emphasize screening, particularly in communities where certain conditions are more prevalent. It all comes down to teamwork—doctors, geneticists, ethicists, and social workers all contribute to shaping care plans that not only address the disorder but also enhance a patient's overall quality of life. In a way, blending medical genetics with social strategies marks a turning point in how we handle the sweeping consequences of these disorders (Peralta et al., 2025) (Figure 8.17).

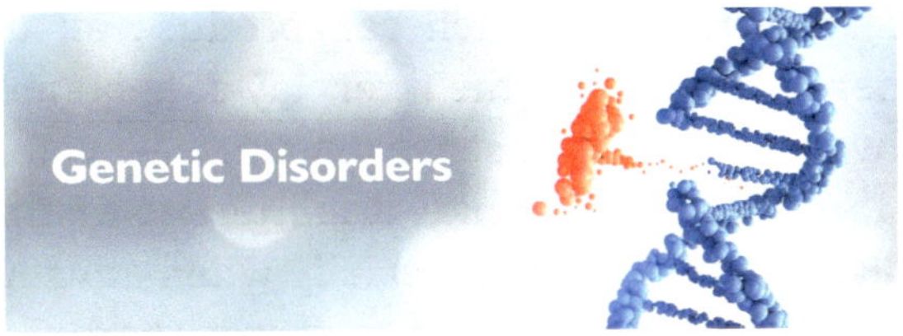

Figure 8.17. Genetic disorder.

Source: https://www.medicoverhospitals.in/images/articles/genetic-disorders.webp.

8.5.1. Types of Genetic Disorders: Single-Gene Versus Multifactorial

Genetic disorders show up in all sorts of ways, hinting at the inner workings that decide how they're passed down. Some of these conditions boil down to a single-gene error – take cystic fibrosis or sickle cell anemia, for instance – where a mutation in one gene typically follows the classic Mendelian cues. This clear link between a faulty gene and the way symptoms appear often makes genetic testing and counseling relatively straightforward; it provides a solid foundation for understanding how traits are passed from one person to the next. In general, the simplicity of these conditions stands in stark contrast to more complex maladies, underscoring how specific genes can have a direct impact on health.

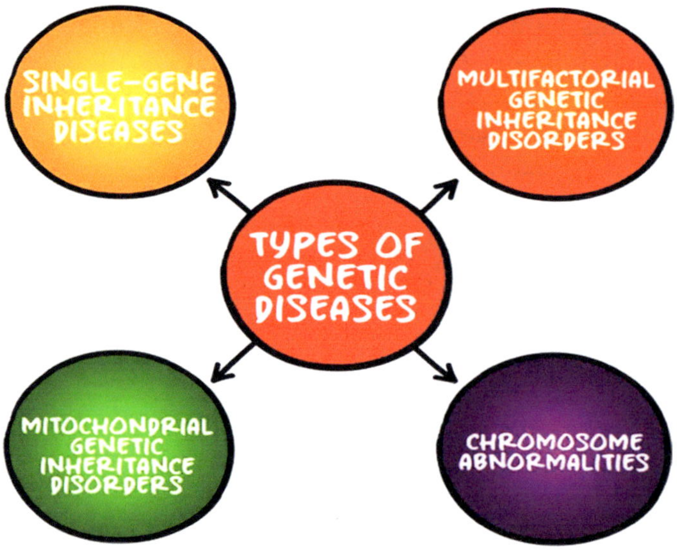

Figure 8.18. Types of genetic diseases.

Source: https://en.pimg.jp/109/689/267/1/109689267.jpg.

On the flip side, multifactorial disorders get messy. They don't arise from just one gene, but from a mix of several genes along with a dose of environmental influence—diabetes and heart disease, for example, spring to mind. In most cases, these disorders don't stick to neat, predictable patterns; instead, a whole array of genetic predispositions ends up mingling with lifestyle and external triggers, which can produce an unpredictable spread of symptoms. Researchers have generally found that the interplay of epigenetics and these gene-environment mashups deepens our view of health and disease dynamics—even if it complicates risk prediction and genetic counseling a bit more than we'd like. It matters to distinguish between a single-gene glitch and these complex, multifactorial issues, especially when advancing in genetic medicine and public health. Single-gene disorders often allow us to target therapies directly at the problem, but tackling multifactorial ones means we have to delve into how genes and our environment interact. For example, the role of the microbiota—tiny communities living in our gut—shows how our natural genetic setup and the world around us can team up in surprising ways, affecting everything from metabolism to the development of cardiovascular troubles (Hou et al., 2022). This kind of insight prompts us to bring in experts from all areas, as blending genetic data with environmental context is crucial to understanding these complex conditions. As genetics continues to evolve, these layered perspectives will likely spark new strategies for early detection, prevention, and targeted care, aiming to boost patient outcomes (Figure 8.18).

8.5.2. Examples of Common Genetic Disorders

Genetic disorders are tricky and show up in all sorts of unexpected ways. Take, for instance, those cases where just one gene goes awry, like with cystic fibrosis. Here, a mutation in the CFTR gene disrupts the normal flow of chloride ions through cell membranes; as a result, thick, sticky mucus accumulates in organs such as the lungs and pancreas, often causing severe breathing and digestive problems. Because this condition runs in families through an autosomal recessive pattern (both parents must usually pass on the faulty gene), the process of identifying and managing it isn't always straightforward. In most cases, delving into these issues not only reveals the complex inner workings of the body but also illuminates the way toward better treatments – a reminder of why nonstop genetic research remains so crucial today. Chromosomal mix-ups form another significant slice of the genetic disorder picture, and Down syndrome is probably the most familiar example. It happens when there's an extra copy of chromosome 21 – a glitch that arises from nondisjunction during meiosis and leads to a condition called trisomy. The outward signs can be pretty varied, with effects that include intellectual disabilities, unique facial traits, and a higher risk for some health problems. Beyond the symptoms themselves, these chromosomal differences stir up a host of family concerns, raising challenging questions about genetic counseling and long-term planning. When a diagnosis eventually comes through, parents often find themselves wrestling with challenging decisions about pregnancy and possible interventions. All in all, the genetic workings behind Down syndrome underscore a broader call for public awareness and honest, informed chats about genetic screening. Bipolar disorder (BD) stands out as one of the more complex genetic puzzles, mainly due to its strong heritability and layered nature. Recent studies have begun to piece together a complex network of risk genes and interconnected pathways – and voltage-gated calcium channels keep emerging as key players. Since BD is marked by erratic mood swings that come and go rather than a steady state, understanding its biological roots is crucial for developing real-world treatment strategies. One could say that this shifting view – seeing BD as a chronic, up-and-down instability rather than a single fixed condition – hits home for those living with it. In many cases, pushing further research in genetics is aimed at refining treatment options and offering more robust support for individuals facing such multifaceted challenges (Paul et al., 2017).

8.5.3. Advances in Genetic Testing and Counseling

Genetics has made significant advancements lately, sparking a notable shift in how doctors detect disorders. Cutting-edge genetic tests now enable healthcare professionals to pinpoint issues with surprising clarity. Often, these new methods don't just identify a diagnosis for an individual showing symptoms—they also shed light on family members who might share a genetic predisposition. In most cases, nearly 90% of clinicians emphasize the importance of examining family history to understand how traits are passed down before deciding on testing and counseling (Kulkarni et al., 2023). This entire process feels both educational and empowering, providing individuals with a clearer understanding of their genetic health, enabling them to make informed choices that impact their lives and those of their loved ones. Genetic counseling, on the other hand, plays a crucial part in easing the effects of these conditions in our communities. Counselors break things down, explaining the genetic basis for certain situations so that patients and families can navigate a maze of options—even preventive ones. There's a kind of back-and-forth vibe in these sessions, as patients learn about recurrence risks and the tests available, which helps smooth out uncertainties while nudging families toward taking charge of their health. This relaxed yet informative chat not only clarifies the often-confusing picture of genetic disorders but also encourages proactive care, gradually easing the overall genetic burden on society (Kulkarni et al., 2023). Bringing genomic medicine into everyday clinical practice presents a mixed bag of opportunities and challenges, particularly when ethics and equitable access are involved. Precision medicine aims to tailor care directly to an individual's genetic profile. Although it has been promising in areas ranging from oncology to rare diseases, its benefits aren't spread evenly. Research generally shows that many healthcare systems and professionals are still not quite ready to adopt, facing obstacles such as staff shortages and suboptimal infrastructure. Addressing these challenges—such as boosting training for non-genetic specialists and advocating for policies that distribute genomic resources more evenly—is key. If we can resolve these issues, the benefits of genetic testing and counseling could reach a broader segment of the population, aligning well with the overall precision medicine vision (Figure 8.19).

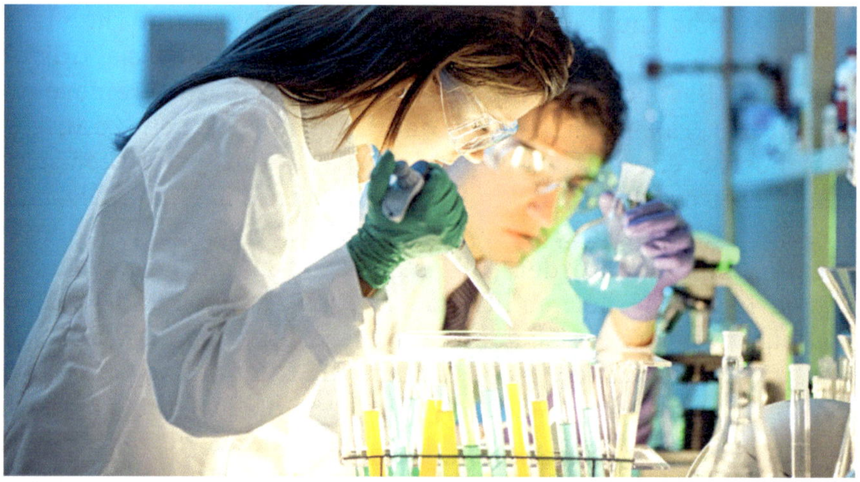

Figure 8.19. ***Genetic Testing.***

Source: https://www.nm.org//-/media/northwestern/healthbeat/images/medical-advances/nm-genetic-counseling-and-testing_feature.jpg.

8.6. Biotechnology and Genetics

Biotechnology and genetics are revolutionizing healthcare and agriculture in ways that might have seemed like science fiction not too long ago. CRISPR, for example, enables researchers to tweak our genetic code with impressive precision, opening the door to treatments that can correct mutations at their source. It's not just neat lab work—this technology also helps produce organisms altered to boost nutrition or fight off pests. In reality, these breakthroughs combine in unexpected ways, illustrating just how complex and interconnected our understanding of biology has become. At the same time, questions about who owns parts of our genetic makeup are growing. The European

Patent Convention advocates for a fair approach; however, upon reviewing the years between 1999 and 2009, it becomes apparent that there were few outside checks, suggesting that the process may require significant reevaluation. Researchers and academics have pointed out that if more voices join in—especially from universities and independent labs—patent reviews could become more transparent, even if it means a few extra steps. This kind of broader participation might slowly build more public trust in how we handle these delicate matters. Then there's nutrigenomics, which combines our understanding of genetics with the impact of our diet on our health. This field is already paving the way for personalized diets and preventive health care, though it isn't without its set of puzzles about data privacy and access. A sound regulatory framework is needed—one that protects personal information while still allowing science to move forward. Overall, individuals from diverse backgrounds, including scientists, lawmakers, and everyday people, need to continue the conversation about striking a balance between innovation and ethics in these rapidly evolving fields (Figure 8.20).

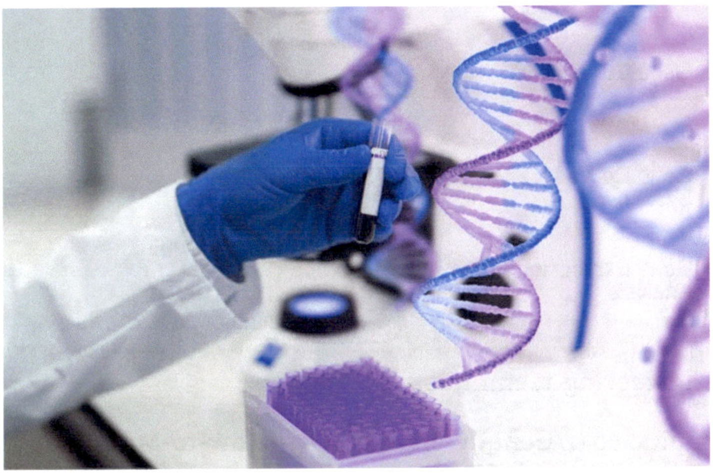

Figure 8.20. Biotechnology and Genetics.

Source: https://www.bennett.edu.in/wp-content/uploads/2023/11/Genatic-Research.jpg.

8.6.1. Overview of Genetic Engineering Techniques

Genetics today is being turned upside down by new ways of tweaking DNA. Researchers now have tools that let them manipulate the genetic code in ways we never dreamed possible—recombinant DNA technology being one of the significant breakthroughs. It essentially allows scientists to mix bits of DNA from different sources, an approach that creates GMOs used in everything from producing insulin and vaccines to enhancing plant growth. Plasmids, which act like tiny carriers, are often used to introduce foreign DNA into a host, allowing researchers to observe specific genes at work. Of course, even as science marches forward, these advances spark debates about biodiversity and food safety, meaning that every breakthrough brings its set of ethical and environmental questions. New gene editing methods, such as CRISPR/Cas9, have also emerged, offering a fresh twist on genetic engineering. This method targets the specific zones within an organism's genome—without necessarily introducing foreign DNA—which generally alleviates some of the ethical concerns associated with older techniques. By causing breaks in the DNA's double strands, CRISPR/Cas9 taps into the cell's natural repair system to incorporate the traits researchers want. This clever hack is already reshaping agriculture, helping crops become tougher in the face of climate change challenges (Nerkar et al., 2022). In most cases, these rapid advances suggest a future where we can reliably produce high-yield, climate-resilient plants to meet global food demands. Even with all these promising innovations, genetic engineering isn't without its headaches. While its benefits are clear, there are numerous challenges and ethical dilemmas that warrant closer examination. Regulatory rules for GMOs and genome-edited organisms tend to differ widely from one region to another, which in turn affects both research projects and market ventures. Environmental worries—from unexpected gene silencing to broader issues about food sovereignty and access—continue to spark debates among scientists and the public alike (Sallam, 2023). Generally speaking, an innovative blend of scientific progress and careful oversight is essential if we're to harness these technologies responsibly, ensuring that moving forward doesn't come at the expense of our ecological or social fabric (Figure 8.21).

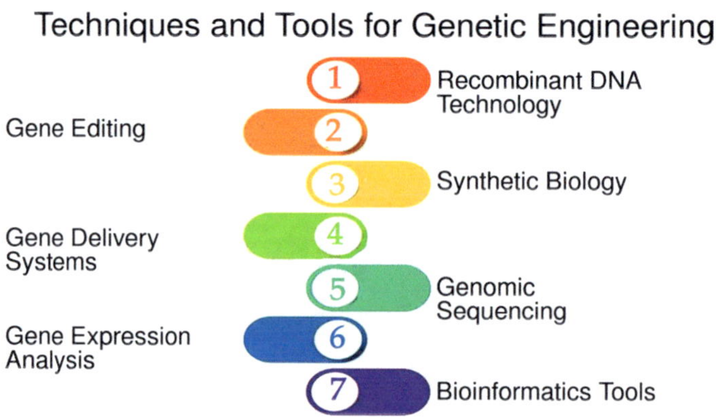

Figure 8.21. Genetic engineering techniques.

Source: https://fastercapital.co/i/Genetic-engineering--How-to-Modify-and-Improve-Your-Genes--Techniques-and-Tools-for-Genetic-Engineering.webp.

8.6.2. Applications of Biotechnology in Medicine and Agriculture

Genetics and biotechnology have revolutionized many areas these days. Medicine, for example, now benefits from genetic tweaks that lead to treatments once thought impossible. CRISPR and similar tools enable us to tweak DNA with a level of precision that is almost pinpoint, opening up options for diseases that previously had no cure. Advances in drug-making are seen—biopharma innovations mean therapies that hit targets harder and with fewer side effects. Generally speaking, this progress in healthcare also sparks a lot of ethical back-and-forth about what long-term changes in our genes might mean for us all. Switching over to farming, modern biotech has been a game-changer for crops. Scientists are now able to tweak plant genes in unexpected ways to make them more resilient against weather extremes and pests. Sometimes, these changes, such as adding drought resistance or extra nutrients, appear in genetically modified organisms (GMOs), reducing the need for chemical pesticides and encouraging farms to adopt more sustainable methods. In most cases, higher yields on less land offer a solid solution to rising food needs—a significant concern as the population continues to grow. It's somewhat surprising how these advancements neatly align with our urgent call for more sustainable food practices, even if it means reevaluating old methods. Then there's the whole new frontier of space. Organizations like NASA have taken an interest in how biotech might play out beyond Earth's boundaries. As Johnston et al. (2025) point out, current farming tricks might not cut it in space, so researchers are exploring new methods to produce food and utilize genetic tools in zero-gravity environments. This move into space brings its bundle of ethical and practical questions, echoing what is seen in both medicine and agriculture. All things considered, as new technologies stir up these debates—and sometimes even prompt new rules—biotech seems set to keep reshaping our lives in unexpected, far-reaching ways (Figure 8.22).

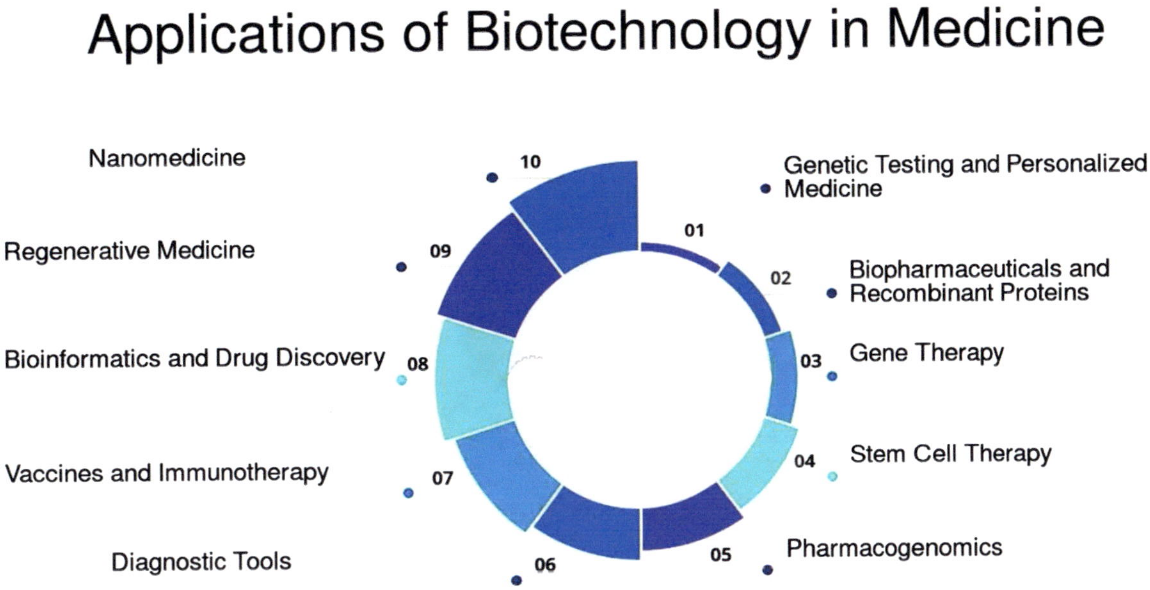

Figure 8.22. Applications of biotechnology in medicine.

Source: https://fastercapital.co/i/Biotechnology-and-life-sciences-Advancements-in-Biotechnology--Revolutionizing-Life-Sciences--Applications-of-Biotechnology-in-Medicine.webp.

8.6.3. Ethical Considerations Surrounding Genetic Manipulation

Genetic manipulation tech has thrown open a Pandora's box of ethical puzzles that one can't just ignore. Changing one creature might, in most cases, trigger unexpected shifts in whole ecosystems—sometimes in ways that were never planned for. Case in point: introducing GMOs can upset delicate natural bonds, those ties that keep the environment stable and, well, sustainable. There's also that chance, however slight, for genes to slip accidentally into wild species, stirring a mix of changes one didn't sign up for. All of these factors point to why there is a need for thorough, comprehensive ecological checks before releasing genetically modified organisms; it's about having a solemn duty to protect the surroundings as technology advances. Social and moral side-effects of genetic manipulation aren't any less worrisome either. Uneven access to these genetic tools often favors wealthier individuals, and this imbalance stokes fears about turning our genetic blueprints into a commodity. In most cases, such inequalities spark significant questions about whether everyone's fundamental rights might be compromised in the pursuit of so-called enhancements. As tweaks and modifications become a regular part of our conversation, society finds itself wrestling with the idea that these changes could set up a whole new order—one where some genetic traits get favored over others, leaving specific individuals out in the cold. When it comes to managing these issues, transparency in research and a solid ethical backbone go hand in hand with genetic manipulation practices. Most scientists agree that clear, trustworthy reporting is key to progress—one survey of outcomes helps ensure that research remains both honest and ethically sound. Guidelines like the revised ARRIVE standards, for example, serve as a crucial playbook for clear reporting in animal studies—although the language can sometimes be inconsistent—and they remind us to maintain fairness in the design of experiments. All in all, addressing the ethical aspects of genetic manipulation requires a combination of environmental stewardship, social responsibility, and effective governance to steer us toward a more balanced and responsible future in genetics.

SUMMARY

Genetics has cracked open many secrets about how our bodies work on a tiny scale. It's not just about genes—it's also about how gene activity, the ways traits get passed along, and even the environment mix to point us toward new health solutions. Adult stem cells, for example, exhibit a form of flexibility (often referred to as lineage plasticity) when they transition into different roles to help repair various tissues. With insights like these, researchers can devise treatments that target the root genetic causes, assisting tissues to heal and slowing disease progression. And, in reality, these ideas prompt us to integrate genetic knowledge into everyday treatments, particularly in regenerative medicine, where they may significantly alter our approach to chronic wounds and cancer (Matthew et al., 2024). Take tubulin isotypes as another case—their study reveals a deep connection between genetics and cell function. Different versions of the TUBB4B gene aren't just repeats; each one plays a distinct part, such as in building cilia and centrioles, which highlights the importance of genetic variation. In most cases, examining patients with primary ciliary dyskinesia makes it clear that mutations can significantly disrupt the body's normal rhythms. This line of research goes beyond laying out basic genetic ideas; it opens up fresh paths to explore how even minor genetic tweaks might lead to broader health issues. These findings also have practical applications, inspiring improved genetic screening and personalized medicine strategies for treating rare disorders (Daniel et al., 2024). To sum it all up, mixing genetics with regenerative medicine creates a unique momentum in healthcare. Understanding how stem cells switch roles and how each gene performs its function provides scientists with a clearer picture of life's complex puzzles. Generally speaking, as one learns more about genetics, the promise of sharper, next-level treatments grows stronger, setting the stage for real breakthroughs. If one studies how genes interact with everything else, they will get a clearer idea of why diseases happen. Ultimately, advancing genetic research not only illuminates the mechanisms of biology but also equips us with the tools necessary to tackle genetic disorders and other complex health challenges (Daniel et al., 2024; Matthew et al., 2024).

Genetics dives into a host of ideas that reveal how life ticks at its core. One prominent focus is genetic drift – researchers lean on the Kolmogorov equation to trace how allele frequencies shift over time. That equation essentially acts as a lens, showing how random sampling nudges variation from one generation to the next. In most cases, recent advances have enabled scientists to pinpoint clear solutions even when multiple alleles are in play, which, frankly, lightens the load compared to older, more complex models. The insights from these models not only deepen our grasp of evolutionary dynamics but also echo classic findings based on fewer alleles—supporting time-tested theories in genetics (Baxter et al., 2005). Collaboration emerges as a key factor in addressing genetic health challenges in domesticated animals. The International Partnership for Dogs, working through the International Dog Health Workshops, reveals that breeders, veterinarians, and many other stakeholders all share the responsibility of keeping canines healthy. These workshops, quite simply, become a hub where vital information and resources are exchanged, sparking breed-specific strategies for improved health. Discussing extreme conformations alongside fresh genetic testing highlights just how much genetics impacts everyday pet care. Ultimately, building these cooperative networks remains crucial to alleviating breed-related health issues and shaping a future where informed breeding practices lead to healthier dogs (Bartels et al., 2017). The reach of these discussions stretches well beyond any one species, hinting at a wider role for genetic principles in conservation and public health. Studying genetic drift isn't merely a theoretical exercise—it finds real-world use in protecting endangered species and in managing genetic diversity in farming systems. Recognizing how variation bolsters a population's resilience sparks plans to maintain diverse and robust ecosystems. And when a mix of stakeholders chime in on genetic debates, it can pave the way for policies that more effectively tackle health issues across different groups. All in all, blending mathematical models with hands-on collaboration not only expands our academic insights but also yields practical ideas that can guide genetic research across many fields (Baxter et al., 2005; Bartels et al., 2017).

CLOSER LOOK

DUCHENNE MUSCULAR DYSTROPHY (DMD)

Duchenne muscular dystrophy (DMD) is a severe, progressive genetic disorder that primarily affects boys and leads to muscle degeneration and weakness. It is caused by mutations in the DMD gene, which encodes the protein dystrophin, a crucial component of the muscle cell membrane that helps stabilize and protect muscle fibers during contraction. Without functional dystrophin, muscle cells become fragile and easily damaged, and they are gradually replaced by fat and fibrous tissue. DMD is inherited in an X-linked recessive pattern, meaning it is passed down through the X chromosome. Since males have only one X chromosome, a single defective gene is enough to cause the disease, while females are usually carriers and may have mild symptoms or none at all. DMD typically manifests in early childhood, with symptoms often appearing between ages 2 and 5. Affected children may have difficulty running, jumping, climbing stairs, or getting up from the floor. They usually display a characteristic waddling gait, frequent falls, and enlarged calf muscles due to pseudohypertrophy, where muscle tissue is replaced by fat and connective tissue.

As the disease progresses, muscle weakness spreads to the arms, neck, and trunk, severely impairing mobility. Most boys with DMD become wheelchair-dependent by their early teens, and without intervention, complications such as scoliosis, respiratory failure, and cardiomyopathy can arise. The heart and respiratory muscles are especially vulnerable, leading to life-threatening issues in the later stages. Despite these challenges, advances in care, particularly in respiratory support and cardiac management, have significantly extended life expectancy into the 20s and 30s for many individuals. Diagnosis of DMD is typically based on clinical signs, elevated levels of creatine kinase (CK) in the blood (a marker of muscle damage), and confirmed through genetic testing to identify mutations in the DMD gene. Muscle biopsy may also be used in some cases to evaluate dystrophin levels. Early diagnosis is critical for initiating treatment and managing complications.

While there is currently no cure for DMD, several treatment approaches are available to slow disease progression and improve quality of life. Corticosteroids, such as prednisone and deflazacort, are the mainstay of treatment, helping to preserve muscle strength and delay the loss of mobility. Physical therapy, orthopedic interventions, and assistive devices also play essential roles in maintaining function and independence. Newer treatments, including exon-skipping drugs like eteplirsen and golodirsen, aim to partially restore dystrophin production in certain subsets of patients with specific genetic mutations. Gene therapy and other experimental treatments are being actively explored, offering hope for future breakthroughs.

Duchenne muscular dystrophy is a devastating but increasingly manageable genetic disorder marked by progressive muscle weakness due to the absence of dystrophin. Though it poses significant physical, emotional, and medical challenges, early intervention, comprehensive care, and ongoing research are improving outcomes and quality of life for those affected. The continued development of targeted therapies and supportive technologies holds promise for altering the course of this once uniformly fatal disease.

REFERENCES

1. Neve, P., Vila-Aiub, M., & Roux, F. (2009). Evolutionary-thinking in agricultural weed management. *New Phytologist, 184*(4), 783–793. https://doi.org/10.1111/j.1469-8137.2009.03034.xAkbari, A., Kasak, L., & Laan, M. (2025). Introduction to androgenetic: Terminology, approaches, and impactful studies across 60 years. *Andrology*. https://www.semanticscholar.org/paper/c10b8e594205cf3ee6de90c24cf25766bb0ff289 (accessed on 26 May 2025).
2. Anderson, H., Studer, A., Holm, K. N., & Suzuki, A. (2021). A case-based active learning session for medical genetics resources. *MedEdPORTAL*. https://doi.org/10.15766/mep_2374-8265.11135.
3. Auton, A., Kong, A., Navarro, A., Necşulea, A., Ratnakumar, A., Siepel, A., et al. (2013). A model-based analysis of GC-biased gene conversion in the human and chimpanzee genomes. https://core.ac.uk/download/17356372.pdf (accessed on 26 May 2025).
4. Bartels, A., Clarke, A. J., Greko, C., et al. (2017). Moving from information and collaboration to action: Report from the 3rd International Dog Health Workshop, Paris in April 2017. https://core.ac.uk/download/141439096.pdf (accessed on 26 May 2025).
5. Baxter, G., Blythe, R. A., & McKane, A. J. (2005). *Exact Solution of the Multi-Allelic Diffusion Model*. http://arxiv.org/abs/q-bio/0508045 (accessed on 26 May 2025).
6. Bloom, J. S., Carlborg, Ö., Forsberg, S. K. G., Kruglyak, L., et al. (2016). *Accounting for Genetic Interactions Improves Modeling of Individual Quantitative Trait Phenotypes in Yeast*. https://core.ac.uk/download/323082139.pdf.
7. Branco, J. A., & Pires, A. M. (2011). *A statistical model to explain the Mendel–Fisher controversy*. http://arxiv.org/abs/1104.2975 (accessed on 26 May 2025).
8. Castle, D. (2007). *Genomic Nutritional Profiling: Innovation and Regulation in Nutrigenomics*. https://core.ac.uk/download/28966982.pdf (accessed on 26 May 2025).
9. Cryan, J. F., O'Riordan, K. J., Cowan, C. S. M., Sandhu, K. V., Bastiaanssen, T. F. S., Boehme, M., Codagnone, M. G., et al. (2019). The microbiota-gut-brain axis. *Physiological Reviews, 99*, 1877–2013. https://doi.org/10.1152/physrev.00018.2018.
10. Danylova, T. (2020). Nobel prize winner Erwin Schrodinger: The physicist, philosopher, and godfather of molecular biology and genetics. *Ukrainian Biochemical Journal, 92*(1), 93–100. https://www.semanticscholar.org/paper/54690a40a8f6dfc8e436b38d42261eb971a161e1 (accessed on 26 May 2025).
11. Dodd, D. O., Mechaussier, S., Yeyati, P., McPhie, F., Anderson, J. R., Khoo, C. J., Shoemark, A., et al. (2024). Ciliopathy patient variants reveal organelle-specific functions for TUBB4B in axonemal microtubules. *Science, 384*. https://www.semanticscholar.org/paper/5ee9bc4e645721f92ca68e0408820717bd1c08be (accessed on 26 May 2025).
12. Dove, O. H. (2005). Ökologische und genetische Differenzierung von Daphnia-galeata-Populationen in Europa. https://core.ac.uk/download/14503040.pdf (accessed on 26 May 2025).
13. ElSayed, N. A., Aleppo, G., Aroda, V. R., Bannuru, R. R., Brown, F. M., Bruemmer, D., Collins, B. S., et al. (2022). Classification and diagnosis of diabetes: *Standards of Care in Diabetes—2023. Diabetes Care, 46*(Supplement_1), S19–S40. https://doi.org/10.2337/dc23-s002.

14. Fady, B., Espósito, E., Abulaila, K., Aleksić, J., Alía, R., Alizoti, P., Apostol, E. N., et al. (2022). Forest genetics research in the Mediterranean Basin: Bibliometric analysis, knowledge gaps, and perspectives. *Current Forestry Reports, 8*, 277–298. https://doi.org/10.1007/s40725-022-00169-8.

15. Fernie, A. R., & Tohge, T. (2017). The genetics of plant metabolism. *Annual Review of Genetics, 51*, 287–310. https://doi.org/10.1146/annurev-genet-120116-024640.

16. Futuyma, D. J. (2017). Evolutionary biology today and the call for an extended synthesis. *Interface Focus, 7*, 20160145. https://doi.org/10.1098/rsfs.2016.0145.

17. Gabriel, W., & Lynch, M. (1992). The selective advantage of reaction norms for environmental tolerance. https://core.ac.uk/download/12165940.pdf (accessed on 26 May 2025).

18. Galluzzi, L., Vitale, I., Aaronson, S. A., Abrams, J., Adam, D., Agostinis, P., Alnemri, E. S., et al. (2018). Molecular mechanisms of cell death: Recommendations of the Nomenclature Committee on Cell Death 2018. *Cell Death and Differentiation, 25*, 486–541. https://doi.org/10.1038/s41418-017-0012-4.

19. Gelman, A., Mena, A., Tomitani, A., Bjorkholm, B., Linz, B., Kusecek, B., Voight, B. F., et al. (2010). *Microevolution of Helicobacter pylori During Prolonged Infection of Single Hosts and Within Families*. https://core.ac.uk/download/46379.pdf (accessed on 26 May 2025).

20. Gliboff, S. (2013). The many sides of Gregor Mendel. https://core.ac.uk/download/213847266.pdf (accessed on 26 May 2025).

21. Gorbalenya, A. E., Baker, S. C., Baric, R. S., de Groot, R. J., Drosten, C., Gulyaeva, A., Haagmans, B. L., et al. (2020). The species *severe acute respiratory syndrome-related coronavirus*: Classifying 2019-nCoV and naming it SARS-CoV-2. *Nature Microbiology, 5*, 536–544. https://doi.org/10.1038/s41564-020-0695-z.

22. Groenendijk, N., Kica, E., & Rodriguez, V. (2010). High-quality patents for emerging science and technology through external actors: community scientific experts and knowledge societies. https://core.ac.uk/download/pdf/11483773.pdf.

23. Harrison, P. J., Geddes, J., & Tunbridge, E. M. (2017). The emerging neurobiology of bipolar disorder. *Trends in Neurosciences, 41*(1), 18–30. https://doi.org/10.1016/j.tins.2017.10.006.

24. Haudry, A., Laurent, S., & Kapun, M. (2020). Population genomics on the fly: Recent advances in *Drosophila*. *Methods in Molecular Biology*. https://doi.org/10.1007/978-1-0716-0199-0_15.

25. Hou, K., Wu, Z. X., Chen, X. Y., Wang, J. Q., Zhang, D., Xiao, C., Zhu, D., et al. (2022). Microbiota in health and diseases. *Signal Transduction and Targeted Therapy, 7*. https://doi.org/10.1038/s41392-022-00974-4.

26. Jack, C. R., Bennett, D. A., Blennow, K., Carrillo, M. C., Dunn, B., Budd Haeberlein, S., Holtzman, D. M., et al. (2018). NIA-AA research framework: Toward a biological definition of Alzheimer's disease. *Alzheimer's & Dementia, 14*, 535–562. https://doi.org/10.1016/j.jalz.2018.02.018.

27. Johnston, R. S., Norton, D. J., & Baldwin, B. H. (2025). Space and biotechnology: An industry profile. https://core.ac.uk/download/pdf/42821064.pdf (accessed on 26 May 2025).

28. Kulkarni, J., Arumugam, S., Subbiah, N. K., & Ghoshal, J. A. (2023). Knowledge, attitude, and practice about the process of genetic counselling among clinicians. *Cureus*. https://doi.org/10.7759/cureus.45883.

29. Li, Z., Liu, B., Jin, W., Wu, X., Zhou, M., Liu, V., Goel, A., et al. (2018). hDNA2 nuclease/helicase promotes centromeric DNA replication and genome stability. *The EMBO Journal, 37*(12), e96729. https://doi.org/10.15252/embj.201796729.

30. Livingston, G., Huntley, J., Sommerlad, A., Ames, D., Ballard, C., Banerjee, S., Brayne, C., et al. (2020). Dementia prevention, intervention, and care: 2020 report of the Lancet Commission. *The Lancet, 396*, 413–446. https://doi.org/10.1016/s0140-6736(20)30367-6.

31. Mach, F., Baigent, C., Catapano, A. L., Koskinas, K. C., Casula, M., Badimón, L., Chapman, M. J., et al. (2019). 2019 ESC/EAS Guidelines for the management of dyslipidemias: lipid modification to reduce cardiovascular risk. *European Heart Journal, 41*, 111–188. https://doi.org/10.1093/eurheartj/ehz455.

32. MacLeod, A., Tait, A., & Turner, C. M. R. (2007). The system of genetic exchange in *Trypanosoma brucei* and other trypanosomatids. https://core.ac.uk/download/1394862.pdf (accessed on 26 May 2025).

33. Mariscal, C., & Petropanagos, A. (2016). *CRISPR as a Driving Force: The Model T of Biotechnology*. https://core.ac.uk/download/131209784.pdf (accessed on 26 May 2025).

34. Matějů, D., Franzmann, T. M., Patel, A., Kopach, A., Boczek, E. E., Maharana, S., Lee, H. O., et al. (2017). An aberrant phase transition of stress granules triggered by misfolded protein and prevented by chaperone function. *The EMBO Journal, 36*, 1669–1687. https://doi.org/10.15252/embj.201695957.

35. McCrory, P., Meeuwisse, W., Dvořák, J., Aubry, M., Bailes, J. E., Broglio, S. P., Cantu, R. C., et al. (2017). Consensus statement on concussion in sport—the 5th international conference on concussion in sport held in Berlin, October 2016. *British Journal of Sports Medicine, 51*, 838–847. https://doi.org/10.1136/bjsports-2017-097699.

36. Morales Peralta, E., González-Argote, J., & Álvarez Fornaris, M. A. (2025). "Las Meninas" in the clinical description of genetic disorders. *Salud, Ciencia y Tecnología–Serie de Conferencias*. https://www.semanticscholar.org/paper/f362f18cd460c4408b82ed532a17f66cd1a9e7f0 (accessed on 26 May 2025).

37. Nagtegaal, I. D., Odze, R. D., Klimstra, D. S., Paradis, V., Rugge, M., Schirmacher, P., Washington, K., et al. (2019). The 2019 WHO classification of tumors of the digestive system. *Histopathology, 76*, 182–188. https://doi.org/10.1111/his.13975.

38. Nerkar, G., Devarumath, S., Purankar, M. V., Kumar, A., Valarmathi, R., Devarumath, R. M., & Appunu, C. (2022). Advances in crop breeding through precision genome editing. *Frontiers in Genetics, 13*. https://doi.org/10.3389/fgene.2022.880195.

39. Nichols, W. W. (2009). New directions in genetics utilizing tissue culture techniques. *Hereditas, 67*(1), 1–14. https://www.semanticscholar.org/paper/7bd9eb80ee4d5cd623fd3f8126e7483 0cfc23bd9 (accessed on 26 May 2025).

40. Novick, A., & Scholl, R. (2017). Presume it not: True causes in the search for the basis of heredity. https://core.ac.uk/download/131214810.pdf (accessed on 26 May 2025).

41. O'Shea, R., Ma, A., Jamieson, R. V., & Rankin, N. (2022). Precision medicine in Australia: Now is the time to get it right. *The Medical Journal of Australia, 217*(11), 559–563. https://doi.org/10.5694/mja2.51777.

42. Percie du Sert, N., Ahluwalia, A., Alam, S., Avey, M. T., Baker, M., Browne, W. J., Clark, A., et al. (2020). Reporting animal research: Explanation and elaboration for the ARRIVE guidelines

2.0. *PLoS Biology, 18*, e3000411. https://doi.org/10.1371/journal.pbio.3000411.

43. Rasmussen, S., & Hamosh, A. (2021). Festschrift for Victor A. McKusick on the centenary of his birth: Introduction. *American Journal of Medical Genetics Part A, 185*(1), 1–3. https://www.semanticscholar.org/paper/430f948482501fcc348aba71eeb7d07f598ab1e0 (accessed on 26 May 2025).

44. Rentzsch, P., Witten, D., Cooper, G. M., Shendure, J., & Kircher, M. (2018). CADD: Predicting the deleteriousness of variants throughout the human genome. *Nucleic Acids Research, 47*(D1), D886–D894. https://doi.org/10.1093/nar/gky1016.

45. Riley, J. S., Quarato, G., Cloix, C., Lopez, J., O'Prey, J., Pearson, M., Chapman, J., et al. (2018). Mitochondrial inner membrane permeabilization enables mtDNA release during apoptosis. *The EMBO Journal, 37*. https://doi.org/10.15252/embj.201899238.

46. Sallam, M. (2023). ChatGPT utility in healthcare education, research, and practice: Systematic review on the promising perspectives and valid concerns. *Healthcare, 11*, 887. https://doi.org/10.3390/healthcare11060887.

47. Stoyanov, G., & Dzhenkov, D. (2018). On the concepts and history of glioblastoma multiforme–morphology, genetics and epigenetics. *Folia Medica, 60*, 48–66. https://www.semanticscholar.org/paper/82ac576e7a88e18ecf5ee2e4947bd4a3f7ceb992 (accessed on 26 May 2025).

48. Tamura, K., Stecher, G., & Kumar, S. (2021). MEGA11: Molecular evolutionary genetics analysis version 11. *Molecular Biology and Evolution, 38*, 3022–3027. https://doi.org/10.1093/molbev/msab120.

49. Tierney, M. T., Polak, L., Yang, Y., Abdusselamoglu, M. D., Baek, I., Stewart, K. S., & Fuchs, E. (2024). Vitamin A resolves lineage plasticity to orchestrate stem cell lineage choices. *Science (New York, N.Y.), 383*, eadi7342. https://www.semanticscholar.org/paper/12729839f1776f6198e472b17ea9555b732a00da (accessed on 26 May 2025).

50. Uffelmann, E., Huang, Q. Q., Munung, N. S., de Vries, J., Okada, Y., Martin, A. R., Martin, H. C., et al. (2021). Genome-wide association studies. *Nature Reviews Methods Primers, 1*. https://doi.org/10.1038/s43586-021-00056-9.

51. V'kovski, P., Kratzel, A., Steiner, S., Stalder, H., & Thiel, V. (2020). Coronavirus biology and replication: Implications for SARS-CoV-2. *Nature Reviews Microbiology, 19*(3), 155–170. https://doi.org/10.1038/s41579-020-00468-6.

52. Vendramin, R., Litchfield, K., & Swanton, C. (2021). Cancer evolution: Darwin and beyond. *The EMBO Journal, 40*(2), e108389. https://doi.org/10.15252/embj.2021108389.

53. Wang, D., Eraslan, B., Wieland, T., Hallström, B. M., Hopf, T. A., Zolg, D. P., Zecha, J., et al. (2019). A deep proteome and transcriptome abundance atlas of 29 healthy human tissues. *Molecular Systems Biology, 15*. https://doi.org/10.15252/msb.20188503.

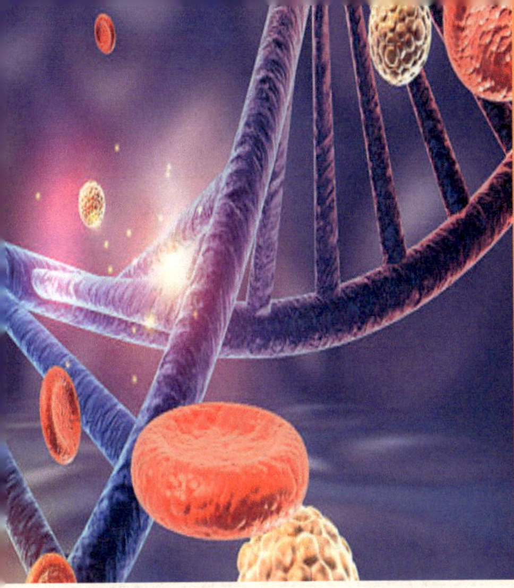

Chapter 9

STRUCTURE AND FUNCTION OF DNA AND RNA

Contents

Introduction

Molecular biology comes to life when nucleic acids, such as DNA and RNA, take center stage. These molecules—the blueprint of life—are central to how genetic info gets passed around. DNA's double helix shape offers a kind of built-in sturdiness, whereas RNA, usually hanging around as a single strand, can take on a bunch of different roles. That clear-cut distinction between them not only hints at their separate roles during processes like transcription and translation, but also showcases the clever ways life keeps on ticking. And as our tools improve—say, with techniques such as fluorescence *in situ* hybridization (FISH)—our understanding of what these molecules do becomes much sharper (Kruti et al., 2021). Focusing on DNA and RNA extends far beyond the basics, even influencing how ecosystems function. For example, DNA sequencing in ecological studies enables scientists to track changes in biodiversity and observe how organisms respond to the effects of human activity. Older, more traditional methods sometimes just don't cut it when fine details are required to understand these tricky biological interactions. On the other hand, techniques like DNA metabarcoding delve deeply into ecosystem functions and help assess how communities respond to various stressors (Lanzén et al., 2016). This turn towards molecular methods not only spices up our discussions about genetic material, but also nudges us toward new ways to think about conservation and environmental health. Understanding how DNA and RNA work is a must—not just for biology's sake, but also when considering their big-time influence on medicine, biotech, and environmental science. Researchers are slowly unearthing layers of complexity, and it's becoming increasingly clear that genetics, ecology, and technology intersect more frequently than previously thought. Additionally, leveraging emerging technologies to harness the potential of these molecules provides us with an opportunity to address significant global challenges, such as genetic disorders and resource depletion. Even if it's a messy process at times, digging into all the nitty-gritty of these structures shows just how crucial they are to life and hints at the amazing ways they could change our future (Figure 9.1).

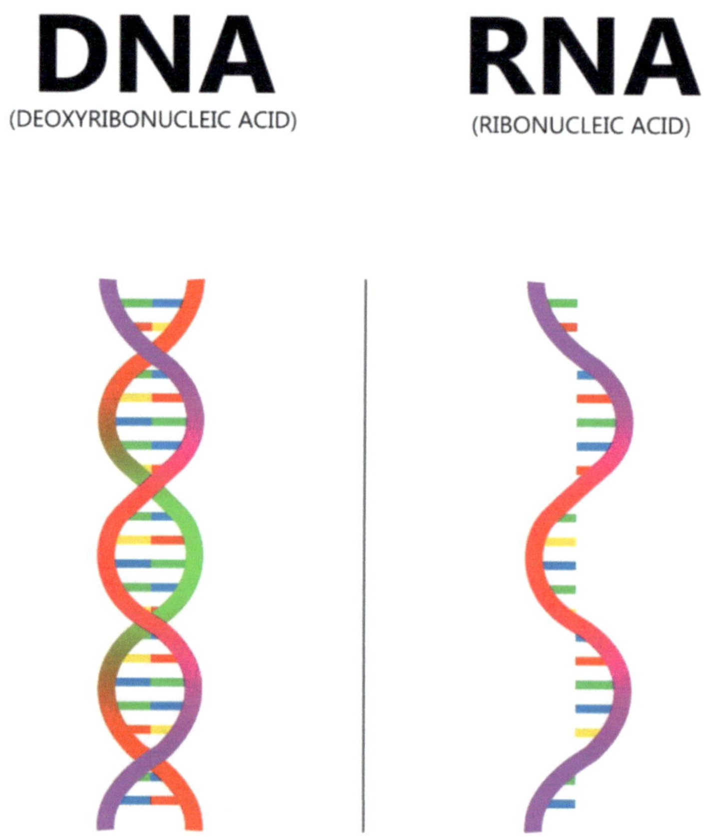

Figure 9.1. Structure and function of DNA and RNA.

Source: https://external-content.duckduckgo.com/iu/?u=https%3A%2F%2Fstatic.vecteezy.com%2Fsystem%2Fresources%2Fpreviews%2F028%2F575%2F214%2Flarge_2x%2Fdna-vs-rna-illustration-educational-genetic-acid-explanation-diagram-nucleobase-structure-labeled-scheme-ribonucleic-and-deoxyribonucleic-molecule-helix-chain-differences-comparison-vector.jpg&f=1&nofb=1&ipt=af2d9955107298d6eb17b8c056433dd66517839e9c0192df710d3d1a7416b16f.

Definition of DNA and RNA

Life's blueprint hides in surprisingly twisty details. DNA and RNA might seem similar at first glance, but they break the mold in their ways—each with its unique construction. DNA, for instance, is built on deoxyribose and typically comes as a sturdy double strand, while RNA runs solo with a ribose base, making it somewhat more flexible at times. Even the nucleotide gang plays a part; DNA sticks with adenine, thymine, cytosine, and guanine, but RNA ditches thymine for uracil. These small choices, such as the type of sugar used and the way bases line up, significantly impact how genetic information is stored and passed along. DNA does a lot more than just as a genetic archive. Often, it's the go-to template that sets off the process of transcription—an event where RNA polymerase, an enzyme with a particular method, reads the DNA and crafts a matching RNA message. In most cases, getting every base pair right is crucial to keeping the cell's instructions intact. This transcription isn't some random scribble; it's a tightly regulated process that underpins everything from cell behavior to protein production. The act of reading DNA and producing RNA is like a well-orchestrated relay, where even a tiny misstep can throw off the entire process. RNA, however, isn't just a simple copycat. It becomes involved in the action by catalyzing chemical reactions—sometimes even acting like an enzyme itself through the use of ribozymes. Generally speaking, such catalytic talent hints at a primordial era where RNA had to multitask, both carrying genetic secrets and starting key reactions. RNA also weaves connections with DNA and proteins, creating a loosely linked network of molecular chatter vital for cellular life. For example, meta-transcriptomic studies have revealed the importance of RNA in mapping out microbial communities—its profiles help us understand not only who's there, but how they function (Urich et al., 2008). This back-and-forth interplay, marked by a few quirks and repeated motifs, effectively demonstrates the versatility and evolutionary importance of RNA (Berti et al., 1997).

Importance of Nucleic Acids in Biology

Nucleic acids aren't just about stashing away genetic blueprints. They're busy little molecules that take on jobs like copying instructions, building proteins, and generally keeping an eye on gene activity. DNA, for example, carries traits from one generation to the next, ensuring that life continues. Inside cells, the way these molecules twist and vary helps them decide which genes to activate or suppress—take DNA methylation, which lightly adjusts gene activity and can even influence an organism's traits. It's this messy, ongoing dance between what's written in our genes and the world around us that shows nucleic acids aren't only the keepers of heredity, but also major players in evolution (Alexandra et al., 2022). Besides just handing down traits, these molecules are crucial for cell health and overall development. RNA – whether it's the familiar mRNA or one of the many non-coding forms – translates genetic instructions into proteins that fuel metabolism, drive enzyme reactions, and hold cells together. With RNA splicing and editing at work, cells produce a surprising variety of proteins, which underscores the many roles nucleic acids play. In most cases, innovations like the RefSeq project have provided researchers with a clearer view of these sequences and their details, making them even more relevant in both science and medicine (Nuala et al., 2015). In the end, nucleic acids become even more interesting when one considers how they alter gene behavior without rewriting the entire DNA script. DNA methylation, for instance, is a classic example of how environmental cues can trigger chemical tweaks that guide development, steer cell differentiation, and shape stress responses. Generally speaking, these subtle epigenetic shifts are key to unraveling complex traits, understanding behaviors, and even figuring out diseases like cancer. As scientists continue to investigate the ever-changing structures and roles of nucleic acids, it becomes increasingly clear how essential they are to biology and medicine (Alexandra et al., 2022) (Figure 9.2).

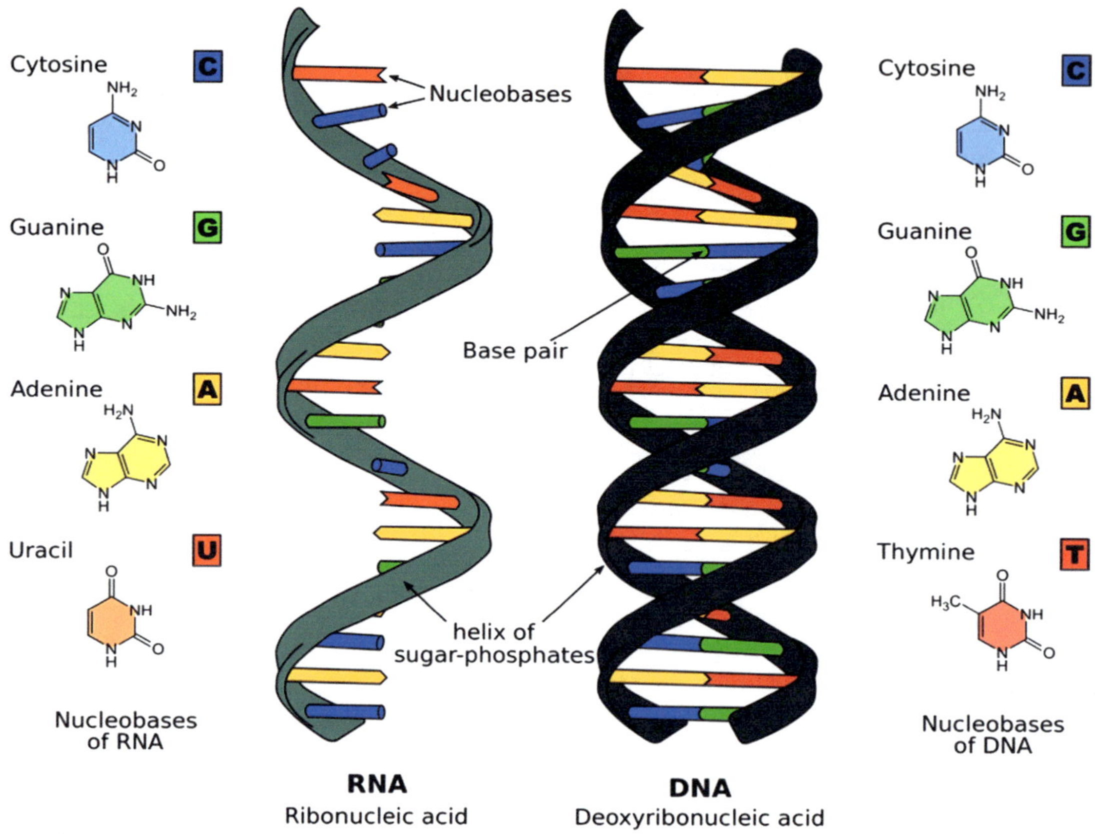

Figure 9.2. Importance of nucleic acids in biology.

Source: https://external-content.duckduckgo.com/iu/?u=https%3A%2F%2Fcdn1.byjus.com%2Fwp-content%2Fuploads%2F2018%2F07%2FNucleic-Acids-Classification-Function-of-Nucleic-Acids.png&f=1&nofb=1&ipt=debdd631dd5f745200e46ac3f01d6060b6a4ca568d8213c2527da397945d96f4.

9.1. Chemical Composition of DNA

Life's inner workings rely on its basic chemical setup – and DNA is a prime example. DNA isn't built on grand designs; it's essentially made up of four basic building blocks – adenine, thymine, cytosine, and guanine – all arranged along a sugar-phosphate strand. This kind of layout gives it the ability to carry the genetic blueprint needed for growth, everyday functioning, and even the process of cell division. Each part consists of a nitrogenous base, a deoxyribose sugar, and a phosphate group; these elements not only store hereditary info but also ensure that copying is done accurately. It's pretty interesting how adenine always ends up with thymine and cytosine with guanine, a pairing that keeps the classic double helix intact across generations. The chemistry of DNA also subtly affects its performance and strength. In most cases, the deoxyribose sugar, which is not found in RNA that uses ribose instead, plays a big part in making the molecule sturdy enough for long-term storage of genetic data; generally speaking, DNA tends to be more stable. Hydrogen bonds between the base pairs help maintain that double helix shape while also easing the copying process during transcription and replication – a neat example of structure working hand in hand with function. Plus, occasional chemical modifications like methylation add another layer by shifting how genes express themselves, so the story of RNA isn't just about the basic sequence but also about these extra, fine-tuning touches. When one studies DNA's chemical design, it also sheds light on larger biological puzzles. Variations in these molecular ingredients contribute to the fantastic diversity seen across species, and some links even point toward a Universal Gene Set shared among many life forms. The molecular toolbox, filled with nucleotides, amino acids, and other biochemicals, is essential for building proteins and running critical metabolic processes. In effect, the chemical makeup of DNA weaves into the broader fabric of life, raising open questions about how chemistry and biology have danced together through evolution (Ahern et al., 2008; Lanier et al., 2017) (Figure 9.3).

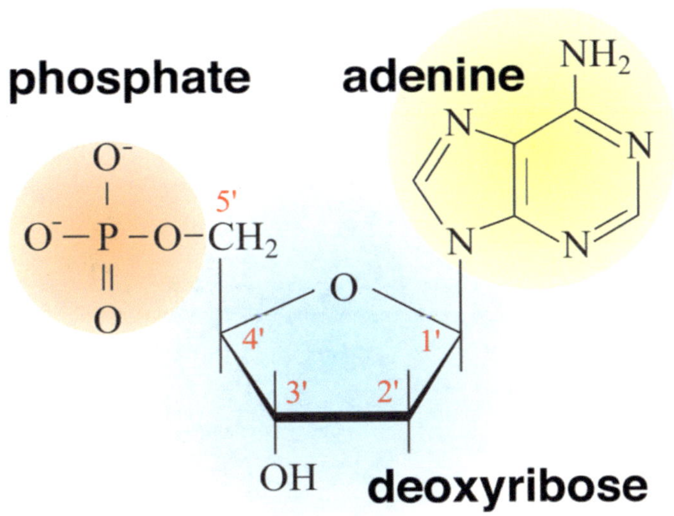

Figure 9.3. The chemical composition of DNA.

Source: https://external-content.duckduckgo.com/iu/?u=http%3A%2F%2Fbrussels-scientific.com%2Fwp-content%2Fuploads%2F2015%2F11%2Fnucleotide-1.jpg&f=1&nofb=1&ipt=6dee8baf5f1d1eb5a6427a6f188200988313bc4f1f9dc34bf4daaf2ced44fe33.

9.1.1. Nucleotide Structure

At the heart of both DNA and RNA lies a simple design—nucleotides made up of a sugar, a phosphate group, and a nitrogenous base. These little building blocks link together with phosphodiester bonds, forming long chains that drive biological processes. Generally speaking, the sugar isn't the same in every case: DNA gets deoxyribose while RNA uses ribose, giving each molecule its chemical twist. The ribose sports an extra hydroxyl group, which helps RNA fold up into unexpected, intricate shapes that matter a lot for things like translation and gene regulation. In most cases, these slight differences not only make the strands more stable but also alter how they interact with other cellular components. Recent breakthroughs in computer modeling have thrown new light on nucleotide behavior. AI-powered techniques are now piecing together nucleotide arrangements with pretty impressive accuracy (Bergonzo et al., 2025). Those flexible regions still pose a real challenge when it comes to base pairing and RNA folding. The changes in these predictions highlight just how complex nucleotide interactions can be. While computational tools are convenient in exploring these structures, experimental validation remains essential before anything can be confirmed. Blending careful experimental observations with these models provides a deeper understanding of how slight changes in structure can ripple through molecular interactions within the cell. Nucleotide structure isn't just about its components; it sets the stage for genetic function. The sequence in which nucleotides come together determines gene coding, influencing protein synthesis and even regulating cellular pathways. One interesting example comes from studies on the nucleotide sequences of medical leeches (Dadashova et al., 2024), which underline how genetic analysis can reveal evolutionary links and the specific roles of certain nucleotides. As research continues to unravel the relationship between structure and function, it's becoming increasingly clear that understanding these details is crucial for advancing genetics and biotechnology. In many cases, the tie between a molecule's solid build and its functional output is fundamental to how nucleotides get down to work in living systems (Figure 9.4).

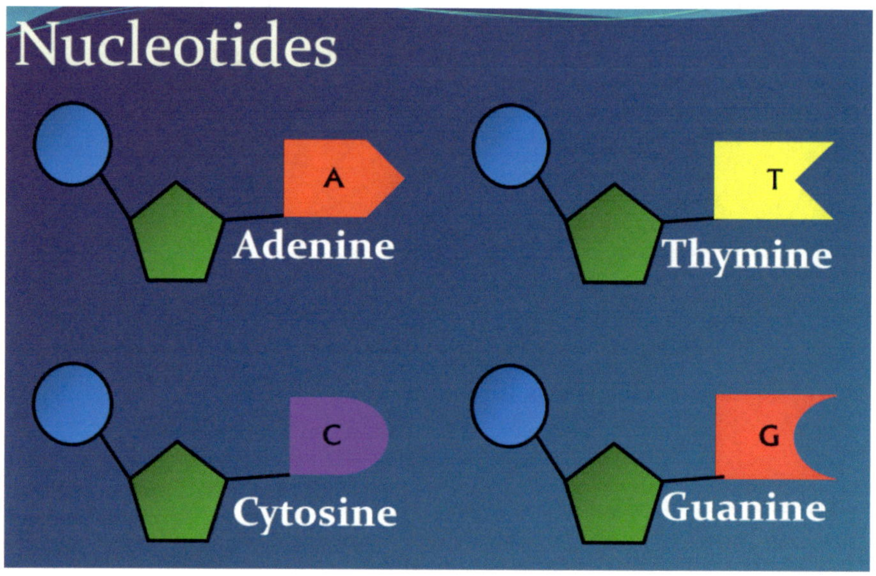

Figure 9.4. Nucleotide structure.

Source: https://external-content.duckduckgo.com/iu/?u=http%3A%2F%2Fwww.sliderbase.com%2Fimages%2Freferats%2F849b%2F(5).PNG&f=1&nofb=1&ipt=b6b6881a0921195b2e78e6edb83c35af95c9013f17ef5edec5fa6c48310bcecb.

9.1.2. Sugar-Phosphate Backbone

At the heart of DNA and RNA lies a backbone composed of sugar and phosphate—a structure that provides these molecules with both stability and shape. Instead of a neat, predictable scaffold, the alternating sugar and phosphate groups join together via phosphodiester bonds, setting a directional tone and even helping twist the molecule into its well-known helix. This arrangement lets nitrogenous bases find one another easily, a vital process for passing on genetic information over time. In most cases, it's this very framework that links the physical structure of nucleic acids to their overall function. Beyond simply holding things together, the sugar-phosphate backbone also sways how DNA and RNA behave by interacting with proteins and other molecules. This shift in activity during key cellular tasks—such as when RNA is busy with protein synthesis or gene regulation—which highlights these interactions. The kind of sugar present—ribose in RNA versus deoxyribose in DNA—not only marks a difference in composition but also shows the differences between how the enzymes such as RNA polymerase and DNA ligase can engage with the strands. All together, these interactions fuel a sort of molecular dance that's central to cell function, with the backbone playing its unsuspecting yet crucial part. Recent advances, both from theoretical work and hands-on experiments, have begun to shed new light on this role. For example, innovative, coarse-grained models have been utilized to explore DNA's stiffness and flexibility. In most cases, these studies suggest that even minor twists in the backbone can alter mechanical properties and even influence phase transitions during processes such as transcription or replication. The persistence length and stacking interactions in this framework can lead to noticeable changes in how nucleic acids fold and behave when conditions shift—an indication of just how versatile this structure is. What's more, these insights extend to our understanding of RNA folding; they suggest that complex interplay within the backbone helps guide the three-dimensional shapes vital for RNA's many roles, as highlighted in some of the newer bioinformatic models examining folding dynamics (Morriss-Andrews et al., 2009; Cragnolini et al., 2014) (Figure 9.5).

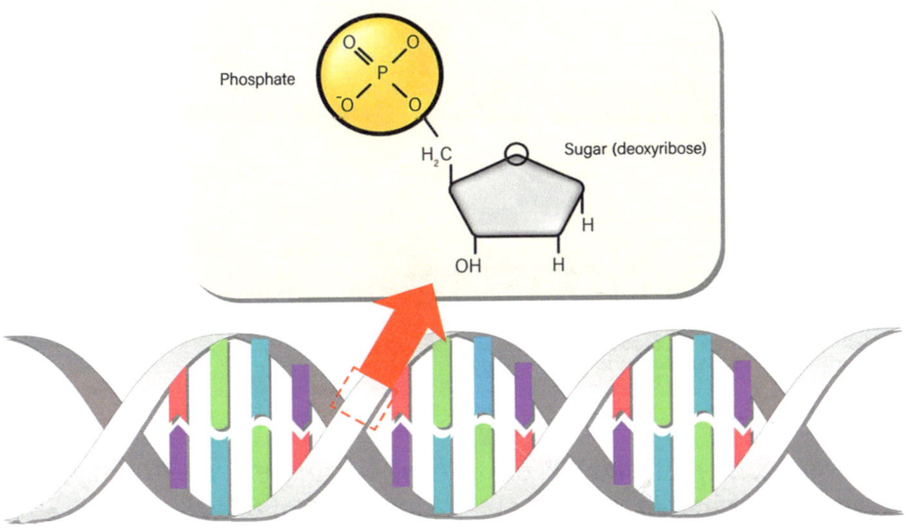

Figure` 9.5. Sugar-phosphate backbone.

Source: https://external-content.duckduckgo.com/iu/?u=https%3A%2F%2Fmedia.istockphoto.com%2Fid%2F1385627601%2Fvector%2Fsugar-phosphate-backbone-structure-dna-double-helix-deoxyribonucleic-acids-nitrogenous-base.jpg%3Fs%3D1024x1024%26w%3Dis%26k%3D20%26c%3Dw51gKogYO0qD-dtQcNe9HEHXtveS5jTkrJfke3O9A7k%3D&f=1&nofb=1&ipt=f08ba408be553e177a5a4d996a72c7b57acafb38ac561787571ab3356504610a.

9.1.3. Nitrogenous Bases and Their Pairing

Nucleic acids have a kind of magic about them—key components inside these molecules interact in ways that make DNA and RNA work properly. Take the bases, for example: adenine (A), thymine (T), guanine (G), and cytosine (C). They tend to pair up in very particular ways, with A linking to T using two hydrogen bonds and G teaming with C via three; it isn't random at all, but a neat consequence of their chemical and structural make-up. These interactions are partly due to the resonant shapes inside the bases, which help form those steady bonds that theoretical models sometimes explain as part of DNA's quirky quantum behavior. This bonding robustness keeps genetic information intact over generations, underscoring its importance for heredity and cell function. Beyond just holding the structure together, the base pairs ultimately play a variety of roles.

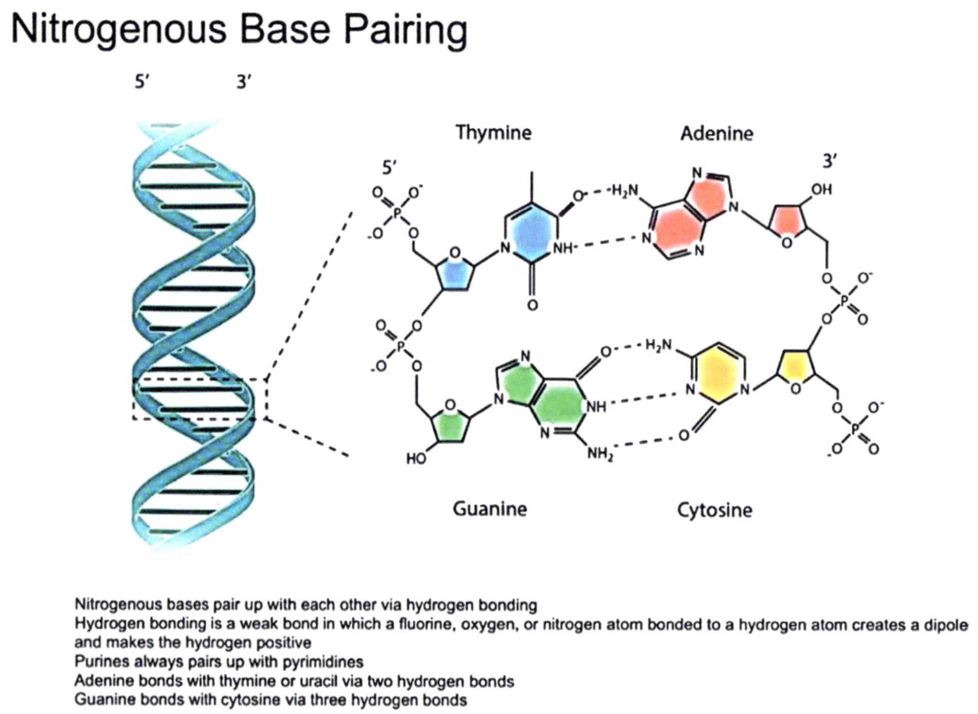

Figure 9.6. Nitrogenous base pairing.

Source: https://external-content.duckduckgo.com/iu/?u=https%3A%2F%2Fi.ytimg.com%2Fvi%2FuBoXP_2vKDE%2Fmaxresdefault.jpg&f=1&nofb=1&ipt=48fd7a567493b59298136708140f6c23f79530fa1eae1316ef82abbebf7603b0.

They help the two strands of DNA align in opposite directions. This twist gives the classic double helix its familiar look, which is vital for processes like replication and transcription. In most cases, the way bases connect also triggers gene expression and sometimes even signals how a cell should respond to oxidative stress from reactive oxygen species (ROS). When cells face these stressors, the stability of DNA can wobble because of minor damage to the bases, thus nudging overall genetic performance off balance. Observing these shifts helps us glimpse the deep relationship between the chemical properties of the bases and overall cellular well-being (Andrés Cés et al., 2021). Interestingly, these nitrogenous bases aren't just about life's blueprints—they're also making waves in the world of quantum computing. In a curious twist, their behavior, when viewed through the lens of quantum physics, bears a striking resemblance to supercurrents that align with qubits in specific computing systems. Those same hydrogen bonds sometimes behave like Josephson junctions, showing how molecular interactions might handle and process information at a delicate and intricate level. In most cases, this quantum angle enriches our understanding of DNA, not only as a builder of life, but also as a potential information-processing marvel—bridging what one knows from traditional genetics with breakthroughs in the realm of quantum computing (Raúl Aroche et al., 2024) (Figure 9.6).

9.2. Chemical Composition of RNA

RNA's chemical makeup plays a significant role in what it does biologically, and that's what sets it apart from DNA. At its core, RNA is built on a backbone of ribose sugars joined by phosphate groups; its structure is further stabilized by nitrogen-rich bases—adenine, guanine, cytosine, and uracil. Unlike DNA, which relies on thymine, RNA substitutes uracil, a change that generally alters its stability and how it reacts. This switch is crucial, as it enables RNA to interact in dynamic ways during processes such as transcription and translation. Also, using ribose instead of deoxyribose makes RNA more reactive and able to handle various catalytic tasks (a quality seen in ribozymes). In most cases, these unique chemical properties shape RNA's role in managing genetic information and regulating cellular mechanisms (Cleaves et al., 2019). RNA also shows off its versatility through the different shapes it takes—a trait that comes straight from its chemistry. While we primarily see RNA as a single-stranded, it can, quite unexpectedly, bend into intricate three-dimensional forms thanks to its base pair interactions. Sometimes, these folding patterns help determine what the molecule can do: mRNA is busy with protein building, while miRNA and siRNA are involved in regulating cell activities. These recurring patterns highlight again how RNA's chemical parts keep reappearing in its many roles. Understanding these properties is crucial in many cases for both ongoing research and the design of RNA-based drugs targeting specific pathways (Xiong et al., 2011). Recent strides in chemical biology have put the spotlight on the vast chemical landscape that RNA inhabits. New sequencing methods, for example, have made it possible to spot novel RNA sequences and pick up on their subtle modifications—offering a fresh look at how minor chemical shifts can affect RNA's stability and its bond with proteins.

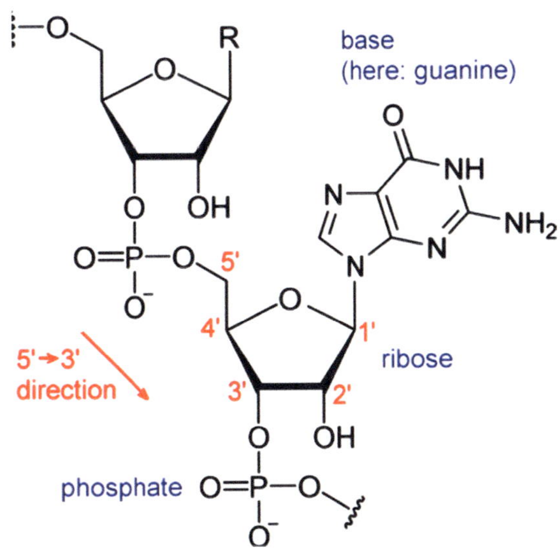

Figure 9.7. Chemical composition of RNA.

Source: https://upload.wikimedia.org/wikipedia/commons/2/2c/RNA_chemical_structure.GIF.

These insights not only enhance our fundamental understanding but also pave the way for creating synthetic molecules that mimic the function of natural RNA. As many researchers continue to test RNA analogs and explore their potential in drug development, the foundational principles of RNA's chemical form remain at the center of bridging pure molecular biology with applied science. In most cases, this connection is sparking new approaches in genomic medicine as well as bioengineering (Cleaves et al., 2019) (Figure 9.7).

9.2.1. Differences Between RNA and DNA Nucleotides

RNA and DNA start quite differently. RNA uses a ribose sugar instead of DNA's deoxyribose – that extra –OH in ribose makes RNA generally more reactive, letting it twist into various roles like protein-making and cell regulation. It's interesting that RNA swaps thymine for uracil (U), joining forces with adenine, cytosine, and guanine in pairings that end up shaping its unique structure; all these little bits add up to make RNA a dynamic player, while DNA tends to stick with its more unchanging, info-keeping role (Kato, 2024).

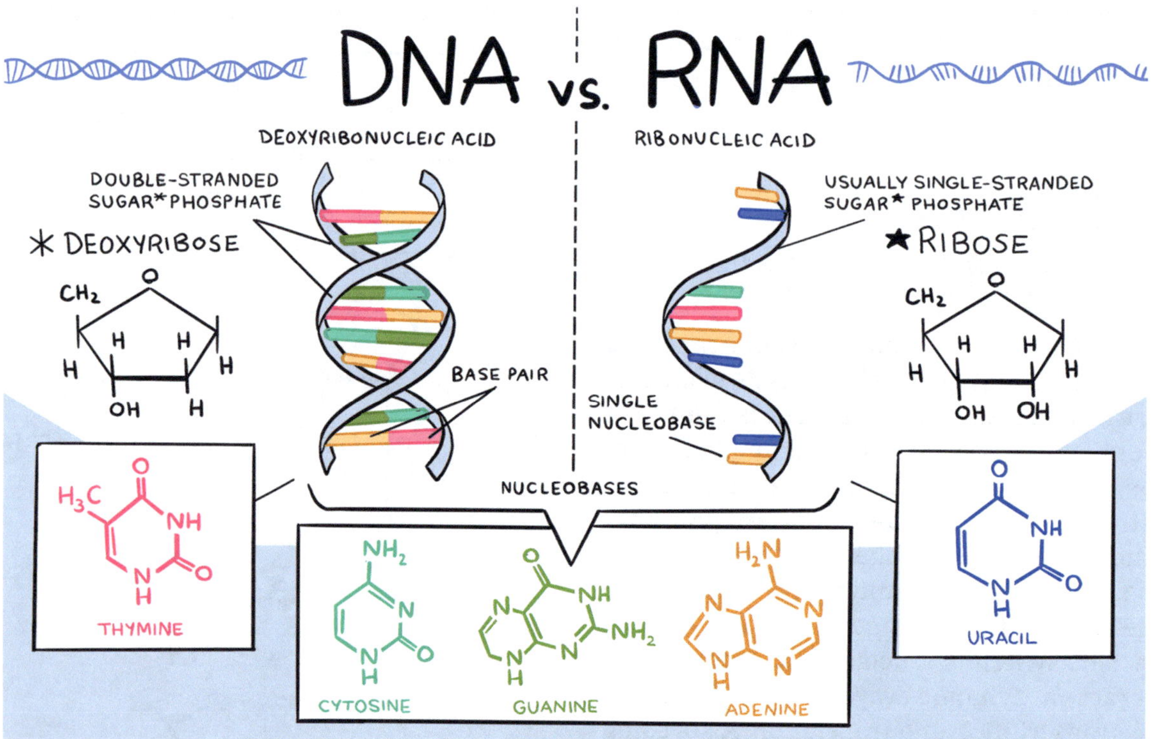

Figure 9.8. The differences between DNA and RNA.

Source: https://www.thoughtco.com/thmb/1TtBt_1NjoC0G2KrtIcuz34PHTk=/1500x0/filters:no_upscale():max_bytes(150000):strip_icc()/dna-versus-rna-608191_sketch_Final-54acdd8f8af04c73817e8811c32905fa.png.

Looking closer at their shapes, RNA's single-stranded nature gives it the chance to bend and fold into all sorts of secondary and tertiary forms, which is crucial for things like catalysis and controlling cellular processes – think ribozymes and other regulatory RNA types. In contrast, DNA's classic double helix, built from neat complementary base pairing and strong hydrogen bonds, serves as a highly reliable vault for genetic material, ensuring high-fidelity replication. The built-in stability of DNA, paired with the flexible and sometimes unpredictable structure of RNA, reveals why both molecules are essential for maintaining the smooth operation of transcription and translation. Sometimes the picture isn't apparent, but overall it's a remarkable balance of rigidity and flexibility at work (Arsdale et al., 2024). When it comes to gene expression and regulation, the differences in their structure highlight their distinct roles. DNA, with its steady, almost unshakeable framework, is responsible mainly for safely storing and accurately copying genetic information. Meanwhile, RNA acts as a kind of messenger — it transcribes genetic blueprints for protein synthesis and plays roles in regulation and even catalysis. There's also that clear contrast in durability: DNA sticks around for the long haul, whereas RNA is more fleeting, which proves handy when cells need to react quickly to changes. All in all, these distinct features demonstrate how the two work in tandem, each with its quirks that shape essential processes within the cell (Kato, 2024) (Figure 9.8).

9.2.2. Types of RNA (mRNA, tRNA, rRNA)

RNA comes in many forms within a cell, with each type performing its unique function. Messenger RNA (mRNA) is the go-between that takes instructions straight from DNA and passes them on to the protein factories. It grabs a DNA message and hands it off so that the string of nucleotides can be turned into a chain of amino acids. After it's made, mRNA can be subtly tweaked by changes that happen later on—post-transcriptional modifications that adjust its stability and performance. Studies have shown that changes, such as pseudo uridylation, can alter mRNA's behavior, especially when a cell is under stress (Cerneckis et al., 2022).

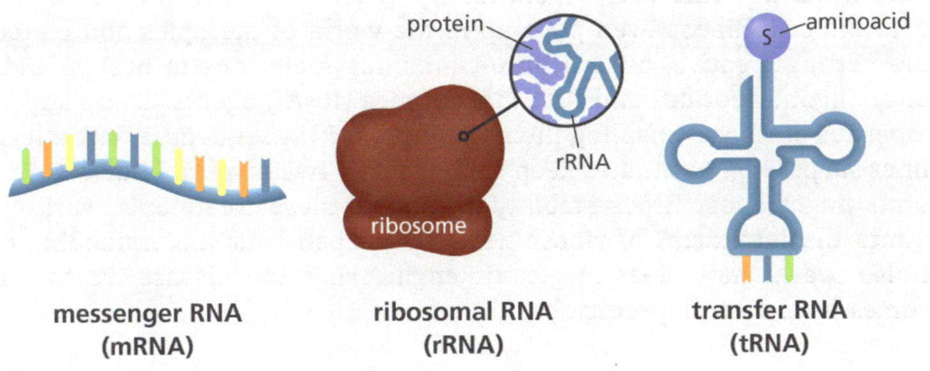

Figure 9.9. Types of RNA.

Source: https://www.yourgenome.org/wp-content/uploads/2023/11/1592-RNA-types.png.

In many cases, this means mRNA isn't just a simple messenger—it's a versatile actor in gene expression. tRNA, or transfer RNA, is another key player, helping to crack the mRNA code during protein assembly. It matches specific amino acids with the corresponding codons on the mRNA, ensuring that the genetic message is translated accurately. Its distinctive cloverleaf shape gives it the edge when mingling with ribosomes and with enzymes called aminoacyl-tRNA synthetases. Sometimes, there are tweaks, such as pseudouridine, that appear on tRNA, and these typically enhance its stability and overall function (Wu et al., 2019). All in all, tRNA's reliable role in choosing and delivering the right amino acids is central to keeping protein synthesis on track. Ribosomal

RNA (rRNA) forms the heart of ribosomes—the cell's protein-making machines. It accounts for roughly 60% of a ribosome's mass, serving not just as a scaffold for ribosomal proteins but also actively helping to form peptide bonds. Modifications, such as pseudo-uridylation, can alter the shape and movement of rRNA, which is crucial for forming stable ribosomes (Cerneckis et al., 2022). Even minor errors in these modifications can disrupt how ribosomes interact with mRNA and tRNA, sometimes leading to conditions such as cancer. rRNA isn't just a structural component; it plays a vital role in keeping cells healthy and functioning properly (Figure 9.9).

9.2.3. Role of Ribose in RNA Structure

Ribose sits right at the heart of RNA's overall setup. This five-carbon sugar—with its extra hydroxyl spots at positions 2 and 3—gives RNA its knack for folding into all kinds of surprising curves and twists. Those hydroxyl groups boost RNA's ability to form hydrogen bonds with neighboring strands and even spur parts of the molecule to interact inside itself, leading to a whole spectrum of shapes. In many cases, these fluctuating forms allow RNA to take on roles such as participating in chemical reactions or maintaining control. Essentially, without ribose doing its thing, RNA wouldn't have the flexibility it needs to play its many parts. It's not just about shape, though. Ribose also affects how RNA interacts with proteins and other biomolecules. The unusual arrangement of its hydroxyl groups gives RNA some pretty distinct binding traits—traits that turn out to be key in settings like ribosome assembly or enzyme-driven reactions. Generally speaking, these bonds can alter the stability of RNA–protein complexes, which in turn affects the efficiency of processes such as translation. And interestingly, the fact that RNA's sugar is ribose while DNA opts for a slightly different partner hints at some early evolutionary twists, marking RNA as a sort of original, versatile actor in the cell. Ribose even pops up in the world of therapies and biotech innovation. Researchers are getting creative, using ribose-containing molecules to design RNA-based drugs, such as antisense oligonucleotides and RNA interference (RNAi) agents. These approaches rely on the unique properties of ribose, enabling them to pinpoint RNA sequences with a level of precision that is sometimes surprising. As studies keep rolling along, tweaking ribonucleotides by modifying their ribose units might boost RNA's stability and make these treatments work even better. All in all, delving into the intricacies of ribose not only deepens our understanding of RNA's inner workings but also sparks new ideas in genetic engineering and disease treatment—even if the journey sometimes feels a bit unpredictable.

9.3. Structure of DNA

DNA's twisty design is key to its role in holding our genetic information. Two long strands of nucleotides wind together into that classic double helix—a shape that Watson and Crick brought into the spotlight back in the 1950s. Each tiny unit packs a phosphate, a sugar, and a nitrogen base, with that base being the game changer for genetic coding. The order of adenine, thymine, cytosine, and guanine establishes the blueprint for how our cells store and read genetic information. The spiral twist also helps keep the molecule steady under everyday conditions, almost like a trusty database of life's instructions. This flexible setup is why DNA plays a crucial role in the replication of cells and the production of proteins. How DNA sits in space is just as important as its building blocks. The two strands run in opposite directions and stick together thanks to a kind of perfect matching—adenine with thymine, and cytosine with guanine. That neat bond not only ensures that the genetic copy job is done correctly but also makes it possible to build more elaborate arrangements, such as chromatin, which tucks DNA into the nucleus. Because of this layout, certain parts of the strand become accessible for transcription, allowing genes to turn on and off naturally. New computational tricks, such as the Molecular Distance Map created using the Chaos Game Representation, reveal that similar twists across various DNA sequences can hint at evolutionary ties and help distinguish between species. In most cases, these methods widen our view of genetic variety and history, reinforcing just how vital DNAs architecture is in biology (Bryans et al., 2014). Understanding DNA goes beyond just knowing its parts—it sets the stage for diving into genetic engineering and synthetic biology. Researchers are now busy crafting artificial cells that mimic natural ones, leveraging DNA's sturdy design for biotechnological uses. These make-believe cells work with real biological membranes and even borrow from the transcription and translation playbook to do specific jobs, much like natural cells would. The success of these setups depends on grasping the nitty-gritty of DNAs structure, which directs cell behavior and interactions. Efforts to merge artificial systems with natural life continue, commonly aimed at enhancing the effectiveness of these constructs (Ding et al., 2014). This hands-on work not only advances biomedical research but also deepens our understanding of the fundamental principles underlying DNA and RNA in various organisms (Figure 9.10).

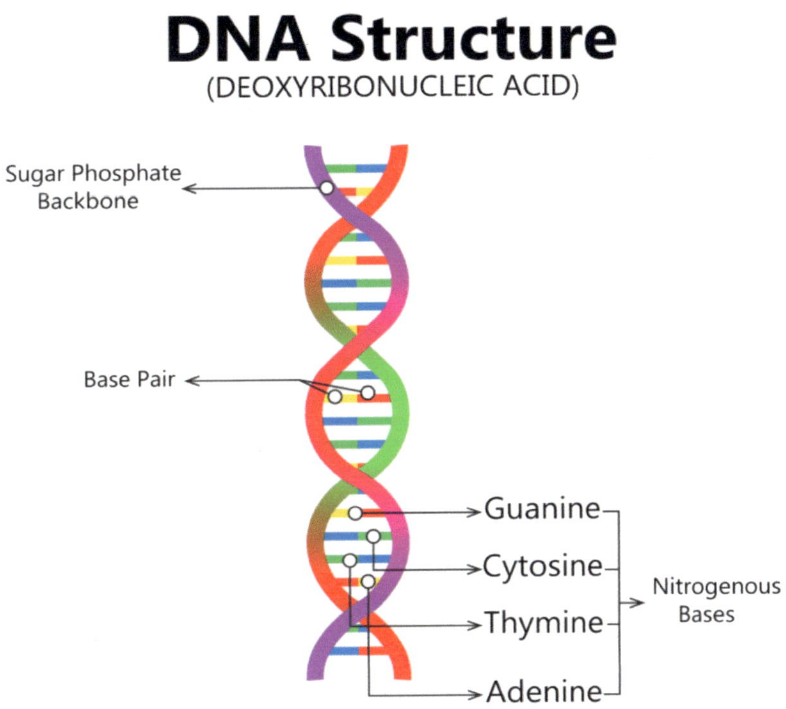

Figure 9.10. Structure of DNA.

Source: https://external-content.duckduckgo.com/iu/?u=https%3A%2F%2Fstatic.vecteezy.com%2Fsystem%2Fresources%2Fpreviews%2F028%2F627%2F407%2Foriginal%2Fscientific-icon-spiral-of-dna-and-rna-an-illustration-of-the-differences-in-the-structure-of-the-dna-and-rna-molecules-image-poster-structure-rna-and-dna-vector.jpg&f=1&nofb=1&ipt=0f3c1c7f420542a6d93f10933b4cbd342620346f6a600ed079f60b21a1c5dfc9.

9.3.1. Double Helix Formation

DNA's twisted, interwoven ladder isn't just a pretty design—it marked a giant evolutionary leap by allowing cells to store and pass on genetic blueprints efficiently. Deep down, there are specific pairings—adenine hangs out with thymine while guanine tends to mix with cytosine—and they stick together mainly through hydrogen bonds. Typically, these bonds build a kind of anti-parallel arrangement that is key for copying DNA and reading its code. This shape also helps the molecule snugly fit inside the cell's nucleus while kickstarting a range of chemical reactions that keep the cell chugging along.

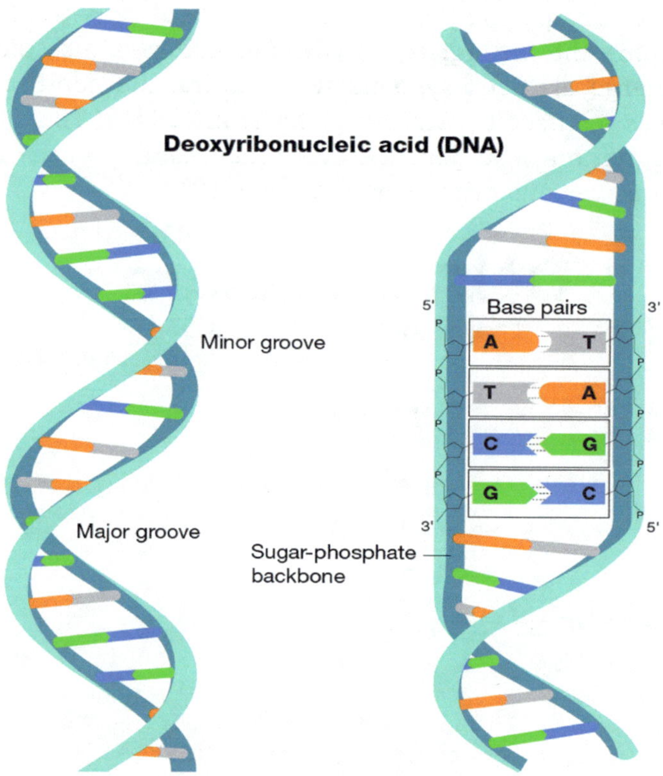

Figure 9.11. Double helix formation of DNA.

Source: https://www.genome.gov/sites/default/files/media/images/tg/Double-helix.jpg.

Understanding this design is, generally speaking, crucial for grasping how nucleic acids behave and interact, highlighting the neat link between how things are built and how they work. Keeping that double helix in tip-top shape is just as important; it acts as a shield against damage that could disrupt our genetic code. When DNA gets hit by environmental hassles or metabolic stresses, robust repair processes usually step in to fix the errors—though sometimes these fixes aren't perfect and might even spark mutations. For example, occasional slip-ups in repair pathways, such as nucleotide excision or homologous recombination, can nudge cells toward premature aging or even push them down a cancerous path. There's this delicate balancing act between the physical structure and the repair systems, and it shapes an organism's resilience to aging and disease, making the study of DNA's makeup and repair mechanisms a must in genetics and cell biology—even if, at times, the details feel a bit messy. Looking at how structure ties in with function, the double helix pretty much steals the show in explaining what happens inside a cell. The unwinding of this spiral allows polymerases to do their job—synthesizing RNA and replicating DNA—which is central not only to cell division but also to turning on genes that manage various biological processes. The complex web of interactions between proteins, DNA and RNA play out as they control cell behavior in unpredictable ways. Examining how these molecular players interact within the helix deepens our understanding of normal physiology and even points to potential abnormalities in diseases such as aging and cancer (Hoeijmakers, 2009). Having a broad look at these interconnections shines a light on the fundamental rules of life at the molecular level, a perspective also mirrored in the guidelines for monitoring biological processes (Daniel et al., 2016) (Figure 9.11).

9.3.2. Antiparallel Strands

Antiparallel strands play a key role in how nucleic acids work. DNA, for example, twists into the classic double helix, where one strand moves in a 5 'to 3' direction and the other in a 3' to 5' direction.

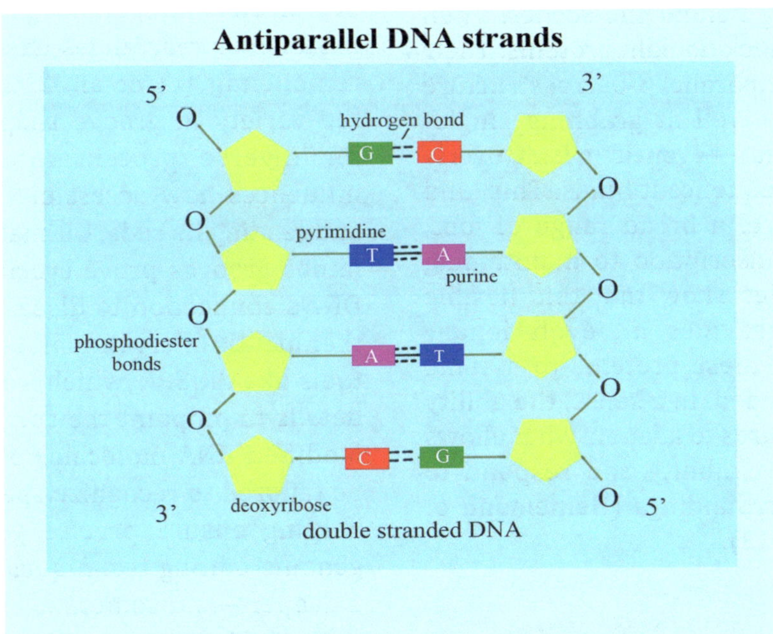

Figure 9.12. Antiparallel strands of DNA.

Source: https://external-content.duckduckgo.com/iu/?u=https%3A%2F%2Fwww.vedantu.com%2Fquestion-sets%2F5b909244-16f0-4f74-a863-26fd7600b8413968907313960664713.png&f=1&nofb=1&ipt=58b3678c039201c1e7017ecccd731792aca28bf7eac43d33b860ff091c8cbf0f.

This setup ensures that adenine is paired with thymine and guanine with cytosine. This arrangement isn't just about keeping things neat; it also protects the genetic code while helping DNA replicate itself correctly during cell division. Complementary base pairing, which relies on this opposite alignment, is essential for maintaining stability and ensuring effective replication. RNA typically appears as a single strand, yet it still exhibits its complexity, with hints of antiparallel design. Sometimes proteins like RBM45 jump in to link RNA and DNA. Its two RNA recognition motifs create binding spots that face in opposite directions and can latch onto different GAC sequences. This unusual pairing not only underpins meaningful biochemical interactions but, in most cases, may also explain why problems in RNA binding can be linked to neurodegenerative diseases (Chen et al., 2021). It's a neat reminder that sometimes, even structures that seem simple are doing a lot of heavy lifting behind the scenes. Then there are the cold-shock domain proteins. Their five-stranded, all-antiparallel β-barrel structure works exceptionally well at grabbing single-stranded nucleic acids—even if it isn't overly picky about which sequence it binds. This kind of formation supports a broad range of jobs, from controlling transcription to maintaining RNA integrity. Studies show that this flexible binding strategy provides an evolutionary advantage, enabling these proteins to assume different roles as needed. In a sense, the ability of antiparallel structures to adapt is what allows cells to to maintain stability and respond to changes in their surroundings (Heinemann et al., 2021) (Figure 9.12).

9.3.3. Major and Minor Grooves

DNA's twisty double helix isn't just a pretty design—it's what drives how genetic info gets used. Inside that spiral, there are two kinds of grooves: a broad, friendly major groove and a tighter, more reserved minor one. These features emerge because the sugar-phosphate backbone aligns unevenly with the nucleotide bases, leaving some areas more open (and others less so) for proteins and enzymes to bind to. Usually, the major groove welcomes DNA-binding proteins with open arms, while the minor groove, being a bit snugger, offers somewhat limited access. This mix of structure turns out to be key for the specificity of protein-DNA interactions, especially in essential processes such as transcription, replication, and repair (Neidle, 2021). Taking a closer look, the way these grooves behave significantly affects how DNA acts under different cellular conditions. DNA's knack for bending and twisting is primarily governed by these groove traits, which in turn shape its rapport with transcription factors and other regulators. For instance, A-tracts—those strings of adenine bases—often nudge the DNA to bend more toward the minor groove.

That subtle twist can reshape DNA's overall structure, altering how it interacts with proteins or rearranges itself during chromatin remodeling (Li et al., 2020). In many cases, the variety in groove shapes not only allows for diverse protein interactions but also influences how accessible DNA is for copying and reading its code. Ultimately, these major and minor grooves prove crucial in understanding DNA's connection to diseases and in designing therapeutic interventions. Consider gene-editing tools like CRISPR, which lean heavily on groove details to pinpoint the correct DNA sequences. Modified RNA molecules or proteins can even be tailored to recognize specific groove shapes, helping ensure precise genomic tweaks. As genome editing techniques continue to evolve, a deeper—and sometimes imperfect—grasp of these DNA features will be crucial for crafting treatments against a host of ailments (Li et al., 2020). Understanding the intricacies of these structural anomalies may pave the way for more effective strategies against genetic disorders.

9.4. Structure of RNA

RNA's twisty design is at the heart of its many jobs inside our cells. Unlike DNA's steady double helix, RNA is far more flexible – it's essentially a chain of nucleotides (each one made of a sugar, a phosphate, and a nitrogen base) that can twist into unexpected shapes. Often, parts of the molecule stick together through internal base pairing, forming quirky elements like hairpins and loops. These varied formations let RNA fold into three-dimensional structures that aren't bound by the classic double helix, opening the door for unique interactions with proteins and other nucleic acids. In most cases, the link between structure and function plays out in remarkable ways. When RNA assumes roles as both a messenger and a catalyst, its secondary and tertiary structures truly shine. For example, tRNA winds itself into a cloverleaf-style shape—a layout that's pretty vital for matching the right amino acids during protein production. This cloverleaf not only helps in recognizing amino acids correctly but also ensures they're appropriately positioned on the ribosome, thereby facilitating the protein-building process. rRNA becomes even more complex in its folds, which help keep the ribosome stable and enhance its catalytic activities.

And mRNA isn't left out either; its stem-loop and pseudoknot configurations often play unexpected but crucial roles in tweaking stability and translation efficiency. As noted in studies on slipped loop structures, the way RNA folds and the way its bases interact ultimately have a significant impact on gene expression and protein synthesis (Lalitha et al., 1994). Beyond translating and catalyzing, RNA's many shapes enable it to play key regulatory roles within the cell. Different kinds—such as small interfering RNA (siRNA) and microRNA (miRNA)—often form specialized configurations tailored to silence or regulate gene activity. These molecules twist and turn so they can pair up with matching mRNA strands, effectively dialing down gene expression when needed. Then there are ribozymes, RNA molecules that get catalytic in a way that's pretty similar to proteins. All of these aspects underscore the idea that RNA's form indeed dictates its function, reinforcing one of the core themes in structural biology: how the very architecture of a molecule translates into its dynamic role in the cell (Zhou et al., 2010) (Figure 9.13).

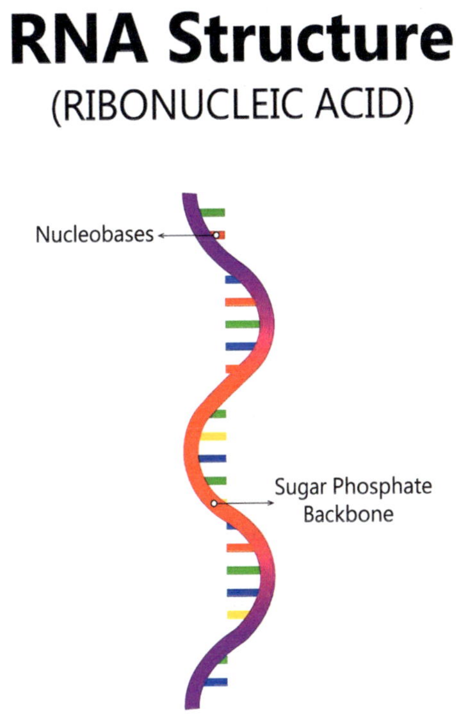

Figure 9.13. Structure of RNA.

Source: https://external-content.duckduckgo.com/iu/?u=https%3A%2F%2Fstatic.vecteezy.com%2Fsystem%2Fresources%2Fpreviews%2F028%2F627%2F406%2Flarge_2x%2Frna-ribonucleic-acid-structural-formula-of-adenine-cytosine-guanine-and-uracil-diagram-for-educational-medical-biological-and-scientific-use-vector.jpg&f=1&nofb=1&ipt=c7df64b6938600f8b4d690325e5c25b0556d5221ba5a3dbd9652ffc11d93614b.

9.4.1. Single-Stranded Nature

Molecular biology reveals its complexity when studying nucleic acids and their differences. RNA, for example, is single-stranded and stands apart from the typical double-stranded DNA. This oddity allows RNA to twist into various shapes, which enables it to participate in tasks such as protein synthesis and regulating gene activity. In many cases, the single-stranded form serves as a ready-made template during translation—ribosomes read it to assemble proteins. Additionally, the twisty, flexible shape allows RNA to interact with other molecules in the cell, thereby giving it a broader range of functions. In RNAi the role of single-stranded RNA becomes even more interesting. Generally, when double-stranded small interfering RNA (ds siRNA) is processed, a single-stranded guide strand emerges to direct the RNA-induced silencing complex (RISC) toward specific mRNA targets. Essentially, the whole process hinges on the idea that the 3' end of the passenger RNA can take on a small DNA extension; this tweak boosts its stability without compromising its function. Constructs like passenger-3-DNA/ds siRNA show that the single-stranded part isn't just a guide—it also helps keep the structure intact. This resistance to being broken down by nucleolytic enzymes underscores the key role single-stranded RNA plays in shaping gene regulation and silencing pathways (Allison et al., 2009). Furthermore, experiments underscore the adaptability of single-stranded RNA in the gene-silencing process. Researchers have experimented with constructs that combine single- and double-stranded elements, and they continue to find that even slight structural changes can alter biological activity. For instance, some single-stranded variants fall prey to serum nucleases, while others prove pretty tough when tied into a double-stranded framework. Studies using guide-3-DNA/ss siRNA have gently reminded us that the way these molecules are built is crucial for keeping RNAi on track—demonstrating the tight link between having a single-stranded setup and overall function. All in all, these insights not only highlight RNA's surprising flexibility but also point to the evolutionary perks of its single-stranded nature, opening doors for future therapeutic ideas (Ahmed et al., 2013) (Figure 9.14).

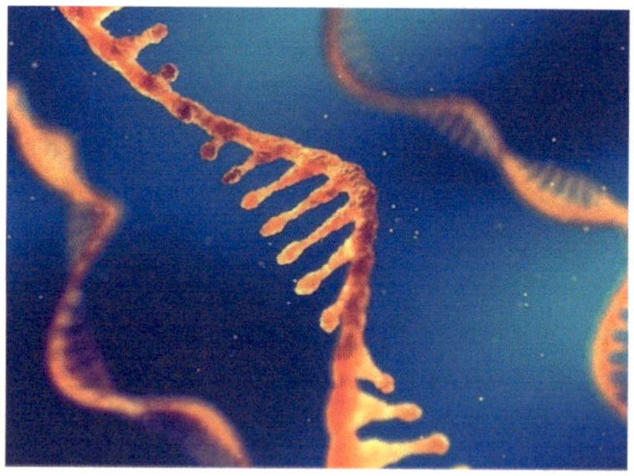

Figure 9.14. ***Single-Stranded Nature.***

Source: https://d2jx2rerrg6sh3.cloudfront.net/image-handler/picture/2021/3/shutterstock_1094792225_(1).jpg.

9.4.2. Secondary Structures (Hairpins, Loops)

Nucleic acids don't simply exist as long strings of code; they fold into shapes that matter, like hairpins and loops, which in many ways dictate how the cell operates. Hairpins, for example, come together when complementary bases bond in just the right way, forming a double-stranded section with a loose, unpaired tip; this isn't just about achieving thermodynamic stability—it actively steers processes such as transcription and translation. In many cases, these hairpin turns end up acting like natural on–off switches for genes, subtly influencing which parts of the genetic blueprint various proteins and other molecules can read. Loops introduce an additional layer of unpredictability. They don't always follow the neat pattern of a hairpin and often emerge from irregular base pairing that leaves clusters of unpaired nucleotides bubbling up. Such loops can spark essential activities—from helping ribozymes form to tweaking how proteins interact with RNA. In long non-coding RNAs (lncRNAs), these loopy bits sometimes weave together with nearby DNA sequences to create complex triplex structures, like those involving DNA:DNA:RNA interactions. Generally speaking, understanding the various ways loops can arrange themselves is crucial to comprehending the full range of lncRNA function. This challenge has led many to advocate for more sophisticated computational prediction methods (Warwick et al., 2023). On the technology side, our computational tools for predicting RNA's secondary shapes are indispensable. Researchers blend bioinformatics with rigorous testing to unravel how even subtle twists in hairpins and loops can affect RNA's behavior inside cells. Given RNA's flexible nature and the wild variety of its expressed sequences, having tools that can catch even minor structural shifts is crucial; these small details can reshape the overall 3D formation and, in turn, the molecule's functionality. The insights gained here significantly help bridge the gap between a molecule's structure and its role in gene regulation, thereby deepening our overall understanding of cellular processes (Matarrese et al., 2022) (Figure 9.15).

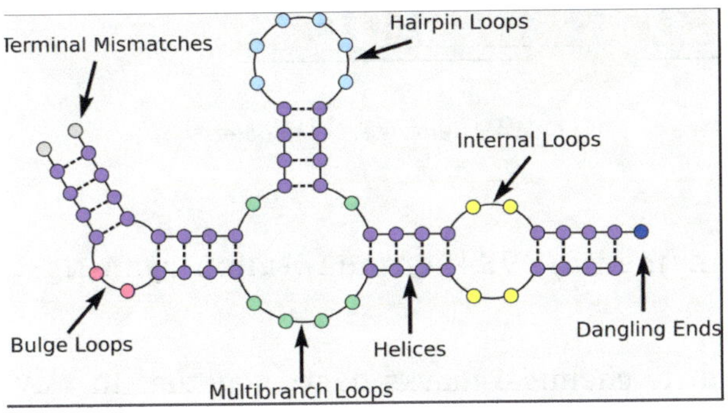

Figure 9.15. RNA secondary structure.

Source: https://external-content.duckduckgo.com/iu/?u=https%3A%2F%2Fgitlab-public.circ.rochester.edu%2Fdmathews%2Fbootcamp%2F-%2Fwikis%2FImages%2FRNA_secondary_structure.png&f=1&nofb=1&ipt=44ff832567316e5a57d58d5223dd59be809aea630cacee4f0b0d3f48d2f99f5a.

9.4.3. Tertiary Structures and Their Significance

RNA molecules often twist into unexpected three-dimensional shapes that play a significant role. One might assume that, like DNA's neat double helix, all genetic material is rigidly organized—but RNA, in most cases, folds into a jumble of loops and knots. These twists aren't just for show; they build sites where reactions take place, whether for translating codes or reading them out. Take circRNAs, for instance—these circular RNAs tend to maintain a stable, unique shape that enhances their ability to regulate genes. Such unique folds enable them to bond with proteins and other RNA strands, suggesting their potential roles in gene regulation and pathways related to cancer research (Shao et al., 2020). Digging a bit deeper, it turns out these structural quirks of RNA play a massive part in how cells manage their business. Often, RNA acts like a rough-and-ready scaffold, gathering other proteins and RNA pieces to tweak gene expression in unpredictable ways. Long noncoding RNAs (lncRNAs) are a good example; they fold into elaborate shapes that mingle with chromatin, transcription factors, and various other cellular components. Generally speaking, this structural diversity makes lncRNAs promising as biomarkers—potentially useful in detecting or treating cancer. Sometimes, when these folds go wrong, it can spell trouble, leading to gene misfires and even tumor growth, which makes further research all the more pressing (Bhan et al., 2017). Looking further ahead, exploring these RNA foldings also provides us with hints about evolution and genetic regulation. Many scientists argue that RNA's shapes have evolved over time, becoming optimized for both stability and versatility in ever-changing environments. This view reminds us that some of these forms are conserved across species, suggesting a fundamental, universally important role. Understanding these shape-driven behaviors may open up new therapeutic avenues, especially when it comes to modulating interactions in disorders where lncRNAs and circRNAs deviate from their usual patterns. So, RNA's twisty forms aren't just an academic curiosity—they might someday guide novel treatments to help bring cellular processes back into balance (Shao et al., 2020).

9.5. Functions of DNA

DNA isn't just a passive manual for life—it's at the heart of what a cell does. It begins by crafting mRNA from its genetic recipe, which then instructs the cell on how to build proteins. Those proteins, by the way, are busy doing everything from fueling metabolism and assembling cellular structures to handling signals in subtle ways. In many cases, there's another twist: chemical tags like methyl groups swing into action, tweaking which parts of the genetic code are active. Research generally points to 5-methylcytosine—a molecule with a somewhat unpredictable spread across our genes—as a significant player in turning some genes off and, in turn, helping shape how a cell behaves as it grows and meets changing environments (Alexandra et al., 2022).

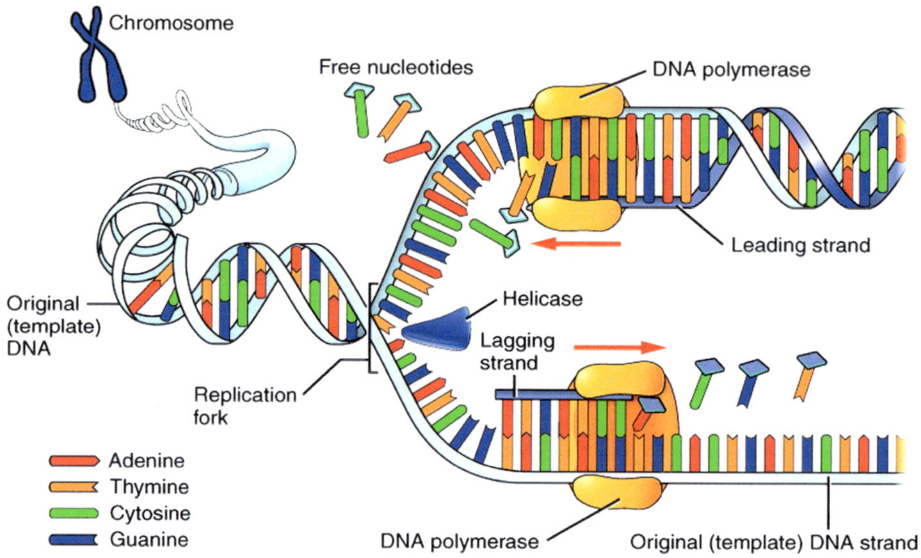

Figure 9.16. Functions of DNA.

Source: https://www.entandaudiologynews.com/media/3934/entnd14-allen-ryan-fig-1.png?width=576;height=349.

All these overlapping layers show that DNA and its chemical marks dance together in ways that guide the cell's every move. Passing down instructions and safeguarding them for future generations is another big job for DNA. When cells get ready to divide, they copy their entire blueprint, making sure every detail sticks around, even though the process isn't always perfect—sometimes a tiny error sneaks in that can lead to mutations with sweeping effects on evolution or even trigger diseases. Additionally, DNA has its built-in repair system: systems like base excision repair and nucleotide excision repair step in when damage from UV light or chemicals is severe. This careful juggling act of copying and mending not only preserves the genome's overall integrity but also ensures that the essential mechanics of life don't come to a grinding halt (Joel et al.,

2020). In a nutshell, DNA weaves together the heritage of the past with the challenges of today and the possibilities of tomorrow. Beyond holding and handing down genetic instructions, DNA also plays a key part in how cells react to what's happening around them. Under stress or during an infection, for example, bits of mitochondrial DNA (mtDNA) might escape into the cell's central area, acting as a sort of early-warning signal that kickstarts the immune system (Joel et al., 2020). This shows that DNA isn't locked away in a static vault; it's right there orchestrating our body's defense strategies. At the same time, cells use specific methylation patterns to determine which genes should be switched on or off to best adapt to their environment. As scientists continue to uncover new details about these processes, it's becoming clear that DNA's influence extends to many areas—shaping everything from development to disease management (Alexandra et al., 2022) (Figure 9.16).

9.5.1. Genetic Information Storage

DNA's intricate structure functions like a precise blueprint for storing genetic information—a fundamental concept underlying every living thing. At its core, DNA twists into a double helix, and if and that the nucleotide bases—adenine (A), thymine (T), cytosine (C), and guanine (G)—pair up in a way that isn't just for show. In most cases, these pairings are crucial for ensuring that replication and transcription occur accurately, keeping the entire process on track. Each bit of DNA houses regulatory segments like promoters—a short stretch where RNA polymerase gets started—which generally determines when and where genes spring into action. Understanding these bits, however, is key; even a minor disruption here can sometimes lead to problems like diabetes or cancer (Pradeepa et al., 2023). RNA then steps in as the go-between, linking DNA with protein synthesis, a role that underscores its significant part in genetic information storage. Transcription is the process by which DNA is converted into mRNA, carrying the code for building proteins, and then a whole host of other RNAs—such as tRNA and rRNA—help out during translation. Generally speaking, RNA's single-stranded nature isn't just a quirk; it folds into specific shapes that boost its function, aiding in the correct conversion of the mRNA script into working proteins. It's interesting how exploring RNA's varied forms continues to open doors to understanding protein synthesis and even points to possible treatments for genetic disorders linked to faulty RNA processing (Naesens et al., 2022). When it comes to keeping genetic information safe, the precision of DNA replication and repair is pretty telling. In most situations, if an error occurs during DNA copying, it must be corrected to preserve genetic integrity. Enzymes like DNA polymerases check the new strands with almost meticulous care, proofreading and helping ensure nothing's out of place. And then there are the elaborate repair mechanisms that jump in when damage occurs, working to patch up anomalies so the blueprint stays intact. A failure in these systems, however, can sometimes have dire consequences—including cancer and other genetic issues. All in all, DNA and RNA, though different in their roles, work together in a loosely interwoven manner that makes accurate genetic storage and transmission a cornerstone of life (Pradeepa et al., 2023).

9.5.2. Replication Process

DNA replication is a complex process that enables cell division, ensuring the transmission of genetic information while also maintaining genetic diversity. It all starts at specific spots on the DNA, often called origins of replication, where the double helix unwinds with helicases doing their part; this exposes a single strand that allows DNA polymerases to roll in and add matching nucleotides. It isn't just a straightforward assembly line, in most cases; factors like R-loops—which form during transcription—can sometimes block the progress by stalling RNA Polymerase II on the chromatin, and that little glitch may lead to genomic instability and, eventually, conditions such as cancer and neurodegeneration (Chakraborty et al., 2018). Keeping the genome intact goes beyond simply copying DNA; it also involves handling the intricate structures it forms. G-quadruplexes (or G4 structures) show up during both replication and transcription, and their role is double-edged. On the one hand, their formation can interfere with the replication process and even cause instability; on the other hand, they may be involved in regulating gene expression or helping to maintain chromosome stability. Their evolutionary persistence suggests they aren't mere accidents but serve fundamental biological roles. Generally speaking, when these G4 formations are disrupted—especially if helicases overreact—the result is increased replication stress and a higher risk of cellular malfunction (Sauer et al., 2017). Replication isn't just a neat, linear sequence of enzyme actions—it's more like a delicate dance where structure and control are constantly jostling with each other. Without the proper checks in place, structures like G4s and R-loops can accumulate, triggering replication stress that renders chromosomes unbearably fragile, eventually opening the door to various diseases. That's why it's so important to understand how these elements interact, even if the picture isn't always obvious. Effective helicases step in as unsung heroes, targeting and resolving these complexities so that replication can continue uninterrupted, reducing the troublesome genetic errors that might compromise cellular health. Ultimately, the intricate interplay between DNA and RNA reveals the importance (and occasionally, the complexity) of precise control in maintaining the smooth operation of our cells (Figure 9.17).

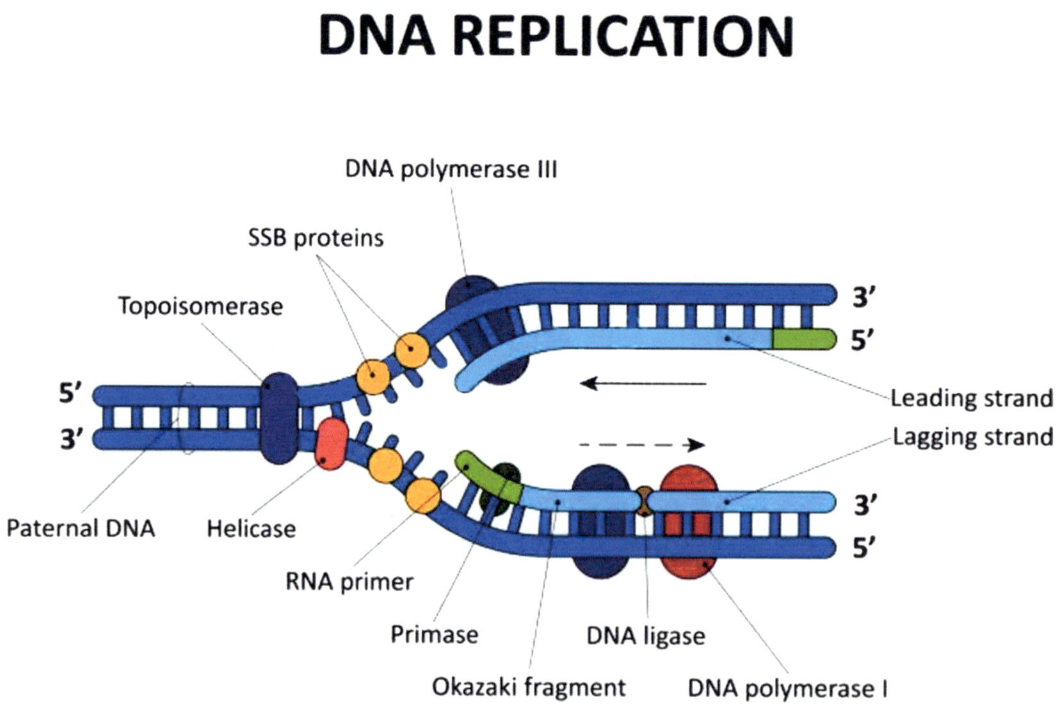

Figure 9.17. DNA replication.

Source: https://thumbs.dreamstime.com/b/dna-replication-process-scientific-diagram-318851786.jpg.

9.5.3. Role in Protein Synthesis

In biology, nucleic acids and proteins are intricately intertwined in ways that can be both surprising and complex. DNA acts as the blueprint, kickstarting the process by being copied into RNA—a step commonly referred to as transcription. That mRNA then sets off on its journey, carrying the instructions to build proteins, which are just strings of amino acids forming the cell's workhorses. This isn't just a neat hand-off; it's an unpredictable process where the details of transcription and translation come together to regulate cellular functions, whether by speeding up reactions or providing cells with structure. Once mRNA is made, it doesn't immediately get to work at the ribosomes. Instead, it goes through a handful of modifications—adding a 5' cap and a poly-A tail, for example—to make the message more stable and signal that it's good to go. Then, during translation, tRNA molecules step in not just to deliver amino acids but also to ensure that their anticodons match the mRNA codons. This detail ups the accuracy of protein synthesis (even if things aren't always perfect). This mix of modifications and careful matching captures the lively, sometimes unpredictable transfer of genetic instructions into the proteins that keep our cells ticking. New technologies have also begun to disrupt the status quo. Lipid nanoparticles (LNPs) are now used to boost protein synthesis by ferrying genetic instructions—like mRNA—directly into cells. Pieter et al. (2017) explain how these particles help mRNA find its way to the ribosomes more efficiently, which in many cases leads to a notable increase in protein production. This innovation shows promise, particularly in addressing diseases associated with protein deficiencies. Meanwhile, Uhl Mén et al. (2015) look at how blending transcriptomics with proteomics, and mapping human tissue proteomes, offers fresh clues about protein expression across different organs. All in all, fusing genetic data with protein profiles might not only reveal more about the complex process of protein synthesis but also pave the way for personalized treatments aimed squarely at repairing protein function (Figure 9.18).

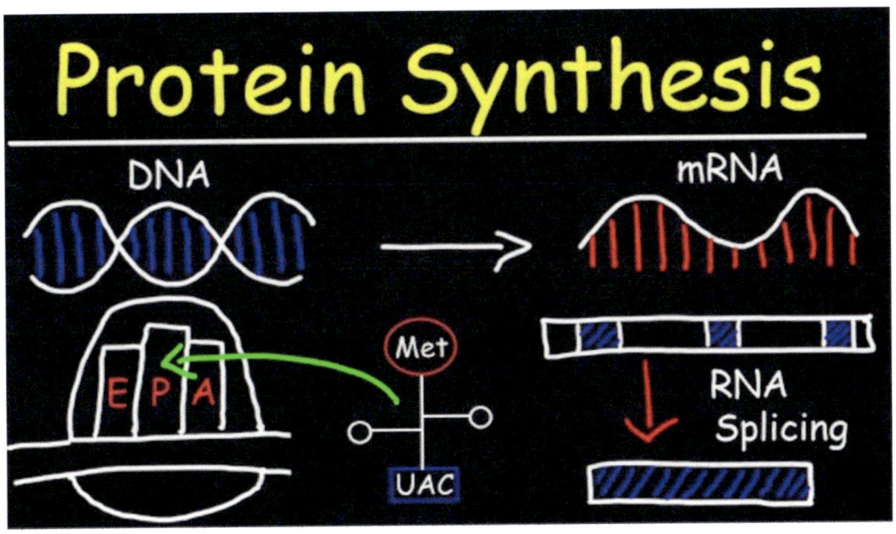

Figure 9.18. Role in protein synthesis.

Source: https://i.ytimg.com/vi/8wAwLwJAGHs/sddefault.jpg.

9.6. Functions of RNA

RNA isn't just a simple messenger in our cells—it does way more than shuttle genetic info around. Deep inside every cell, this molecule takes a blueprint from DNA and helps produce actual proteins, much like a busy translator turning ideas into action. In most cases, mRNA leaves the nucleus carrying instructions over to ribosomes, where it's read and turned into chains of amino acids, which then fold into proteins that the cell needs. Managing mRNA effectively is also crucial; those minor tweaks after transcription can significantly impact its lifespan, destination, and translation efficiency. And if mRNA goes awry, cells sometimes hit the panic button, which shows RNA's role goes beyond merely coding—it helps keep everything running smoothly (Joel et al., 2020). Yet there's more to RNA than just mRNA. Different types of non-coding RNA (ncRNA) play distinct roles in cellular processes. For example, tRNA is essential for reading the genetic code by bringing the right amino acids to ribosomes, matching them to the mRNA's instructions. Meanwhile, rRNA isn't just taking up space—it forms the structural core of the ribosome and helps link amino acids together. The back-and-forth between these RNA types may sound a bit complex, but it ensures that proteins are assembled correctly. Also, siRNA and miRNA step in to fine-tune things by influencing the stability and translation of mRNA, underscoring just how many roles RNA can play (Monahan et al., 2017). Furthermore, RNA also participates in cellular signaling and control networks. Take ribozymes, for instance—these catalytic RNA molecules demonstrate that RNA can sometimes initiate chemical reactions on its own, without relying on proteins. They can promote interactions with other nucleic acids or even small molecules, hinting at RNA's deep evolutionary roots. RNA also appears; specific pattern recognition receptors are tuned in to RNA from viruses, which then trigger defensive reactions. In most cases, the many faces and functions of RNA—from guiding protein construction to fine-tuning gene expression and stirring up chemical activity—make it an indispensable part of life (Joel et al., 2020) (Figure 9.19).

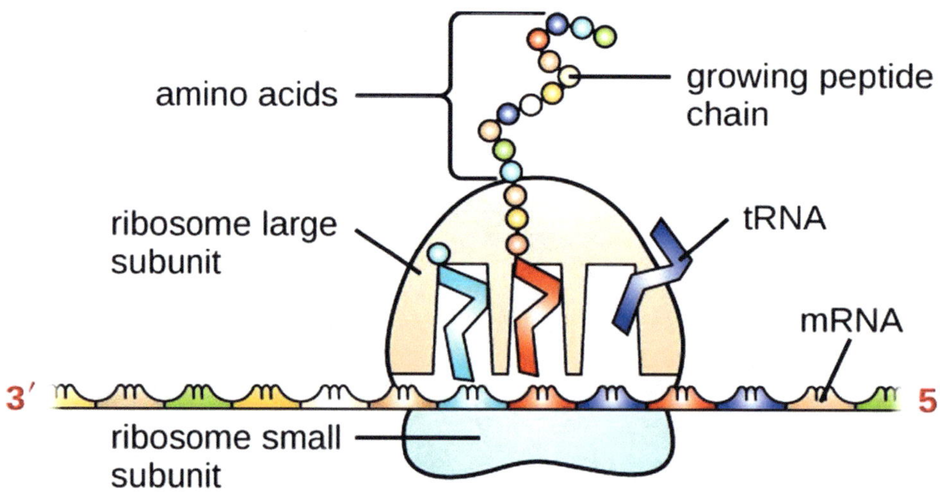

Figure 9.19. Functions of RNA.

Source: https://s3-us-west-2.amazonaws.com/courses-images/wp-content/uploads/sites/1094/2016/11/03164525/OSC_Microbio_10_03_RNAFunct.jpg.

9.6.1. Messenger Role in Protein Synthesis

DNA and RNA work together in a surprisingly intricate way that forms the backbone of life. In our cells, mRNA acts as the messenger linking the genetic blueprint stored in DNA to the protein factories within the ribosome. When RNA polymerase reads the DNA template, it creates an mRNA transcript that mirrors the original instructions; even a minor mistake at this stage can lead to proteins that don't perform as they should, potentially disrupting essential cell tasks. In most cases, this need for extreme accuracy shows that mRNA isn't just a simple courier—it also plays a part in subtly regulating other cellular activities, underscoring its vital role in molecular biology. After mRNA receives its processing and minor modifications, it leaves the nucleus and enters the cytoplasm, where it associates with rRNA and tRNA at the ribosome. The ribosome then reads the mRNA sequence in groups of three bases—each triplet, or codon, specifying one particular amino acid. As tRNA molecules drop off their matching amino acids, a polypeptide chain gradually forms until it blossoms into a functional protein. This isn't just a mechanical assembly line; a mix of factors fine-tunes both the pace and the precision of the process. Even segments of the mRNA itself, such as the untranslated regions (UTRs), help determine its stability and efficiency, illustrating the dynamic nature of protein synthesis. mRNA's influence goes well beyond sparking protein synthesis. It also plays a significant role in the broader regulatory networks that keep cells running smoothly. Recent studies generally suggest that many signaling pathways utilize mRNA as a form of raw material for regulation, much like second messenger molecules do. For example, cyclic adenosine monophosphate (cAMP) and cyclic guanosine monophosphate (cGMP) can alter gene expression by interacting with RNA, linking signal transduction directly to protein production (Cho et al., 2017). This capacity to adapt protein output on the fly is crucial for maintaining balance and reacting to environmental shifts (Horowitz et al., 1965). In short, mRNA isn't merely a messenger; it's a fundamental piece of the intricate puzzle that governs cellular life (Figure 9.20).

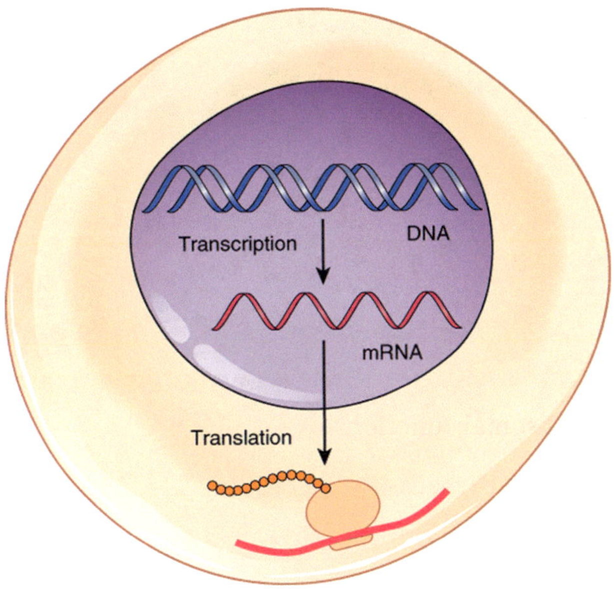

Figure 9.20. Messenger role in protein synthesis.

Source: https://open.oregonstate.education/app/uploads/sites/157/2021/02/0328_Transcription-translation_Summary.jpg.

9.6.2. Transfer and Ribosomal Functions

Proteins come to life when tRNA and ribosomes mix their skills in a surprisingly jumbled yet effective way. tRNA acts like a handy courier, hauling specific amino acids directly to ribosomes; each one sports a unique anticodon that finds its matching mRNA codon almost like a secret handshake. This match-up is key for the cell to decode its genetic script correctly. Sometimes, a tweak at what's known as the wobble spot lets one tRNA cover different codons. That extra bit of flexibility helps keep protein synthesis running smoothly, even under shifting conditions—recent studies (Joel et al., 2020) have noticed this clever trick. Ribosomes are like busy little factories that pull together the amino acids brought in by tRNA. They line up these building blocks according to the mRNA's instructions, and along the way, the ribosomal subunits (made up of rRNA and assorted proteins) twist and turn, shifting shape to snap new peptide bonds into place. In most cases, as they move from one state to the next—from elongation right through to termination—they also team up with a variety of helper factors; this fluid structure turns out to be essential for keeping the entire translation process on track (Joel et al., 2020). tRNA and ribosomes depend on each other in a kind of intricate dance that keeps the cell's inner workings balanced. Take it that ribosomes operate best when tRNA is in tip-top shape – a state often achieved through minor modifications, with enzymes like NSUN3 playing a crucial role. It might sound like a minor detail, but these adjustments stabilize the whole translation process and help the cell maintain its often finicky equilibrium. Understanding these twists in the system not only sheds light on the nuts and bolts of gene expression but also suggests fresh approaches to tackling genetic disorders and even battling microbial resistance (Haag et al., 2016) (Figure 9.21).

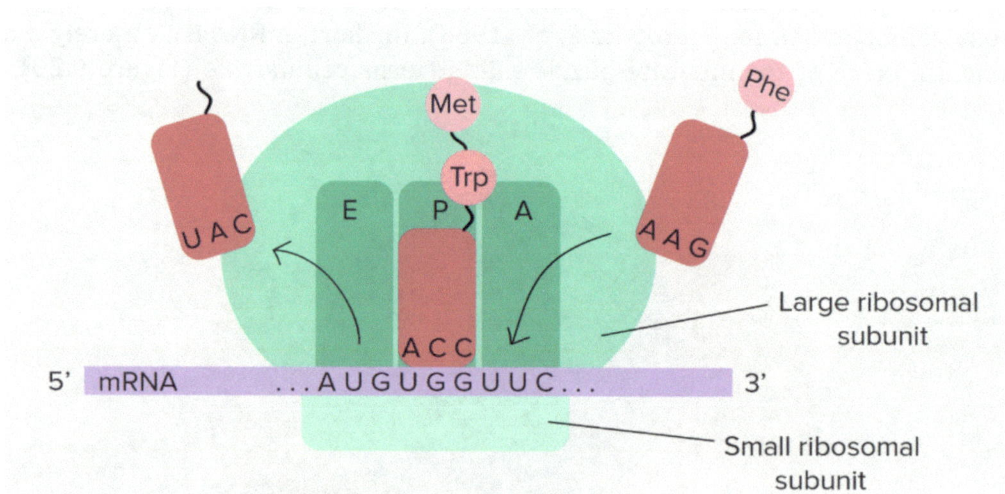

Figure 9.21. Transfer and ribosomal functions.

Source: https://cdn.kastatic.org/ka-perseus-images/282fd6184d65eaf8e8284edccf3aa650ad11d774.png.

9.6.3. Regulatory Roles in Gene Expression

Inside cells, molecules interact in a sort of spontaneous dance that drives many of life's essential processes. Gene expression takes center stage here—it's the process that turns the DNA's blueprint into proteins the cell uses. Transcription factors bind to specific stretches of DNA, either enhancing or inhibiting transcription, depending on internal signals or subtle environmental changes. Their presence often spells the difference between a gene being active or not, and in most cases, this is critical for a cell to develop its identity or respond to shifts around it. Sometimes, these proteins are tweaked after they're made, acting as a kind of connector between signals from outside the nucleus and the genome itself. This highlights how flexible and ever-changing gene regulation can be, ultimately influencing both cellular functions and overall development. RNA molecules add another fascinating layer to this story. Beyond transcription factors, regulatory RNAs—such as miRNAs and long non-coding RNAs (lncRNAs)—have come to play a crucial role in fine-tuning which genes are expressed. For example, miRNAs are known to bind to mRNAs and either prevent them from being translated into proteins or direct them toward degradation, which means specific proteins may never be produced. This form of post-transcriptional control enables cells to respond rapidly when conditions change, a crucial process during events such as growth or programmed cell death. At the same time, lncRNAs can interact with chromatin or work in conjunction with the transcription machinery, influencing the accessibility of DNA and the ease with which transcription factors can bind. Ultimately, these overlapping controls between DNA and RNA highlight the complexity of the entire gene regulation landscape. Then there's the twist involving mtDNA and the immune response. Research suggests that during various stress events, mtDNA can leak into the cytoplasm and essentially act as an alarm, triggering immune receptors like cGAS and TLR9. This alarm, in many cases, triggers the production of pro-inflammatory cytokines and type I interferons—a clear indication of how gene regulation is directly tied to immune activation. It's also been noted that mtDNA tends to be less methylated compared to its nuclear counterpart, hinting that the rules of regulation might differ between these two DNA types. Oddly enough, even the quirks of DNA structure, such as the formation of G-quadruplexes in regions that control gene activity, seem to matter a great deal—especially under stress conditions (Spiegel et al., 2019; Joel et al., 2020).

SUMMARY

DNA and RNA are closely tied in their roles, each playing a key part in how our genes are expressed and regulated. Lately, breakthroughs have given us a peek into DNA methylation—it's not just a simple genetic code, but a process that adds another layer of control. Scientists have been examining modifications like 5-methylcytosine, and, generally speaking, these changes are shedding light on gene regulation and cell differentiation in unexpected ways. This growing pool of insights deepens our understanding of molecular biology while also sparking debates around new treatments for various diseases. The quest to unravel DNA's structure and function remains a lively and often unpredictable journey in genetic research (Alexandra et al., 2022). RNA, with its diverse shapes and functions, serves as more than just a messenger in the cell. Recent work on the SARS-CoV-2 nucleocapsid protein, for example, has revealed surprising interactions between viral RNA and the host's cell systems—a twist that goes beyond the usual expectations. RNA casually interacts with various biomolecules, including DNA and proteins, placing it at the heart of cellular activity. Its involvement in everything from viral replication to gene control means that RNA continues to challenge and expand our current understanding, prompting further exploration into its broad and varied contributions (Zhou et al., 2020). In conclusion, the functions and forms of DNA and RNA weave together a complex narrative about gene management and evolution. Ongoing research increasingly demands an interdisciplinary approach—drawing from genetics, molecular biology, and computational analysis—to truly capture the essence of genetic inheritance and expression, and to explore how we might modify these molecules for therapeutic purposes. The future of genetic studies looks promising, hinting at even deeper links between these molecules that could be vital for combating diseases and fueling biotechnological innovations. With each discovery, the unfolding saga of DNA and RNA continues to push the boundaries of what we know about life itself (Alexandra et al., 2022).

Understanding how DNA and RNA are constructed is crucial when examining the processes that occur within a cell. DNA's famous for keeping our genetic instructions safe—its double helix isn't just an elegant twist; it also serves as a solid pattern for copying itself and making RNA. Meanwhile, RNA primarily exists as a single strand that can fold in unexpected ways to accomplish its tasks. These design differences aren't just academic details; they openly reveal how each molecule has its distinct role, from storing genetic information to guiding protein production and even contributing to gene regulation. This mix of roles sets a playful stage for digging deeper into how both types of nucleic acids power our cellular systems and influence health in most cases. Inside our cells, DNA and RNA are constantly engaged in a dynamic process that keeps things moving along. Transcription, for example, takes a bit of DNA and converts it into mRNA, which then provides ribosomes with the rough blueprint needed to build proteins. It's a pretty crucial step—one that, in most cases, makes sure that genes are expressed and the right proteins show up to keep the cell functioning. Not to be left out, molecules like tRNA and rRNA step in during translation, piecing together amino acids into chains, almost like various workers on an assembly line (even if the process can feel a bit haphazard at times). This flow from a written code to actual biological products captures the essence of molecular biology and reminds us how life springs to action from tiny sequences of letters. In recent years, breakthroughs in molecular techniques have opened up a new level of detail about nucleic acids. For instance, research into coronaviruses has shown how viral RNA can interact with host cell machinery—information that's proving helpful in developing better treatments for infections. And then there are new computer tools, like Phenix, that make it much easier to visualize the inner workings of these molecules on almost an atomic level, which is, frankly, quite remarkable. Generally speaking, being able to unravel these microscopic details doesn't just fuel therapy development; it also helps in spotting potential disease outbreaks, as seen with those lineage B beta coronaviruses. These insights go a long way toward demonstrating how the fine structure of DNA and RNA directly ties into everything from everyday cell life to the development of diseases, cementing their key role in today's science (Dorothée Liebschner et al., 2019; Letko et al., 2020).

CLOSER LOOK

DEOXYRIBOSE SUGAR

Deoxyribose sugar is a five-carbon monosaccharide (simple sugar) that plays a critical role in the structure and function of deoxyribonucleic acid (DNA). This molecule carries genetic information in almost all living organisms. Chemically known as 2-deoxyribose, it is a type of pentose sugar, meaning it contains five carbon atoms. What distinguishes deoxyribose from its close relative ribose (found in RNA) is the absence of an oxygen atom on the second carbon (C2') of its sugar ring. In ribose, this carbon has a hydroxyl group (-OH), whereas in deoxyribose, it has only a hydrogen atom (-H), hence the name "deoxy," meaning "without oxygen." This seemingly small structural difference has profound implications for the stability, structure, and function of DNA compared to RNA.

Deoxyribose exists predominantly in a cyclic furanose form in DNA, where four carbon atoms and one oxygen atom form a five-membered ring. This sugar forms the backbone of the DNA molecule by linking with phosphate groups and nitrogenous bases to create nucleotides, the building blocks of DNA. In a nucleotide, deoxyribose is covalently bonded to a phosphate group at its 5' carbon and to a nitrogenous base (adenine, guanine, cytosine, or thymine) at its 1' carbon. Nucleotides are joined together by phosphodiester bonds between the 3' carbon of one sugar and the 5' carbon of the next, creating a sugar-phosphate backbone that gives DNA its directionality and structural integrity. The deoxyribose sugar helps maintain the double helical structure of DNA by promoting a stable, less reactive environment compared to RNA.

One of the key reasons why DNA is more stable than RNA is due to the absence of the 2'-OH group in deoxyribose. In RNA, the hydroxyl group at the 2' position can participate in chemical reactions that can lead to strand cleavage, making RNA more susceptible to degradation. DNA's deoxyribose, lacking this reactive group, contributes to the molecule's chemical stability, which is essential for the long-term storage of genetic information. This is especially important in cells, where DNA must remain intact for the organism's lifetime and be accurately replicated during cell division.

Deoxyribose is synthesized in cells through a reduction process involving ribose-5-phosphate, a product of the pentose phosphate pathway. This process is catalyzed by the enzyme ribonucleotide reductase, which removes the 2'-hydroxyl group from ribonucleotides to produce deoxyribonucleotides. These deoxyribonucleotides are then used in the synthesis of DNA during replication and repair. The correct functioning of these biochemical pathways is critical for maintaining the accuracy and fidelity of DNA replication.

Deoxyribose sugar is a fundamental component of DNA, providing the scaffold for genetic coding and transmission. Its unique structure, especially the lack of a 2'-hydroxyl group, imparts chemical stability that is essential for DNA's role in heredity and molecular biology. As a core element of nucleotides, deoxyribose plays a vital role in the continuity of life by enabling the secure storage and faithful replication of genetic information across generations.

REFERENCES

1. Georgakopoulos, D. G., Després, V., Fröhlich-Nowoisky, J., Psenner, R., Ariya, P. A., Pósfai, M., Ahern, H. E., Moffett, B. F., & Hill, T. C. J. (2009). Microbiology and atmospheric processes: biological, physical and chemical characterization of aerosol particles. *Biogeosciences*, *6*(4), 721–737. https://doi.org/10.5194/bg-6-721-2009Ahmed, A., Beckerman, B., Burnett, C., Carthew, R., Castanotto, D., et al. (2013). RNA interference by single- and double-stranded siRNA with a DNA extension containing a 3′ nuclease-resistant mini-hairpin structure. https://core.ac.uk/download/30734768.pdf (accessed on 26 May 2025).
2. Allison, S. J., & Milner, J. (2009). RNA interference by single- and double-stranded siRNA with a DNA extension containing a 3′ nuclease-resistant mini-hairpin structure. https://core.ac.uk/download/pdf/30734768.pdf (accessed on 26 May 2025).
3. Andrés, C., Pérez de la Lastra, J. M., Plou, F. J., & Pérez-Lebeña, E. (2021). The chemistry of reactive oxygen species (ROS) revisited: Outlining their role in biological macromolecules (DNA, lipids and proteins) and induced pathologies. *International Journal of Molecular Sciences, 22*(9), 4642. https://doi.org/10.3390/ijms22094642.
4. Bergonzo, C., & Grishaev, A. V. (2025). Critical assessment of RNA and DNA structure predictions via artificial intelligence: The imitation game. *Journal of Chemical Information and Modeling, 65*(8), 3544–3554. https://www.semanticscholar.org/paper/dca5279c8cc65048f0f33919501f3f8c1152b0a1 (accessed on 26 May 2025).
5. Berti, D., Franchi, L., Baglioni, P., & Luisi, P. (1997). Molecular recognition in monolayers: Complementary base pairing in dioleoylphosphatidyl derivatives of adenosine, uridine, and cytidine. *Langmuir, 13*(12), 3438–3444. https://www.semanticscholar.org/paper/1c83d4b9d06abf4a5babc3a6a9eb549a33e8e545 (accessed on 26 May 2025).
6. Bhan, A., Soleimani, M., & Mandal, S. S. (2017). Long noncoding RNA and cancer: A new paradigm. *Cancer Research, 77*(14), 3965–3981. https://doi.org/10.1158/0008-5472.CAN-16-2634.
7. Bryans, N., Dattani, N. S., Davis, K., Hill, J., et al. (2014). Mapping the space of genomic signatures. *arXiv*. http://arxiv.org/abs/1406.4105 (accessed on 26 May 2025).
8. Cerneckis, J., Cui, Q., He, C., Yi, C., & Shi, Y. (2022). Decoding pseudo uridine: An emerging target for therapeutic development. *Trends in Pharmacological Sciences, 43*(7), 522–535. https://doi.org/10.1016/j.tips.2022.03.008.
9. Chakraborty, P., Huang, J., & Hiom, K. (2018). DHX9 helicase promotes R-loop formation in cells with impaired RNA splicing. *Nature Communications, 9*. https://doi.org/10.1038/s41467-018-06677-1.
10. Chen, X., Yang, Z., Wang, W., Qian, K., Liu, M., Wang, J., & Wang, M. (2021). Structural basis for RNA recognition by the N-terminal tandem RRM domains of human RBM45. *Nucleic Acids Research, 49*, 2946–2958. https://doi.org/10.1093/nar/gkab075.
11. Cho, K. H., Fahmi, T., & Port, G. C. (2017). c-di-AMP: An essential molecule in the signaling pathways that regulate the viability and virulence of gram-positive bacteria. https://core.ac.uk/download/129069092.pdf (accessed on 26 May 2025).
12. Cleaves, H., Butch, C. J., Burger, P., Goodwin, J., & Meringer, M. (2019). One among millions: The chemical space of nucleic acid-like molecules. *Journal of Chemical Information and*

Modeling. https://www.semanticscholar.org/paper/28800cce38a8dd3205e5663151b7370b4aff4104 (accessed on 26 May 2026).

13. Cragnolini, T., Derreumaux, P., & Pasquali, S. (2014). Ab initio RNA folding. *arXiv*. http://arxiv.org/abs/1501.00022 (accessed on 26 May 2025).
14. Cullis, P. R., & Hope, M. J. (2017). Lipid nanoparticle systems for enabling gene therapies. *Molecular Therapy, 25*(6), 1467–1475. https://doi.org/10.1016/j.ymthe.2017.03.013.
15. Dadashova, L., & Mammadov, A. (2024). Intraspecies molecular DNA polymorphism and threat of *Hirudo orientalis*. *Bulletin of Science and Practice*. https://www.semanticscholar.org/paper/0206d8060dfa649aab0c288404727f1ed96040d3 (accessed on 26 May 2025).
16. Ding, Y., Tan, C., & Wu, F. (2014). Synthetic biology: A bridge between artificial and natural cells. https://core.ac.uk/download/323068426.pdf.
17. Galluzzi, L., Vitale, I., Aaronson, S. A., Abrams, J., Adam, D., Agostinis, P., Alnemri, E. S., et al. (2018). Molecular mechanisms of cell death: Recommendations of the Nomenclature Committee on Cell Death 2018. *Cell Death and Differentiation, 25*(3), 486–541. https://doi.org/10.1038/s41418-017-0012-4.
18. Haag, S., Sloan, K. E., Ranjan, N., Warda, A. S., Kretschmer, J., Blessing, C., Hübner, B., et al. (2016). NSUN3 and ABH1 modify the wobble position of mt-tRNA^{Met} to expand codon recognition in mitochondrial translation. *The EMBO Journal, 35*, 2104–2119. https://doi.org/10.15252/embj.201694885.
19. Heinemann, U., & Roske, Y. (2021). Cold-shock domains—Abundance, structure, properties, and nucleic-acid binding. *Cancers, 13*, 190. https://doi.org/10.3390/cancers13020190.
20. Hoeijmakers, J. H. J. (2009). DNA damage, aging, and cancer. *New England Journal of Medicine, 361*(15), 1475–1485. https://doi.org/10.1056/nejmra0804615.
21. Horowitz, N. H., & Metzenberg, R. L. (1965). Biochemical aspects of genetics. https://core.ac.uk/download/4869315.pdf.
22. Kato, D. K. (2024). Exploring the dynamic world of DNA and RNA: From structure to function and beyond. *INOSR Applied Sciences*. https://www.semanticscholar.org/paper/cf6ff9fdf2209610511f78731142ad6ff6cf334f (accessed on 26 May 2025).
23. Klionsky, D. J., Abdelmohsen, K., Abe, A., Abedin, M. J., Abeliovich, H., Acevedo-Arozena, A., Adachi, H., et al. (2016). Guidelines for the use and interpretation of assays for monitoring autophagy (3rd edition). *Autophagy, 12*(1), 1–222. https://doi.org/10.1080/15548627.2015.1100356.
24. Kruti, D., Prajapati, M., Deepika, P., Luluaa, A., & Suthar, K. (2021). Fluorescence *in-situ* hybridization: Technology to detect genetic mutation. *International Journal of Current Research and Review*. https://www.semanticscholar.org/paper/28a3992a557ab9c971fbbddb485c272695967f53 (accessed on 26 May 2025).
25. Lalitha, V., & Yathindra, N. (1994). Visualization of inter loop tertiary base pairing and stacking interactions in an unusual slipped loop DNA structure. https://core.ac.uk/download/pdf/291553339.pdf (accessed on 26 May 2025).
26. Lanier, K. A., & Williams, L. D. (2017). The origin of life: Models and data. https://core.ac.uk/download/323062617.pdf.

27. Lanzén, A., Lekang, K., Jonassen, I., Thompson, E., & Troedsson, C. (2016). High-throughput metabarcoding of eukaryotic diversity for environmental monitoring of offshore oil-drilling activities. *Molecular Ecology, 25*. https://www.semanticscholar.org/paper/21126499906d8ace60e9bb6a9d06e26c2c78465b (accessed on 26 May 2025).

28. Letko, M., Marzi, A., & Munster, V. J. (2020). Functional assessment of cell entry and receptor usage for SARS-CoV-2 and other lineage B beta coronaviruses. *Nature Microbiology, 5*(4), 562–569. https://doi.org/10.1038/s41564-020-0688-y.

29. Li, H., Yang, Y., Hong, W., Huang, M., Wu, M., & Zhao, X. (2020). Applications of genome editing technology in the targeted therapy of human diseases: Mechanisms, advances and prospects. *Signal Transduction and Targeted Therapy, 5*. https://doi.org/10.1038/s41392-019-0089-y.

30. Liebschner, D., Afonine, P. V., Baker, M. L., Bunkóczi, G., Chen, V. B., Croll, T. I., Hintze, B. J., et al. (2019). Macromolecular structure determination using X-rays, neutrons and electrons: Recent developments in *Phenix*. *Acta Crystallographic Section D Structural Biology, 75*(9), 861–877. https://doi.org/10.1107/s2059798319011471.

31. Matarrese, M., Loppini, A., Nicoletti, M., Filippi, S., & Chiodo, L. (2022). Assessment of tools for RNA secondary structure prediction and extraction: A final-user perspective. *Journal of Biomolecular Structure and Dynamics, 41*(21), 6917–6936. https://www.semanticscholar.org/paper/29dfaaef852acf894a29afe097063482494659fd (accessed on 26 May 2025).

32. Mattei, A. L., Bailly, N., & Meissner, A. (2022). DNA methylation: A historical perspective. *Trends in Genetics, 38*(8), 676–707. https://doi.org/10.1016/j.tig.2022.03.010.

33. Monahan, Z., Ryan, V. H., Janke, A. M., Burke, K. A., Rhoads, S. N., Zerze, G. H., O'Meally, R. N., et al. (2017). Phosphorylation of the FUS low-complexity domain disrupts phase separation, aggregation, and toxicity. *The EMBO Journal, 36*, 2951–2967. https://doi.org/10.15252/embj.201696394.

34. Morriss-Andrews, A., Ashcroft, N. W., Branden, C., de Gennes, P. G., Rottler, J., Kuipers, J., Lamb, H., et al. (2009). A systematically coarse-grained model for DNA, and its predictions for persistence length, stacking, twist, and chirality. *arXiv*. http://arxiv.org/abs/0911.4226 (accessed on 26 May 2025).

35. Naesens, L., Nemegeer, J., Roelens, F., Vallaeys, L., Meuwissen, M., Janssens, K., Verloo, P., et al. (2022). Mutations in RNU7-1 weaken secondary RNA structure, induce MCP-1 and CXCL10 in CSF, and result in Aicardi-Goutières syndrome with severe end-organ involvement. *Journal of Clinical Immunology, 42*(4), 962–974. https://www.semanticscholar.org/paper/7e7889d87c8d76e7471659ebaf3e692c76cc4e6d (accessed on 26 May 2025).

36. Neidle, S. (2021). Beyond the double helix: DNA structural diversity and the PDB. *Journal of Biological Chemistry, 296*, 100553. https://doi.org/10.1016/j.jbc.2021.100553.

37. O'Leary, N. A., Wright, M. W., Brister, J. R., Ciufo, S., Haddad, D., McVeigh, R., Rajput, B., et al. (2015). Reference sequence (RefSeq) database at NCBI: Current status, taxonomic expansion, and functional annotation. *Nucleic Acids Research, 44*(D1), D733–D745. https://doi.org/10.1093/nar/gkv1189.

38. Pradeepa, S., Gaspar, N., Shanmuganathan, V., Subbulakshmi, P., Alkhayyat, A., & Kaliappan, M. (2023). Classifying promoters by interpreting the hidden information of DNA sequences for disease prediction in clinical laboratories using Gaussian decision boundary estimation.

Intelligent Decision Technologies, 18(4), 613–631. https://www.semanticscholar.org/paper/e104c097da43fa3a330cd4c240a044a317123356 (accessed on 26 May 2025).

39. Riera Aroche, R., Ortiz-García, Y. M., Martínez Arellano, M. A., & Riera Leal, A. (2024). DNA as a perfect quantum computer based on the quantum physics principles. *Scientific Reports, 14*. https://doi.org/10.1038/s41598-024-62539-5.
40. Riley, J. S., & Tait, S. W. G. (2020). Mitochondrial DNA in inflammation and immunity. *EMBO Reports, 21*(4). https://doi.org/10.15252/embr.201949799.
41. Sauer, M., & Paeschke, K. (2017). G-quadruplex unwinding helicases and their function *in vivo*. *Biochemical Society Transactions, 45*(5), 1173–1182. https://doi.org/10.1042/bst20170097.
42. Shao, T., Pan, Y., & Xiong, X. (2020). Circular RNA: An important player with multiple facets to regulate its parental gene expression. *Molecular Therapy–Nucleic Acids, 23*, 369–376. https://doi.org/10.1016/j.omtn.2020.11.008.
43. Spiegel, J., Adhikari, S., & Balasubramanian, S. (2019). The structure and function of DNA G-quadruplexes. *Trends in Chemistry, 2*(2), 123–136. https://doi.org/10.1016/j.trechm.2019.07.002.
44. Uhlén, M., Fagerberg, L., Hallström, B. M., Lindskog, C., Oksvold, P., Mardinoğlu, A., Sivertsson, Å., et al. (2015). Tissue-based map of the human proteome. *Science, 347*(6220), 1260419. https://doi.org/10.1126/science.1260419.
45. Urich, T., Lanzén, A., Qi, J., Huson, D., Schleper, C., & Schuster, S. (2008). Simultaneous assessment of soil microbial community structure and function through analysis of the meta-transcriptome. *PLoS ONE, 3*. https://www.semanticscholar.org/paper/1e0929930008d239b345194dcf8d221a6fbfd1ec (accessed on 26 May 2025).
46. Van Arsdale, A., Turker, L., Chang, Y. C., Gould, J., Harmon, B., Maggi, E., Meshcheryakova, O., et al. (2024). Structure and transcription of integrated HPV DNA in vulvar carcinomas. *NPJ Genomic Medicine, 9*. https://www.semanticscholar.org/paper/1a040a0cb95cb5f3026b82c4853a3fbf7dc09e9f (accessed on 26 May 2025).
47. Warwick, T., Brandes, R., & Leisegang, M. (2023). Computational methods to study DNA: DNA: RNA triplex formation by lncRNAs. *Non-Coding RNA, 9*. https://www.semanticscholar.org/paper/7b7b875dbd696d1195b44494dea3c641a44c75e4 (accessed on 26 May 2025).
48. Wu, J., Qi, X., Liu, L., Hu, X., Liu, J., Yang, J., Yang, J., et al. (2019). Emerging epigenetic regulation of circular RNAs in human cancer. *Molecular Therapy–Nucleic Acids, 16*, 589–596. https://doi.org/10.1016/j.omtn.2019.04.011.
49. Xiong, M., Zhao, Z., Arnold, J., & Yu, F. (2011). Next-generation sequencing. *Journal of Biomedicine and Biotechnology, 2010*, Article ID 730418. https://www.semanticscholar.org/paper/ebd0db19e450d5941695afd860ed1f94123e8d5d (accessed on 26 May 2025).
50. Zhou, R., Zeng, R., von Brunn, A., & Lei, J. (2020). Structural characterization of the C-terminal domain of SARS-CoV-2 nucleocapsid protein. *Molecular Biomedicine, 1*. https://doi.org/10.1186/s43556-020-00001-4.
51. Zhou, Y. (2010). From sequence to structure, to function, and back again: Integrating knowledge-based approaches with physical intuitions for protein folding, binding, and design. https://core.ac.uk/download/46964282.pdf (accessed on 26 May 2025).

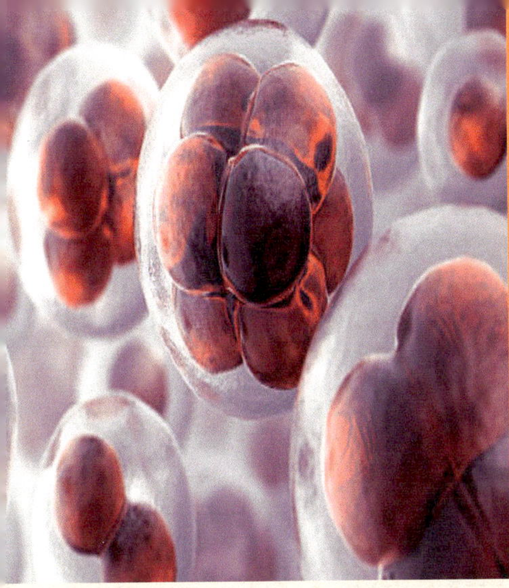

Chapter 10

CHROMOSOMES AND CELL DIVISION

Contents

Introduction

Cellular life ties closely to how chromosomes are built and behave—they're the carriers of our genetic blueprint. When a cell splits, it copies its DNA and shuffles it into daughter cells, and if that process stumbles, this may result in mutations or even cancer. It's interesting to note that watching these events unfold can reveal a great deal about genetic vulnerabilities; indeed, research often shows that maintaining chromosome stability is crucial. For example, human chromosomes 1, 4, and 7 appear to play a significant role in managing cell aging, which not only provides insight into the aging process but also helps suppress tumors (Leung et al., 2001). Recent breakthroughs in molecular genetics have shifted our understanding of gene expression—an area deeply linked to cell division. RNA transcription and subsequent translation into proteins are facilitated by a host of factors; some act directly within the chromatin, while others play a more remote role. In most cases, these processes are crucial for maintaining cell health and preserving genetic integrity. Current literature tells us that the complex world of eukaryotic gene expression isn't just about chromosomes doing their thing, but also about the whole genome's layout. Odd chromosomal behaviors, like uniparental disomy, remind us that even slight imbalances can have significant effects on health and disease (Stephenson, 1997). As research evolves, the methods used to study chromosomes and cell division have become increasingly sharper and more refined—think PCR-based cloning and hybridization techniques, which have significantly opened up the complex details of our genome. With these tools, scientists can better elucidate how specific genes interact within larger nucleoprotein complexes, which in turn play a major role in gene expression and control. It appears that by exploring the intricacies of somatic mutations and complex disorders, we gain a clearer understanding of the various roles chromosomes play in our overall well-being. This multi-angle approach not only sheds light on fundamental biological puzzles but also fuels the development of new therapies, as seen in gene therapy research that aims to fix genetic issues (Stephenson, 1997; Leung et al., 2001) (Figure 10.1).

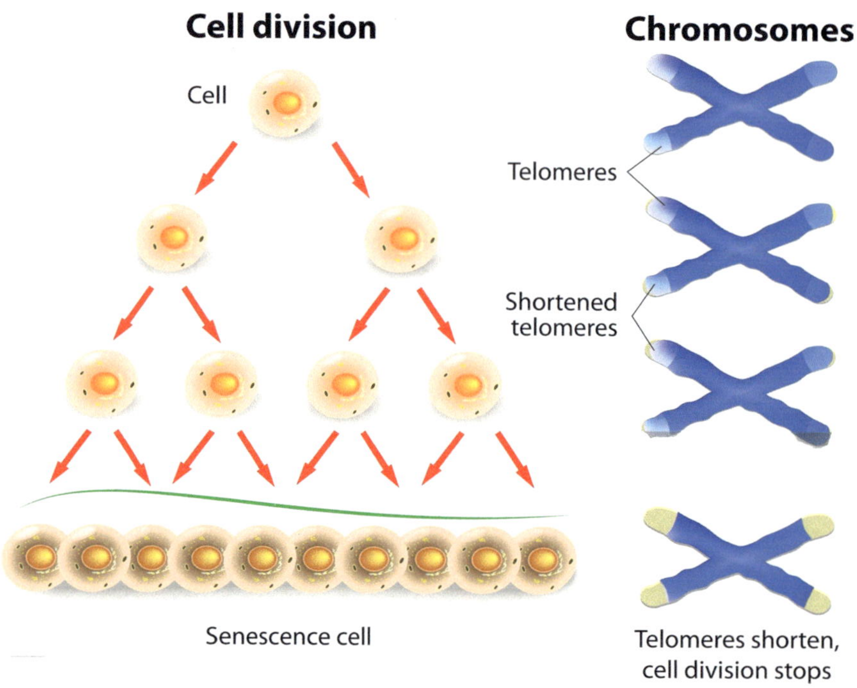

Figure 10.1. Chromosomes and cell division.

Source: https://external-content.duckduckgo.com/iu/?u=http%3A%2F%2Fthumbs.dreamstime.com%2Fz%2Ftelomere-cell-division-human-chromosomes-telomeres-ends-serve-to-protect-coding-dna-genome-telomeres-shorten-36972246.jpg&f=1&nofb=1&ipt=d122b3a23f3721860ddbe0a6f49622af7ac78264e0b517800719176932f10ae7.

Definition of Chromosomes

Cellular biology revolves around how genetic material is organized and moves around, mostly tucked inside chromosomes. Think of them as tightly packaged bundles where DNA coils around histone proteins, making it easy to fit inside the cell's nucleus. When cells split, one may notice chromosomes each taking on their shape that helps ensure a fair share goes to the new cells. In simple terms, chromosomes carry life's blueprint—they house the genes that shape cell traits and functions. Intriguingly, every species has a unique count; for instance, humans carry 46 chromosomes in 23 pairs. Generally speaking, this setup plays a massive role in maintaining genetic diversity and evolution, since even minor tweaks in these bundles can spark mutations that affect how organisms grow and thrive. A closer look at chromosomes reveals that they're not static boxes of information but active players in the cell cycle. During interphase, they relax into what we call chromatin, making it easier for the cell to access the genetic instructions needed for protein synthesis. Then, as division looms, chromatin slowly shifts gears—by prophase, it condenses into tighter forms that not only facilitate even distribution during cell division but also protect the DNA from harm. Along the way, several proteins regulate gene activity, deciding which sections of DNA get read at any moment. In most cases, this dynamic behavior is crucial for maintaining the genetic system's stability while navigating the numerous twists and turns of the cell cycle. The link between chromosomes and cell division is a bit like a well-choreographed dance. When a cell is about to divide, every chromosome duplicates, creating sister chromatids that stick together at a region called the centromere until they're pulled apart in anaphase. This careful process typically ensures that both daughter cells receive an exact copy of the original genetic material, thereby maintaining the genome's integrity and preventing issues such as aneuploidy, where chromosome numbers become distorted. New methods, such as pA-DamID, even allow scientists to visualize and map how chromosomes interact with the nuclear lamina during division, providing fresh insights into their behavior. Altogether, understanding these intricate moves not only sheds light on the core principles of biology but also hints at how errors in this process might connect to hereditary diseases and developmental disorders, linking form and function in living things (Figure 10.2).

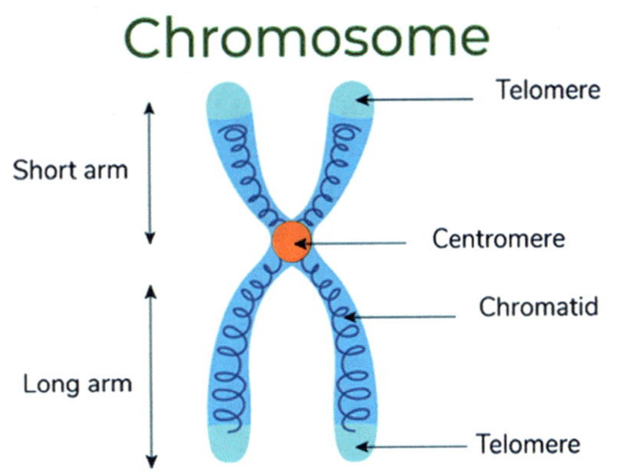

Figure 10.2. Definition of chromosomes.

Source: https://external-content.duckduckgo.com/iu/?u=https%3A%2F%2Fmedia.geeksforgeeks.org%2Fwp-content%2Fuploads%2F20240212133717%2FChromosome-660.png&f=1&nofb=1&ipt=466328c407eb09b8021ee3f51a13a1d91f6b5e1acd3f00325f53cb9094f73cd5.

Importance of Cell Division

Cell division is at the heart of how multicellular life keeps going. When a cell divides, it produces new cells that assume roles such as growth, tissue repair, and reproduction. This can be seen in parts of the body like the skin or gut lining, where cells are replaced faster than one might expect – a sign that keeping everything balanced depends on these tiny divisions. If things go haywire and cells lose control, it results in issues like cancer, where unchecked proliferation takes over. It's a clear reminder that keeping cell division in check is vital, especially since it's so closely tied to the genetic instructions nestled in our chromosomes. Understanding how cells divide isn't just an academic exercise—it also helps us tackle real-world challenges. Recent studies generally show that non-living stressors, such as heat and drought, can significantly impact crop growth. These environmental pressures disrupt cell functions in ways that initiate a cascade of physiological and biochemical disruptions, which in turn can lower overall plant health and yield. By gaining a more nuanced understanding of how cell division responds to stress, researchers can develop more effective crop management practices and targeted breeding programs to enhance resilience. In most cases, this insight weaves together basic science and practical applications that are crucial for food security and long-term sustainability. Then there's the intriguing layer of epigenetics, where gene expression is tweaked without changing the DNA sequence itself. Researchers have begun to notice that these epigenetic shifts can influence cell behavior during division, sometimes causing cells to assume slightly different roles or identities across tissues. Even subtle modifications can affect developmental processes and may even open up pathways to diseases like cancer. Understanding how these epigenetic factors influence cell division isn't just about decoding one process—it broadens our understanding of development and disease alike, tying together multiple strands of biological research in a remarkably unexpected way.

10.1. Structure of Chromosomes

Genetic material in a cell is arranged in a way that's crucial to keeping things stable during division. Chromosomes, for example, aren't just neat packages of DNA; they're built from strands of DNA wound around proteins called histones, forming what we call chromatin.

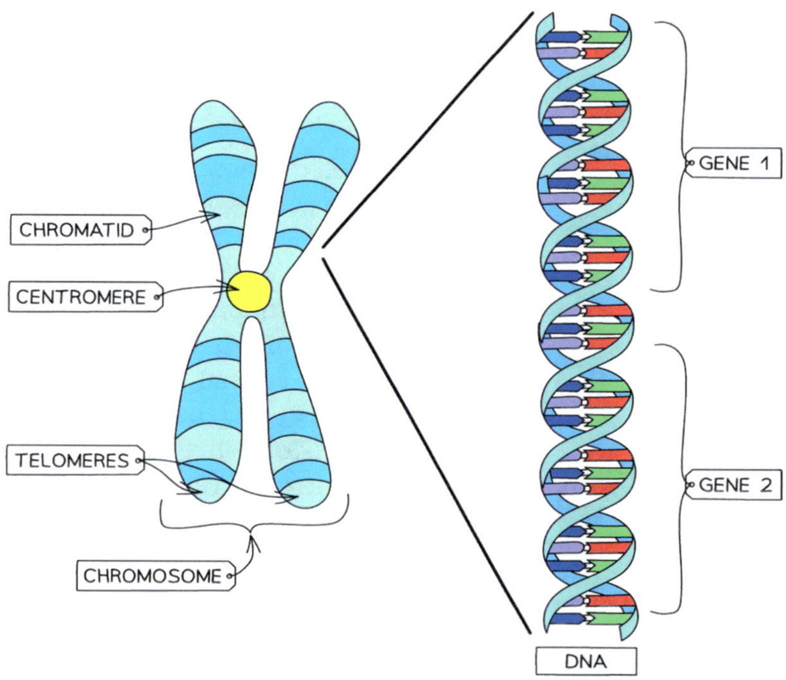

Figure 10.3. Chromosome structure.

Source: https://external-content.duckduckgo.com/iu/?u=https%3A%2F%2Fcdn.savemyexams.com%2Fcdn-cgi%2Fimage%2Fw%3D1920%2Cf%3Dauto%2Fuploads%2F2021%2F01%2FStructure-of-chromosome.png&f=1&nofb=1&ipt=5a01e0b9b2e4ee99fe3e7ac48344810f6eafca870fe96a4078ad1f0a3ddb7c45.

This chromatin isn't merely a storage box—it gets involved in reading, copying, and even repairing our genetic script. As cells prepare to divide, chromatin shrinks into clumps that we recognize as visible chromosomes, making sure every new cell inherits the same set of instructions. The innovative design of these chromosomes lets cells not only copy their genetic blueprint reliably but also split sister chromatids perfectly, which is vital for healthy cell growth. Examining prokaryotic organisms reveals that things work a little differently, yet they often manage to be as efficient. Generally speaking, these simpler cells usually have one circular chromosome, hosted in a region called the nucleoid. Even with this straightforward setup, a range of proteins are involved in making sure the DNA gets duplicated and appropriately divided. For instance, proteins like ParA and ParB play a key role—they help position and even pull chromosomes apart, ensuring the genetic material is split correctly. This flexible arrangement in prokaryotes highlights the basic principles of heredity and cellular function, demonstrating that whether the cell is simple or complex, the core ideas remain remarkably consistent. When it comes time for chromosomes to get ready for division, keeping sister chromatids together is essential. Proteins known as cohesins wrap around the DNA like belts, holding the sister copies together until the right moment. Then, during the transition from metaphase to anaphase, these cohesin bonds break down in a highly coordinated manner, allowing the copies to separate evenly. If this step doesn't work correctly, it might lead to aneuploidy—a condition that's often seen in cancer cases. In most cases, exploring how chromosome structure, cohesion, and overall genomic stability interact isn't just an academic exercise; it might open the door to new cancer treatments targeting these genetic missteps (Pati, 2024) (Figure 10.3).

10.1.1. Composition of DNA and Proteins

DNA and proteins team up in ways that are both surprising and essential to how genes are expressed and how cells function. DNA, built from nucleotides, is akin to a natural storage system for hereditary information that shapes everything from development to appearance. Every nucleotide comes with a sugar, a phosphate chunk, and one of several nitrogen bases—it's the way these pieces line up that sets the instructions for a cell's behavior. On the other hand, proteins—essentially chains of amino acids—perform a wide array of tasks crucial for life, in most cases doing a remarkably effective job. The basic structure of these proteins kicks off when ribosomes transform mRNA (which, by the way, is copied from DNA) into a specific amino acid sequence. Generally speaking, this translation process is tightly controlled, affecting how cells grow, split, and even change over time. So, gaining a good understanding of what makes up DNA and proteins turns out to be key for understanding how chromosomes carry genetic information during both mitosis and meiosis. DNA's bond with proteins takes on another role when it comes to shaping chromatin, especially as cells prepare to divide. When DNA wraps around histone proteins, it forms a compact coil that fits neatly into the nucleus; this tight packing not only preserves the genetic material but also plays a role in determining which genes are turned on or off. Protein complexes sometimes step in to remodel chromatin in ways that can either activate or silence genes based on what the cell needs at the moment. This kind of flexible response is super vital throughout the various stages of cell division—ensuring that gene copies are made correctly and passed along fairly to the new cells. Further research reveals that minor adjustments, such as methylation and acetylation, can alter the accessibility of DNA—underscoring the intricate and nuanced nature of this biological process. Beyond holding the structure together, proteins that stick with DNA also handle repair and replication duties. For instance, enzymes like DNA polymerases are vital for synthesizing a new DNA strand during replication, while others—ligases—help join the Okazaki fragments on the lagging strand. These partnerships are especially significant during cell division, as maintaining error-free DNA replication is crucial to prevent mutations that can lead to diseases such as cancer. Additionally, repair proteins play a significant role in maintaining genomic stability by correcting mistakes that occur during replication or due to environmental damage. The way DNA's makeup and protein activity mesh together not only ensures that genetic information is reliably passed on but also maintains the overall health of the organism. In short, delving into the details of DNA and proteins is absolutely central to understanding chromosomes and how cell division works, highlighting their core role in the ongoing, complex process of life (Figure 10.4).

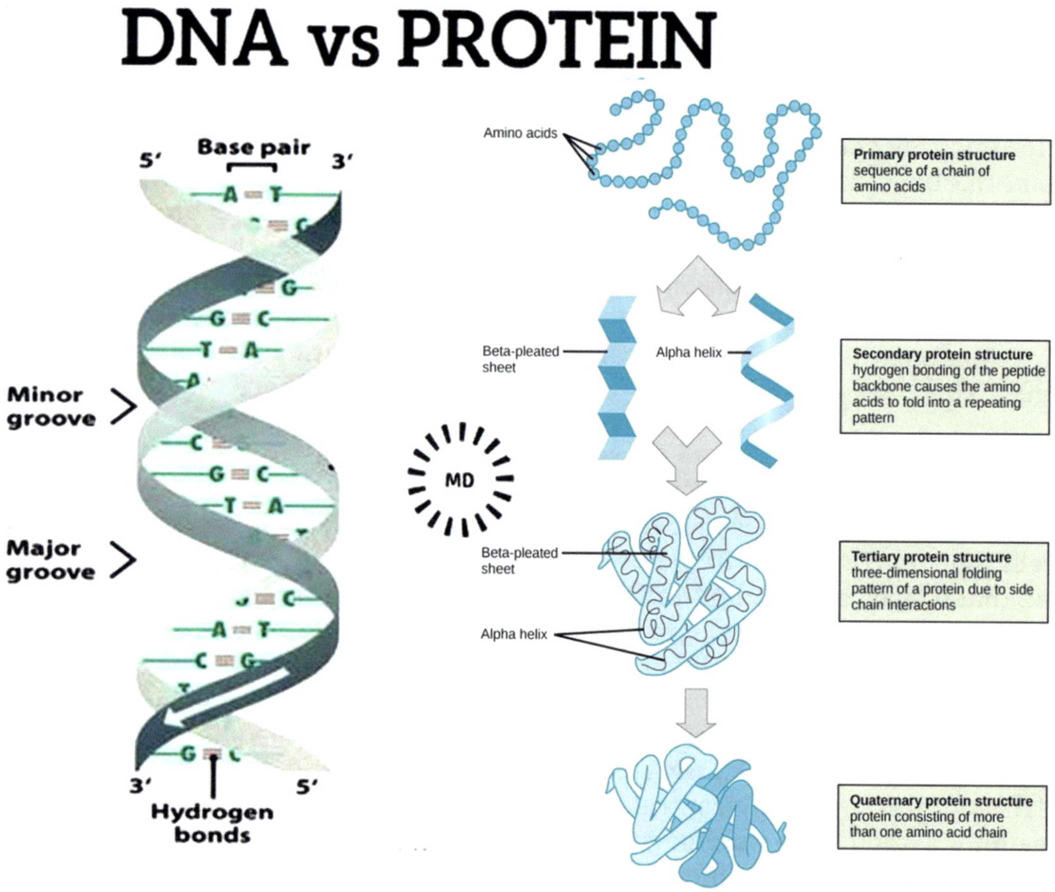

Figure 10.4. Composition of DNA and proteins.

Source: https://blogger.googleusercontent.com/img/b/R29vZ2xl/AVvXsEj2Hile2B7S2igo6PmoyYwmMhrroa-oo_F1H12dPvQMu4gE9oWeMxrXXkZgZ3qcY M7tPw8J3hZSEJlgZLmJVN2JrJQmbx03x2KzIUPSJ3KWmsibtrf HJXyQezFiLnwPwf9PVoUJl2WVEqMI/s1600/DNA+vs+Protein.png.

10.1.2. Chromatin Versus Chromosome

Cells manage their genetic material in a way that's pretty crucial to how they work and divide. Chromatin, which is essentially a combination of DNA and proteins, is responsible for organizing all that information compactly. There are two kinds here—euchromatin and heterochromatin. Generally speaking, euchromatin is not tightly wound, making it easier for genes to be read and used, while heterochromatin is packed closely together, providing both structure and a means to regulate gene activity. This variation in the way chromatin is organized matters a lot because it affects how accessible the DNA is for processes like replication, repair, and, by extension, the cell's overall health when it divides. When a cell is preparing to divide, changes begin to occur. The structure of chromatin undergoes significant changes, ultimately forming the structures we call chromosomes. In most cases, each chromosome is a condensed version of the original chromatin, and it's made up of two sister chromatids connected at the centromere. This compacting process is crucial because it ensures that genetic material is shared evenly between daughter cells, whether during mitosis or meiosis. Sometimes—if issues arise from things like heavy metals, say chromium or cadmium—the transformation can go awry, leading to genomic instability that might even trigger cancer. Knowing the subtle nuances between chromatin and chromosomes is crucial for understanding how cells maintain their genetic integrity. Beyond just the packing and repacking business, both chromatin and chromosomes play a role in how cells respond to environmental stress. Take oxidative stress as an example; it can disrupt the chromatin layout and, in doing so, affect genes involved in survival and repair. There are shifts in the cell's surroundings—like what happens during wound healing—that are linked to changes in chromatin. There's a kind of natural redundancy here; the way chromatin adapts is always tied back to overall cell function. New single-cell analysis methods are even starting to uncover the diverse ways chromatin behaves in healthy versus diseased states. These insights, in most cases, help us gain a better understanding of cell division mechanisms and their impact on human health and disease (Mélanie Rodrigues et al., 2018; Balali et al., 2021) (Figure 10.5).

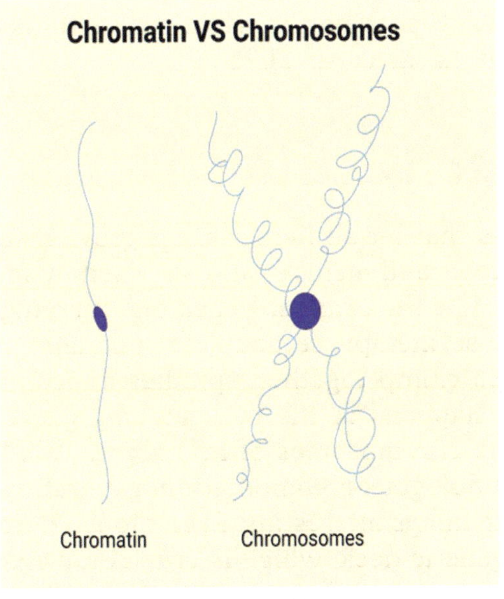

Figure 10.5. Chromatin versus chromosome.

Source: https://knyamed.com/cdn/shop/articles/Chromatin-VS-Chromosomes.jpg?v=1706099120.

10.1.3. Karyotype and Chromosome Organization

Chromosome organization and karyotype form a complex, almost intertwined relationship that helps us understand what's happening when cells divide. Eukaryotic genomes, for instance, differ wildly in both size and the number of chromosomes they carry, and these differences shape their overall layout in interesting ways. A study using fused karyotypes in budding yeast even hinted that when chromosomes come in matching sizes, they tend to stretch out and cover more of the nuclear space. Hi-C mapping picked up these three-dimensional shifts when centromeres and telomeres were switched off—showing, in most cases, that chromosomes aren't just static blocks but play a part in replication timing and genome stability. This all points to the need for a solid chromosomal arrangement during cell division (Lazar et al., 2022). A significant piece of this puzzle is heterochromatin. It's found mostly around pericentromeric and telomeric regions and turns out to be key for maintaining genome stability. Loaded with repetitive sequences, heterochromatin practically demands its special way of being compartmentalized and silenced so that things don't fall apart. Its dynamic behavior is especially noticeable during critical moments like mitosis and DNA repair. Even a slight slip in maintaining this balance can lead to errors in chromosome segregation or cause replication stress, which may ripple into genetic instability and even contribute to aging and tumor formation (Janssen et al., 2018). The influence of karyotype and chromosome layout extends beyond forming a physical structure—it also profoundly affects how cells function. Throughout the cell cycle, the positioning and interactions of chromosomes within the nucleus change in somewhat unpredictable ways. For example, during anaphase, the reorganization of chromatin seems to ensure that vital components like rDNA contacts and centromeres wind up exactly where they belong. Should these spatial dynamics become disrupted, it might compromise replication timing and overall cell viability. Generally speaking, exploring how karyotypes and chromosome arrangements function provides insights into key cellular events, linking these physical structures to both normal cellular functions and the origins of pathological conditions (Janssen et al., 2018; Lazar et al., 2022).

10.2. Types of Cell Division

Cells split and multiply in ways that let all living things grow, heal, and keep going. Most people discuss two main methods: mitosis and meiosis. Mitosis, used by most body cells, creates two new cells that end up almost exactly like the original – each one carrying the same set of chromosomes. It goes through steps like prophase, metaphase, anaphase, and telophase, with each stage performing its specific tasks (chromosomes clump together, spindles appear, etc.). Meiosis, by contrast, is a more specialized process that happens in the cells making gametes—sperm and eggs—so that each new cell gets only half the chromosomes of its parent. This halving, combined with a form of genetic shuffling through homologous recombination, generally adds variety to the mix, fueling sexual reproduction and keeping things interesting. Even though mitosis is mostly about maintaining stability, meiosis shuffles the genetic deck, which is crucial for evolution and adaptation. In most cases, meiosis happens in two rounds—meiosis I and then meiosis II. In the first round, homologous chromosomes pair up and exchange segments of genetic code, a process that increases the odds for diverse alleles in the gametes. Then, the second round resembles mitosis, splitting the sister chromatids into separate cells. This entire balancing act is typically maintained under tight control by molecules such as cyclin-dependent kinases (Cdks) and their partners, cyclins, which help guide the cell cycle. Recent studies—even though they're sometimes a bit tentative—have pointed out the role of proteins such as ASY1 in lining up chromosomes, adding yet another layer to the already complex world of cell division (Yang et al., 2019). Apart from mitosis and meiosis, there are other ways cells divide. For example, binary fission, seen in bacteria and other single-celled creatures, involves a cell copying its genetic material and then splitting roughly into two equal halves. This more straightforward method can allow populations to grow very rapidly when conditions are just right, sidestepping the more complex routines of mitosis or meiosis. Other strategies, such as budding and fragmentation, also emerge in various organisms, each adapted to its life cycle and environmental demands. All these varied routes provide life forms with different tools for maintaining genetic stability and adapting to change, offering us crucial insights into evolution and adaptability across the board (Kamil et al., 2016) (Figure 10.6).

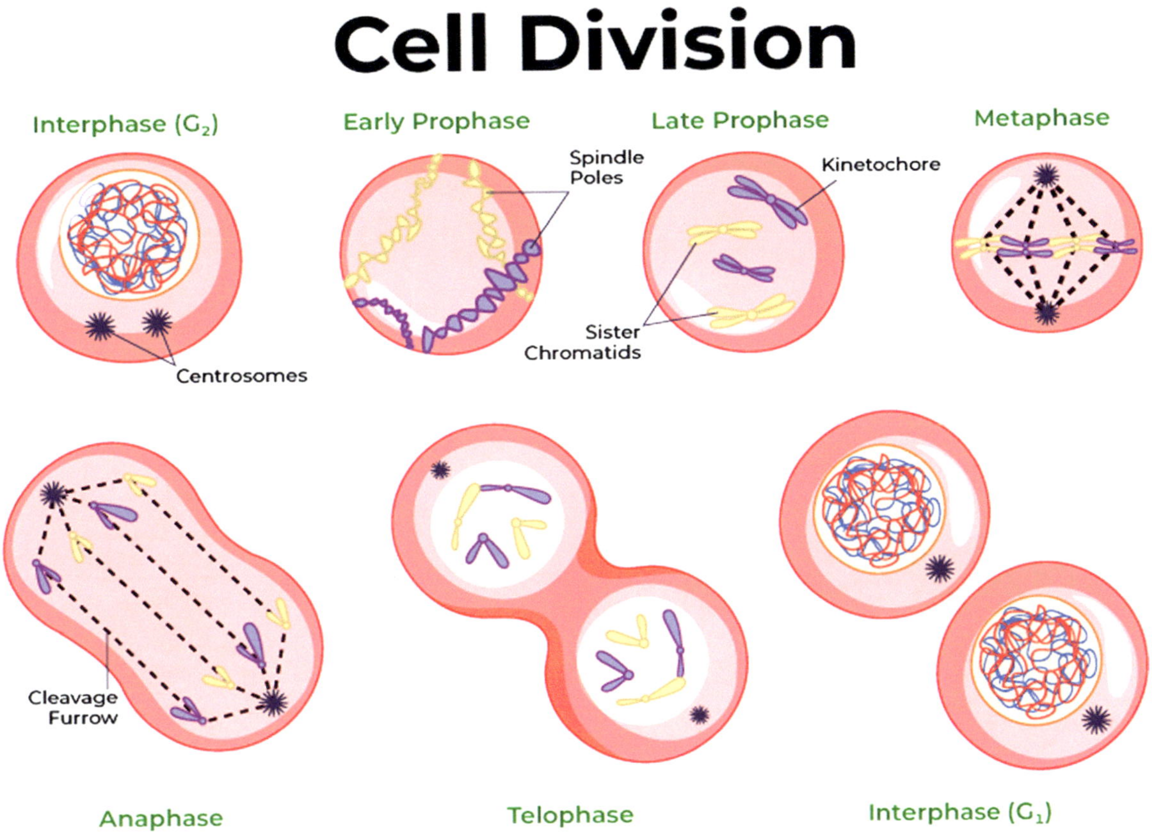

Figure 10.6. Types of cell division.

Source: https://media.geeksforgeeks.org/wp-content/uploads/20230320155637/Cell-Division.png.

10.2.1. Mitosis: Definition and Purpose

Mitosis is the unsung mechanism behind cell splitting—it's the way a cell divides and passes along its genetic blueprint. One cell, in a surprisingly dynamic moment, splits into two with nearly identical sets of genes, fueling everything from growth to everyday repairs. Chromosomes take center stage here; when they bundle up into distinct shapes, it helps ensure nothing gets lost in the shuffle. Even a tiny misstep during this wrangling phase can trigger major issues like aneuploidy or sometimes even cancer, which shows just how crucial this process is for keeping our genetic code stable. Cells wander through several steps as they divide, almost like they're following a set of loosely ordered instructions. In prophase, for example, the messy chromatin bundles into what we recognize as chromosomes, while spindle fibers—those tiny rope-like structures—start stretching out from the centrosomes.

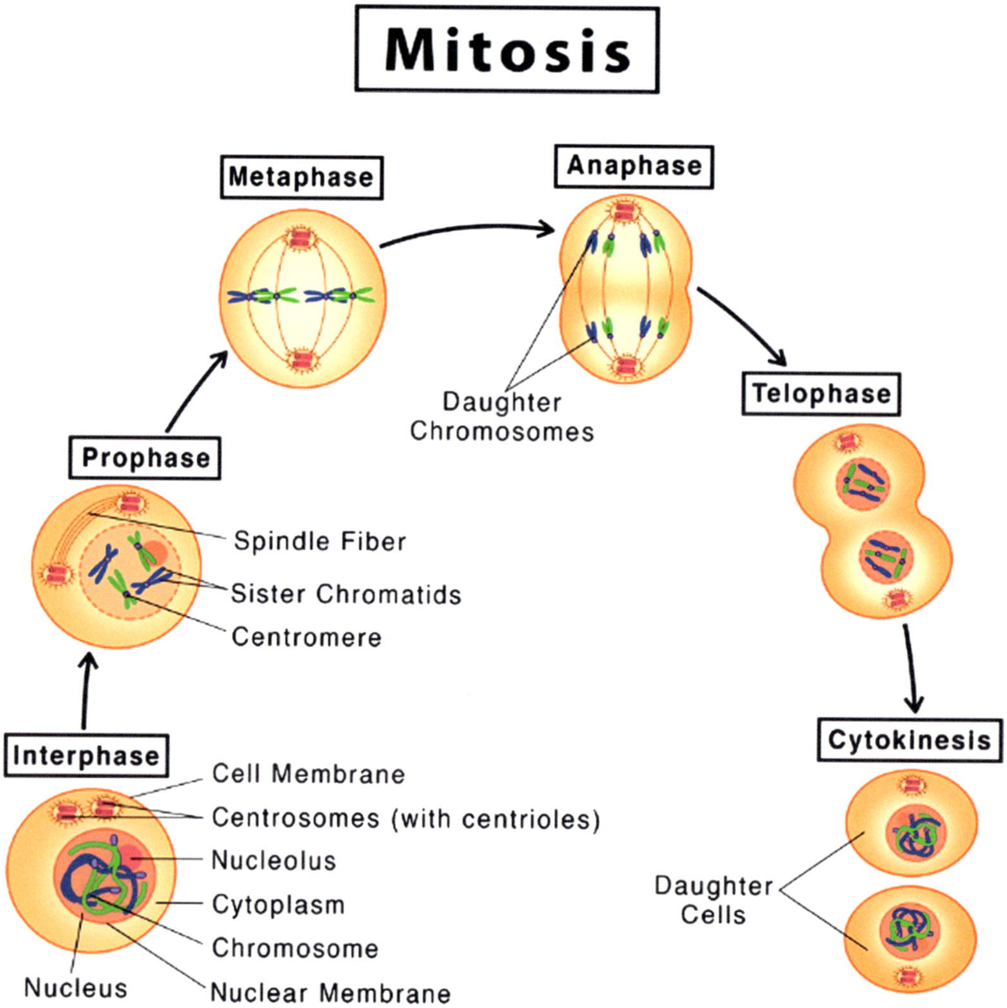

Figure 10.7. Mitosis.

Source: https://www.sciencefacts.net/wp-content/uploads/2020/08/Mitosis-Phases-Diagram.jpg.

Then, in metaphase, the chromosomes line up in a row that seems almost too neat, each waiting for its turn. Soon after, anaphase takes over as the two copies are pulled apart, and telophase concludes with new membranes forming around the separate groups. A series of subtle signals nudges everything into place along the way, ensuring that every bit of genetic material finds its proper home. The impact of mitosis extends far beyond simple cell multiplication. It's the quiet workhorse behind wound healing, stepping in to repair tissue when damage occurs, and in some single-celled organisms, it even serves as their way of reproducing under the right conditions. On a less promising note, if things go off course during mitosis, errors can eventually lead to tumor formation. Generally speaking, understanding these cellular steps is not only key to grasping the basics of biology, but it also helps shape medical approaches to diseases that arise when cell division goes awry. All these layers, from the behavior of chromosomes to the overall choreography of the cell, remind us why mitosis remains a central pillar in both biology and medical research (Galluzzi et al., 2018; Sina et al., 2018) (Figure 10.7).

10.2.2. Meiosis: Definition and Purpose

Meiosis initiates a multitude of vital processes in numerous living organisms—from animals to plants and even fungi. It reduces the chromosome count in half to produce haploid gametes (such as eggs and sperm) that ultimately shuffle genetic traits. In early stages, such as prophase I, chromosomes exchange small bits of information—a crossover here, an independent assortment there—which generally results in a mix of genes. This mix isn't just for show; it fuels natural selection, letting populations adapt when the environment changes. , delving into how meiosis works reveals why evolution continues to progress, even if a few errors in the process sometimes lead to genetic disorders.

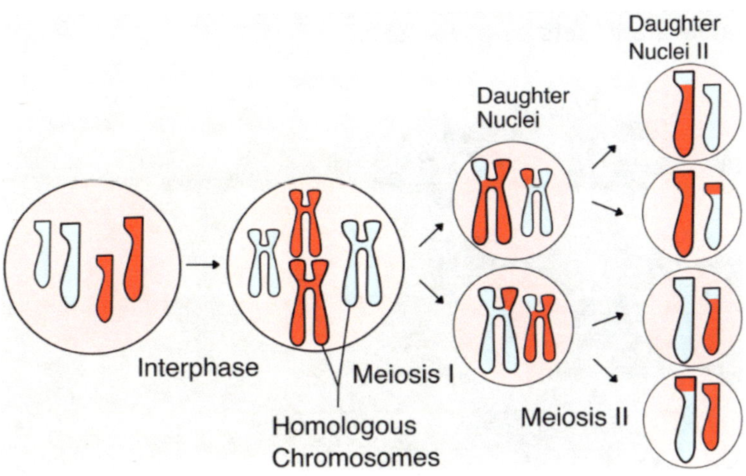

Figure 10.8. Meiosis.

Source: https://upload.wikimedia.org/wikipedia/commons/thumb/9/96/Meiosis_Overview_new.svg/1200px-Meiosis_Overview_new.svg.png.

At the same time, meiosis isn't solely about mixing up genetic ingredients for reproduction—it also stands as a bedrock for keeping our genome stable. Each move during meiosis is pretty critical: during metaphase I, for instance, homologous chromosomes line up along the cell's middle, ensuring that every gamete gets its fair share of chromosomes. If this lineup gets a bit off-kilter, errors like aneuploidy can occur (conditions where cells have the wrong chromosome number, as in Down syndrome). Even if the system isn't always flawless, the delicate balance between preserving order and fostering diversity emphasizes how essential meiosis is to cellular integrity and overall development. The tangled, intriguing aspects of meiosis and its repercussions on genome evolution have become much more apparent to us thanks to more recent discoveries in genomics and molecular biology. Some studies, for example, have taken a close look at transposable elements (TEs) (Bourque et al., 2018)—those mobile pieces of DNA that, in many cases, can tweak recombination and mutation rates in surprising ways. This fresh look helps us see how genetic material gets reworked generation after generation, subtly shifting evolutionary paths. Genomic insights have even nudged us toward a more refined classification of eukaryotes by revealing how environmental factors and genetic diversity interact (Sina et al., 2018). As researchers peel back more layers, these findings not only point to new ways of tackling genetic diseases but also underscore the inherent, fundamental role of meiosis in life's grand blueprint (Figure 10.8).

10.2.3. Comparison Between Mitosis and Meiosis

Cell division—whether it happens through mitosis or meiosis—is a core part of life that keeps things running. Mitosis splits regular body cells into two clones that carry the same set of chromosomes as the original cell. This neat process is crucial for repairing tissues and maintaining overall balance. Then there's meiosis, which kicks in for reproductive cells. It takes one diploid cell and, in a two-step dance, produces four haploid cells that each carry a unique mix of genetic material. In most cases, this drop in chromosome count, along with the shuffling brought about by independent assortment and crossing over, helps maintain stability while still stirring up genetic diversity. Both mitosis and meiosis have their sets of processes.

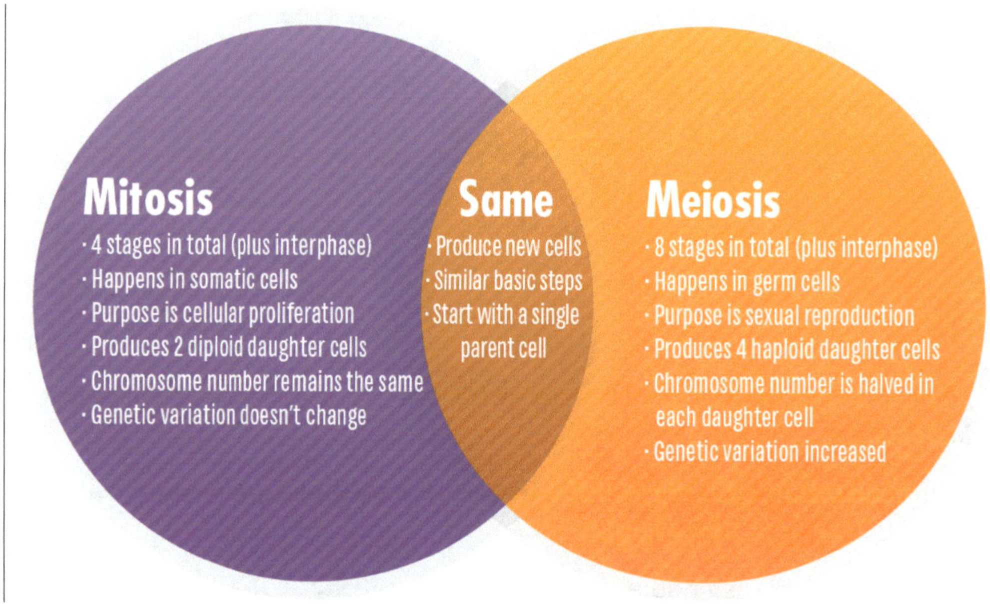

Figure 10.9. Comparison between mitosis and meiosis.

Source: https://cdn.technologynetworks.com/tn/images/body/venndiagram-v41543416662799.png.

Mitosis proceeds through its familiar stages—prophase, metaphase, anaphase, and telophase—ensuring that every new cell ends up with an identical set of chromosomes. Meanwhile, a safeguard like the p53–DREAM pathway remains vigilant to monitor events throughout all the steps from

DNA synthesis to cytokinesis (Engeland, 2017). Meiosis is a more complex process, involving two distinct phases. In the first phase, homologous chromosomes pair up and then split apart. The second round plays out much like mitosis, separating the sister chromatids. This combination, generally speaking, is the engine behind the unique genetic mixes that fuel evolution. It all comes down to keeping things on track, although the process isn't always flawless. When errors creep into mitosis, they can lead to aneuploidy or other chromosomal mix-ups that raise the risk of cancer and various diseases. Pathways controlled by p53, for example, work to correct these errors, which is crucial for maintaining the genome integrity (John et al., 2017). Similarly, when errors occur during meiosis—for instance, during homologous recombination—the resulting gametes might end up with the wrong number of chromosomes, potentially setting the stage for conditions such as Down syndrome. The careful yet sometimes unpredictable choreography of mitosis and meiosis not only keeps our bodies maintained but also drives the variation and adaptability that underpin evolution (Figure 10.9).

10.3. The Cell Cycle

Cells perform delicate work that enables living things to grow, repair, and maintain their tissues. Deep inside each cell is a process known simply as the cell cycle—a series of surprising stages where a cell copies itself and its genetic blueprint. Instead of following a strict order, the cycle splits into two broad parts. First comes interphase, which we typically break down into G1, S, and G2 phases. In this phase, the cell is busy growing, duplicating chromosomes, and reorganizing vital organelles so that when division occurs, each new cell ends up with everything it needs. Understanding this setup is key since it paves the way for what follows, and as Bhattacharya et al. (2024) point out, the way these changes happen shows how each little twist ensures DNA stays right.

Then, things shift into what we often call the mitotic phase, where the cell embarks on a series of steps that eventually culminate in cytokinesis—the final division into two daughter cells. Mitosis is a process that, generally speaking, leaves no room for error; each new cell gets an identical set of chromosomes, thanks in part to a host of proteins that manage these transitions. As Bhattacharya et al. (2024) notes, important cell-body parts—like the nuclear envelope and even the endoplasmic reticulum—are broken down and rebuilt during this time. At the same time, a rearrangement of the cell's internal framework, the cytoskeleton, helps position chromosomes in just the right spots. If any step stumbles, it can throw off the whole process, showing that every small detail counts in keeping the division on track. Lastly, the role of telomeres is significant in the whole process. These tiny, protective caps at the ends of chromosomes act like shields to prevent the genetic material from wearing down as cells repeat the process. With each division, telomeres shorten a bit, influencing how cells age and function. This gradual change ties back into the overall dynamics of the cell cycle, and studies on telomere length (TL) across different species have shown that both environmental conditions and genetic factors can play a part () in these shifts. In most cases, examining how telomeres behave provides a comprehensive view of the connection between cellular longevity and well-being, highlighting the intricate interplay among our genes, our environment, and the inner workings of our cells (Figure 10.10).

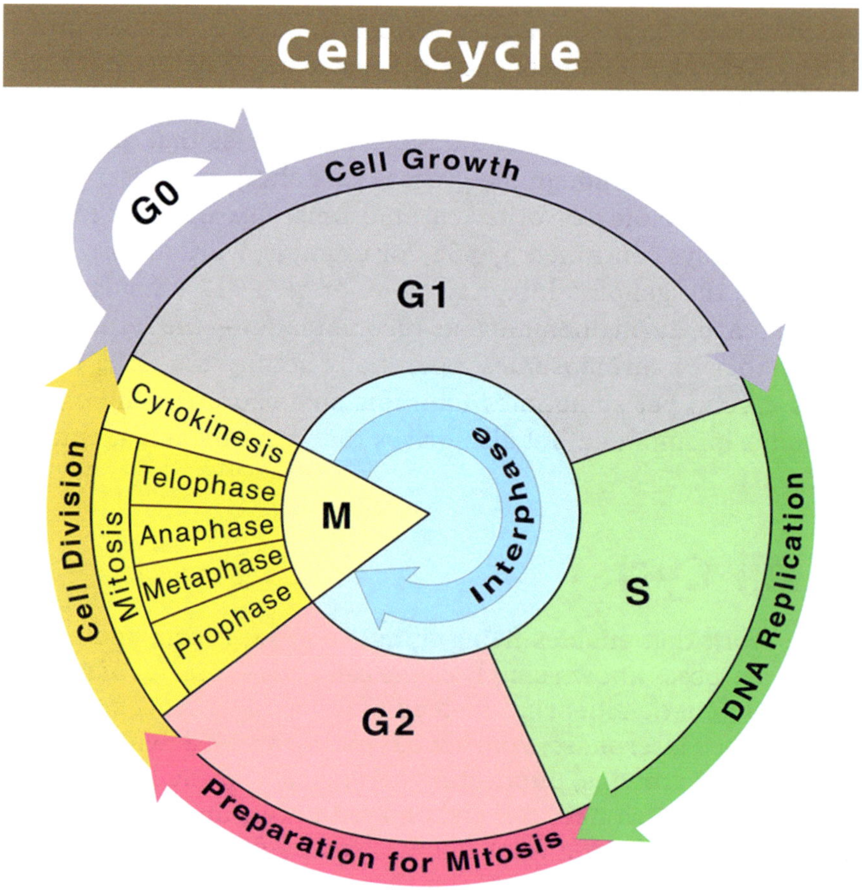

Figure 10.10. The cell cycle.

Source: https://www.sciencefacts.net/wp-content/uploads/2020/11/Cell-Cycle-Diagram.jpg.

10.3.1. Phases of the Cell Cycle

Cell division is a bit like a well-rehearsed, if unpredictable, dance that shapes both individual cell function and the growth of an entire organism. Most of the time, we break it down into four parts—G1 (Gap 1), S (Synthesis), G2 (Gap 2) and M (Mitosis)—even though in practice these steps can feel more fluid than a neat checklist. In G1, a cell grows larger and begins producing the proteins necessary to replicate its DNA, which then sets the stage for the S phase. There, chromosomes are replicated, so each one ends up with two sister copies—an essential step for maintaining the genetic blueprint intact. And, generally speaking, a series of checkpoints quietly assesses that everything's on track, stopping progress if there's even a hint of trouble. Next up is the G2 phase, where cells prepare for the ultimate showdown of division. During this phase, cells not only stockpile the proteins required to separate their chromosomes, they also perform a kind of last-minute DNA quality check. If any errors or damage from earlier replication are detected, the cycle can be paused long enough for repair crews to intervene—crucial for ensuring that the genetic information remains reliable for future generations. It's interesting to note that, under conditions where nutrients and energy are in short supply, some cells with extra chromosome sets seem to behave more aggressively, hinting at a link between cellular energy states and cycle progression (Andor et al., 2019). Then comes the M phase, where everything is organized and split apart in a carefully coordinated sequence. It all starts with prophase, when the formerly loose chromatin condenses into clear, distinct chromosomes. Almost imperceptibly, the scene shifts in metaphase as these chromosomes line up across the cell's middle. Next, during anaphase, spindle fibers help yank the sister chromatids toward opposite ends of the cell. Finally, in telophase, new nuclear membranes form around the separated groups, setting the stage for cytokinesis—the final divider of the cell's physical contents into two nearly identical daughter cells. Every step here is critical; missing a beat can lead to conditions like aneuploidy, which has been connected with various cancers and genetic disorders. Gaining insight into these phases provides a better understanding of how cell division unfolds and what can go wrong when the process isn't precise (Olsson-Strömberg et al., 2006) (Figure 10.11).

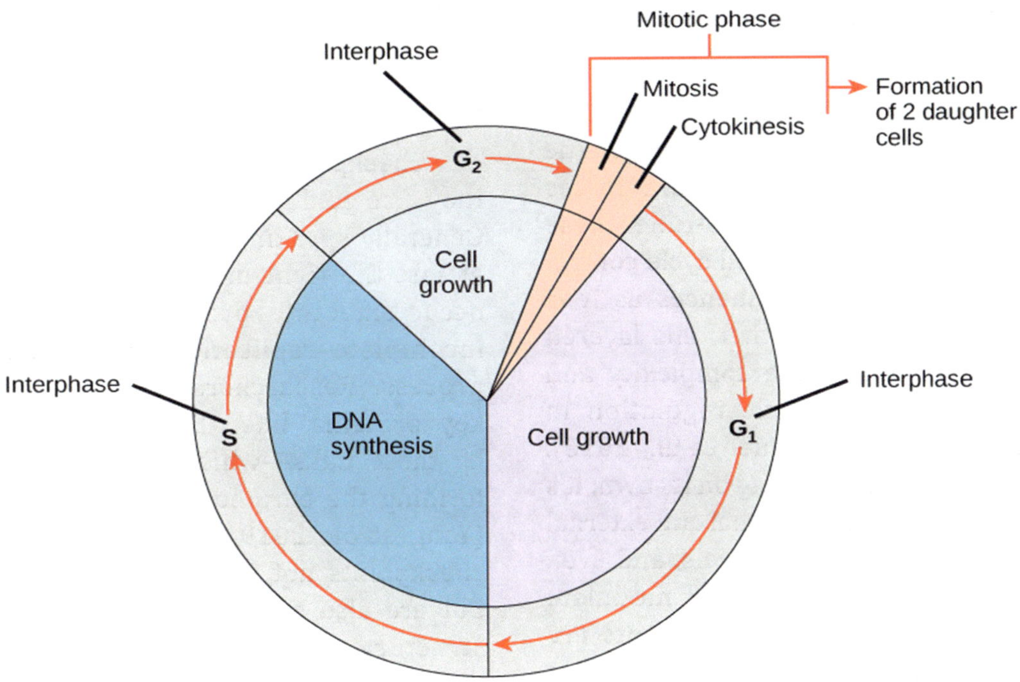

Figure 10.11. Phases of the cell cycle.

Source: https://cdn.kastatic.org/ka-perseus-images/6afac0fce62ec8a30c86f3e02c457224339bb697.png.

10.3.2. Regulation of the Cell Cycle

Maintaining proper cell division depends on an unexpectedly intricate dance of cellular processes. Checkpoints appear during the cycle, ensuring cells only move forward when conditions are just right. Proteins such as cyclins and CDKs are the key players here – they essentially drive the transition from one phase to the next. Their precise location and amount are crucial; if things go wrong, it can lead to runaway cell growth, which, in most cases, sets the stage for cancer. Understanding exactly how these proteins shift over time and space expands our view of cell operations, and it can even help in crafting targeted treatments. Research efforts, such as those behind the Cell Atlas (Thul et al., 2017), underscore the importance of mapping protein interactions for a more comprehensive understanding of cell biology. Cells don't move through division in a predictable, step-by-step fashion; instead, each phase—G1, S, G2, and M—carries its set of checks. For instance, the G1 checkpoint typically reviews cell size and DNA quality before replication starts in S phase. If any DNA damage occurs, the whole process pauses briefly, allowing repair systems to intervene and correct the issue, preventing mistakes from being passed on.

Clearly, these checkpoints do more than manage division - they safeguard our genetic blueprint. External signals, too, join forces with internal regulators to fine-tune these transitions, reminding us that cell cycle control is as much about outside influences as it is about internal checks. Altogether, this layered control system highlights the complexity and criticality of proper cell-cycle regulation in keeping diseases at bay (Daniel et al., 2016). Cell cycle regulation isn't running on its own; it's constantly juggling a mix of internal and external cues. Growth factors, nutrient levels, and even cellular stress responses all help modulate the process. Sometimes, when nutrients are plentiful, metabolic pathways adjust to fine-tune cyclin-CDK activity, which can alter the timing of cell division. And don't forget autophagy—a recycling process that makes sure damaged bits don't end up in new cells. Research on autophagy and its role in cell-cycle management highlights the intricate interconnection of these pathways. By unraveling these complex relationships, scientists hope to uncover innovative new strategies for tackling disorders that arise when cell division loses its tight control (Daniel et al., 2016; Thul et al., 2017).

10.3.3. Importance of Checkpoints

Cell division isn't just a neat, step-by-step routine; it can be a rather cumbersome affair that relies on a number of checkpoints staying in sync to keep chromosomes behaving correctly. In most cases, different mechanisms emerge unexpectedly to catch mistakes before they develop into full-blown aneuploidy. For example, consider the spindle assembly checkpoint (SAC) —it monitors how chromosomes attach to spindle fibers and holds back anaphase until every kinetochore is properly in place. This entire mix-up of checkpoint proteins working side by side effectively demonstrates how cells maintain their genomic integrity, a process reflected across different species (Yang et al., 2019).

Checkpoints do more than just fix errors; they also guide the cell cycle along its pathway. Generally speaking, CDKs need to be activated at just the right moments so that transitions occur smoothly, preventing DNA damage or incomplete replication from disrupting the process. Researchers have even noted that key proteins, like ASY1, get phosphorylated by these Cdks—which in turn contributes to forming the chromosome axis during meiosis (Yang et al., 2019). These clues suggest that checkpoints not only serve as quality control but are also actively engaged in steering the structural events necessary for proper cell division, inherently balancing both stability and forward momentum. Ignoring such checkpoints can have serious consequences. When the usual chromosomal regulations go off track, aneuploid cells can begin to appear—cells that are either too heavy or too light in genetic information, often associated with cancers or developmental abnormalities. Sometimes, when chromosome checks fail, even gametes end up imbalanced, which can hurt both reproductive outcomes and fetal health (Marchetti et al., 2010). Overall, these checkpoints serve as our cellular safety nets, guarding against the misdistribution of genetic material while also subtly regulating the pace of developmental processes—a dual role that makes them indispensable in biology (Figure 10.12).

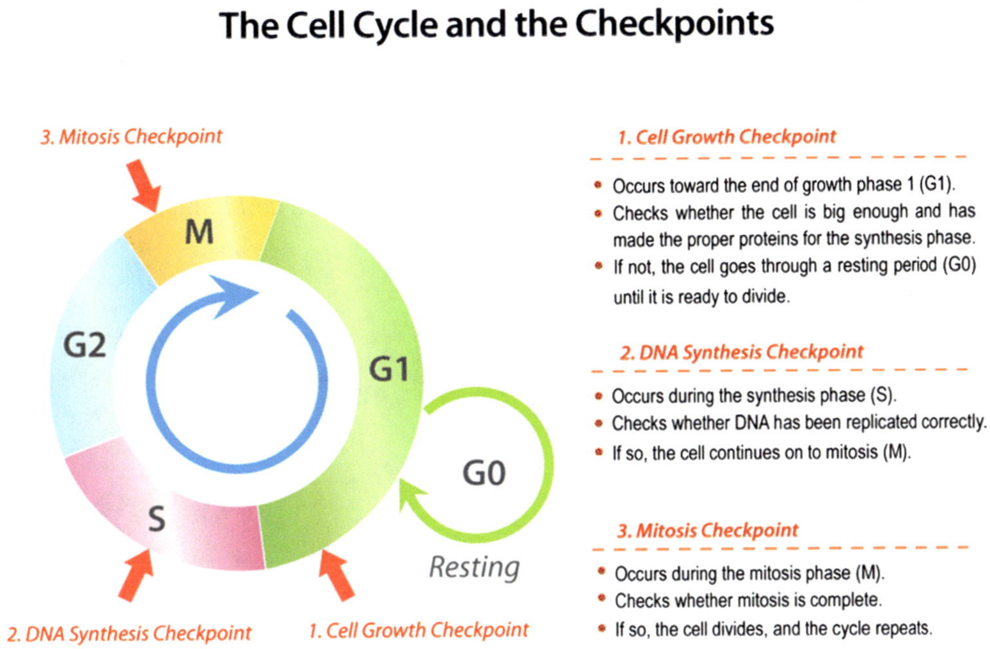

Figure 10.12. Cell cycle checkpoints.

Source: https://assets.coursehero.com/study-guides/lumen/images/wmopen-nmbiology1/cell-cycle-checkpoints/CellCycleCheckpoints1.png.

10.4. Mitosis in Detail

Cell division relies on mitosis to accurately pass on our genetic blueprint, and it all starts when duplicated chromosomes—or chromatids, for short—gather near the middle of the cell. At that point, the spindle apparatus helps them line up just right, but if things go wrong, it may result in aneuploidy, which significantly disrupts cell function. Super-resolution microscopy and other advanced imaging tools have given us new ways to see these processes in action, letting researchers catch not only the spindle's part in the show but also some odd behaviors from the chromosomes during different stages of division. These methods have revealed unusual changes, such as lagging or mis-segregated chromosomes, which can significantly impair cell viability, as recent studies have noted (Garg et al., 2024). Digging a bit deeper, there's a whole set of regulatory systems that make sure chromosomes segregate correctly – it's not random at all. A significant part of this control stems from the condition of the chromatin, the material that holds our DNA together. Cell checkpoints closely monitor whether chromosomes attach to spindle fibers properly, and if anything appears amiss, the process is halted until the issue is resolved. For example, treatments like paclitaxel can upset the normal microtubule dynamics, causing unusual chromosomal behavior. Research generally shows that when the spindle's function is interfered with, it can trigger significant changes in chromatin structure—often condensing it too much—and this can even lead to cell death. All of these observations underscore the complexity of mitosis and highlight the importance of chromatin interactions in maintaining genomic stability (Garg et al., 2024). Then there's the early phase of embryonic development, which highlights just how finely tuned the timing of mitosis must be. Even the brief intervals between key moments—say, the fading of the pronucleus and that very first cell split—appear to set the stage for later developmental competence. Studies suggest that when these gaps persist for too long, errors such as unequal cleavage can occur, impairing the chromosomal setup of the developing embryo. Even minor delays in the mitotic process appear capable of disrupting the delicate balance necessary for proper chromosome separation, often resulting in significant developmental consequences. Recognizing these small yet impactful timing changes provides valuable insights into both normal and abnormal cell behaviors, as recent research has revealed (Garg et al., 2024) (Figure 10.13).

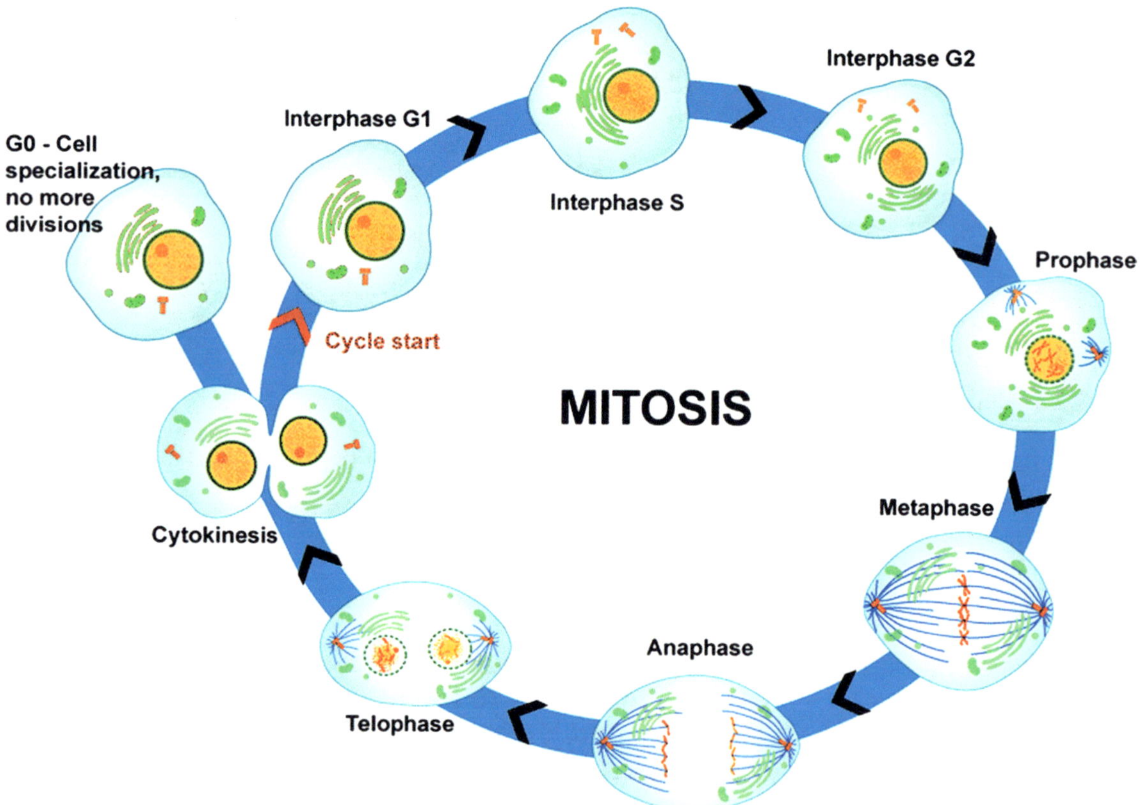

Figure 10.13. Mitosis in detail.

Source: https://bio.libretexts.org/@api/deki/files/18986/f-d%253A2611548d82f15409dfa0558a89cb81ae4ac2f4853857993918f39514_IMAGE_TINY_IMAGE_TINY.1?revision=1.

10.4.1. Prophase: Key Events

Prophase marks the onset of a significant change within the cell. Chromatin, once a loose tangle, starts bunching up into distinct chromosomes that can be seen under a microscope. This clumping isn't just for show—it's key to keeping the genetic blueprint solid so that when the cell divides, each new cell gets the correct set of chromosomes. At this point, homologous chromosomes unexpectedly pair with one another, thanks to a process known as synapsis. Proteins that usually handle DNA repair and recombination kind of step in to help line up these pairs. As they do so, the chromosomes group together into tight clusters called tetrads, which ultimately become critical for exchanging segments of genetic material—an exchange often referred to as crossing over (Rachel et al., 2023). A striking step in prophase is the deliberate formation of double-strand breaks (DSBs) in the DNA. In most cases, these breaks set the stage for a recombination process essential to meiosis. The cell carefully regulates both the formation and repair of these breaks, so that crossovers between homologs occur precisely, spurring genetic variation. That said, if repairs go wrong, this may result in aneuploid gametes, which the cell wants to avoid. Proteins like CDK2 play a central, phosphorylation-driven role, with differential modifications at specific sites governing their activity throughout the phase. Early in prophase, there's an inhibitory phosphorylation of CDK2 at tyrosine 15—a checkpoint measure to keep the genome steady before the cell moves further into meiosis. One might even say it's like a carefully tuned orchestra, with each protein note adjusting to the shifting rhythm of chromosome dynamics (Rachel et al., 2023). As prophase progresses, multiple processes are simultaneously reaching their peak. Beyond the genetic shuffle happening from pairing and recombination, the cell begins laying down the framework for future chromosome movement by organizing microtubules. The spindle apparatus, which will eventually separate the chromosomes, starts to take shape as microtubules radiate from the centrosomes. This mix of structural changes and regulatory signals—especially those from kinase pathways—highlights the intricate interplay between processes during cell division. The ongoing phosphorylation of CDK2 marks a passage into later prophase stages, ushering in vital structural adjustments. All these interwoven, sometimes messy events come together to set the stage for a successful meiotic split, which is essential for producing viable gametes (Funda et al., 2021).

10.4.2. Metaphase: Chromosome Alignment

Cell division is cumbersome, but one key moment is the metaphase when chromosomes line up—a crucial step that helps each daughter cell pick up just the right mix of genetic material. It's the mitotic spindle—a web of microtubules—that gets things in order by latching onto tiny markers called kinetochores at the chromosomes' centromeres. These kinetochores don't just grab the spindle fibers; they also help build tension on each chromosome, keeping them stable and making sure they settle along the metaphase plate. If things go sideways and the alignment isn't spot on, chromosomes can end up misallocated, usually leading to aneuploidy, which in many cases is linked to diseases like cancer (Jolien et al., 2017). The entire process of lining up relies on a constant back-and-forth exchange between kinetochores and microtubules—attachments forming and breaking under precise control. As chromosomes settle into place, microtubules reach out from opposing spindle poles, handling the balance like a tightrope walker. This setup is under the watchful eye of the SAC, which keeps tabs on whether every kinetochore is snugly connected before giving the green light to move into anaphase. This safeguard minimizes errors in separation; if it fails, the fallout can be pretty severe (Polak et al., 2016). New research now suggests a more dynamic role for kinetochores than previously thought. These structures appear less like static anchors and more like active signaling hubs that adjust their behavior as mitosis progresses. Their signals help shift positions and fine-tune microtubule connections, ensuring a balanced pull on each chromosome. Specific proteins at the kinetochores, by the way, adjust themselves in response to shifting conditions, generally working to preserve genomic integrity. All in all, the intricate partnership between kinetochores and spindle microtubules remains fundamental for reliable cell division, laying the groundwork for healthy organismal development (Jolien et al., 2017) (Figure 10.14).

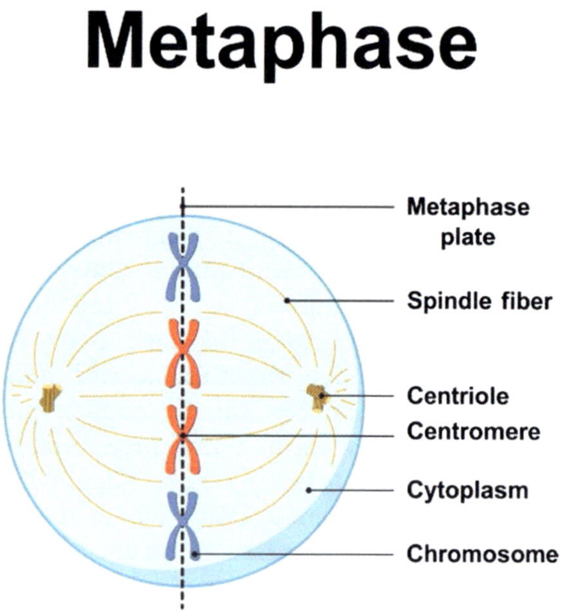

Figure 10.14. Metaphase: Chromosome alignment.

Source: https://nursehub.com/wp-content/uploads/2023/11/shutterstock_2125958618-1024x1024.jpg.

10.4.3. Anaphase and Telophase: Separation and Reformation

Cells divide in a somewhat unpredictable dance, where anaphase and telophase both jump in to keep chromosome numbers spot on. After chromosomes find their way to the middle stage (the metaphase plate), anaphase kicks off by snapping apart the bond between sister chromatids. Tiny spindle fibers, pushed along by motor proteins, tug the chromatids in opposite directions toward the cell's ends. This whole tugging act is crucial – if it slips up, aneuploidy can occur, which in most cases is linked to several cancers. Lately, some studies have suggested that lamina-associated domains (LADs) play a role in how chromosomes are arranged, indicating a complex interplay between chromosomal movement and the nucleus's layout (Tom van Schaik et al., 2020). Then, as the cell enters telophase, the now-separated chromatids, which have become individual chromosomes, begin to uncoil and regain their interphase structure. It's more than just a physical unwind; it's about readying the chromosomes for the next round, when genes need to fire up and the cell gets busy again. The reassembly of the nuclear lamina around these softening chromosomes helps rebuild a working nucleus, and at the same time, proteins that had hung on to chromatin during mitosis are tweaked and let go just at the right moment, allowing the nucleus form properly (Marie et al., 2015).

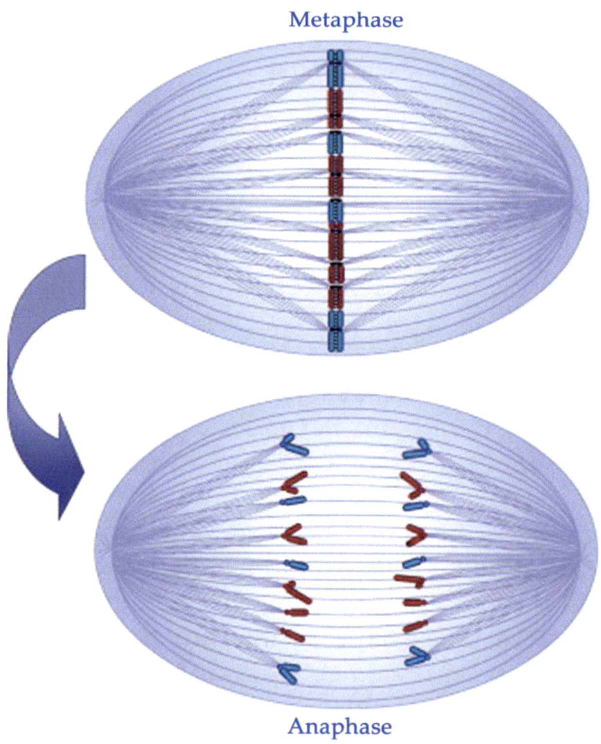

Figure 10.15. Anaphase and telophase.

Source: https://ars.els-cdn.com/content/image/3-s2.0-B9780080918655000060-f06-11-9780080918655.jpg.

Therefore, keeping chromatin and nuclear reorganization in sync proves to be absolutely crucial for genetic stability. We can see that the smooth run through anaphase and telophase underscores how intricate cell division is. Recent work into proteins such as DEK has shown—interestingly—that these molecules are essential for managing chromatin dynamics, and when they're off their game, trouble can brew. Mutations or abnormal levels of DEK may prevent chromatin from separating correctly, which in turn can disrupt chromosome segregation and result in daughter cells with genetic defects (Marie et al., 2015). In the broader context, examining the intricacies of anaphase and telophase extends beyond simple cell division; it provides insights into processes that may contribute to cancer, highlighting the crucial role of careful regulation throughout cell division (Figure 10.15).

10.5. Meiosis in Detail

Meiosis sits at the heart of biological reproduction, mixing up genetic material in ways that support diversity. Once germ cells finish an initial mitotic division, they jump into two rounds of division—commonly called meiosis I and meiosis II.

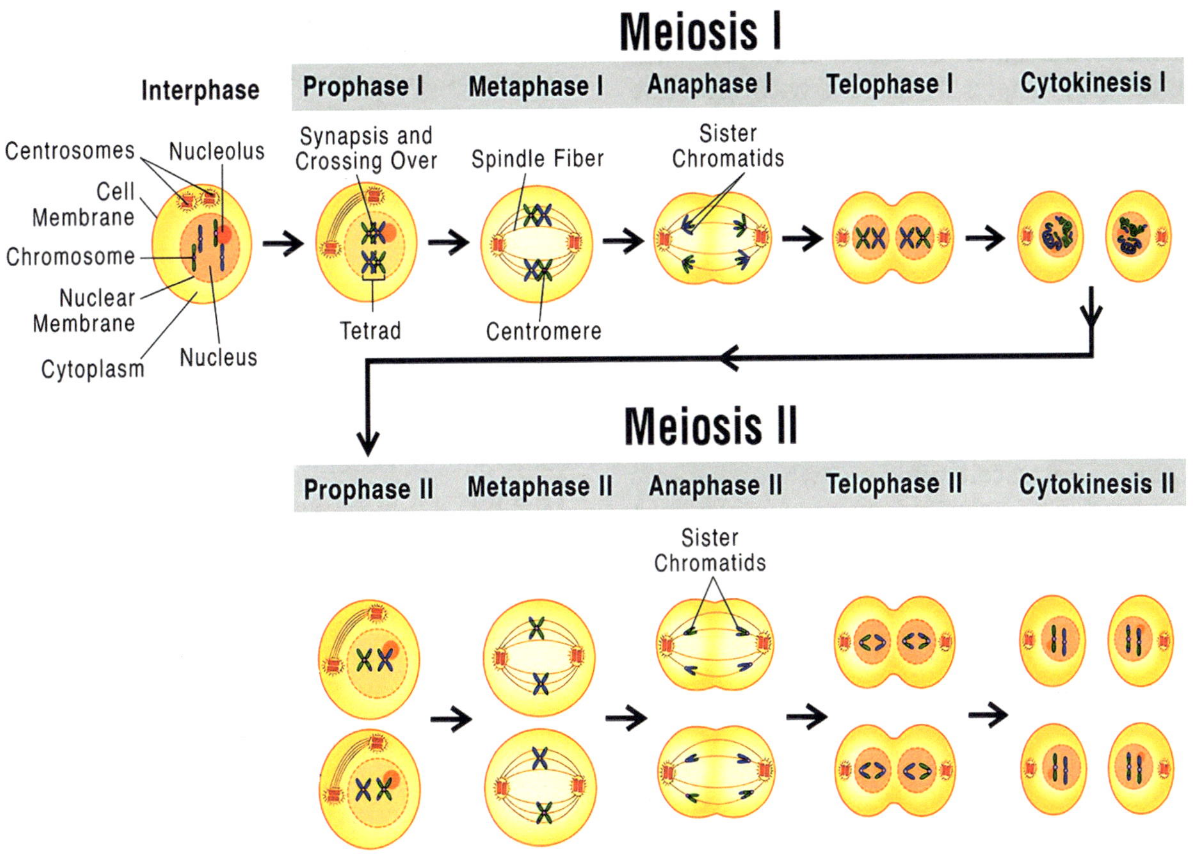

Figure 10.16. Meiosis in detail.

Source: https://external-content.duckduckgo.com/iu/?u=https%3A%2F%2Fwww.sciencefacts.net%2Fwp-content%2Fuploads%2F2020%2F09%2FMeiosis-Stages-Diagram-768x567.jpg&f=1&nofb=1&ipt=d4f6d38a0f8f7f8ff51a62a6246df443a8813bac8e4f987ae76f8bbe636a8331.

In these stages, the cell not only halves its chromosome count but also exchanges pieces of genetic information through crossing over. This shuffling, which ups the variety among gametes, lays the groundwork for organisms to adapt and evolve in changing conditions. Multiple phases like prophase, metaphase, anaphase, and telophase each brings different processes as to how chromosomes get arranged, preparing haploid cells nearly ready for fertilization. Keeping meiosis on track requires tight regulation of many cellular processes—processes that are, generally speaking, indispensable for a faultless process. For instance, oocytes; they begin their journey through meiosis, including uneven, asymmetric divisions that ensure the cell's cytoplasmic organelles end up in the right place to support early embryo development. Actin filaments, small GTPases, and even actin nucleators get roped in to help with jobs like moving the spindle and getting the polar body out, especially as the oocyte matures. These operations, with their remarkable intricacies, suggest at a finely tuned system that manages to maintain genetic integrity while boosting reproductive success, even if sometimes it feels a bit unpredictable (Duan et al., 2018). During spermatogenesis, meiosis plays a crucial role in shaping spermatozoa. It all begins with germ cells multiplying via mitosis; then they jump into the meiosis cell division, where genetic recombination and chromosome reduction both take center stage. After this phase, haploid round spermatids transform into fully functional sperm, a process known as spermiogenesis. The seminiferous tubules are remarkably ordered, if not always exactly linear, structures that resemble a busy workshop where multiple generations of germ cells grow up simultaneously. The timing for these steps can vary slightly from species to species—researchers are still fine-tuning their understanding of exactly how long each part takes. All in all, as we delve deeper into these mechanisms, it becomes even clearer how crucial meiosis is for maintaining male fertility (Staub et al., 2018) (Figure 10.16).

10.5.1. Meiosis I: Homologous Chromosome Separation

Meiosis I initiates cell division by reshuffling the genetic deck and ensuring that chromosomes separate correctly. Homologous chromosomes line up, then pull apart so that haploid gametes can eventually form. During synapsis, each chromosome finds a mate, and they swap little bits of DNA at spots called chiasmata. This exchange not only boosts genetic variety but also gives the chromosomes a temporary "glue" hold until it's time to let go. Removing cohesin proteins from the arms allows the chromosomes to reshape for the next round. Generally speaking, this stepwise dismantling is carefully controlled, ensuring that things work out just right during meiosis I (Gryaznova et al., 2021). Chromosome splitting isn't all about the chromosomes alone—it also relies on structures called kinetochores. Each chromosome sports a bundle of proteins right at its center, and these kinetochores serve as the landing pads for spindle fibers. Early on, chromosomes line up at the metaphase plate where the spindle fibers attach in a uniquely mono-oriented way, which, in most cases, stops them from parting ways too early. Then, in anaphase I, the cohesin gets nibbled away from the arms while a portion stubbornly clings around the centromeres, keeping sister chromatids together. This uneven breakup is crucial for maintaining genome integrity and ensures that parental genes are sorted into gametes correctly, thereby preventing mishaps such as aneuploidy (Alfaro et al., 2021). As things progress in meiosis I, the structure of chromosomes is given an extra push by special proteins that keep the whole separation process in order. Take separase, for example; this enzyme cuts the cohesins holding sister chromatids in a sort of "till-next-time" embrace, setting the stage for their final split in meiosis II. Interestingly, some recent work suggests that kinetochores may pull apart on their during anaphase I, largely independent of the usual spindle forces. This suggests that detaching the kinetochores may be a necessary prerequisite for subsequent steps. Keeping cohesin snug around the centromeres until later appears to reduce mix-ups during division, ensuring the gametes have the correct genetic load. All in all, gaining a better understanding of these twists and turns provides insight into how chromosomes behave and why reproductive genetics can be so remarkably complex (Gryaznova et al., 2021) (Figure 10.17).

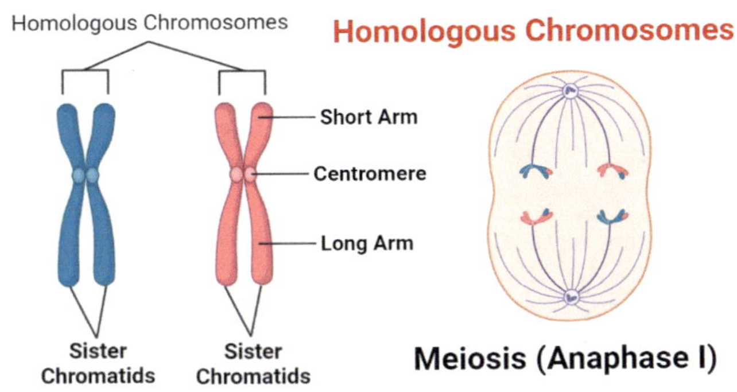

Figure 10.17. Meiosis I: Homologous chromosome separation.

Source: https://microbenotes.com/wp-content/uploads/2023/09/Homologous-Chromosomes.jpeg.

10.5.2. Meiosis II: Sister Chromatid Separation

The transition from meiosis I to meiosis II is a significant turning point in cellular division. In the first round, chromosomes pair up and sort themselves out, but it's during the second phase that sister chromatids split apart—often kind of unexpectedly. The spindle apparatus plays a crucial role here; it aligns the chromatids along a rough central line (the metaphase plate) before opposing microtubules tug them in different directions. Kinetochores must align in just the right position so that each new cell ends up with the correct mix of DNA. This subtle balancing act, which impacts genetic diversity and maintains genome integrity for future generations, demonstrates the intricate nature of meiotic division (Storme et al., 2014). Another piece of this puzzle is how the cell releases its sister chromatids by breaking down the cohesin complexes—those proteins that generally keep the twin chromatids attached after DNA replication. In many cases, the careful cutting (proteolytic cleavage) of cohesin as cells transition from metaphase to anaphase physically frees the chromatids to move apart. Meanwhile, the spindle checkpoint is busy double-checking that kinetochores stick to microtubules properly. A mistake here might cause aneuploidy, which underlines why getting these processes right is so important. Research generally indicates that when spindle orientation and checkpoint functions are accurate, chromosomal segregation remains accurate during the final phase of meiosis (Biswas et al., 2020). It isn't just the mechanical forces at play either—molecular factors add another layer of complexity. Proteins like ESCO2 and SMC3, for example, help maintain the bond between sister chromatids during the various stages of meiosis. Their involvement suggests an additional regulatory twist, subtly enhancing the role of cohesin during chromosome pairing and subsequent separation. As meiosis progresses, the balance between these molecular elements and the cell's structural dynamics becomes ever more crucial for proper cell division. Studies have shown that even minor disruptions in the cohesin pathway can lead to serious issues in gamete formation, making it clear that meiosis II isn't a simple mechanical process but a carefully orchestrated event reliant on intricate, sometimes unpredictable, molecular interactions.

This complexity highlights the crucial role of faithful chromatid separation in maintaining overall chromosomal stability (Storme et al., 2014) (Figure 10.18).

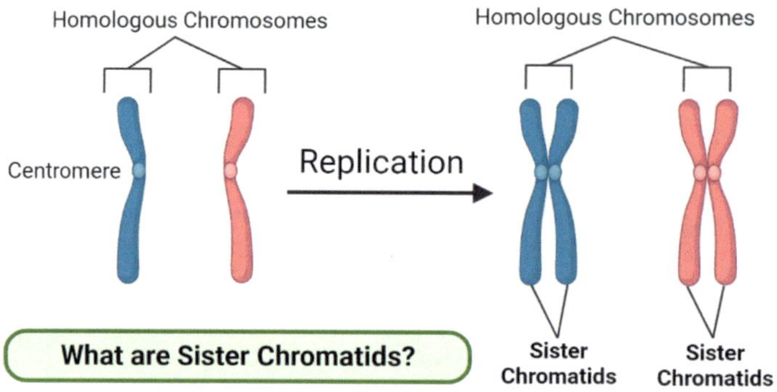

Figure 10.18. Sister chromatids.

Source: https://microbenotes.com/wp-content/uploads/2022/07/Sister-Chromatids.jpg.

10.5.3. Genetic Variation Through Crossing Over

Genetic recombination in meiosis gives life its colorful mix. Crossing over—where matching chromosomes swap snippets of their DNA—is the engine behind most of that diversity. In prophase, chromosomes line up and slip into a state called synapsis, forming structures folks refer to as tetrads. Inside these clusters, chromatids trade fragments of code, so offspring end up with a new blend of alleles. This gene swapping not only boosts variety, but in most cases, it also helps populations adjust to unexpected changes in their surroundings. The inner workings of crossing over underline its vital role in the ongoing story of heredity and evolution. During the process of crossing over, chemical pathways work diligently to ensure that the DNA mix-up proceeds smoothly. Enzymes like recombinases jump in to help exchange strands right at the crossover spots.

They act on the DNA, allowing similar sequences to come together and trade bits of genetic material. The resulting chromosomes carry a fresh set of instructions that can shape traits in future generations. This kind of genetic variation proves especially crucial when environmental pressures mount, as the ability to adapt can make all the difference between survival and struggle. By studying these molecular details, we gain insight into how such processes feed into larger ecological and evolutionary trends. Genetic variation from crossing over isn't just a neat natural trick—it has real-world perks, too, especially in agriculture. Farmers and breeders tap into this process to develop crop varieties with traits that stand up to harsh conditions, like drought or poor soil. By taking advantage of natural genetic variations, they select for plants that deliver higher yields or exhibit greater resilience, which is crucial for sustainable farming in our changing climate. Methods similar to those discussed regarding plant responses to stress (Fahad et al., 2017) and mechanisms for salt tolerance (Munns et al., 2006) are often put to work to boost crop productivity and protect food security. All in all, combining genetics, environmental shifts, and practical farming demonstrates just how central crossing over is in the broader context of cell division and life itself.

10.6. Chromosomal Abnormalities

Mitosis and meiosis play a significant role in keeping the cell's DNA in check during development. Cells split in these ways, and – naturally – mistakes can slip in, sometimes causing unusual chromosome counts that can affect an organism's well-being. Aneuploidy, for example, occurs when a cell has too many or too few chromosomes; this type of error is commonly observed in early embryos, where chromosome sorting can go wrong from the first few divisions, resulting in a mosaic effect. Studies have shown that many embryos already exhibit signs of these chromosome errors before implantation, raising questions about their likelihood of developing normally in the future. Overall, it appears that preventing genetic diseases and reproductive problems requires precisely regulating the alignment and division of chromosomes at these critical stages.. The consequences of these chromosomal abnormalities extend well beyond minor genetic adjustments; they are linked to complex reproductive issues such as early embryo loss. Chromosomes can occasionally fragment and generate tiny additional bodies called micronuclei when they are missorted, which further blurs the genetic picture. Studies using nonhuman primate models have shown that the broken fragments can even come from both the mother and the father, which underscores why cells need a way to spot and handle these errors. In most cases, cells try to cope by bundling of these fragments into micronuclei and by weeding out the abnormal cells. This strategy stops too many aneuploid cells from messing up the developing blastocyst and, ultimately, helps keep the future baby's genome intact. It's interesting to explore how these chromosome problems crop up during early development. Advanced imaging techniques have now shown that zygotic events like multipolar divisions – even as early as at the two-cell stage – can throw the whole system off, mixing normal and abnormal blastomeres in one place. This patchwork of cells reveals just how flexible and unpredictable the cellular response to errors can be. One neat, albeit messy, tactic is that mis segregated chromosomes end up tucked away in micronuclei, which seems to serve as a kind of safety net against the full impact of aneuploidy, while the embryo also tends to cull cells that are too far gone. All this, generally speaking, enhances the understanding of reproductive biology and contributes to the ongoing discussion about the broader effects of chromosomal errors on human health (Brittany et al., 2019; Cerys et al., 2022) (Figure 10.19).

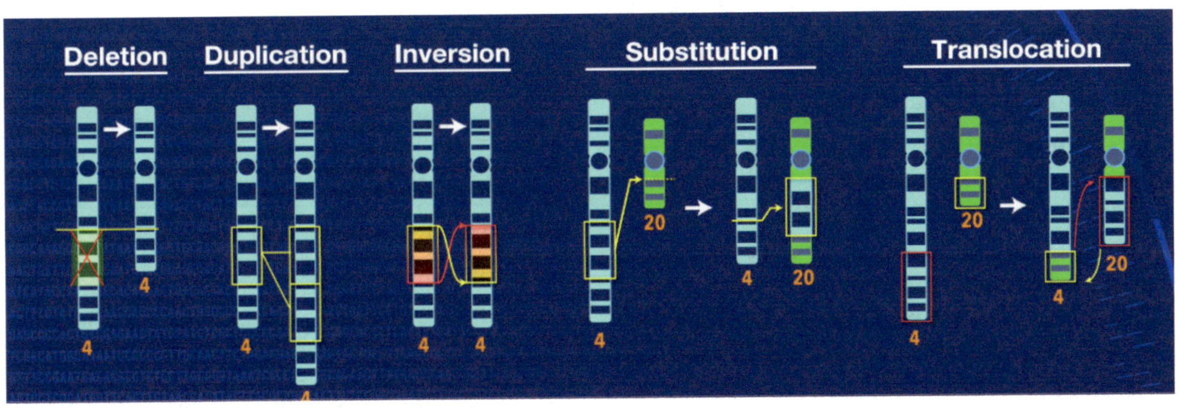

Figure 10.19. Chromosomal abnormalities.

Source: https://www.genome.gov/sites/default/files/inline-images/ChrAbnormalities_Fact-sheet2020.jpg.

10.6.1. Types of Chromosomal Abnormalities

Chromosomal changes can shed light on many genetic disorders that impact our everyday health. Sometimes, errors in cell division leave us with too many—or sometimes too few—chromosomes; this kind of mix-up, known as aneuploidy, is behind conditions like Down syndrome, which happens when there's an extra copy of chromosome 21 (trisomy 21). Interestingly, similar extra copies can also manifest as trisomy 18 (Edwards syndrome) or trisomy 13 (Patau syndrome), conditions that typically present with significant developmental challenges and a reduced life expectancy. Detailed prenatal scans often detect these anomalies early, underscoring the importance of timely checks and sensible counseling for expectant parents (Grati, 2016). Then there's another side to the story involving structural changes in chromosomes. At times, chromosomes can lose pieces, get duplicated, even flip or swap segments in an almost haphazard way—yet these changes can seriously interrupt how genes function. For example, a deletion on chromosome 5 might trigger Cri du Chat syndrome, a disorder characterized by distinctive physical features and cognitive challenges. On the other hand, when chromosome segments exchange places (like parts trading between chromosomes 9 and 22 to form the BCR-ABL fusion gene), it can set off cancers such as chronic myeloid leukemia. Generally speaking, untangling these rearrangements helps provide a better understanding of how diseases work and are passed through generations (Walter et al., 2008). Adding another twist is chromosomal mosaicism, where not all cells in an individual share the same genetic makeup. This situation often arises when errors occur during the early cell divisions that follow fertilization, resulting in some cells carrying abnormalities while others don't. The patchy nature of this condition can lead to a range of physical outcomes, sometimes even making prenatal tests a bit confusing. For instance, fetoplacental mosaicism—where the placenta's chromosomes differ from those of the fetus—can sometimes yield false-positive results in non-invasive prenatal screenings. All of these complexities highlight why, in many cases, a careful and personalized approach to genetic counseling and diagnosis is indispensable (Grati, 2016).

10.6.2. Effects on Cell Division and Organism

Cells are busy in ways that are not always obvious at first glance. Chromosomes during cell splitting, there ser series of steps that tie directly into how organisms develop. One striking piece of this puzzle is polyploidy—a situation where a cell ends up with an extra copy (or more) of its complete genome. This whole doubling process tends to increase the genetic diversity within each cell and, in most cases, subtly alters the traits of the entire organism. Interestingly, in some species, having extra genetic material seems to help them deal with stressors like high salt levels. Examining how these polyploid processes operate across a range of organisms, from plants to animals, reveals unexpected insights into biodiversity and the resilience of ecosystems (Donald et al., 2020). It even appears that these cellular changes ripple outward, nudging evolutionary paths through both internal dynamics and external challenges. Now, consider chromosome segregation while cells divide - it's a process that just can't be overlooked if genetic material is to be correctly passed on. The key player here is what many call the mitotic spindle; it not only aligns chromosomes but also helps them separate, and it does so through a mix of force generation and attachment stability. Newer computer models, experimenting with fission yeast systems, have shown that if these forces or attachments slip, the result can be a genome off course—one of the common routes to instability that ties into many diseases, including cancer. With each study, it becomes increasingly clear that understanding the intricacies of spindle behavior is vital, not only for academic curiosity but also for developing therapies to counteract segregation errors and enhance overall cell health (Edelmaier et al., 2020). When the influence of polyploidy is combined with dynamic chromosome behavior, things get even more interesting. The effects of whole-genome duplication often manifest as larger cell sizes and unexpected shifts in metabolic pathways, which in turn can influence tissue development and overall organism health. And as these polyploid cells face environmental challenges, they sometimes develop traits that, albeit subtly, lead to improvements in agricultural practices or even innovative biomedical applications. In this way, the intersection of genome doubling and cell mechanics opens a door for research that transcends traditional scientific boundaries. Bringing together minds from genetics, ecology, and beyond may offer fresh strategies to enhance species resilience, improve crop yields, and combat diseases linked to chromosome misalignments (Donald et al., 2020) (Figure 10.20).

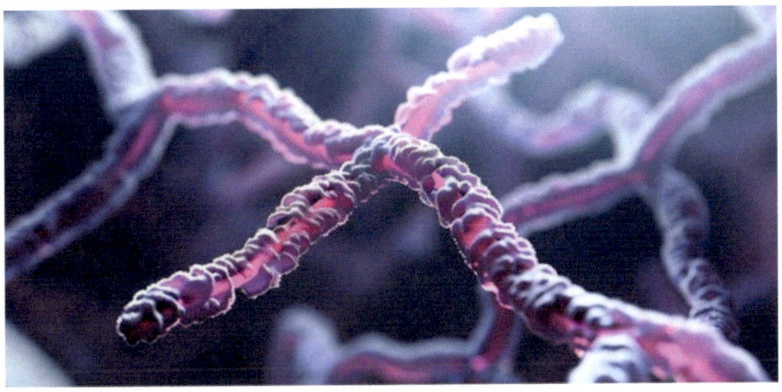

Figure 10.20. ***Cell Division and Organism.***

Source: https://external-content.duckduckgo.com/iu/?u=https%3A%2F%2Fimg.freepik.com%2Fpremium-photo%2Fexploring-vibrancy-human-chromosomes-cell-division-concept-genetic-studies-cell-division-process-dna-replication-chromosomal-abnormalities-mitosis-stages_864588-263414.jpg&f=1&nofb=1&ipt=2107a35d61c738d0e968013541f9f5dc3435500e5479612c56e717c96cdfed64.

10.6.3. Examples of Diseases Caused by Abnormalities

Chromosomal mishaps are closely linked to many illnesses, highlighting the importance of cell division in the correct manner. Aneuploidy – when cells end up with a strange number of chromosomes – can set the stage for conditions like Turner syndrome or even Down syndrome. Down syndrome, for instance, comes about when there's an extra copy of chromosome 21, which generally brings along intellectual delays and a range of physical differences. Often, these issues stem from errors during meiosis that disrupt the normal flow of chromosomal integrity, thereby paving the way for these unusual genetic arrangements. Getting a grip on such irregularities lets researchers explore new ways to help and support patients, which can, in most cases, make a real difference in their quality of life. Some substances that harm cells can also shed light on how these chromosomal abnormalities manifest in diseases. For example, work on *Mammea africana* has revealed that its extract, applied to *Allium cepa* root cells, may trigger chromosomal mistakes and even cause the formation of micronuclei (Okokon et al., 2024). These kinds of genotoxic effects stir up concerns over everyday exposures from the environment or even medicines, as they might eventually lead to chromosomal damage in humans. This cellular toxicity can sometimes lead to significant problems like cancer, where unreliable cell division and genomic instability are big culprits behind tumors. Investigating these biochemical interactions and their impact on cellular systems is crucial for understanding broader public health risks. On another note, cohesin complexes play a crucial role in maintaining the proper alignment of chromosomes during cell division. Generally speaking, flaws in cohesin come with serious fallout, such as infertility and developmental oddities (Liu et al., 2024). Studies with organisms like *Caenorhabditis elegans* have shown that even small mutations in cohesin proteins can mess up the bonding between sister chromatids – a step that's critical for correct chromosome separation. Interestingly, when the specialized areas of cohesin are altered, age-related chromosomal issues can also occur. In short, untangling how cohesin sometimes goes awry not only deepens our insight into various genetic diseases but also suggests possible targets for treatments aimed at getting chromosomes back on track.

SUMMARY

Chromosomes and cell division keep life ticking, even if we rarely stop to think about it. They're not only in charge of copying our genetic info correctly but also seem to flex when organisms need to adapt. In many mammalian cells—take the liver, for instance—there are some instances of polyploidy. It isn't just a structural abnormality; it appears generally linked to subtle regulatory cues, like those from miRNAs. In most cases, miR-122 appears to play a role in how liver cells regulate their chromosome counts (Shu-Hsu et al., 2016). This quirky connection raises the question of whether we should delve deeper into how chromosomal twists impact overall cell well-being. Chromosomes don't merely split and replicate; they mingle with what's happening outside the cell as well. Volume-regulated anion channels—VRACs, as they are sometimes called—join the party when cells react to chemotherapeutic agents. Recent work suggests that these channels facilitate the transport of drugs while also promoting cell death, a process known as apoptosis. It's a messy, fascinating dance that—if we learn to tweak it—might someday open up new ways to fight cancer (Planells et al., 2015). Sometimes, the interplay between these elements gives our understanding of cellular behavior an entirely new perspective. Ultimately, merging knowledge about chromosomes and cell division blurs the lines between genetics, cancer research, and cell physiology. As we keep poking around, it's hard not to wonder how these microscopic processes tie into larger health issues. The combination of chromosome dynamics and cellular signaling may ultimately rewrite our understanding of disorders and even lead to novel therapeutic ideas. Keeping an eye on miRNAs, chromosome upkeep, and drug responses remains crucial, even if things sometimes get a bit tangled in the details.

Chromosomes play a significant role in life—they house our DNA, wound tightly around proteins called histones, which helps keep everything neatly organized. When cells prepare to divide, whether through processes like mitosis or meiosis, these bundles of genetic information undergo essential changes so that every new cell receives an exact copy of what's needed, there are these check points—sort of like built-in quality checks driven by a mix of proteins and enzymes—that generally help keep the genetic blueprint intact, and if something goes awry here, problems like cancer might crop up. Telomeres, the protective caps on chromosome ends, are also gaining attention lately because their gradual shortening appears to be linked to signs of cellular aging and other health issues (Corbett et al., 2015). Cell division isn't just a mandatory biological event—it's an intricately regulated process, almost like a well-rehearsed dance with multiple cues and signals. After the chromosomes have been duplicated, mitosis takes charge by splitting them equally between the resulting cells.

At the same time, meiosis works differently by shuffling the genes, introducing unexpected variations that are necessary for diversity. In most cases, these mechanisms are crucial not only for growth and development but also for maintaining a balanced genetic ledger over many generations. Telomeres continue to play a crucial role in this process, guarding the ends of chromosomes against decay. Interestingly, research indicates that factors such as oxidative stress and inflammation can erode these structures, accelerating cellular aging and impacting overall well-being (Corbett et al., 2015). When it comes to disease, any disruptions in chromosome integrity and telomere dynamics appear to matter significantly. For example, conditions like astrocytomas—a type of brain tumor—have been linked to these disruptions. Experiments, often using mouse models, have shed light on the complex networks that drive the initiation and progression of aggressive astrocytomas, highlighting pathways involved in cell cycle control and DNA repair. This messy yet fascinating interplay between genetic stability and cancer development makes it clear that more probing is needed. Digging into these relationships not only broadens our understanding of how tumors form, but it also sets the stage for honing treatments that might better target these molecular misfirings. The overall complexity of how cells manage their chromosomes and protect against disease underscores why we still have so many unanswered questions in genetics and cell biology.

CLOSER LOOK

ANEUPLOIDY

Aneuploidy is a chromosomal abnormality characterized by an abnormal number of chromosomes within a cell, deviating from the normal diploid number. In humans, this means having more or fewer than the typical 46 chromosomes. Aneuploidy arises due to errors in chromosome segregation during cell division, particularly during meiosis (the process that produces gametes) or mitosis. The most common cause of aneuploidy is nondisjunction, a failure of homologous chromosomes or sister chromatids to separate properly. This results in gametes that either lack a chromosome or contain an extra one. When such gametes are involved in fertilization, they give rise to zygotes with an abnormal chromosomal count. Aneuploidy can involve autosomes or sex chromosomes and may result in monosomy (loss of a single chromosome, such as Turner syndrome, 45,X) or trisomy (gain of a single chromosome, such as Down syndrome, 47,XX+21 or 47,XY+21). While some forms of aneuploidy are compatible with life, many others are lethal, leading to miscarriage or early embryonic death.

Among viable aneuploidies, Down syndrome (trisomy 21) is the most common and well-known, associated with developmental delays, characteristic facial features, and a higher risk of certain medical conditions. Other notable trisomies include Edwards syndrome (trisomy 18) and Patau syndrome (trisomy 13), both of which are associated with severe developmental and health problems and typically result in early infant mortality. Aneuploidy involving sex chromosomes tends to have milder physical consequences. For instance, Klinefelter syndrome (47XXY) affects males and may lead to reduced fertility and some physical differences, while Turner syndrome affects females and is characterized by short stature and infertility. Interestingly, individuals with extra sex chromosomes (such as 47,XXX or 47,XYY) may exhibit only mild symptoms or even remain undiagnosed throughout life.

Aneuploidy is a significant cause of pregnancy loss, especially in the first trimester, and its incidence increases significantly with maternal age. This age-related risk is thought to be due to the decline in cohesin proteins and SAC efficiency in aging oocytes, which increases the likelihood of nondisjunction. Diagnostic tools such as karyotyping, fluorescence in situ hybridization (FISH), and newer technologies like chromosomal microarray analysis and non-invasive prenatal testing (NIPT) can detect aneuploidy in embryos or fetuses, aiding in early diagnosis and informed decision-making. In addition to its implications in prenatal development, aneuploidy is also a hallmark of many cancers, where chromosomal instability contributes to tumor progression and resistance to therapy.

Understanding aneuploidy is crucial not only for managing genetic disorders and reproductive health but also for advancing cancer biology and regenerative medicine. Research into the molecular mechanisms underlying chromosome missegregation continues to reveal potential targets for therapeutic intervention. Although currently there are no cures for aneuploidy syndromes, supportive care and early interventions can significantly improve the quality of life for affected individuals. Thus, aneuploidy represents both a fundamental biological phenomenon and a significant clinical challenge in modern medicine.

REFERENCES

1. Adl, S. M., Bass, D., Lane, C. E., Lukeš, J., Schoch, C. L., Смирнов, A. B., Agatha, S., et al. (2018). Revisions to the classification, nomenclature, and diversity of eukaryotes. *Journal of Eukaryotic Microbiology, 66*(1), 4–119. https://doi.org/10.1111/jeu.12691.
2. Alfaro, E., López-Jiménez, P., González-Martínez, J., Malumbres, M., Suja, J. Á., & Gómez, R. (2021). PLK1 regulates centrosome migration and spindle dynamics in male mouse meiosis. *EMBO Reports, 22*(2), e51030. https://doi.org/10.15252/embr.202051030.
3. Andor, N., Barnholtz-Sloan, J., & Ji, H. (2019). COMP-01. MODELING THE EVOLUTION OF PLOIDY IN a RESOURCE RESTRICTED ENVIRONMENT. *Neuro-Oncology, 21*(Supplement_6), vi61. https://doi.org/10.1093/neuonc/noz175.244Balali-Mood, M., Naseri, K., Tahergorabi, Z., Khazdair, M. R., & Sadeghi, M. (2021). Toxic mechanisms of five heavy metals: Mercury, lead, chromium, cadmium, and arsenic. *Frontiers in Pharmacology, 12*, Article 643972. https://doi.org/10.3389/fphar.2021.643972.
4. Bhattacharya, S., Dutta, S., Chowrasia, S., & Das, S. (2024). Unveiling the dynamics: A comprehensive review of biological membrane kinetics during cell division. *Asian Journal of Biological Sciences*. https://www.semanticscholar.org/paper/d9e896c8b8e69db24d52c96cfca2d076f7cf9ff8 (accessed on 26 May 2025).
5. Biswas, U., Eichele, G., Hempel, K., et al. (2020). Meiotic sex chromosome cohesion and autosomal synapsis are supported by Esco2.
6. Bodmer, W. F., Bielas, J. H., & Beckman, R. A. (2008). Genetic instability is not a requirement for tumor development. *Cancer Research, 68*(9), 3558–3561. https://doi.org/10.1158/0008-5472.can-07-6544.
7. Bourque, G., Burns, K. H., Gehring, M., Gorbunova, V., Seluanov, A., Hammell, M., Imbeault, M., et al. (2018). Ten things you should know about transposable elements. *Genome Biology, 19*, 199. https://doi.org/10.1186/s13059-018-1577-z.
8. Bowman, J. L., Kohchi, T., Yamato, K. T., Jenkins, J., Shu, S., Ishizaki, K., Yamaoka, S., et al. (2017). Insights into land plant evolution garnered from the *Marchantia polymorpha* genome. *Cell, 171*(2), 287–304.e15. https://doi.org/10.1016/j.cell.2017.09.030.
9. Bradley, R. A., Wolff, I. D., Cohen, P., & Gray, S. (2023). Dynamic regulatory phosphorylation of mouse CDK2 occurs during meiotic prophase I. *bioRxiv*. https://www.semanticscholar.org/paper/9186a72d78e2d9f84c24e6b7b6fd8de6308cbf9c (accessed on 26 May 2025).
10. Corbett, N., & Alda, M. (2015). On telomeres long and short. *Journal of Psychiatry & Neuroscience, 40*(1), 3–4. https://www.semanticscholar.org/paper/0936682e947acb19c74b079102d1f690f003ecc0 (accessed on 26 May 2025).
11. Currie, C. E., Ford, E., Benham Whyte, L., Taylor, D. M., Mihalas, B. P., Erent, M., Marston, A. L., et al. (2022). The first mitotic division of human embryos is highly error prone. *Nature Communications, 13*, Article 1234. https://doi.org/10.1038/s41467-022-34294-6.
12. Daughtry, B. L., Rosenkrantz, J. L., Lazar, N. H., Fei, S. S., Redmayne, N., Torkenczy, K. A., Adey, A., et al. (2019). Single-cell sequencing of primate preimplantation embryos reveals chromosome elimination via cellular fragmentation and blastomere exclusion. *Genome Research, 29*(3), 367–382. https://doi.org/10.1101/gr.239830.118.

13. De Storme, N., Geelen, D., Pawlowski, W., & Tiang, C. L. (2014). Chromosome segregation in plant meiosis. https://core.ac.uk/download/55854046.pdf (accessed on 26 May 2025).

14. Deans, C., & Maggert, K. A. (2015). What do you mean, "epigenetic"? *Genetics, 199*(3), 887–896. https://doi.org/10.1534/genetics.114.173492.

15. Duan, X., & Sun, S. C. (2018). Actin cytoskeleton dynamics in mammalian oocyte meiosis. *Biology of Reproduction, 100*(1), 15–24. https://doi.org/10.1093/biolre/ioy163.

16. Edelmaier, C. J., Lamson, A., Gergely, Z. R., Ansari, S., Blackwell, R., McIntosh, J. R., Glaser, M. A., et al. (2020). Mechanisms of chromosome biorientation and bipolar spindle assembly analyzed by computational modeling. *eLife, 9*, e48787. https://doi.org/10.7554/eLife.48787.

17. Engeland, K. (2017). Cell cycle arrest through indirect transcriptional repression by p53: I have a DREAM. *Cell Death and Differentiation, 25*(1), 114–132. https://doi.org/10.1038/cdd.2017.172.

18. Fahad, S., Bajwa, A. A., Nazir, U., Anjum, S. A., Farooq, A., Zohaib, A., Sadia, S., et al. (2017). Crop production under drought and heat stress: Plant responses and management options. *Frontiers in Plant Science, 8*. https://doi.org/10.3389/fpls.2017.01147.

19. Fox, D. T., Soltis, P. S., Ashman, T. L., & Van de Peer, Y. (2020). Polyploidy: A biological force from cells to ecosystems. *Trends in Cell Biology, 30*(8), 688–694. https://doi.org/10.1016/j.tcb.2020.06.006.

20. Galluzzi, L., Vitale, I., Aaronson, S. A., Abrams, J., Adam, D., Agostinis, P., Alnemri, E. S., et al. (2018). Molecular mechanisms of cell death: Recommendations of the Nomenclature Committee on Cell Death 2018. *Cell Death and Differentiation, 25*(3), 486–541. https://doi.org/10.1038/s41418-017-0012-4.

21. Garg, R., Kaushik, K., Salam, A., Kundu, R., Chandra, S., & Nandi, C. K. (2024). Carbon nanodots as a red emissive fluorescent probe for the super-resolution microscopy of DNA dynamics during paclitaxel treatment. *bioRxiv*. https://www.semanticscholar.org/paper/9e69b3bc905f093165c3956ea79b59c00bd1896c (accessed on 26 May 2025).

22. Glover, N., Redestig, H., & Dessimoz, C. (2016). Homeologs: What are they and how do we infer them? *Trends in Plant Science, 21*(8), 609–621. https://doi.org/10.1016/j.tplants.2016.02.005.

23. Grati, F. R. (2016). Implications of fetoplacental mosaicism on cell-free DNA testing: A review of a common biological phenomenon. *Ultrasound in Obstetrics & Gynecology, 48*(4), 415–423. https://doi.org/10.1002/uog.15975.

24. Gryaznova, Y., Keating, L., Touati, S. A., Cladière, D., El Yakoubi, W., Buffin, E., & Wassmann, K. (2021). Kinetochore individualization in meiosis I is required for centromeric cohesion removal in meiosis II. *The EMBO Journal, 40*(15). https://doi.org/10.15252/embj.2020106797.

25. Hsu, S. H., Delgado, E. R., Otero, P. A., Teng, K. Y., Kutay, H., Meehan, K. M., Moroney, J. B., et al. (2016). MicroRNA-122 regulates polyploidization in the murine liver. *Hepatology, 64*(2), 599–615. https://doi.org/10.1002/hep.28573.

26. Janssen, A., Colmenares, S. U., & Karpen, G. H. (2018). Heterochromatin: Guardian of the genome. *Annual Review of Cell and Developmental Biology, 34*, 265–288. https://doi.org/10.1146/annurev-cellbio-100617-062653.

27. Kar, F. M., & Hochwagen, A. (2021). Phospho-regulation of meiotic prophase. *Frontiers in*

Cell and Developmental Biology, 9, Article 653118. https://www.semanticscholar.org/paper/ab41a0caa24e145fbf953f115881103f74431559 (accessed on 26 May 2025).

28. Klionsky, D. J., Abdelmohsen, K., Abe, A., Abedin, M. J., Abeliovich, H., Acevedo-Arozena, A., Adachi, H., et al. (2016). Guidelines for the use and interpretation of assays for monitoring autophagy (3rd edition). *Autophagy, 12*(1), 1–222. https://doi.org/10.1080/15548627.2015.1100356.
29. Lagalla, C., Marchio, L., Bartolacci, A., Piccioni, C., Zacà, C., Tarozzi, N., Spadoni, V., et al. (2023). Larger time intervals between pronuclear fading and the first mitosis are strongly associated with trichotomous mitoses and cleavage arrest in human embryos. *Human Reproduction*. Advance online publication. https://www.semanticscholar.org/paper/0749b70883170daa90a87291e9ba4c30cdf9b37b (accessed on 26 May 2025).
30. Lazar-Stefanita, L., Luo, J., Montagne, R., Thierry, A., Sun, X., Mercy, G., Mozziconacci, J., et al. (2022). Karyotype engineering reveals spatio-temporal control of replication firing and gene contacts. *Cell Genomics, 2*(1), 100163. https://doi.org/10.1016/j.xgen.2022.100163.
31. Leung, J., Pardo, P., & Pereira-Smith, O. (2001). The role of the MRG gene family in replicative senescence and immortalization. *The Scientific World Journal, 1*, 66. https://www.semanticscholar.org/paper/8d70198e79e9916a609adb10eeb9eb1b74c6a303 (accessed on 26 May 2025).
32. Lipinski, K. A., Barber, L. J., Davies, M. N., Ashenden, M., Sottoriva, A., & Gerlinger, M. (2016). Cancer evolution and the limits of predictability in precision cancer medicine. *Trends in Cancer, 2*(1), 49–63. https://doi.org/10.1016/j.trecan.2015.11.003.
33. Liu, Y., Liu, B., Zhang, R., Zhu, Z., Zhao, L., Jiang, R., Wang, Y., et al. (2024). Cohesion ring gates are specialized for meiotic cell division. *Journal of Molecular Cell Biology*. https://www.semanticscholar.org/paper/fce6941f9e5300efab26e852fd6c1b675c63a904 (accessed on 26 May 2025).
34. Marchetti, F., & Venkatachalam, S. (2010). The multiple roles of Bub1 in chromosome segregation during mitosis and meiosis. *Cell Cycle, 9*(1), 58–63. https://doi.org/10.4161/cc.9.1.10348.
35. Matrka, M. C., Hennigan, R. F., Kappes, F., DeLay, M., Lambert, P. F., Aronow, B. J., & Wells, S. I. (2015). DEK over-expression promotes mitotic defects and micronucleus formation. *Cell Cycle, 14*(22), 3939–3953. https://doi.org/10.1080/15384101.2015.1044177.
36. Munns, R., James, R. A., & Läuchli, A. (2006). Approaches to increasing the salt tolerance of wheat and other cereals. *Journal of Experimental Botany, 57*(5), 1025–1043. https://doi.org/10.1093/jxb/erj100.
37. Nannipieri, P., Ascher-Jenull, J., Ceccherini, M. T., Landi, L., Pietramellara, G., & Renella, G. (2017). Microbial diversity and soil functions. *European Journal of Soil Science, 68*(1), 12–26. https://doi.org/10.1111/ejss.4_12398.
38. Okokon, J., Edet, E. O., Iyanyi, U., Ebong, N., Anagboso, M. O., & Johhny, I. I. (2024). Genotoxicity and cytotoxicity activities of stembark extract of *Mammea africana*. *Asian Journal of Biochemistry, Genetics and Molecular Biology*. https://www.semanticscholar.org/paper/d09b5bdcc1f5b6df90ad92b437716497111a0ce0 (accessed on 26 May 2025).
39. Olsson-Strömberg, U., Höglund, M., Björkholm, M., Braide, I., Carlson, K., Gahrton, G., Grimfors, G., et al. (2006). Successful mobilization of Ph-negative blood stem cells with intensive

chemotherapy + G-CSF in patients with chronic myelogenous leukemia in first chronic phase. *Leukemia & Lymphoma, 47*(9), 1768–1773. https://www.semanticscholar.org/paper/c20a775b7e0d1157061e9f620b0d491723584ca6 (accessed on 26 May 2025).

40. Parwin, S., & Srivastava, P. (2024). Role of orphan ParA proteins in replication and cell division in *Rhodococcus erythropolis* PR4. *Journal of Basic Microbiology*. https://www.semanticscholar.org/paper/295bc9f87d84c96ff60d0cf044280a5e45505bfb (accessed on 26 May 2025).

41. Pati, D. (2024). Role of chromosomal cohesion and separation in aneuploidy and tumorigenesis. *Cellular and Molecular Life Sciences, 81*, Article 12345. https://www.semanticscholar.org/paper/9091149cd2ae0d48e0791af432a0e5f775d8a563 (accessed on 26 May 2025).

42. Pepke, M. L., Kvalnes, T., Wright, J., Araya-Ajoy, Y., Ranke, P., Boner, W., Monaghan, P., et al. (2023). Longitudinal telomere dynamics within natural lifespans of a wild bird. *Scientific Reports, 13*, Article 100163. https://www.semanticscholar.org/paper/a3be9f69d522fad9dedb337b6c8bc3f9c8ccf389 (accessed on 26 May 2025).

43. Planells-Cases, R., Lutter, D., Guyader, C., Gerhards, N. M., Ullrich, F., Elger, D. A., Küçükosmanoğlu, A., et al. (2015). Subunit composition of VRAC channels determines substrate specificity and cellular resistance to Pt-based anti-cancer drugs. *The EMBO Journal, 34*(23), 2993–3008. https://doi.org/10.15252/embj.201592409.

44. Polak, B., Risteski, P., Lesjak, S., & Tolić, I. M. (2016). PRC1-labeled microtubule bundles and kinetochore pairs show one-to-one association in metaphase. *EMBO Reports, 18*(2), 217–230. https://doi.org/10.15252/embr.201642650.

45. Rodrigues, M., Kosaric, N., Bonham, C. A., & Gurtner, G. C. (2018). Wound healing: A cellular perspective. *Physiological Reviews, 99*(1), 665–706. https://doi.org/10.1152/physrev.00067.2017.

46. Ruzankina, Y., Kutlu, B., Wang, S. S. W., Song, Y., Householder, D., Martin, P. L., Baran, M., et al. (2013). Abstract 1809: Analysis of molecular networks that drive astrocytoma initiation and progression. *Cancer Research, 73*(8 Supplement), 1809–1809. https://www.semanticscholar.org/paper/3491a00b705f2dd993517f652a85c5a58980642c (accessed on 26 May 2025).

47. Staub, C., & Johnson, L. (2018). Review: Spermatogenesis in the bull. *animal, 12*(s1), s27–s35. https://doi.org/10.1017/s1751731118000435.

48. Stephenson, D. (1997). Genetics variants and strains of the laboratory mouse (3rd ed.). In M. F. Lyon, S. Rastan, & S. D. M. Brown (Eds.), *Annals of Human Genetics* (Vol. 61, pp. 1807). Oxford University Press. https://www.semanticscholar.org/paper/ee17f2adb94714ac4bbda3f324d825a7055fa5d3 (accessed on 26 May 2025).

49. Thul, P., Åkesson, L., Wiking, M., Mahdessian, D., Geladaki, A., Ait Blal, H., Alm, T., et al. (2017). A subcellular map of the human proteome. *Science, 356*(6340), eaal3321. https://doi.org/10.1126/science.aal3321.

50. van Hooff, J. J. E., Tromer, E. C., van Wijk, L. M., Snel, B., & Kops, G. J. P. L. (2017). Evolutionary dynamics of the kinetochore network in eukaryotes as revealed by comparative genomics. *EMBO Reports, 18*(10), 1559–1571. https://doi.org/10.15252/embr.201744102.

51. van Schaik, T., Vos, M., Peric-Hupkes, D., Celie, P. H. N., & van Steensel, B. (2020). Cell cycle dynamics of lamina-associated DNA. *EMBO Reports, 21*(6). https://doi.org/10.15252/embr.202050636.

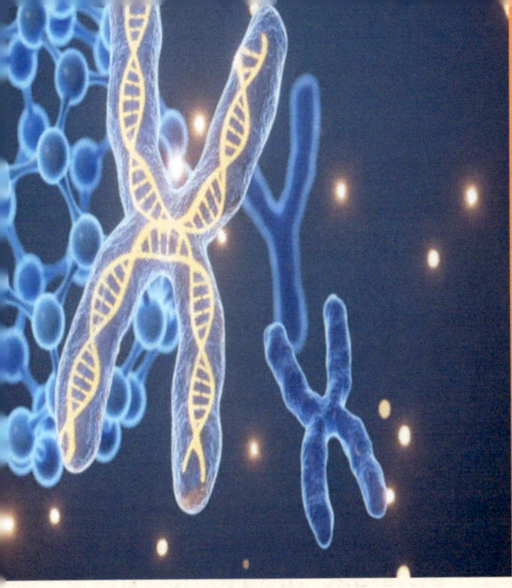

Chapter 11
MENDELIAN GENETICS

Contents

Introduction

Gregor Mendel's pea plant work in the mid-1800s kick-started modern genetics in ways that still surprise us today. He dove right in, carefully experimenting with how traits pass from one generation to the next. His discovery—that traits tend to separate and mix independently—changed the game. Mendel's approach, with its insistence on counting and careful observation (yes, even a bit of number-crunching), set a pattern that would later be known as Mendelian genetics. This chapter will delve into these early insights, examining how they integrate into the broader story of genetics and continue to influence research and real-world applications. In understanding these basics, not only does the story of science get a little richer, but we also start to see more clearly how biology works in everyday life. As genetics moved into the 20th century, Mendel's work took on an almost legendary role—a story that laboratories and textbooks revisited again and again. Generally speaking, scientists began rethinking their ideas in light of newer discoveries, sparking a lively chat between old theories and fresh insights about heredity. A peek at textbooks and period literature reveals that this blending of ideas helped train the next generation of geneticists, shaping the way they thought about science. It's interesting how these historical accounts, often repeated with minor twists, ended up framing the subject's boundaries while also opening doors to entirely new questions (Skopek et al., 2008). Even today, Mendel's insights show up in unexpected places like genetic engineering and biotech, fields that lean heavily on a solid grasp of inheritance. His basic ideas still give us clues on how genetic traits can be nudged or mixed—whether it's about boosting crop resistance or fine-tuning livestock traits. At the same time, his work sparks a fair share of debate on ethical issues, especially when it comes to topics such as genetic modification and human genetics. The ongoing clash between early findings and modern bioethical questions makes it clear that, as our scientific understanding grows, we must keep ethics in the picture. As this discussion unfolds, expect a deep dive into both the cornerstone ideas of Mendelian genetics and the ripple effects they continue to have on scientific thought and society at large (Costa et al., 2014) (Figure 11.1).

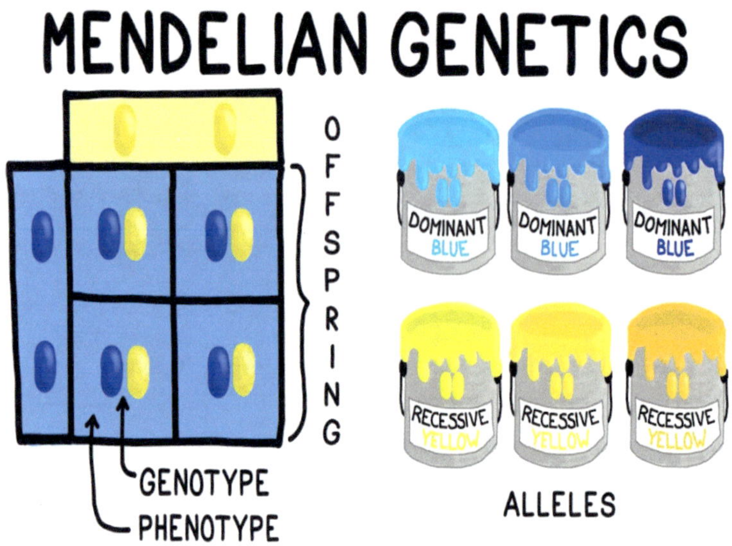

Figure 11.1. Mendelian genetics.

Source: https://external-content.duckduckgo.com/iu/?u=https%3A%2F%2Fi.ytimg.com%2Fvi%2F_478UemZ-2E%2Fmaxresdefault.jpg&f=1&nofb=1&ipt=20750e03f090fda46ce565ad05a68f23bd5a93c76dab32ad42cd8da0d596ac80.

Definition of Mendelian Genetics

Genetic inheritance provides a natural framework for understanding how traits are passed along over generations. Mendelian genetics – named after Gregor Mendel, that 19th-century trailblazer – kickstarted our grasp of trait transmission when he experimented with pea plants. His work revealed concepts such as segregation and independent assortment, demonstrating that alleles tend to separate and recombine during gamete formation, which in most cases leads to fairly predictable traits in the offspring. This early, groundbreaking work laid the groundwork for modern genetics and still offers valuable insights into both straightforward and more complex inheritance patterns in living beings. Modern research builds on these Mendelian basics in unexpected ways. Generally speaking, traits aren't always transferred through simple dominant-or-recessive rules. Sometimes, instances of incomplete dominance, co-dominance, or even multi-allelic situations add layers of complexity to what we once thought was a clear-cut process. When scientists examine small creatures like Drosophila melanogaster, they often encounter cases that defy straightforward classification. At Arizona State University, for example, students dive into hands-on experiments, tackling phenotypes that don't neatly fit the usual boxes. This interactive approach not only clarifies aspects of molecular genetics but also enhances their ability to assess and even manipulate these more complex genetic traits (Marshall, 2008). Mendelian ideas even echo in modern agriculture. Take rice lesion mimic mutants (LMMs) – here, spontaneous leaf lesions follow Mendelian rules, offering clues about how breeding strategies might boost crop resilience and yield. Research shows that these mutants possess natural self-defense mechanisms against environmental stresses, which in turn can impact photosynthesis and overall plant health. When geneticists apply these classic principles to the challenges of today's crops, they often uncover new proteins and physiological processes that lead to improved performance. In this sense, Mendelian genetics isn't just an outdated textbook theory – it provides practical strategies for enhancing agricultural productivity and food security (Kang et al., 2021).

Historical Context and Significance

Back in the late 1800s and early 1900s, science was buzzing with new ideas about how traits passed down—but it wasn't all neat at first. Gregor Mendel's pioneering experiments with pea plants might have been ignored initially, yet they soon turned into the beating heart of genetics. His work on segregation and independent assortment basically showed us that traits jump from generation to generation in a way that challenged those old "everything blends together" ideas. When his research was rediscovered in the early 1900s, it bridged the old-school views of classical biology with this fresh, up-and-coming field we now call genetics. His discoveries not only sparked more questions about heredity, but they also set off a chain reaction that eventually led to the modern synthesis—a creative melding of Mendelian rules with Darwinian evolution that firmly established genetic theory as a core component of biology. Mendelian genetics quickly began to reach far beyond simple theories. Today, its impact spills over into medicine, agriculture, and even biotechnology. Figuring out how traits are passed on has powered advances in genetic engineering, allowing scientists to tweak genes in crops and livestock for improved yields. This type of work helps boost food security and the efficiency of farming efforts. Additionally, these same principles have driven breakthroughs in medical genetics, particularly in identifying genetic disorders early and developing targeted treatments. For example, applying Mendel's insights to study rare genetic diseases has helped with earlier diagnoses and quicker interventions, which in turn improve patient outcomes. All this demonstrates that his work is more than just an academic milestone—it's a practical toolkit that addresses modern challenges in healthcare and food production. Meanwhile, our understanding of basic biology continues to evolve with new discoveries, particularly in the realm of microbial genetics. Recent work is full of surprises about how the microbiome—those tiny organisms living with us—can shape gene expression and overall health in ways that go beyond simple Mendelian patterns. The concept of holobionts, which bundles a host with its microscopic partners, throws a wrench into the old notion that genes operate independently; it hints at a much more linked and lively view of life. As researchers incorporate these fresh perspectives into genetic studies, Mendelian ideas are expanding into conversations that extend into ecology and microbiology. This ever-changing dialogue not only paints a richer picture of heredity but also continually reaffirms the historical and practical significance of Mendel's early work—even if, at times, its presentation might feel a bit off-kilter or redundant, just like natural human thought (Figure 11.2).

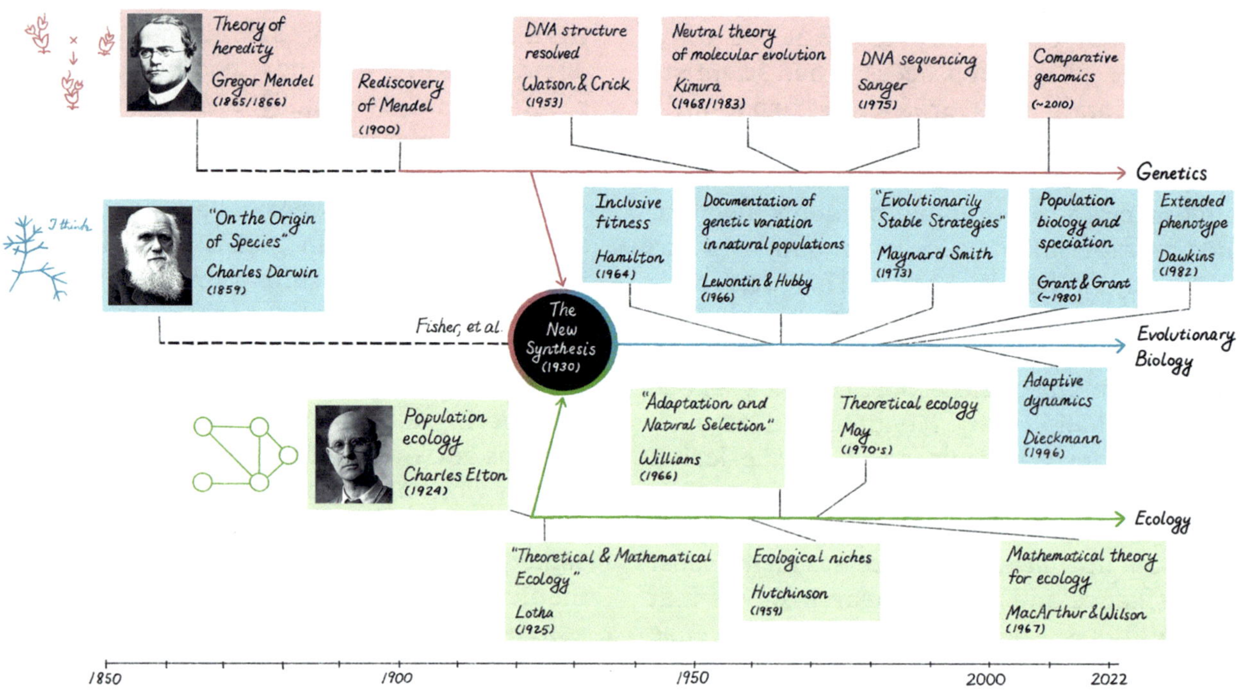

Figure 11.2. Historical context of Mendelian genetics.

Source: https://external-content.duckduckgo.com/iu/?u=https%3A%2F%2Fwww.pnas.org%2Fcms%2F10.1073%2Fpnas.2201327119%2Fasset%2Fb42a64b9-a6d0-4b41-b792-880ecb928a18%2Fassets%2Fimages%2Flarge%2Fpnas.2201327119fig04.jpg&f=1&nofb=1&ipt=1e93107fd8b4857df040a6a029d4d260f8bc241ca164762f25f138cf2144d713.

Overview of Key Concepts

Gregor Mendel's work kick-started our view of how traits are passed down through generations, a concept first explored back in the 1800s. His idea was simple: when reproductive cells form, the gene variants—alleles, as we call them—split up, which explains the ratios we eventually see in offspring. In most cases, one trait doesn't mess with another because of what's now known as independent assortment. These basic notions help us get why so much genetic variety exists; they're not just academic—they matter in everyday fields like farming and medicine, where breeding and genetic tweaks shape practical outcomes. Another piece of the puzzle is alleles, the different versions of a gene that each person inherits—one from their mother and one from their father. This can lead to countless possibilities. Often, a dominant allele will completely hide the recessive one, so the outward trait (or phenotype) might show only the strong aspect. This kind of back-and-forth contributes heavily to the mix of characteristics we see in populations, and, in most cases, it's crucial for predicting what gets passed on. Increasingly, even in clinics, genetic testing is being used to diagnose better and treat issues, sharpening our view of genetic disorders

(Kessler, 2025). Population genetics takes these fundamentals a step further by examining how allele counts change over many generations. Here, factors such as mutation, migration, and natural selection—yes, all in a bit of a jumbled interplay—keep the genetic pool lively and ever-changing. These shifting patterns, in most cases, help shape the overall genetic landscape and even nudge evolution along. Mendelian inheritance, then, isn't just a neat idea from a textbook; it stands as a building block for understanding the messy complexity of biological systems. Many educators and researchers emphasize the importance of understanding these concepts, thereby bridging the gap between classical genetic principles and modern applications in both evolutionary biology and medicine (Iglesias-Ramas et al., 2024).

11.1. Gregor Mendel's Experiments

Gregor Mendel's experiments are often oversimplified in classrooms, leaving a distorted view of his trailblazing work in genetics. Instead of showing the messy, real-life process of inheritance, students typically see a neat version where traits snap to alleles—as if heredity were that simple. This overly tidy picture overlooks the complex historical mix of ideas that Mendel uncovered and the profound depth of genetic inheritance. In most cases, such simplifications have been twisted further, even used by early 20th-century ideologues to back eugenics movements (Kampourakis, 2024). As a result, learners miss out on the genuine, if tangled, nature of scientific inquiry and the full scope of how traits develop. Mendel wasn't simply fussing over pea plants to expose heredity; his work was also laced with a deeper wonder about how new species might come about. Today, some revisionist historians argue that labeling him solely as a geneticist misses the point—his research explored hybridization and even flirted with the idea of creating new species, a concept that early botanists like Linnaeus had already considered. Generally speaking, Mendel was navigating a complex world where defining a species wasn't straightforward, especially when comparing varieties to entirely new species (van Dijk et al., 2023).

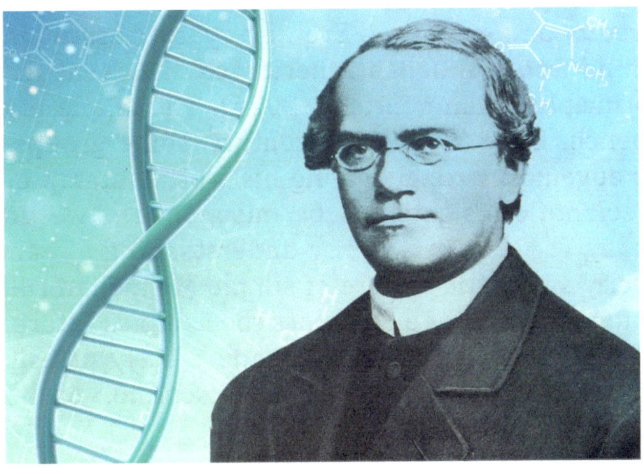

Figure 11.3. Gregor Mendel's experiments.

Source: https://external-content.duckduckgo.com/iu/?u=https%3A%2F%2Fnrgene.com%2Fwp-content%2Fuploads%2F2022%2F07%2FWhatsApp-Image-2022-07-21-at-2.12.12-PM.jpeg&f=1&nofb=1&ipt=1f2312959c855e9c412168dc9f81f4309ffd7308b9fe43420483b69784d8cb9f.

By playing around with different pea hybrids and even observing the steady patterns in hawkweeds, he peeled back layers of genetic complexity while asking far bigger questions than simple inheritance. There's also a fair amount of debate over what Mendel intended and how he set up his experiments, which tells us that context matters—a lot. Although many celebrate his contributions, his research is often lumped together in ways that overlook the unique characteristics of different species' reproductive systems. When his findings on peas are combined with later work on hawkweeds, the story becomes oversimplified, and much of the nuance is lost. Recent historical insights suggest that Mendel's original goals were more nuanced than previously believed, challenging the conventional narrative (van Dijk et al., 2023). In a way, reexamining his work reminds us that genetic research is multifaceted and that understanding science fully entails examining it within its proper, and sometimes messy, historical context (Figure 11.3).

11.1.1. Background on Gregor Mendel

Back in the mid-19th century, heredity didn't seem as random as many once assumed. An Austrian monk, Gregor Mendel, spent long hours tending to his pea plants, and his patient work quietly reshaped our grasp of how traits are passed along generations. He examined aspects such as flower color and seed shape, and in doing so, he unearthed recurring patterns that no one had previously noticed. His insights eventually pointed to ideas we now call segregation and independent assortment—simple ways to explain how bits of genetic info get sorted into gametes during reproduction. Although most of his contemporaries barely took note, his experiments later became a bedrock in biology and medical science, a lesson in how hands-on research can change our understanding of life itself (Strome et al., 2024). Mendel's work wasn't just about spotting a few clear-cut patterns; it opened up a window into the tangled nature of genetic inheritance. When he mixed and matched traits in his plants, it became apparent that characteristics arise not from a single parental gene alone but from a nuanced interplay between them. Sadly, many educational overviews have condensed his discoveries into tidy, overly simplified boxes, which somewhat obscures the whole picture. This oversimplification isn't trivial—it leads to widespread misunderstandings that warp our view of heredity and evolution. Even everyday classroom conversations sometimes miss the bigger story behind non-Mendelian inheritance, which, at its core, still rests on those original, more intricate principles (Kampourakis, 2024). The ripple effects of Mendel's research go well beyond the lab bench. Early in the 20th century, some groups cropped up who twisted his ideas into support for eugenics, wrongly giving his work a stamp of scientific authority. Such events demonstrate that scientific insights can be misapplied if we don't examine them with a broad, thoughtful lens. Today, as we gain a better understanding of genetics, there's a clear push to move away from the overly simplistic picture of simple Mendelian rules. Instead, educators and scientists alike are calling for lessons that encompass the complex interplay between development, environment, and natural selection. In this light, Mendel's early principles aren't just basic facts to be memorized—they're starting points for a richer discussion on both science and the ethics of applying it in our society (Kampourakis, 2024).

11.1.2. Methodology of Mendel's Pea Plant Experiments

Gregor Mendel's work with pea plants still stands out as a mix of strict experimentation and practical observation. He kept a tight rein on his breeding experiment, controlling every step so that even small details, such as flower color and seed shape, could be observed. Purebred lines—

usually the go-to method—helped him see that any variation in the offspring was more about genetics than the environment. Instead of following a predictable routine, he employed unexpected cross-pollination methods that allowed him to track traits over generations; over roughly eight years, this unconventional yet thorough experiment delved into the concepts of dominance and recessiveness. In most cases, his approach revealed that simple, hands-on methods can open doors to big discoveries in biology. This concept still echoes in modern studies of plant breeding and genetics (Friedt et al., 2022). Mendel also mixed a surprising amount of quantitative work into his research. He diligently counted the number of plants exhibiting specific traits from generation to generation, building a statistical case for his ideas.

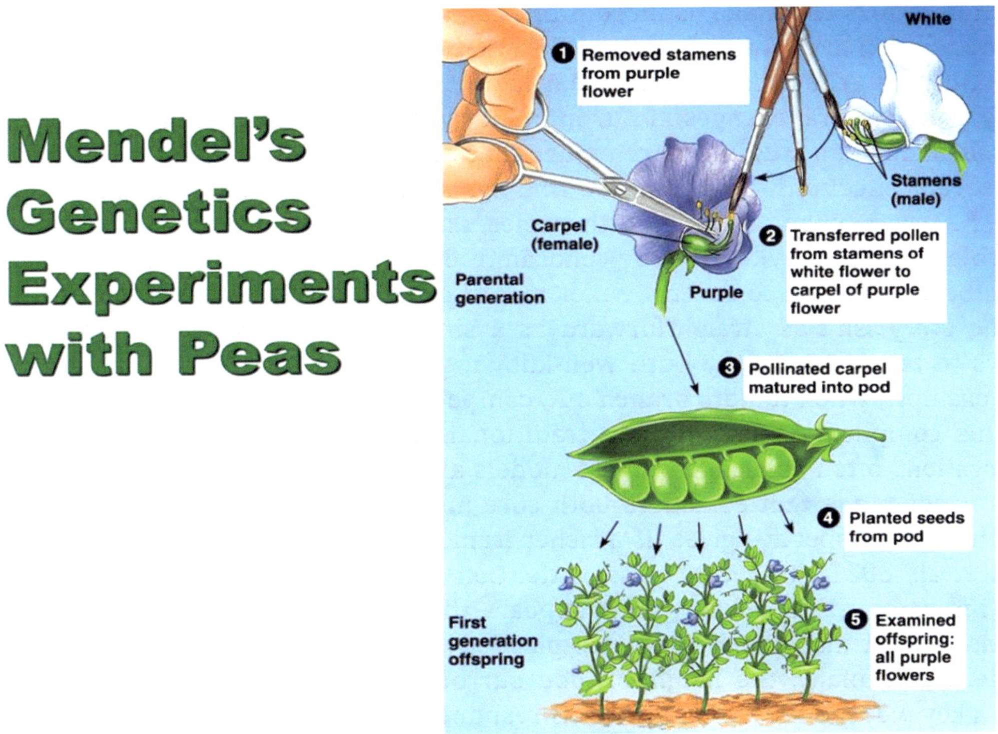

Figure 11.4. Methodology of Mendel's pea plant experiments.

Source: https://external-content.duckduckgo.com/iu/?u=https%3A%2F%2Fimage1.slideserve.com%2F3210865%2Fmendel-s-genetics-experiments-with-peas-l.jpg&f=1&nofb=1&ipt=88ab765511130534aecf650ad420115b35e012a99e36c247182d40973adcb5d8.

This careful tallying led him to ratios that practically spoke for themselves, like the classic 3:1 split of dominant to recessive traits in the F2 generation. Generally speaking, bringing math into biology not only helped solidify genetics as a real science but also paved the way for future researchers to adopt similar hands-on counting techniques. His methods, in effect, laid the groundwork for breeding techniques that now boost agricultural genetics, playing a role in crop improvement and food security (Leitão et al., 2021). It wasn't just the experiments that counted—how Mendel wrote down and shared his findings was equally influential. In his work Experiments on Plant Hybridization, he explains inherited traits in a clear, if sometimes unexpectedly casual, manner that underlined their predictability. Even though his insights weren't widely celebrated during his lifetime, the sheer rigor of his investigations inspired a rediscovery of these principles in the early 20th century, sparking further research far and wide. His painstaking planning and sometimes repetitive data recording have influenced generations of scientists. Modern genetics, while continuously evolving, still leans on the basic methods he laid out, a testament to the enduring spirit of his pioneering work (Friedt et al., 2022) (Figure 11.4).

11.1.3. Key Findings and Observations

Scientists have long been fascinated by the messy link between genetics and disease—even if it sometimes feels like untangling a knotted ball of yarn. People have discovered that, in many cases, inherited factors can make us more prone to certain illnesses, especially those troublesome infectious ones. Researchers, using both traditional methods and modern molecular techniques, have uncovered a range of genetic clues that appear to determine how our bodies respond to pathogens. Interestingly, some natural changes in our immune system show up as traits similar to those first seen in classic Mendelian studies – a reminder that tiny shifts in our genetic blueprint can nudge our risk of severe infections. Overall, these findings influence our understanding of public health and inform the development of targeted therapies, underscoring once again that our genes play a significant role in shaping who we are (Vendramin et al., 2021). Lately, the picture of Mendelian genetics has been stretched to cover a wider mix of processes driving cancer evolution. Generally speaking, the story isn't as straightforward as a simple inheritance chart; tumor development now appears to be influenced by both well-known genetic variations and other, non-Mendelian factors. For example, when tumors branch out, competing groups of cells spark unexpected genetic diversity. This complication renders the traditional, linear view of inheritance a bit too neat. These observations often challenge our old models and suggest that a more layered, multifaceted approach is needed, one that considers both core mutations and environmental factors. In most cases, this blended perspective gives us a richer framework for understanding how tumors behave (Vendramin et al., 2021). In recent years, attention has also shifted toward non-genetic factors that subtly influence cancer evolution. It appears that cancer cells can sometimes change their characteristics—what many refer to as cell plasticity—without actually altering their underlying genetic code. Additionally, the neighborhood surrounding a tumor, its microenvironment, has emerged as a key player, influencing how cells respond to mutations and even treatments. This mix of heritable and non-heritable factors prompts us to pause and reconsider the old, rigid boundaries drawn by Mendelian genetics. Taking both genetic and epigenetic influences into account may unlock new paths for diagnosis and therapy, ultimately enhancing patient care and deepening our understanding of these intricate disease mechanisms (Jean-Casanova et al., 2020).

11.2. Mendel's Laws of Inheritance

Gregor Mendel's early work with pea plants turned out to be much more influential than one might have expected. His experiments not only illuminated how traits are passed down in living things but also set the stage for what we now call Mendelian genetics. He introduced two fundamental concepts—the Law of Segregation and the Law of Independent Assortment—that, in most cases, explain how traits are transmitted from parents to offspring. These seemingly simple rules carried profound, far-reaching implications and, for many generations, guided the course of genetic research. It's interesting to note that, despite their eventual universal acceptance, these principles were mainly disregarded during Mendel's lifetime, prompting us to question how new scientific discoveries are acknowledged—or not (Muller-Wille et al., 2018). This gap between discovery and acknowledgment highlights the complexity of the dynamics within the scientific community when it comes to new theories. By the early 20th century, as the study of heredity began to evolve in unexpected ways, Mendel's ideas came back into focus. The rediscovery of his work ignited a newfound curiosity about how traits get passed on, coinciding with breakthroughs in various areas of biology. Yet even as these ideas gained traction, they also revealed some limitations. For instance, traits like human height don't fit neatly into the discrete categories Mendel originally described. Such continuous characteristics prompted scientists, generally speaking, to rethink traditional categories, eventually leading to the rise of quantitative genetics—a field that recognized the role of many genes working together. By blending Mendelian insights with statistical approaches, researchers enriched our understanding of trait inheritance, opening up new avenues in both agricultural practices and medical research (Pallares et al., 2020). Today, Mendel's contributions are undergoing a fresh round of scrutiny. Modern genome-wide studies show that, more often than not, most traits are controlled by a host of genes rather than by a single, neat factor. Models like the omnigenic framework suggest that nearly every expressed gene may contribute to a particular trait, which significantly challenges our earlier, simpler ideas about gene action. As this shift in perspective unfolds, the ripple effects of Mendel's early experiments extend into fields such as molecular biology and evolutionary theory, prompting scientists to reexamine established notions of genetic expression and adaptation. In many ways, the evolving take on heredity—a process that continues to surprise us—can still be traced back to those initial, foundational ideas introduced by Mendel (Pallares et al., 2020) (Figure 11.5).

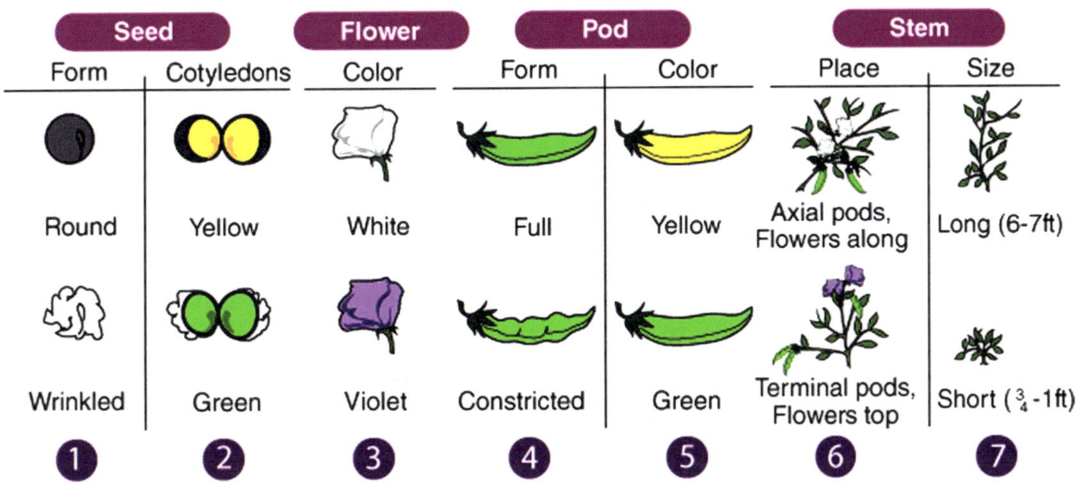

Figure 11.5. Mendel's laws of inheritance.

Source: https://cdn1.byjus.com/wp-content/uploads/2022/05/Mendels-Law-of-Inheritance.png.

11.2.1. Law of Segregation

Genetic inheritance matters a lot—think back to Mendel's pea plant trials. He noticed that certain traits kept appearing in a distinct pattern, which suggested the existence of some fundamental building blocks (we now call them alleles). Every living thing seems to come equipped with two of these, one handed down from each parent. Then, when gametes form through meiosis, these alleles split up so that each gamete only gets one copy per trait. This splitting is key for keeping genetic diversity alive; it's what gives offspring random mixes of alleles, adding that crucial variety to populations. Beyond just promoting diversity, the Law of Segregation helps to gain a better understanding of genetic disorders. When one studies how alleles separate, researchers can identify patterns in inherited diseases.

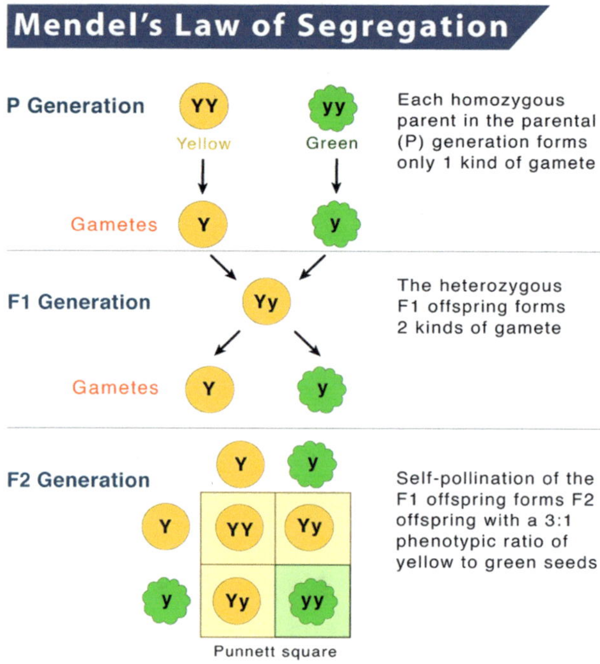

Figure 11.6. Mendel's laws of segregation.

Source: https://www.sciencefacts.net/wp-content/uploads/2022/10/Law-of-Segregation.jpg.

For example, some disorders are tied to recessive alleles, meaning one inherits a copy from both parents for symptoms to show. Generally speaking, this understanding not only supports genetic counseling but also boosts the ability to forecast these conditions within families. One could even point to recent studies on *Trypanosoma brucei*—which, interestingly enough, confirm that even in complex genetic systems, segregation still happens—thereby reinforcing Mendelian ideas across many species (Tweedie et al., 2005). Furthermore, this principle underpins many genetic research methods, particularly in designing breeding experiments. By exploiting the almost predictable way alleles separate, scientists can create tests to see specific genetic outcomes. This method enables them to fine-tune traits in both plants and animals, advancing farming and animal care. In most cases, as techniques like CRISPR evolve, a solid understanding of segregation offers vital insights for gene editing and other biotechnological endeavors. While researchers aim to modify genes with pinpoint accuracy, the basic idea of allele splitting remains relevant, guiding our understanding of how these changes unfold within groups. So, the Law of Segregation isn't just the backbone of classic Mendelian genetics—it also remains a cornerstone for new breakthroughs in genetic science (Ferguson-Smith et al., 2022) (Figure 11.6).

11.2.2. Law of Independent Assortment

Gregor Mendel's pea plant experiments turned everything upside down. His work shone a light on how traits sneak their way from one generation to the next—what we now call the Law of Independent Assortment. Instead of traits being blindly bundled together, genes for different features sort themselves out separately when gametes form. Mendel noticed this by casually tracking differences such as seed shape and flower color, and that each trait behaves independently from generation to generation.

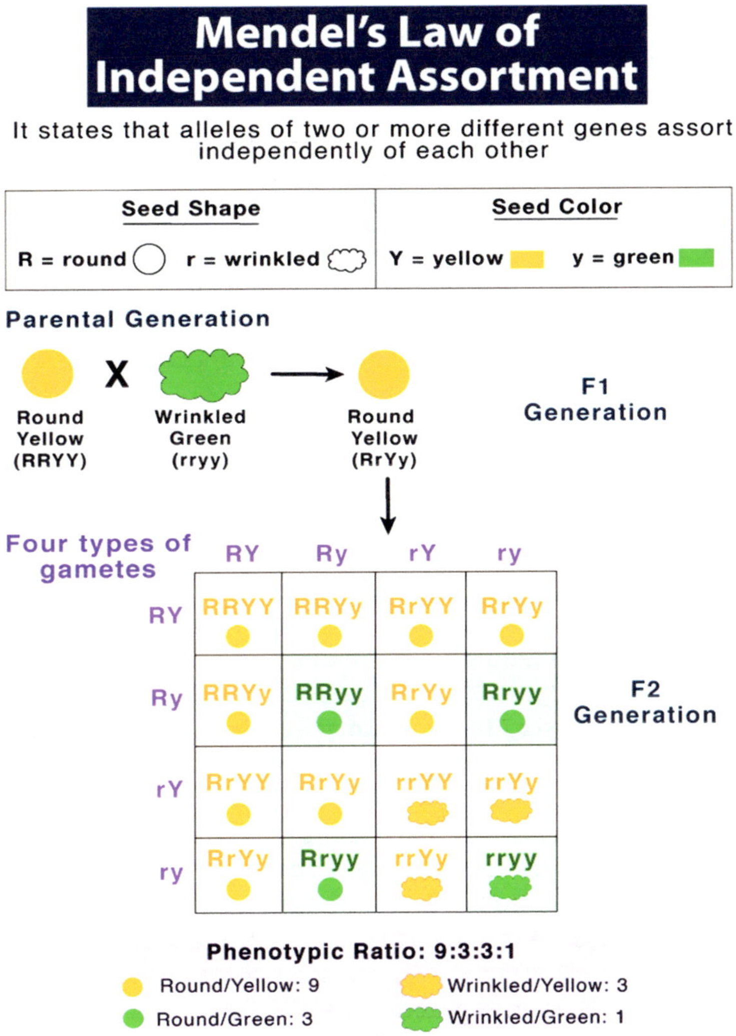

Figure 11.7. Mendel's law of independent assortment.

Source: https://www.sciencefacts.net/wp-content/uploads/2022/10/Law-of-Independent-Assortment.jpg.

This idea opened up a whole new way to look at genetic variety and laid the groundwork for understanding why we're all so different. It has also become a key part of gene mapping and breeding methods, reflecting the wild mix of hereditary combinations in sexually reproducing organisms. When studied in more depth, the Law of Independent Assortment becomes a bit more tangled. It's not just about classic Mendelian ideas; the concept has nudged scientists into exploring more complex scenarios, including gene linkage and epistasis, where genes don't always follow simple rules. In most cases, studies show that while the notion holds under neat laboratory conditions, natural genetic linkage can throw in a twist, making the whole picture a lot more nuanced. Family studies, for instance, have provided clues that our standard view may need a slight adjustment when multiple factors are at work. Generally speaking, this means we have to blend old-school Mendelian principles with fresh insights to finger the whole story behind inheritance. The impact of this law extends far beyond basic genetics, even touching on evolutionary theory. It not only helps us guess which traits might emerge, but it also aligns with broader ideas in evolutionary biology that examine how genetic differences influence survival in unpredictable environments. In most investigations, researchers find that genetic variation can influence fitness—a nod, in a sense, to those early ideas of natural selection. As new studies hint at processes such as niche construction and phenotypic plasticity, the interplay between genes and their surroundings becomes even more intriguing. So, understanding the Law of Independent Assortment isn't just a job for geneticists; it's a must for evolutionary biologists trying to unravel the messy, adaptive dance of life—as Mendel's legacy continues to surprise us all (Figure 11.7).

11.2.3. Law of Dominance

Mendel's work kickstarted a whole new way of understanding how traits are passed from one generation to the next. His pea plant experiments weren't exactly well planned; he just noticed that when different gene versions showed up together, one usually ended up hiding the other. If an organism carries two different alleles, one tends to mask its partner – a simple idea that soon came to be known as the Law of Dominance. Early on, this notion changed how many thought about the link between genetic makeup and what one sees. Over time, people working in fields such as farming and medicine adopted these ideas, using them to predict traits more easily in future generations. Beyond that basic idea, the story gets a bit more tangled. Sometimes, instead of one trait completely overruling the other, traits end up blending in a way that doesn't fit the old rules – what we now call incomplete dominance or codominance. In certain instances, heterozygous individuals can exhibit a mix of features rather than a clear dominant or recessive trait, and this subtle variation invites a lot more questioning about how genes actually interact. In most cases, as research progressed, scientists began to see hints that factors beyond simple dominance – such as epigenetic influences – might also be at play. It turns out the traditional view of one allele always taking charge isn't the whole story after all. As the science of genetics marched on, the influence of what Mendel discovered stretched into practical realms, too. Selectively breeding plants for their dominant traits led to crops that were not only high-yielding but also more resistant to disease – a pretty big deal for sustainable agriculture. Similarly, in medical genetics, understanding how dominant mutations cause disorders has enabled researchers to develop more targeted treatments and improved genetic counseling approaches for families. While Mendel's early work may seem like ancient history, his ideas continue to resonate today, blending with new discoveries and continually shaping our understanding and management of genetic inheritance in fields as diverse as biotechnology and medicine (Figure 11.8).

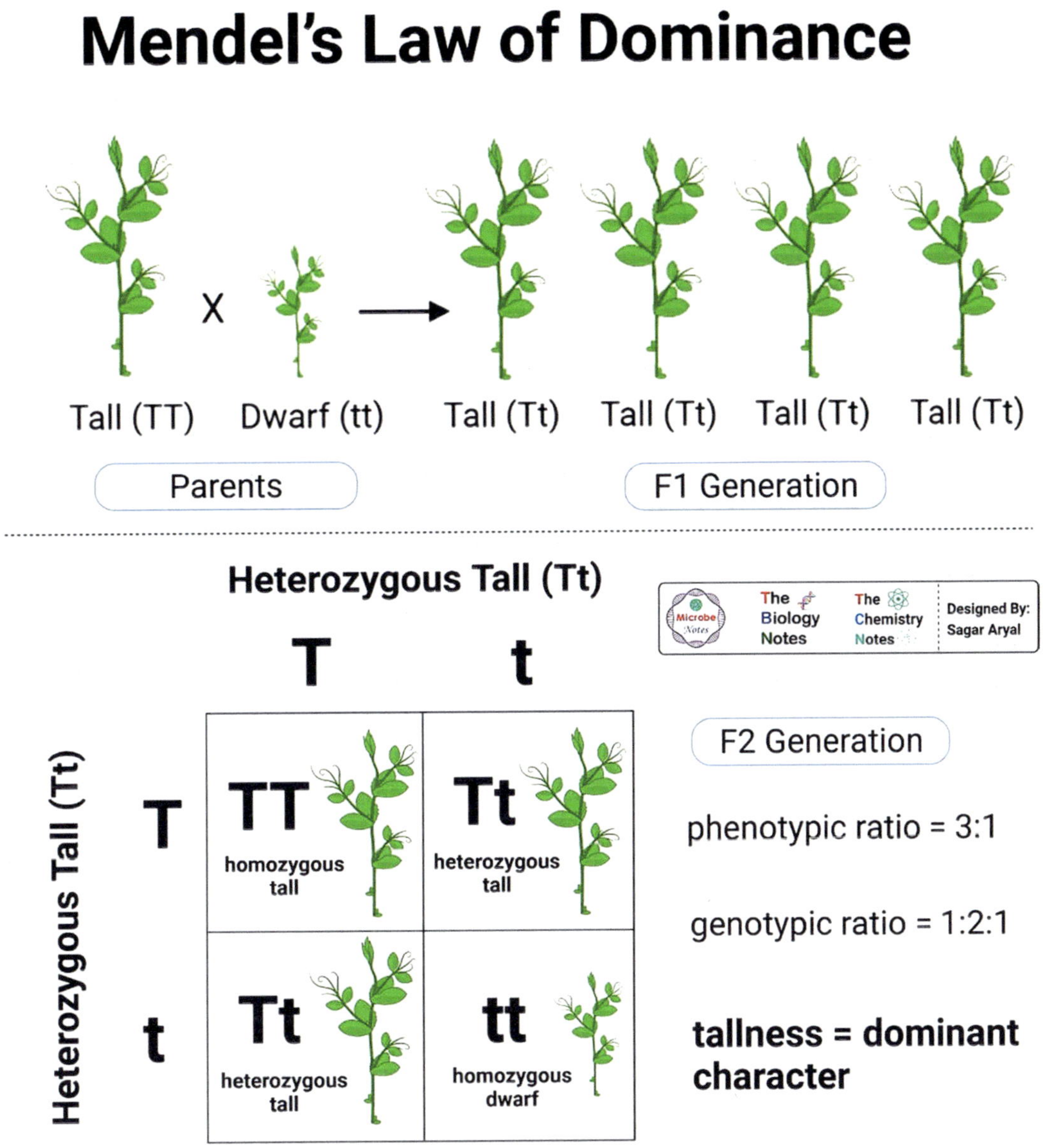

Figure 11.8. Mendel's law of dominance.

Source: https://microbenotes.com/wp-content/uploads/2021/06/Mendels-Law-of-Dominance-Pea-Plant.jpeg.

11.3. Genetic Terminology

Genetics has come a long way in how we talk about genes. Back in the early 1900s, a gene was just some fuzzy bit—a vague unit of inheritance. Then, as experiments rolled on (classical and neoclassical genetics, to be exact), that hazy idea began to sharpen. At first, scientists viewed a gene as nothing more than a dimensionless dot on a chromosome; later, they started treating it as a distinct stretch of DNA that encodes polypeptides, much like a recipe for making proteins. This entire shift demonstrates how we've transitioned from vague notions to a clearer understanding of heredity. Still, in most cases, today's high-tech research reveals that even our refined definition struggles to capture the gene's full role within the messy, larger context of the genome (Portin et al., 2017). Heterosis, often referred to as hybrid vigor, is another notable example that frequently appears, particularly in agriculture. Simply put, hybrids tend to beat their parent strains—displaying faster growth, higher yields, and a kind of extra resilience. Farmers have long cherished this trait, and it has become a linchpin in modern crop breeding. Scientists believe that the magic happens due to a combination of dominance and overdominance; in other words, being heterozygous often confers a certain advantage. Generally speaking, the lessons we learn from heterosis don't just stay on the farm. They spill over to deepen our grasp of genetic interactions and even evolutionary dynamics that shape biodiversity. It's a multifaceted idea that invites us to explore further into how genes work together—and sometimes contradict each other—in surprising ways (Mélisande et al., 2015). Trying to nail down genetic terminology means we have to look at alleles, genotypes, and phenotypes as well. Think of alleles as the different flavors a gene might take, while a genotype is more like the complete ingredient list unique to an individual. Then there's the phenotype, which is the visible outcome of that mix—the traits one can see from all those genetic ingredients interacting with the environment. This trio forms the bedrock of Mendelian genetics; classic experiments with single and double hybrids drove this point home. If they can't be differentiated, it's tough to grasp how inheritance patterns are woven together fully. And, as research continually evolves, even these definitions get revisited, underscoring just how dynamic and, dare I say, imperfect the language of genetics is (Portin et al., 2017) (Figure 11.9).

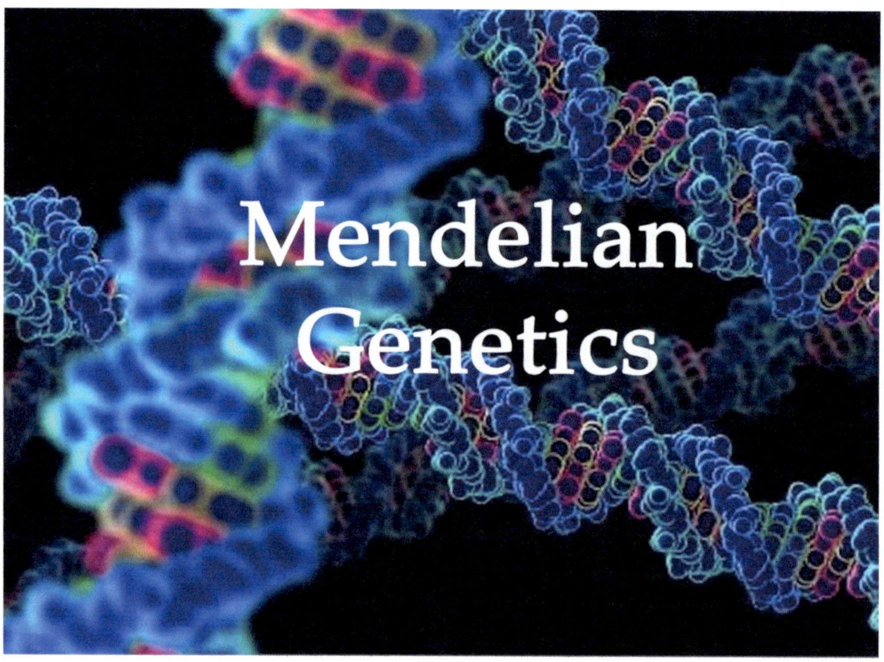

Figure 11.9.Mendelian Genetics.

Source: https://external-content.duckduckgo.com/iu/?u=https%3A%2F%2Fslideplayer.com%2F35%2F10465164%2Fbig_thumb.jpg&f=1&nofb=1&ipt=decd86a66564b17f4b773b16d19e7ad345261dcfb938adf284c86df4ad51514d.

11.3.1. Alleles and Their Types

Alleles lie at the heart of genetics, shaping how traits show up. Each person ends up with two alleles per gene—one from each parent—even though these are just slightly different versions of the same instruction. Sometimes one allele seems to overshadow the other, so that a dominant one hides its recessive mate; Mendel's classic pea plant work, for instance, made it clear that features like flower color come out because of these allele pairings. Understanding these basic variants isn't just an academic exercise—it sets the stage for breakthroughs in genetic research and biotech (Wilde et al., 2022). When studied in depth, the picture gets even more interesting. There are dominant, recessive, and co-dominant alleles. A dominant allele only needs to show up once to influence the trait, while recessive ones only have their say if there are two copies. Co-dominant alleles, however, play a different game altogether: both alleles make themselves known at the same time. It's a bit like seeing both flavors in one, something one can spot in the AB blood type, where both A and B alleles are present (Wilde et al., 2022). This mix-and-match of effects helps shed light on how traits are passed down and even on the origins of certain disorders. But genetics isn't always as tidy as simple Mendelian rules. Sometimes, a gene shows up in more than just two forms, which opens up a wider range of traits—think of the ABO blood group system that juggles A, B, and O alleles into various combinations. There are also cases where one gene interferes with another—what we often call epistasis—so that one gene's expression can dull or mask another's. These subtle but essential interactions not only boost our understanding of genetic variation and evolution but also point us toward new therapeutic paths in modern genetics (Wilde et al., 2022) (Figure 11.10).

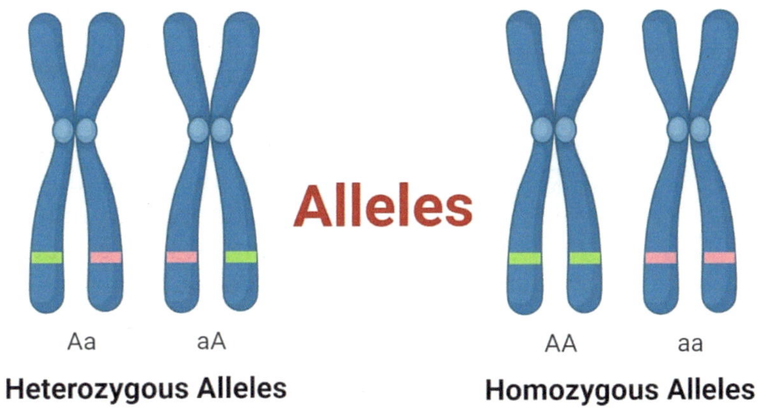

Figure 11.10. Alleles and their types.

Source: https://microbenotes.com/wp-content/uploads/2023/05/Alleles.jpg.

11.3.2. Genotype Versus Phenotype

Genetic expression is a tangled affair—a mix between inherited blueprint and the traits one ends up showing. One's genotype, which is simply the complete set of one's genetic material, sets the stage for what might appear, yet what one sees on the surface is also shaped by everyday life. Sometimes the same set of genes can lead to different outcomes when environmental conditions change; for example, an individual carrying a gene linked to a disorder might not exhibit any symptoms at all, a scenario explained by concepts such as penetrance and expressivity. In many cases, it's clear that things aren't always straightforward: beyond just the genes, the environment also leaves its mark on what traits emerge. In addition to the basic Mendelian view, things become even more interesting with the introduction of modifier genes and oligogenic factors. These modifier genes can alter the influence of other genes, so that even individuals with identical genetic blueprints may exhibit different traits. And then, everyday factors—what one eats, how one lives, and even exposure to pollutants—can also play a significant, sometimes unexpected, role. A recent study even pinpointed various loci associated with daytime napping and linked these genetic findings to aspects of cardiometabolic health (Hassan et al., 2021). This mix of influences suggests that genes don't decide everything; instead, the combination of one's DNA and their environment plays a crucial role.

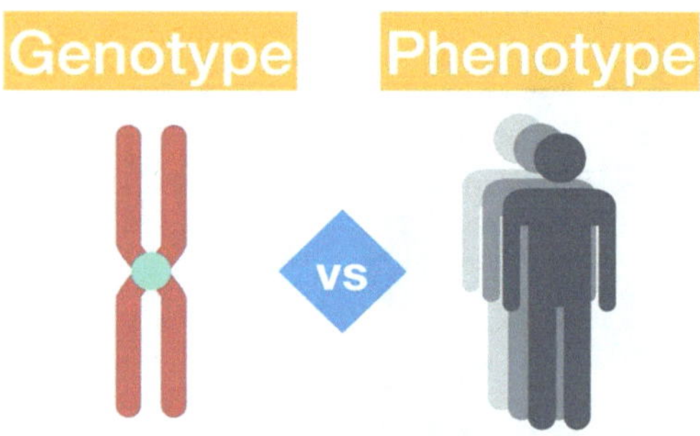

Figure 11.11. Genotype versus phenotype.

Source: https://geneticeducation.co.in/wp-content/uploads/2020/05/Genotype-vs-phenotype-.003.jpeg.

The practical side of this gets pretty important in clinical genetics and risk assessment. Genetic tests look for variants that might suggest a predisposition to disease, but finding a so-called pathogenic variant doesn't automatically mean the disease will develop, thanks to the interplay of other genetic and environmental factors. Consider inherited cardiovascular disorders: even if the genetic risk seems high, many individuals surprisingly remain unaffected. Researchers have recognized that genetic modifiers, which can sometimes worsen and at other times lessen symptoms, are key players in this scenario (Wilde et al., 2022). In most cases, understanding both the genetic setup and the external influences is crucial for creating personalized approaches to treatment and prevention, paving the way for fundamental advances in precision medicine (Figure 11.11).

11.3.3. Homozygous and Heterozygous Conditions

Traits in organisms owe a great deal to their underlying genetic makeup, which naturally falls into two categories—one where individuals have two matching copies of a gene, and another where the copies differ. When an individual has matching alleles, whether dominant or recessive, the traits typically manifest predictably, echoing traditional Mendelian principles. Yet, if the alleles differ, the dominant one usually takes center stage, and this subtle twist adds a layer of complexity to how traits manifest. In short, the mix-up between these allelic forms sets the stage for understanding how traits get passed on, why there's so much genetic variety, and even hints at how evolution might roll along. It isn't just about straightforward trait expression either—these genetic states spill over into how populations function. Generally speaking, individuals with different alleles often have a natural edge in varied environments, thanks to what one might call a broader genetic toolkit that fuels adaptability. For example, studies on the malaria vector *Anopheles gambiae* have shown that when gene drives disrupt both copies of a gene, such as *doublesex*, it can lead to reproductive troubles in females (Kyrou et al., 2018). These insights emphasize that while having identical alleles can make things a bit more predictable, having a mix usually enhances resilience and evolutionary potential in a changing world. Upon closer examination, the distinction between homozygous and heterozygous conditions reveals why maintaining a diverse gene pool is essential for long-term species survival. In agriculture and conservation, this type of genetic knowledge guides breeding strategies aimed at creating more robust and adaptable populations. For instance, if one is trying to grow crops that fight off disease, using plants with different alleles might help them cope better with challenges. On the flip side, a heavy dose of identical alleles can sometimes lead to inbreeding depression—slightly lowering overall fitness and leaving populations more open to environmental pressures. Balancing these genetic states, then, is key for intelligent management and conservation, making a strong case for ongoing research in Mendelian genetics to fine-tune our strategies (François Mach et al., 2019) (Figure 11.12).

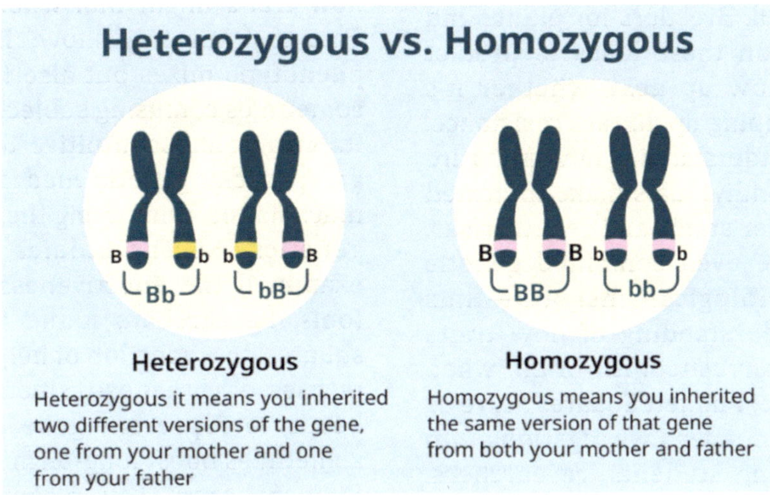

Figure 11.12. Homozygous and heterozygous conditions.

Source: https://www.verywellhealth.com/thmb/UjJ6pepg2ZmUVYptgUizL52-WE4=/1500x0/filters:no_upscale():max_bytes(150000):strip_icc()/EVERGREEN-Heterozygousvs.HomozygousWhat_stheDifference_txt-1-75c4ae6000a946b4969935d21686171e.jpg.

11.4. Punnett Squares and Genetic Predictions

Genetics begins with understanding how traits are passed down, and Punnett Squares are a helpful tool that helps us visualize potential outcomes. They work by crossing alleles from parents in a step-by-step fashion, allowing both researchers and students to predict outcomes in terms of genotypes and phenotypes. It's pretty straightforward—whether one is looking at one-trait (monohybrid) situations or juggling two traits (dihybrid)—and studies generally show that tools like these can boost how well students stick with the tougher ideas in Mendelian genetics (Akpan et al., 2025). That easy-to-see picture of genetic ratios ends up laying the groundwork for diving into even more tangled genetic patterns, so it's no wonder they're still a big deal in both school and lab discussions. At the same time, the strength of Punnett Squares isn't just about the basics. They shed light on key concepts such as dominance, recessiveness, and independent assortment. This visual method helps students get a good feel for tricky concepts like heterozygosity and homozygosity—stuff that can sometimes seem a bit abstract. For example, when there is a classic

3:1 ratio that appears in a monohybrid cross, it makes the entire genetic setup a bit more tangible. Some recent findings even suggest that incorporating hands-on tools with these squares might better solidify Mendelian principles (Akpan et al., 2025). Generally speaking, these fresh twists help educators spark a deeper understanding of how traits come together, setting the stage for more advanced biology adventures. Beyond classrooms and textbooks, these squares have practical applications in the real world as well. Breeders for plants and animals often lean on these ideas to predict which traits will show up next, whether it's boosting yield or ramping up disease resistance. In human genetics, understanding how traits are passed on can help individuals make informed decisions about carrier status and genetic risks. Several studies have even combined genetic data with epidemiological insights—thus broadening our understanding of how traits and diseases are interrelated. All in all, when theory meets practice, Punnett Squares serve as a launching pad for deeper investigations into inheritance, providing students, researchers, and professionals alike with the tools they need to navigate the often complex web of genetic prediction (Figure 11.13).

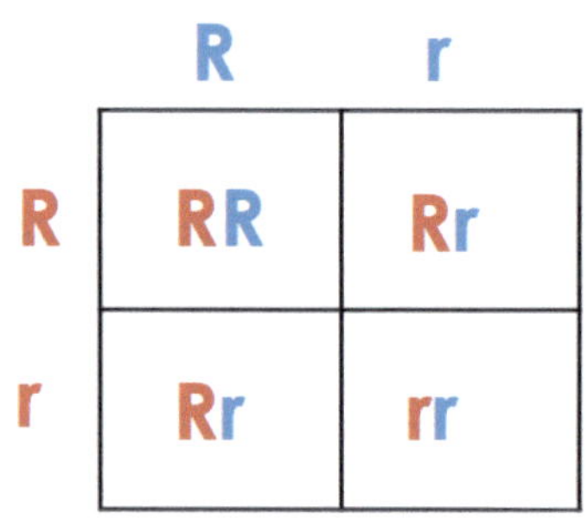

Figure 11.13. Punnett squares and genetic predictions.

Source: https://i0.wp.com/allinonehighschool.com/wp-content/uploads/2018/01/geneticsseedprobsoln.png?resize=369%2C326&ssl=1.

11.4.1. Introduction to Punnett Squares

Gregor Mendel's work with pea plants kickstarted our journey into understanding inheritance. He wasn't fussing over complicated models—instead, his simple experiments revealed core ideas that still shape how we look at genetics. His clever approach eventually led to the creation of what we now call the Punnett square, a handy diagram for seeing how traits might mix when organisms breed. This tool not only shows likely genotype and phenotype mixes but also helps break down a sometimes confusing subject into digestible bits. Its clear, almost intuitive design lets students grasp tricky genetic mechanisms without too much hassle, reinforcing the basics of Mendelian genetics. Recent studies, in general, have examined the effectiveness of these teaching tools. Researchers found that while Punnett squares do a good job of helping to solve genetic puzzles, other hands-on methods—such as using beads to represent gene combinations—can sometimes boost long-term memory even more. In many cases, this means that even though the squares provide a solid foundation, they may not be sufficient for every student over time. This mix of outcomes encourages teachers to blend different strategies in the classroom, accommodating varied learning styles and keeping students engaged in this ever-evolving field of genetics (Akpan et al., 2025). Beyond crunching numbers, the Punnett square pushes budding scientists to think critically and solve problems creatively. When learners experiment with different gene pairings, they slowly begin to notice subtle nuances in how traits get passed on. Although relying mainly on single-gene models can oversimplify things at times, these foundational ideas still serve as a gateway for deeper exploration. With the modern world of genetics presenting increasingly complex challenges that, in many cases, ruffle Mendel's traditional views, it's more important than ever for educators to weave together classic concepts and recent advances carefully. This balanced approach ensures that students gradually build a well-rounded, evolving picture of genetic inheritance (Robert, 2023) (Figure 11.14).

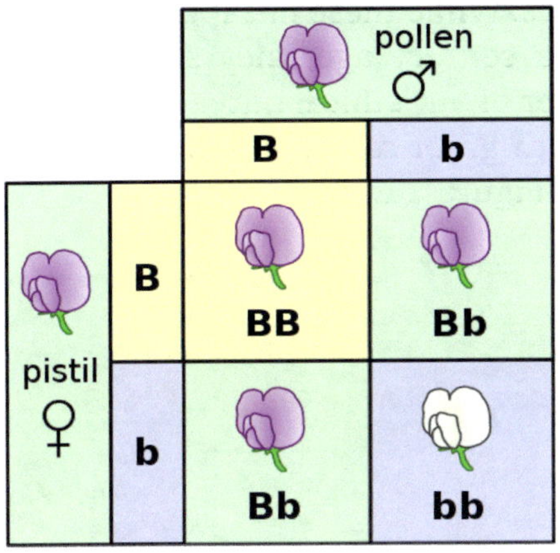

Figure 11.14. Punnett squares intro.

Source: https://kaiserscience.wordpress.com/wp-content/uploads/2018/01/punnett-square-mendel-wikipedia.png.

11.4.2. Examples of Monohybrid Crosses

Mendelian genetics comes alive when a simple monohybrid cross is seen—just one trait tracked over a few generations. Take a case where a completely dominant pea plant (TT) meets a purely recessive one (tt); the first group of offspring, or F1 generation, all turn out to be heterozygous (Tt). Then, when these F1 plants self-fertilize, an F2 group is seen in which roughly three plants show the dominant trait and one shows the recessive, a ratio that neatly mirrors basic genetic transmission. This straightforward pattern, showcasing dominant and recessive alleles, captures, in a practical way, the heart of Mendel's ideas. Shifting the scene a bit, similar ideas come up in other species—maize, for instance. One study examined the genetic relationship between silkless and tassel seed traits by crossing specific mutant genes with subtropical inbreds. The findings generally confirmed that the characteristics followed a single-gene, or monogenic, pattern, with F2 progenies segregating as expected. However, the research also uncovered hints of more complex interactions, such as recessive epistasis in certain allele combinations. In effect, these mono-hybrid crosses not only echo classical inheritance patterns but also reveal extra layers of complexity that help breeders refine crop traits (Zunjare et al., 2024).

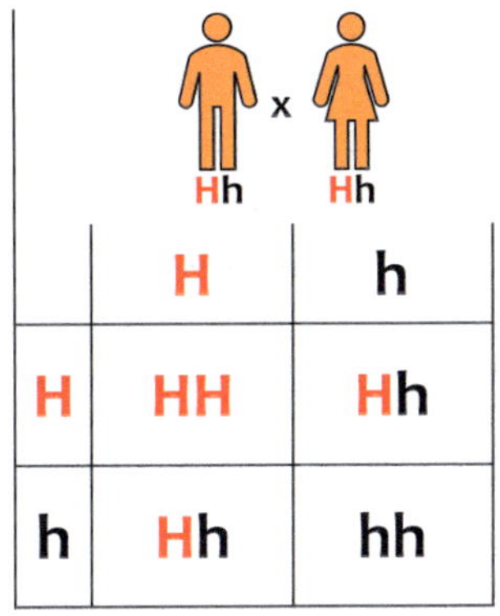

Figure 11.15. Monohybrid crosses.

Source: https://external-content.duckduckgo.com/iu/?u=https%3A%2F%2Fstudy.com%2Fcimages%2Fmultimages%2F16%2Fhet_x_het_4502983340502508845725.png&f=1&nofb=1&ipt=f055a41f89214aeaf7bf35b98d53637a37815fe508aec6d2f84f0c8d60aeabd1.

At the same time, it's important to remember that these neat models only scratch the surface of how genes work in the real world. Most traits in many organisms are influenced by several genes—a scenario known as polygenic inheritance—which disrupts the straightforward 3:1 ratio we observe in these basic crosses. This kind of oversimplification, while useful for getting started, can lead some (or even students) to think that a single gene drives complex traits mistakenly. As noted in some pedagogical critiques, focusing too much on these simple crosses might unintentionally promote a deterministic view of genetics, sometimes overlooking the real impact of environmental factors (Robert, 2023). In most cases, a richer, more layered perspective is needed to truly appreciate the messiness of biological inheritance (Figure 11.15).

11.4.3. Examples of Dihybrid Crosses

Genetic inheritance has been studied by many researchers over time, and one approach that stands out is the dihybrid cross. It illustrates how two different traits are passed along simultaneously, providing insight into how genes combine their alleles. Take pea plants, for example—Mendel kept a careful watch on features like seed shape and color. He observed that these traits ultimately combined in a way that produced a fairly predictable pattern; in most cases, the F2 generation exhibits the classic 9:3:3:1 ratio. This ratio comes from alleles sorting themselves out independently during gamete formation, rather than sticking together in a fixed pattern. Even though the experiment looks simple, it set the stage for all the more complicated genetic studies that followed. Scientists didn't stop at peas, either. They later applied dihybrid crosses to other organisms, with fruit flies (*Drosophila melanogaster*) becoming a favorite model. Thanks to their fast life cycles and relatively straightforward genetics, these little critters let researchers explore traits like eye color and wing shape in a very hands-on way. Often, the results mirror what Mendel originally predicted, which only serves to boost confidence in this method. By combining the traditional approaches of classical genetics with modern molecular tools, these studies demonstrate both the strength of Mendelian principles and their application in addressing complex genetic questions (Gramates et al., 2022). There's, however, a darker side to the history of dihybrid crosses. Back in the early 20th century, certain folks twisted these genetic ideas to support biased and discriminatory ideologies. For instance, figures like Charles B. Davenport misused the concept of dihybrid crosses to back unfounded claims about supposed disharmony in interracial unions. This misuse of genetic theory—often glossed over in textbooks—serves as a cautionary tale about how scientific ideas can be corrupted when mixed with social prejudice. While these misapplications occurred nearly a century ago, they serve as a general reminder of our ethical duty to interpret genetic data with great care and responsibility (Mark, 2018) (Figure 11.16).

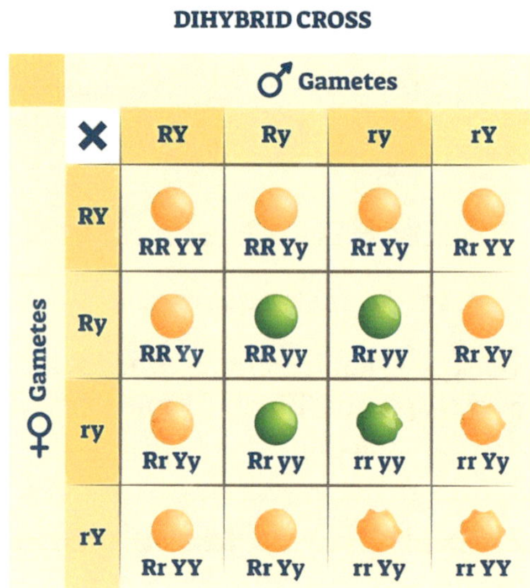

Figure 11.16. Dihybrid crosses.

Source: https://external-content.duckduckgo.com/iu/?u=https%3A%2F%2Fas1.ftcdn.net%2Fv2%2Fjpg%2F03%2F40%2F61%2F40%2F1000_F_340614035_1FjXsxkQqokmm9WK5C3qN0R1zrYd03as.jpg&f=1&nofb=1&ipt=d235391b14c13ce978ae255166cd7acb48e403bf11d7321419a71e7fd5170434.

11.5. Extensions of Mendelian Genetics

Genetic inheritance isn't what it used to be. Old Mendelian rules—simple, one-gene ideas—have taken a back seat to a more complex picture, where several alleles interact to shape complex traits. In most cases, traits and diseases aren't ruled by a single gene; instead, they come from a jumble of genetic cues that make each case a little different. High-throughput genotyping now enables scientists to delve into genome-wide association studies (GWAS) that explore these complexities. This work, which has ramped up our insight into pinpointing specific variants behind complex traits, is a game-changer for personalized medicine. Look at resources like the GWAS Catalog—they're sometimes messy but remain a vital resource in ongoing research (Buniello et al., 2018). New methods have further advanced our understanding of genetic links—often through a technique known as Mendelian randomization. Using data pulled from GWAS, researchers can apply what's known as two-sample Mendelian randomization (2SMR) to tease out cause-and-effect between traits, sidestepping the need for individual-level data. This clever approach helps avoid biases that often arise in observational work and delves deeper into genuine associations. That said, its success hinges on the quality of the GWAS data, which can be hit or miss. Platforms like MR-Base step in to bundle curated results, allowing scientists to sift through millions of potential links while running sensitivity tests that, in most cases, strengthen the entire analysis (Hemani et al., 2018). All in all, these twisty extensions of Mendelian genetics mark a shift in the field, melding good old genetic ideas with modern computing power. The way genetic variants get wedded to complex traits highlights a need for a team effort—bringing together data science, biology, and computer modeling in a refreshingly unpredictable way. As these innovations continue to evolve, their impact on clinical practice becomes increasingly pronounced, hinting at a future where therapies are tailored to an individual's unique genetic makeup. Blending traditional genetics with today's technology and massive databases, scientists are chipping away at the tangled web of heredity, reshaping how we see disease and design treatment strategies.

11.5.1. Incomplete Dominance

Genetic inheritance isn't as straightforward as old textbooks might have us believe—take incomplete dominance, for instance. Often, instead of one trait completely masking the other, heterozygous genes produce a sort of intermediate result, a blend of both extremes. A red flower can be crossed with a white flower and unexpectedly end up with pink blooms; both alleles chip in rather than one taking over completely. This mixed outcome not only muddles our predictions about appearance but also highlights the varied gene expression that can occur among plants and animals, sometimes hinting at evolutionary adaptations that help species adjust to shifting environments. Incomplete dominance also tends to blur the neat lines of traditional Mendelian rules. Generally speaking, while Mendel's early work set up a solid starting point, it didn't capture every twist of inheritance. Researchers eventually noticed that what we call "dominance" isn't etched in stone—it can change when different genetic backgrounds come into play, with several loci working together in unpredictable ways. Studies on variable dominance even suggest that epistatic interactions can alter how a trait ultimately manifests (Bank et al., 2023). In this messy real-world scenario, the tidy models of classical genetics give way to a far more intertwined narrative. Realizing that traits sometimes mix in unexpected ways forces us to reconsider the foundations of heredity. Critics of strict Mendelian genetics once pointed out that these odd cases were proof of its limits (Gliboff et al., 2015). In a sense, those nonconforming examples sparked fresh avenues of research, prompting scientists to expand on Mendel's initial ideas rather than dismiss them outright. As modern genetics steadily uncovers new layers, recognizing incomplete dominance encourages a deeper and more nuanced understanding of how life adapts. Although the path isn't perfectly linear—and, true to form, there are a few rough edges—it ultimately helps us understand the dynamic forces behind evolution and speciation (Figure 11.17).

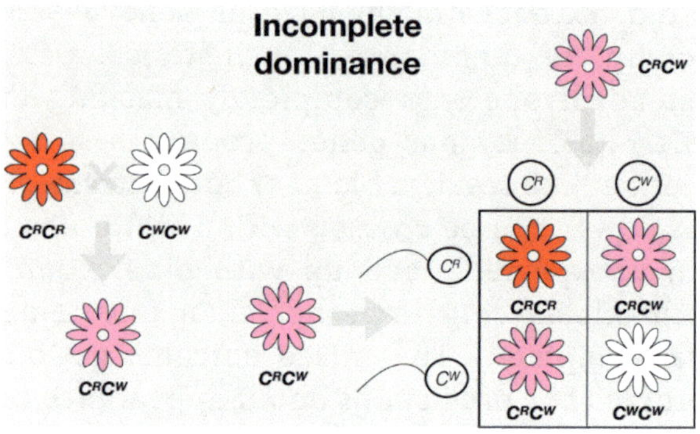

Figure 11.17. Incomplete dominance.

Source: https://external-content.duckduckgo.com/iu/?u=https%3A%2F%2Fslcc.pressbooks.pub%2Fapp%2Fuploads%2Fsites%2F20%2F2021%2F02%2FIncomplete-Dominance-1536x952.png&f=1&nofb=1&ipt=798e46b74c99dc3756908d1b5b32a62e0a34542cddbbd7187d169e78045e5ddb.

11.5.2. Codominance

Codominance is a notable concept in Mendelian genetics. Instead of the usual picture where one allele overshadows the other, both alleles end up showing up in the final trait. like in blood types. For instance, consider the ABO system: if an individual has both IA and IB, their blood type is classified as AB, which has both A and B antigens on their red blood cells. This type of dual display prompts us to reconsider the notion that genes always act in a straightforward, binary manner. Even though codominance rarely gives us the classic Mendelian ratios, it still runs under the same basic rules of segregation and independent assortment during gamete formation (Strome et al., 2024). To understand codominance, it's helpful to distinguish it from concepts like incomplete dominance and polygenic inheritance. In many cases, codominance deepens our understanding of genetic expression because it shows how each allele can contribute equally, rather than one allele remaining in the background. This idea aligns well with discussions in molecular biology, where interactions occur at various levels, ranging from molecules to whole genomes – a combination that effectively influences the traits we observe. Generally speaking, peeling back these layers reveals how finely balanced our genetic setup is. As a result, codominance highlights the multi-layered nature of inheritance, making it clear that we need ongoing updates to our teaching resources to keep the picture accurate (Selcen, 2023). Beyond theory, codominance has real, hands-on impacts in areas like medicine and agriculture. In medicine, understanding codominance can significantly impact determining blood compatibility for transfusions or organ transplants, as the presence of both blood antigens can affect patient outcomes. In agriculture, a solid grasp of codominance helps in developing crops that harness beneficial features from both parent lines—leading to hybrids that may be more resistant to diseases or richer in nutrients. This practical edge highlights why accurately capturing the details of genetic expression is crucial for real-world applications. In short, codominance fits neatly within the broader framework of Mendelian genetics, while also advancing both scientific research and everyday practices (Strome et al., 2024) (Figure 11.18).

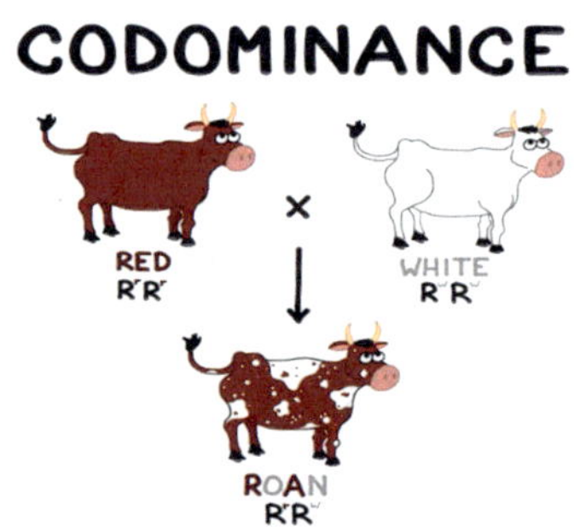

Figure 11.18. Codominance.

Source: https://external-content.duckduckgo.com/iu/?u=https%3A%2F%2Fi.pinimg.com%2Foriginals%2F0f%2Faa%2F1f%2F0faa1fe0395809172c6ee5627215c606.jpg&f=1&nofb=1&ipt=5b5f808210b3f045b4c94bfb2c26fa38b6b5a5d8a7b33fbb11fbe69f92800094.

11.5.3. Multiple Alleles

In genetics, a tiny change at a single gene spot can yield a bunch of different alleles, and that spices up our overall genetic mix. Instead of the old two-allele rule from Mendel, there's a messier scene at play where several alleles mix things up. The ABO blood system, for instance, alleles IA, IB, and i can combine in various ways to give rise to A, B, AB, or even O blood types. Often, the traits that show up depend on the blend inherited from both parents. This process makes those multiple alleles even more interesting by deepening our understanding of trait passage, as outlined by classical Mendelian ideas. Having several alleles circulating tends to complicate the inheritance map and the way traits manifest, which, generally speaking, provides a better insight into developmental biology. Different allelic forms sometimes result in scenarios such as incomplete dominance or codominance, where no single allele always prevails. One might notice that occasionally unexpected trait combinations show up– just as the varied color schemes of snapdragon flowers hint at. This kind of complexity underscores why we often need to draw on different fields, combining molecular biology insights with studies of visible characteristics. Ultimately, when multiple alleles interact, they disrupt the tidy Mendelian classification system and prompt researchers to explore the roles of polygenic inheritance and environmental cues. Recently, the dance between multiple alleles has gained even more significance in modern genetics, particularly in studies of populations and evolutionary trends. Variants spread across genes can help groups adapt to ever-changing environments – a key driver of natural selection. For example, allele frequencies in human populations often mirror local adaptations, such as how some individuals cope with malaria. The sickle cell allele, in particular, exhibits a complex and fascinating interplay between our genes and our surroundings. Recent genomic breakthroughs, such as whole-exome sequencing, have made it easier to examine these shifts closely, thereby sharpening our understanding of how complex traits function. As we continue to unravel the story behind multiple alleles, it becomes clear that they're not just markers on a page, but crucial players in health and disease, linking back to the roots of Mendelian genetics in many profound ways (Wilde et al., 2022).

11.6. Applications of Mendelian Genetics

Mendelian genetics has advanced our understanding of genetic variation in some surprising ways that ripple throughout modern science. GWAS are a clear example—they enable researchers to pinpoint genetic markers associated with specific traits or diseases. Testing large groups against hundreds of thousands of variants suddenly reveals robust links that shed light on how traits are passed on and what they might mean for our overall health. In most cases, these findings not only refine genetic risk assessments but also suggest possible cause-and-effect relationships that inform drug discovery efforts. As GWAS continually get fine-tuned, they remind us that the good old Mendelian ideas still play a significant role in unraveling the complex biology behind various diseases and traits (Uffelmann et al., 2021). Then there's DisGeNET, which reveals another aspect of how classical genetics intersects with today's genomic medicine. This platform combines data on disease-linked genes and their variants, essentially creating a one-stop resource that brings genetic research closer to real-world medical applications. It covers a wide range of human diseases and traits by blending expert insights with automated reviews of scientific literature, sometimes in ways that feel almost serendipitous. Generally speaking, this type of integration leads to a better understanding of how genes contribute to disease processes, helping us connect those genetic dots to clearer clinical outcomes. Plus, the tools DisGeNET offers simplify the whole process—from pulling in data to analyzing it for use in genomic medicine and drug research and development (Jñero et al., 2019). These advances shake things up, especially in personalized medicine where knowing a patient's unique genetic makeup can tailor treatments on the fly. By leveraging Mendelian genetics, doctors are better equipped to plan treatments, predict how an individual might react to a drug, and even avoid unwanted side effects. This individualized approach not only enhances patient outcomes but also encourages healthcare to become more proactive. As we peel back more layers of how our genes influence health, it's becoming clear that those time-tested genetic principles are key to revamping medical practice. In a blend of solid foundational ideas and modern technology, the promise of personalized care is poised to reshape our understanding of health and disease management.

11.6.1. Plant and Animal Breeding

Plant and animal breeding has a long, complex history that owes a great deal to those early insights into genetics—Mendel's ideas, even if no one knew it at the time. Early breeders, without all the fancy terminology, just kept picking plants and animals for traits that seemed to work, almost by accident. In most cases, they were following what later came to be understood as Mendel's laws. Once scientific minds began to accept these genetic clues, a more orderly way of breeding started taking shape, even if the shift wasn't sudden or perfectly neat. Mendel's discoveries, in a way, cleared up the mess about how traits show up in offspring and gave farmers and ranchers a bit more confidence to work with nature. That old, hands-on experience not only molded traditional breeding practices but also set the stage for modern biotechnical tricks that tweak genetic blueprints to achieve the desired results. New genomic technologies have significantly shaken up the breeding scene in plants and animals. These days, genomic prediction comes into play—an approach that directly determines an individual's genetic potential from their genome. This means there's no need to dig deep into endless pedigrees. In large groups, such as the well-studied Soay sheep (for instance), this method has proven its worth by pinpointing traits linked to key genetic loci, even when some genes appear to have little or no effect at all. Breeders now piece together the entire picture by weighing both major players and minor contributors, making the process more efficient overall. As these techniques mature—albeit not without a few quirks—their reach is even extending into wild populations, offering fresh angles on genetic research.

In short, combining genomic prediction with traditional methods accelerates breeding while maintaining a balanced mix of genetic diversity and ecosystem health (Ashraf et al., 2020; Ashraf et al., 2021). Looking at things from an evolutionary perspective, these advances stretch far beyond the farm. Researchers are increasingly applying genomic prediction to wild organisms to gain a better understanding of the genetic factors that influence survival and reproduction. Generally speaking, this move towards molecular quantitative genetics is a game-changer because it cuts down on the need for vast amounts of field data or deep family histories, which used to hold studies back. The ability to quickly check genetic traits—even if it sometimes feels a bit rough—allows scientists to delve into adaptive evolution under shifting environments. And when one considers how breeding practices interact with natural ecosystems, it becomes clear that there's room for innovative conservation tactics. Ultimately, whether it involves farmland or wildlife reserves, managing genetic resources now relies on a combination of traditional practices and modern molecular insights (Ashraf et al., 2020; Ashraf et al., 2021) (Figure 11.19).

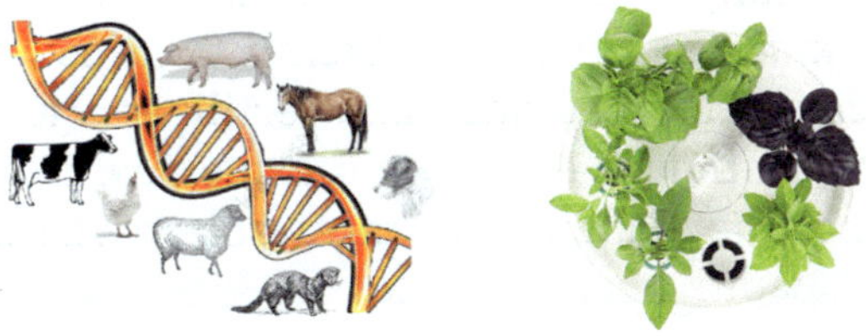

Figure 11.19. ***Plant and Animal Breeding.***

Source: https://www.bookmyessay.com/wp-content/uploads/2018/10/Selective-Breeding-in-Animals-and-Plants.png.

11.6.2. Human Genetic Disorders

Genetic mutations and inherited disorders get tangled in ways that aren't always obvious—even though Mendelian genetics still seems to offer a helpful clue. Take non-obstructive azoospermia (NOA) for example; this condition, where no sperm show up in the ejaculate, is a clear sign of underlying genetic issues. In approximately 20% of cases, specific recessive mutations can be identified as the culprits (Nagirnaja et al., 2022). It's interesting how these cases hint at a far more complicated genetic picture than we once thought, which, generally speaking, might call for a fresh look at how we classify these conditions. When studied in depth, genetic disorders, particularly loss-of-function variants, start to emerge as strong signals that some genes are indispensable. Researchers, by pooling vast amounts of genomic data, have uncovered a host of these predicted loss-of-function changes—each one offering another piece of the Mendelian puzzle. By examining genetic information from large groups of individuals, scientists identify which genes are essential for normal function and which ones can tolerate a certain level of variability without noticeable side effects (Konrad et al., 2020). This method not only sharpens our insight into well-known disorders but also opens up unexpected avenues for discovering new genetic influences behind both common and rare diseases. These findings extend far beyond categorizing disorders into tidy categories; they pave the way for targeted treatments and more nuanced genetic counseling. When clinicians gain a solid understanding of the Mendelian patterns underlying these conditions, they're better equipped to explain risks and even the possibility that certain conditions may be inherited within families. And with breakthroughs in gene editing and the rise of personalized medicine, there's hope for interventions that tackle the genetic roots head-on. As researchers gradually untangle the intricate interplay between environment and our genes, it's becoming clear that this mix is vital for an individual's health, underscoring the importance of Mendelian genetics in both everyday clinical decisions and broader health policies (Figure 11.20).

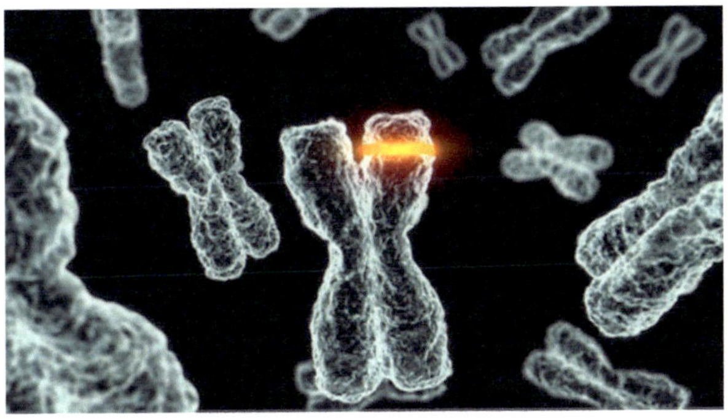

Figure 11.20. ***Human Genetic Disorders.***

Source: https://www.genome.gov/sites/default/files/4.2.5.19_Fragile_X_Syndrome.jpg.

11.6.3. Biotechnology and Genetic Engineering

Agriculture has undergone significant changes over the years—it's no longer just about adhering to traditional Mendelian genetics. Scientists today work right at the gene level, tweaking bits of DNA with a kind of precision that wasn't even imagined a few decades back. They're now able to build resistance against pests and tough weather, leading to crops that often emerge stronger and higher yielding. A mix of methods, from straightforward gene tweaks to using molecular selection markers, has given birth to many transgenic crops. In most cases, this shift means that biotech is taking center stage in tackling significant problems, such as food shortages and sustainability, while reducing the use of chemical pesticides and fertilizers (KC et al., 2021). Still, with all this promise comes some tough questions—ethical and ecological issues that just can't be swept under the rug. GMOs, for instance, have stirred debates about whether they're safe in the long run for both our environment and our health. While many believe that these modified organisms might help alleviate food scarcity and even reduce greenhouse gas emissions, others worry about a loss of biodiversity and potential health risks that could go unnoticed. Commercial interests in transgenic crops only add fuel to debates over who controls our genetic resources. It has become essential for the scientific community and decision-makers to conduct thorough risk assessments and engage in honest, open discussions about these concerns (KC et al., 2021). Lately, the picture's getting even more interesting with digital tech joining the mix. Ideas like Digital Twins are emerging—an approach that gathers detailed information about our bodies and lifestyles to create ever-changing models of individuals, effectively redrawing what "health" means on a personal scale. With these data-driven methods at work, tailored treatments seem more likely than ever, nudging us toward a new era in personalized healthcare. That said, this whole shift isn't without its complications, especially when it comes to protecting data privacy and ensuring fair access for everyone. As biotech and digital models advance, it's crucial—if not downright necessary—to balance these innovations with thoughtful discussions about ethics and equity, ultimately reshaping how we approach healthcare delivery.

SUMMARY

Mendelian genetics has long been more than just a set of rules about inheritance—it's become a gateway into practical applications in medicine and research today. Traits are passed down through generations via small genetic bits, and understanding this process allows scientists sometimes to use a method called Mendelian randomization to know how genetic quirks contribute to disease risk. This approach emerges when attempting to decipher the complex genetic origins of illnesses that result from multiple factors. In several studies, solid genetic data supporting the role of everyday lifestyle choices—such as being active or mostly sedentary—have even pointed to links with outcomes like COVID-19 hospitalization (Chen et al., 2022). All in all, the work in Mendelian genetics interweaves pure scientific inquiry with the complex challenges of real-world health issues. Blending traditional observational work with these genetic techniques provides a fresh approach to distinguishing between cause and correlation in health research. Researchers have looked into how body fat ties into heart disease risk, and in many cases, the evidence strongly suggests that obesity goes hand in hand with higher chances of various heart ailments (Kim et al., 2021). What makes this whole genetic approach stand out is its ability to tease apart associations from true cause-and-effect—a game-changer when it comes to planning public health moves and shaping policy. As the field continues to evolve, it's clear that tapping into these genetic tools is key to developing preventive strategies that can alleviate the burden of diseases rooted in our genes. The reach of Mendelian genetics stretches way beyond textbook theory. It provides today's researchers and clinicians with a solid framework for understanding how our genes influence health, paving the way toward personalized medicine and treatments tailored to individual needs. Ongoing exploration of genetic clues is steadily refining our understanding of complex disorders, sparking a richer dialogue between what happens in the lab and what unfolds in real-world clinics. Even as new health challenges emerge unexpectedly, these genetics-based methods continue to illuminate the path toward innovative ideas and improved outcomes, underscoring their vital role in the future landscape of medical research and public health strategies.

Gregor Mendel started what we now call genetics with some simple experiments using pea plants in the mid-1800s. His work uncovered a sort of natural rulebook for how traits get passed along—almost like a chance meeting order in nature. One key concept is that gene parts, or alleles, separate during gamete formation; this separation, known as segregation, means each parent contributes only one allele per trait, which explains the ratios observed in basic crosses. Then there's the idea that different characteristics, sort of on their schedule, get shuffled independently as gametes form—independent assortment, —adding a dash of variety to every new generation. All in all, these early insights form the backbone of classical genetics, allowing researchers to predict trait patterns in everything from peas to more complex organisms. There's another piece of the puzzle known as dominance. In a heterozygous mix, only the dominant allele is seen carrying out its function, totally overshadowing the recessive one—even when both alleles are there. It's kind of like a genetic tug-of-war, and in most cases, the dominant side wins, which is why some traits stay hidden. Understanding this back-and-forth opens up our view of genetic diversity. It's a concept that not only deepens our biological insights but also gets put to work in fields like agriculture, where breeders exploit these patterns to boost desired qualities in crops and livestock. Mendel's early discoveries, with all these layers, helped set the stage for today's advances in genetic research. Recently, modern studies have revitalized these classic Mendelian ideas. Research using methods like Mendelian randomization now explores how both our genes and the environment interact to shape health outcomes. For example, some investigations look at how a mother's genetic setup can subtly affect traits in her kids—proving that Mendel's basic rules still echo in today's science. This line of work is even helping to untangle complex diseases like Alzheimer's, where specific gene mutations follow those very patterns Mendel described. The blend of age-old ideas and new techniques not only deepens our understanding of genetic risk factors but also informs efforts to develop more targeted and personalized treatments, as demonstrated in recent studies (Freudenberg-Hua et al., 2018; David et al., 2019).

CLOSER LOOK

MENDELIAN RANDOMIZATION

Mendelian randomization (MR) is a method used in epidemiology and genetics to assess the causal relationship between an exposure (such as a lifestyle factor or biomarker) and an outcome (such as a disease) using genetic variants as instrumental variables. The approach relies on the principle that alleles are randomly assorted during gamete formation, by Mendel's laws, and are thus generally independent of confounding environmental factors that can bias observational studies. By leveraging this natural genetic randomization, MR aims to mimic the design of a randomized controlled trial, offering a way to infer causality from observational data where controlled experiments may not be feasible or ethical. Genetic variants, typically single-nucleotide polymorphisms (SNPs), that are robustly associated with the exposure of interest are identified through GWAS and then used as proxies to examine their effect on the outcome.

For MR to provide valid causal estimates, three core assumptions must be met: first, the genetic variants used as instruments must be strongly associated with the exposure (relevance); second, the variants must not be related to confounders of the exposure-outcome relationship (independence); and third, the variants must influence the outcome solely through their effect on the exposure, not through alternative biological pathways (exclusion restriction). Violations of these assumptions, particularly through pleiotropy (when a genetic variant affects multiple traits), can lead to biased or misleading results. To address these challenges, various MR methods and sensitivity analyses have been developed, including MR-Egger regression, weighted median approaches, and multivariable MR, all designed to detect and correct for potential violations of assumptions.

Mendelian randomization has become an increasingly popular tool in public health and biomedical research due to its ability to strengthen causal inference. For example, MR studies have been instrumental in establishing that elevated levels of low-density lipoprotein (LDL) cholesterol are causally linked to coronary artery disease, validating cholesterol as a therapeutic target. Similarly, MR has been used to challenge previously assumed causal relationships, such as questioning the protective effects of high-density lipoprotein (HDL) cholesterol on heart disease, which observational studies had suggested but MR did not support. This method has also been applied to a wide range of exposures and outcomes, from alcohol consumption and smoking to vitamin D levels, obesity, and mental health disorders.

In recent years, the availability of large-scale biobank data and high-powered GWAS has significantly enhanced the scope and precision of MR analyses. Two-sample MR, which utilizes summary statistics from separate GWAS for the exposure and outcome, has further expanded the applicability of the method, enabling researchers to investigate causal links across diverse populations and traits. Despite its strengths, Mendelian randomization is not without limitations, and careful study design and interpretation are essential to ensure valid conclusions. Nonetheless, it remains a powerful tool for advancing our understanding of the causal pathways underlying disease, guiding public health interventions, and informing drug development by identifying and validating potential therapeutic targets.

REFERENCES

1. Akpan, M. E., & Ekpo, M. O. (2025). Effects of Punnett Square and Beads teaching resources on students' retention in mendelian genetics in secondary schools in Uyo, Nigeria. *British Journal of Education, 13*(5), 84–94. https://doi.org/10.37745/bje.2013/vol13n58494Ashraf, B., Hunter, D. C., Bérénos, C., Ellis, P. A., Johnston, S. E., Pilkington, J. G., Pemberton, J. M., et al. (2021). Genomic prediction in the wild: A case study in Soay sheep. *Molecular Ecology, 31*, 6541–6555. https://doi.org/10.1111/mec.16262.
2. Ashraf, B., Hunter, D. C., Bérénos, C., Ellis, P. A., Johnston, S. E., Pilkington, J. G., Pemberton, J. M., et al. (2020). Genomic prediction in the wild: A case study in Soay sheep. *bioRxiv*. https://doi.org/10.1101/2020.07.15.205385.
3. Bank, C., & Li, J. (2023). Dominance and multi-locus interaction. *arXiv*. http://arxiv.org/abs/2310.04730 (accessed on 26 May 2025).
4. Blein-Nicolas, M., Albertin, W., da Silva, T., Valot, B., Balliau, T., Masneuf-Pomarède, I., Bely, M., et al. (2015). A systems approach to elucidate heterosis of protein abundances in yeast. *Molecular & Cellular Proteomics, 14*, 2056–2071. https://doi.org/10.1074/mcp.M115.048058.
5. Bordenstein, S. R., & Theis, K. R. (2015). Host biology in light of the microbiome: Ten principles of holobionts and hologenomes. *PLoS Biology, 13*(8), e1002226. https://doi.org/10.1371/journal.pbio.1002226.
6. Bowden, J., & Holmes, M. V. (2019). Meta-analysis and Mendelian randomization: A review. *Research Synthesis Methods, 10*, 486–496. https://doi.org/10.1002/jrsm.1346.
7. Brumpton, B., Sanderson, E., Heilbron, K., Hartwig, F. P., Harrison, S., Åberge Vie, G., Cho, Y., et al. (2020). Avoiding dynastic, assortative mating, and population stratification biases in Mendelian randomization through within-family analyses. *Nature Communications, 11*. https://doi.org/10.1038/s41467-020-17117-4.
8. Bruynseels, K., Santoni de Sio, F., & van den Hoven, J. (2018). Digital twins in health care: Ethical implications of an emerging engineering paradigm. *Frontiers in Genetics, 9*, Article 31. https://doi.org/10.3389/fgene.2018.00031.
9. Buniello, A., MacArthur, J., Cerezo, M., Harris, L. W., Hayhurst, J., Malangone, C., McMahon, A., et al. (2018). The NHGRI-EBI GWAS Catalog of published genome-wide association studies, targeted arrays and summary statistics 2019. *Nucleic Acids Research, 47*, D1005–D1012. https://doi.org/10.1093/nar/gky1120.
10. Casanova, J. L., & Abel, L. (2020). Lethal infectious diseases as inborn errors of immunity: Toward a synthesis of the germ and genetic theories. *Annual Review of Pathology: Mechanisms of Disease, 16*, 23–50. https://doi.org/10.1146/annurev-pathol-031920-101429.
11. Çelik Uzuner, S. (2023). Fine-tuning argument from the perspective of molecular biology in human. *FLSF Felsefe ve Sosyal Bilimler Dergisi*. https://doi.org/10.53844/flsf.1301688.
12. Chen, X., Hong, X., Gao, W., Luo, S., Cai, J., Liu, G., & Huang, Y. (2022). Causal relationship between physical activity, leisure sedentary behaviors and COVID-19 risk: A Mendelian randomization study. *Journal of Translational Medicine, 20*, 1–11. https://doi.org/10.1186/s12967-022-03407-6.

13. Costa, R., & Frezza, G. (2014). Crossovers between epigenesis and epigenetics. A multicenter approach to the history of epigenetics (1901–1975). https://core.ac.uk/download/144472860.pdf (accessed on 26 May 2025).

14. Dashti, H. S., Daghlas, I., Lane, J. M., Huang, Y., Udler, M. S., Wang, H., Ollila, H. M., et al. (2021). Genetic determinants of daytime napping and effects on cardiometabolic health. *Nature Communications, 12*, Article 900. https://doi.org/10.1038/s41467-020-20585-3.

15. Evans, D. M., Moen, G., Hwang, L. D., Lawlor, D., & Warrington, N. (2019). Elucidating the role of maternal environmental exposures on offspring health and disease using two-sample Mendelian randomization. *International Journal of Epidemiology, 48*, 861–875. https://www.semanticscholar.org/paper/7e5c6eadf3a8114224ce9de2a9295ce564781f0e (accessed on 26 May 2025).

16. Ferguson-Smith, A. C., Lorenz, A., & Wolf, J. B. (2022). Mendel's laws of heredity on his 200th birthday: What have we learned by considering exceptions? https://core.ac.uk/download/559320617.pdf (accessed on 26 May 2025).

17. Freudenberg-Hua, Y., Li, W., & Davies, P. (2018). The role of genetics in advancing precision medicine for Alzheimer's disease—A narrative review. *Frontiers in Medicine, 5*, Article 108. https://www.semanticscholar.org/paper/dc79c691d638bd8e5a6b03b8151ee2fedb071236 (accessed on 26 May 2025).

18. Friedt, W., & Ordon, F. (2022). Mendel's laws and their impact on plant breeding. https://core.ac.uk/download/551440467.pdf (accessed on 26 May 2025).

19. Futuyma, D. J. (2017). Evolutionary biology today and the call for an extended synthesis. *Interface Focus, 7*, 20160145. https://doi.org/10.1098/rsfs.2016.0145.

20. Gibran, H., Zheng, J., Elsworth, B., Wade, K. H., Haberland, V., Baird, D., Laurin, C., et al. (2018). The MR-Base platform supports systematic causal inference across the human phenome. *eLife, 7*, e34408. https://doi.org/10.7554/eLife.34408.

21. Gliboff, S. (2015). *The Mendelian and Non-Mendelian Origins of Genetics*. https://core.ac.uk/download/213847263.pdf (accessed on 26 May 2025).

22. Gramates, L. S., Agapite, J., Attrill, H., Calvi, B. R., Crosby, M. A., dos Santos, G., Goodman, J. L., et al. (2022). FlyBase: A guided tour of highlighted features. *Genetics, 220*. https://doi.org/10.1093/genetics/iyac035.

23. Iglesias-Ramas, A., Lipani, S. P., & Allen, R. J. (2024). Population genetics: An introduction for physicists. *SciPost Physics Lecture Notes*. https://www.semanticscholar.org/paper/77b21a77e77f971530835efbd2adeee8747b5d78 (accessed on 26 May 2025).

24. Johnston, R. C. (2023). Is it time to remove Mendel from the school curriculum? *Journal of Biological Education, 57*(6), 707–708. https://www.semanticscholar.org/paper/c305cce1f7bcb99b855b86a817c64fbeb7ffda9d (accessed on 26 May 2025).

25. K. C., M., & Lamichhane, A. (2021). Advances in agricultural biotechnology. *Nepal Journal of Biotechnology, 9*(1), 85–92. https://doi.org/10.3126/njb.v9i1.38643.

26. Kampourakis, K. (2024). Teaching school genetics in the 2020s: Why "naive" Mendelian genetics has to go. *Cold Spring Harbor Perspectives in Biology*. https://www.semanticscholar.org/paper/7be74ed2c8854a475f70a087274e8d77a97c5d78 (accessed on 26 May 2025).

27. Kang, S., Lee, K. E., Singh, M., Kumar, P., & Matin, M. (2021). Rice lesion mimic mutants (LMM): The current understanding of genetic mutations in the failure of ROS scavenging during lesion formation. *Plants, 10*(9), 1–17. https://www.semanticscholar.org/paper/3d4b8696b1c5488b04dfd50554128d00b00dbeea (accessed on 26 May 2025).

28. Karczewski, K. J., Francioli, L. C., Tiao, G., Cummings, B. B., Alföldi, J., Wang, Q., Collins, R. L., et al. (2020). The mutational constraint spectrum quantified from variation in 141,456 humans. *Nature, 581*, 434–443. https://doi.org/10.1038/s41586-020-2308-7.

29. Kessler, S. K. (2025). Epilepsy genetics. *Continuum, 31*(1), 81–94. https://www.semanticscholar.org/paper/3d6c98de175af9cc496dcccc6f729f3109524ac0 (accessed on 26 May 2025).

30. Kim, M. S., Kim, W. J., Khera, A. V., Kim, J. Y., Yon, D. K., Lee, S. W., Shin, J. I., et al. (2021). Association between adiposity and cardiovascular outcomes: An umbrella review and meta-analysis of observational and Mendelian randomization studies. *European Heart Journal, 42*, 3388–3403. https://doi.org/10.1093/eurheartj/ehab454.

31. Kyrou, K., Hammond, A., Galizi, R., Kranjc, N., Burt, A., Beaghton, A., Nolan, T., et al. (2018). A CRISPR–Cas9 gene drive targeting doublesex causes complete population suppression in caged *Anopheles gambiae* mosquitoes. *Nature Biotechnology, 36*, 1062–1066. https://doi.org/10.1038/nbt.4245.

32. Leitão, J., & Pereira, R. (2021). *A Non-Rogue Mutant Line Induced by ENU Mutagenesis in Paramutated Rogue Peas (Pisum sativum L.) is Still Sensitive to the Rogue Paramutation*. https://core.ac.uk/download/489471831.pdf (accessed on 26 May 2025).

33. Mach, F., Baigent, C., Catapano, A. L., Koskinas, K. C., Casula, M., Badimón, L., Chapman, M. J., et al. (2019). 2019 ESC/EAS Guidelines for the management of dyslipidemia's: Lipid modification to reduce cardiovascular risk. *European Heart Journal, 41*, 111–188. https://doi.org/10.1093/eurheartj/ehz455.

34. Marshall, P. (2008). Development of higher-level cognitive skills in a learner-centered lab on extensions of Mendelian inheritance using *Drosophila*. *Journal of Microbiology & Biology Education, 9*(1), 12–24. https://www.semanticscholar.org/paper/79da43564dfdee1628113a7fe64f31496b83b8ec (accessed on 26 May 2025).

35. Meng, C., Ren, J., Gu, H., Shi, H., Luo, H., Wang, Z., Li, C., et al. (2024). Association between genetically plasma proteins and osteonecrosis: A proteome-wide Mendelian randomization analysis. *Frontiers in Genetics, 15*. https://www.semanticscholar.org/paper/a00f926a038c6769747b83f7e0aa59d9993709b5 (accessed on 26 May 2025).

36. Muller-Wille, S. E. W. (2018). *Gregor Mendel and the History of Heredity*. https://core.ac.uk/download/161939777.pdf (accessed on 26 May 2025).

37. Nagirnaja, L., Lopes, A. M., Charng, W. L., Miller, B., Stakaitis, R., Golubickaitė, I., Stendahl, A. M., et al. (2022). Diverse monogenic sub forms of human spermatogenic failure. *Nature Communications, 13*, Article 1836. https://doi.org/10.1038/s41467-022-35661-z.

38. Pallares, L., Reeves, G., & Tautz, D. (2020). *The New (old) Genetics, Version 1.0*. https://core.ac.uk/download/387895912.pdf (accessed on 26 May 2025).

39. Piñero, J., Ramírez-Anguita, J. M., Saüch-Pitarch, J., Ronzano, F., Centeno, E., Sanz, F., & Furlong, L. I. (2019). The DisGeNET knowledge platform for disease genomics: 2019 update. *Nucleic Acids Research*. https://doi.org/10.1093/nar/gkz1021.

40. Portin, P., & Wilkins, A. S. (2017). The evolving definition of the term "gene." *Genetics, 205*(4), 1353–1364. https://doi.org/10.1534/genetics.116.196956.

41. Shan, Y. (2019). A new functional approach to scientific progress. *Philosophy of Science, 86*(4), 739–758. https://doi.org/10.1086/704980.

42. Shotwell, M. A. (2018). The misuse of genetics: The dihybrid cross & the threat of "race crossing." *The American Biology Teacher, 81*(1), 3–10. https://doi.org/10.1525/abt.2019.81.1.3.

43. Skopek, J. M. (2008). *Shaping Science with the Past: Textbooks, History, and the Disciplining of Genetics.* https://core.ac.uk/download/2734232.pdf (accessed on 26 May 2025).

44. Strome, S., Bhalla, N., Kamakaka, R. T., Sharma, U., & Sullivan, W. (2024). Clarifying Mendelian vs non-Mendelian inheritance. *Genetics, 227*(1). https://doi.org/10.1093/genetics/iyae078.

45. Tweedie, A., Tait, A., Cooper, A., MacLeod, A., Benson, C., Turner, M. R., et al. (2005). Allelic segregation and independent assortment in *T. brucei* crosses: Proof that the genetic system is Mendelian and involves meiosis. https://core.ac.uk/download/1394865.pdf (accessed on 26 May 2025).

46. Uffelmann, E., Huang, Q. Q., Munung, N. S., de Vries, J., Okada, Y., Martin, A. R., Martin, H. C., et al. (2021). Genome-wide association studies. *Nature Reviews Methods Primers, 1.* https://doi.org/10.1038/s43586-021-00056-9.

47. van Dijk, P. V., & Ellis, T. H. (2023). Gregor Mendel and the theory of species multiplication. *Genetics.* https://www.semanticscholar.org/paper/73bea5c5cd69ecafeadb91c3a06e59eb990aa488 (accessed on 26 May 2025).

48. Vendramin, R., Litchfield, K., & Swanton, C. (2021). Cancer evolution: Darwin and beyond. *The EMBO Journal, 40*(15), e108389. https://doi.org/10.15252/embj.2021108389.

49. Wilde, A. A. M., Semsarian, C., Márquez, M. F., Sepehri Shamloo, A., Ackerman, M. J., Ashley, E. A., Back Sternick, E., et al. (2022). European Heart Rhythm Association (EHRA)/Heart Rhythm Society (HRS)/Asia Pacific Heart Rhythm Society (APHRS)/Latin American Heart Rhythm Society (LAHRS) expert consensus statement on the state of genetic testing for cardiac diseases. *Heart Rhythm, 19*, e1–e60. https://doi.org/10.1016/j.hrthm.2022.03.1225.

50. Wilde, A. A. M., Semsarian, C., Márquez, M. F., Sepehri Shamloo, A., Ackerman, M. J., Ashley, E. A., Sternick, E. B., et al. (2022). European Heart Rhythm Association (EHRA)/Heart Rhythm Society (HRS)/Asia Pacific Heart Rhythm Society (APHRS)/Latin American Heart Rhythm Society (LAHRS) expert consensus statement on the state of genetic testing for cardiac diseases. *Journal of Arrhythmia, 38*, 491–553. https://doi.org/10.1002/joa3.12717.

51. Zunjare, R., Muthusamy, V., Chand, G., Chauhan, P., Rathore, A. S., Katral, A., Mishra, S. J., et al. (2024). Genetic evidence of recessive epistasis among sex determining *silkless1* (*sk1*), *tasselseed1* (*ts1*) and *tasselseed2* (*ts2*) genes and its utility in maize (*Zea mays* L.) breeding. *Plant Breeding.* https://www.semanticscholar.org/paper/b43a4f180f4c8199ba0d9d0d51bdad2a73282669 (accessed on 26 May 2025).

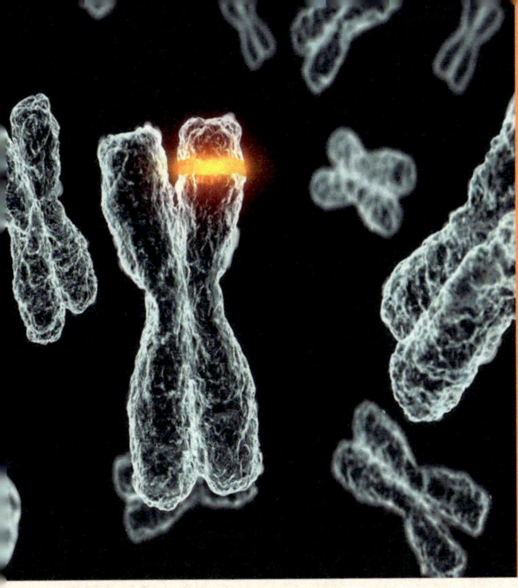

Chapter 12
GENETIC MUTATIONS AND DISORDERS

Contents

Introduction

Genetic information forms the backbone of how living things are built and function—it's a subject that has always drawn the attention of biology and medicine enthusiasts alike. There's this essential split in our DNA between bits that code for proteins and parts that don't, even though those noncoding regions—about 98.5% of our genetic makeup—still steer gene regulation in subtle ways. Roughly 1.5% of our genome makes proteins, but don't get it twisted; the rest quietly plays its part. Researchers generally focus on new, spontaneously appearing changes – de novo mutations – which show up without being passed down and can be a key, if sometimes puzzling, link in disorders like autism spectrum disorder (ASD) (Joon-An et al., 2018). Whole-genome sequencing has significantly enhanced our ability to identify genetic variations associated with diseases. In a study with 1902 families – where a child with ASD was compared with their unaffected siblings – scientists noticed a surprising excess of spontaneous mutations in particular segments of the coding regions. This kind of outcome suggests that not all mutations affect equally; some parts of our coding sequence bear the brunt more than others, prompting us toward more holistic methods for disorder analysis. By merging data on gene function with clues from our evolutionary past, researchers gain a deeper understanding of these variations. Additionally, the notion that even noncoding mutations, especially those in areas controlling gene activity, contribute to ASD flips the old idea that only coding parts matter. This gradual change in focus is pretty pivotal for both better diagnostics and refined treatment approaches (Joon-An et al., 2018). Big genetic databases—such as the Exome Aggregation Consortium (ExAC)—have also emerged as indispensable resources. When scientists sift through high-quality exome data from more than 60,000 people, common mutations start to stand out and researchers can better gauge if specific variants are likely to cause trouble. This massive catalog not only sheds light on which genes appear to be under selective pressure but also helps narrow down candidates when searching for disease-causing mutations. Moreover, such collections of genetic diversity continually advance our understanding of human diseases, constantly refining the clinical tools we rely on. As ongoing research gradually reveals more about both coding and noncoding changes, our understanding of genetic disorders deepens, guiding the way toward more targeted treatments (Figure 12.1).

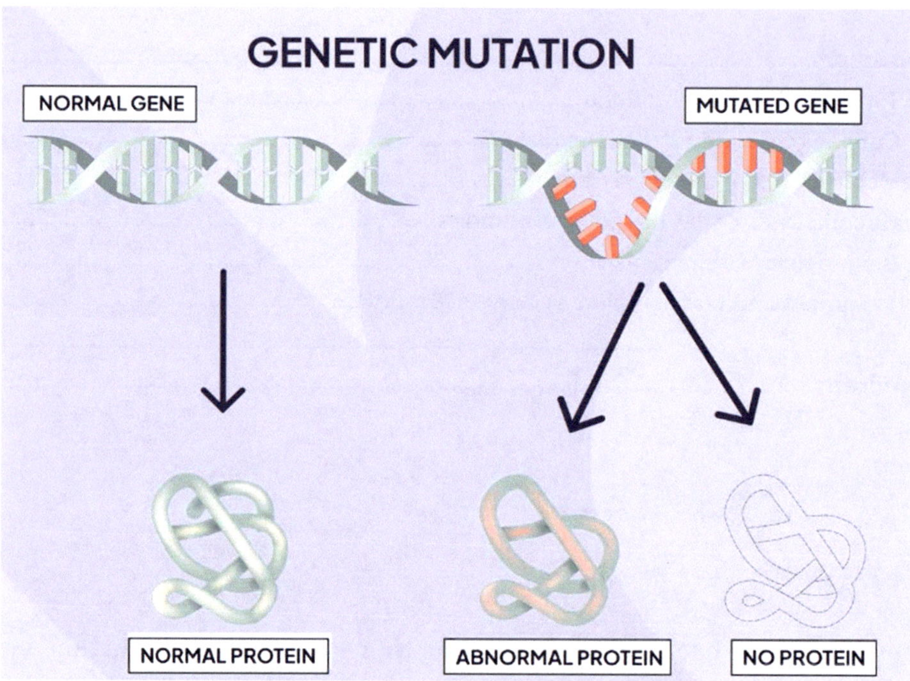

Figure 12.1. Genetic mutation.

Source: https://www.health.com/thmb/7UPmUcOC32y23eEXnKKjbbDzOjk=/1500x0/filters:no_upscale():max_bytes(150000):strip_icc()/Health-Genetic-Mutation-background-light-purple-a6ad7969c03e4780ae174b4c9f705c0c.jpg.

Definition of Genetic Mutations

Genetic mutations play a role in driving both the emergence of new biological traits and various diseases. Mutations come in many forms, like when a single nucleotide changes (that's a point mutation), or when bits of DNA get added or dropped, sometimes even involving entire chunks of chromosomes. A single-letter swap in DNA could dramatically change a protein if it happens in a coding region—seemingly small but sometimes having huge effects. Meanwhile, insertions and deletions tend to disrupt the entire reading frame of a gene, meaning the resulting protein may not function properly. And then there's the scenario where large chunks of chromosomes are altered, leading to the loss or gain of entire gene sections, which can significantly disrupt the cell's balance. Generally speaking, these types of changes keep evolution messy and unpredictable, and they significantly impact our health; many of these mutations directly relate to hereditary disorders and even some forms of cancer, making it clear why genetic counseling and medical intervention are so important. Mutations don't just sit in a lab classification scheme—they have real-world health impacts. For instance, mutations in the BRCA1 and BRCA2 genes are now recognized as significant risk factors for breast and ovarian cancer. In most cases, identifying these changes has led to better preventive measures, such as regular genetic screening and more personalized treatment options. It's like healthcare professionals are given a heads-up when they understand that a particular mutation might predispose an individual or even a whole family to certain diseases. Consequently, testing for these genetic quirks becomes a crucial part of early diagnosis and tailoring medical care, allowing for more proactive interventions when harmful mutations are present. Researchers, by digging into these specific mutations and how they tie to different disorders, are slowly opening the door to targeted therapies and even gene-editing tools that aim to fix the underlying issues. The field of genetics has shifted gears significantly with new technology, especially next-generation sequencing, which has, in most cases, completely reshaped our understanding of genetic variation. This progress, although complex, demonstrates that mutations can arise from both nuclear and mitochondrial DNA (mtDNA), resulting in a surprising variety of physical traits. Studies indicate that some disease-causing variants disrupt standard metabolic pathways, often triggering symptoms that affect multiple systems and complicating diagnosis for clinicians. Even though we have better diagnostics these days, determining conditions linked to mutations remains a challenging task, partly because many genetic disorders share similar symptoms and involve multiple contributing factors. Overall, this complex web of genetic change means that researchers must continue to gather data and refine methods—not only to support more accurate clinical diagnoses but also to explore innovative therapies that address the root causes of these mutations.

Importance of Studying Genetic Disorders

Genetic disorders hit people and families hard, and it's clear we need to get what's going on behind these conditions. Science continues to unravel the complex web of human genetics, and in most cases, this only underscores why exploring these issues is so crucial. Gene changes sometimes spark a range of health troubles that extend beyond the body, affecting minds and social lives as well. For example, cystic fibrosis or Huntington's disease remind us again and again that a small glitch in our genes can significantly impact the quality of life. When researchers unravel these complex gene puzzles, they open doors to treatments that directly address the problem, leading to better outcomes and a glimmer of hope for affected families. All in all, exploring our genetic makeup stokes fresh ideas in medicine and, generally speaking, makes a strong case for keeping genetic studies at the heart of clinical work. There's also something to be said about showing the public what these genetic issues are all about. When more people have access to genetics, the chance of catching things early and acting on them increases significantly. Often, by taking a closer look at how genes misbehave, healthcare experts can identify individuals who might be at risk and even guide them toward treatments that fit a person's unique genetic profile. This means a more hands-on and tailored approach that seems to work better for each individual. Consider recent strides, such as gene therapies for some rare conditions—the breakthrough treatments we're discussing rely heavily on the deep understanding gained from studying genes. In essence, investing energy and money in educating people about genetic disorders isn't just a nice idea; it empowers individuals to take charge of their health, which, in turn, enhances the overall well-being of our communities. We also can't ignore the social side of things when it comes to gene troubles. Often, gene mutations are linked with broader public health issues, pointing us toward new ways to tackle challenges both at the personal level and within whole communities.

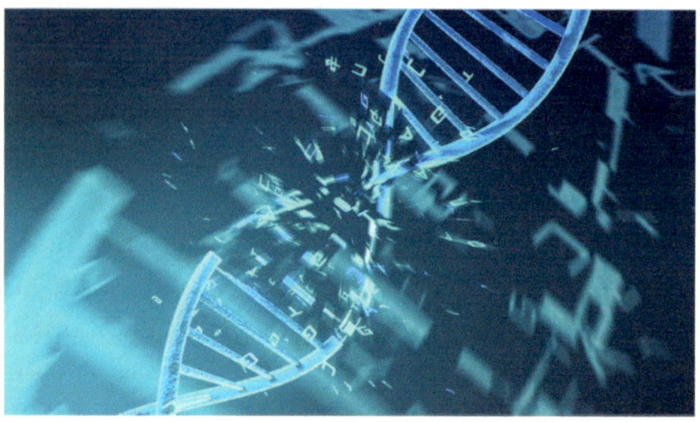

Figure 12.2. Genetic disorders.

Source: https://www.cdc.gov/genomics-and-health/media/images/double_helix_broken.jpg.

For instance, a genetic predisposition to diabetes or certain cancers provides us with valuable insights into preventing these diseases. Unraveling the messy genetic backdrop of complex disorders even helps us see how everyday factors like lifestyle and environment might widen health gaps among different groups. Understanding that genes and socio-economic conditions interact helps policymakers design health plans that truly meet the needs. In this setting, studying these disorders does more than spark scientific curiosity—it also shapes public policy, ensuring that decisions are based on a well-rounded understanding of both genetic triats and everyday influences on our health (Chalasani et al., 2017; Lilley et al., 2020) (Figure 12.2).

12.1. Types of Genetic Mutations

Genetic mutations manifest in various ways, each with its unique characteristics when it comes to causing disorders. Point mutations, for example, usually mean that one tiny nucleotide gets swapped out – a change that might seem small but can mess things up. In sickle cell disease, a single nucleotide tweak alters hemoglobin so drastically that the effects are severe. Then there are insertions and deletions (indels), where a few nucleotides either emerge or vanish unexpectedly. These changes can disrupt the entire reading frame, resulting in the protein-making process producing a faulty or incomplete product, and highlighting just how crucial these subtle errors can sometimes be. Looking at things on a larger scale, chromosomal mutations offer an even broader spectrum of alterations. Sometimes vast segments of DNA become involved; duplications can lead to extra gene copies that may overexert their function, while deletions—such as the one seen on chromosome 5 in cri du chat syndrome—remove critical bits of information. Translocations also occur when a segment of one chromosome ends up relocated to another, potentially derailing gene function and even sparking oncogenesis in specific cases. Generally speaking, these kinds of changes underline the far-reaching and unpredictable consequences that can arise when the blueprint of life is rearranged. Beyond these obvious structural tweaks, researchers find the evolutionary aspect of mutations particularly compelling—especially in the complex world of cancer. Tumors are like a patchwork quilt of various mutation types, thanks to factors such as random mutation events, genetic drift, and even some clonal selection thrown into the mix; this creates a kind of intratumoral heterogeneity that's hard to pin down. As tumors evolve, identifying different mutation forms—from minor point changes to wild chromosomal rearrangements—becomes essential for understanding how they grow and respond to therapy. Significantly, the unpredictable, almost stochastic nature of these changes complicates predictions about tumor behavior and treatment success; thus, advanced genomic tools are, in most cases, indispensable for teasing apart these complex interactions, and they highlight the deep connection between genetic mutations and disorders such as cancer (Kamil et al., 2016; Verhaart et al., 2017).

12.1.1. Point Mutations

Genes can be unpredictable. Often, understanding these tiny shifts means examining point mutations—a small switch in one DNA letter that can sometimes disrupt the entire system. A point mutation is just that, a single nucleotide change in our long genetic script, and in most cases, it can interfere with protein assembly and function. Sometimes nothing happens—what is termed as a silent change—but other times, a missense error crops up, swapping one amino acid for another, or a nonsense mistake happens that cuts a protein short with an early stop.

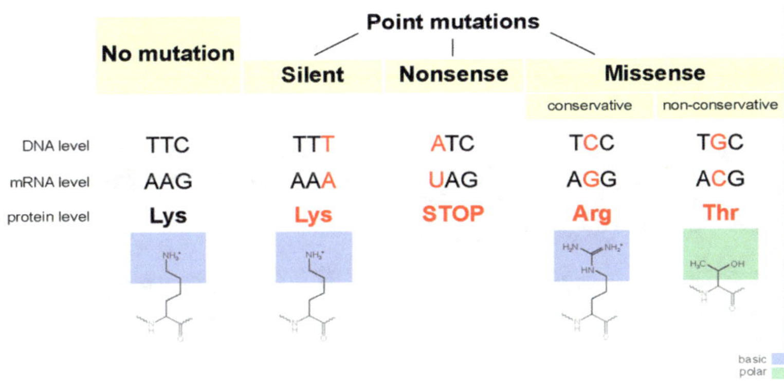

Figure 12.3. Point mutations.

Source: https://files.mtstatic.com/site_4463/52576/1?Expires=1747022838&Signature=CB2KUVFXxZfzoox0TrhpceWjD5uGofbWyQl6uSKknsijAR6JX03Ig0uLvuBWp9JCtZjY~-CvJRSn77ZWUwjCTF2X3uKLkHUE3rpLo5iEIR09JOcTwyJMHqS~K7br8ta-Pv5JinSF02oWBG~VcM05aJKKb1RTb5OkbHHsqeFcHZg_&Key-Pair-Id=APKAJ5Y6AV4GI7A555NA.

Even though it may seem like a trivial glitch, a single switch can upset the delicate balance in our genetic code and pave the way for various disorders (Lilley et al., 2020). Point mutations also appear on the clinic's radar in a significant way. Many brain development disorders, for example, where thinking and moving get affected, have been linked to these tiny genetic blips. Consider SHANK3: this gene, which plays a crucial role in maintaining brain signal connections, often exhibits mutations in conditions such as Phelan-McDermid syndrome. It goes to show that our neurodevelopment isn't just a straight road—it's a muddled amalgamation of genetic traits and environmental influences. And generally speaking, once these subtle changes are identified, they provide doctors with clues for more accurate diagnoses and more targeted treatment plans, underscoring the importance of detecting even the smallest genetic missteps (Lilley et al., 2020). Molecular genetics continues to reveal new insights into how a single-letter error can ripple through an organism. Thanks to breakthrough technologies like next-generation sequencing (NGS), identifying these pathogenic changes has become significantly more efficient. In most cases, digging deeper into the common routes that these point mutations disturb can lead to new, unexpected strategies for treating disorders, especially those affecting brain function. For instance, when a mutation disrupts the usual flow of synaptic plasticity or interferes with signaling pathways, such as mTOR, it often reveals a potential new target for therapy. This muddled overlap between lab discoveries and real-life treatments underscores the need to integrate our growing genetic knowledge into improved methods of understanding and managing genetic disorders (Parenti et al., 2020) (Figure 12.3).

12.1.2. Insertions and Deletions

Sometimes, an organism's genetic blueprint shifts in unexpected ways—little bits of its code might slip in or vanish, and this random tinkering is what folks often call "indels." When extra nucleotides join the DNA chain or when some are suddenly missing, it throws off the regular reading of genes. This simple change can reorder the entire string of amino acids that follow, and if it occurs in a crucial coding spot, the resulting protein may not function properly at all. In most cases, these missteps end up leading to a host of genetic issues that, frankly, can have a serious impact on health and development.

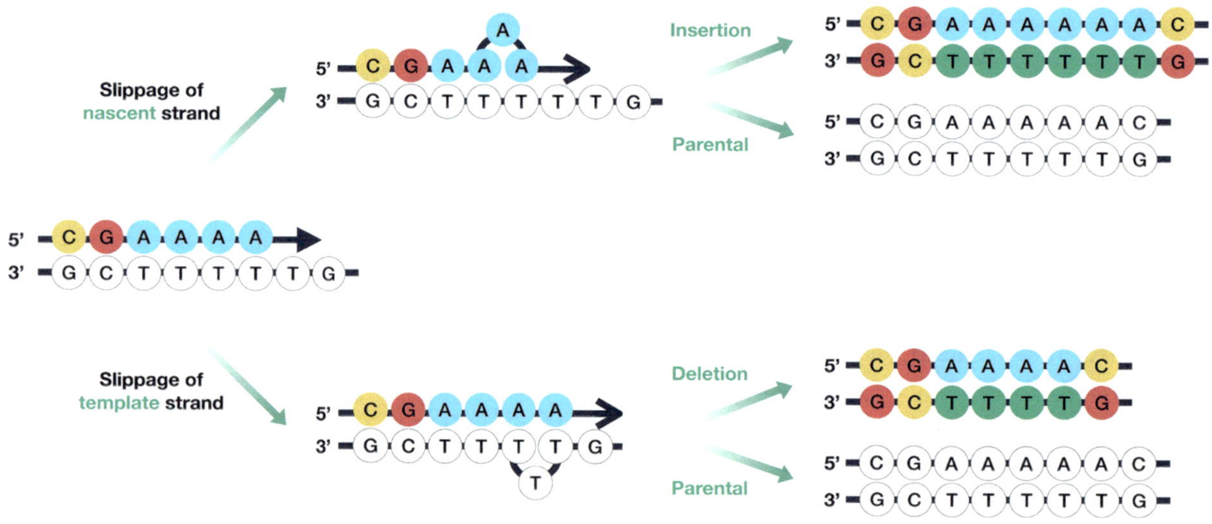

Figure 12.4. Insertions and deletions mutations.

Source: https://ars.els-cdn.com/content/image/1-s2.0-S0734975022001069-gr1.jpg.

Take cystic fibrosis and certain types of muscular dystrophy, for example. There's a well-known case of three nucleotides being deleted from the CFTR gene—a strike that knocks out a phenylalanine at position 508. This tiny deletion disrupts protein folding, which in turn affects ion transport across cell membranes, ultimately triggering the classic symptoms associated with the disease. Similarly, a deletion in the dystrophin gene is linked to Duchenne muscular dystrophy, where missing a key structural piece causes muscles to break down gradually. It's interesting how these small changes keep reminding us that maintaining the integrity of our genome is no small feat. Lately, breakthroughs like CRISPR-Cas9 have emerged as promising solutions to these DNA issues. This tool functions like a precise repair kit, enabling scientists to target and correct the exact locations where insertions or deletions have disrupted the balance. Researchers, generally speaking, are optimistic about the potential to correct these faults at their source, and early clinical trials are already investigating treatments for hereditary conditions (Hu et al., 2020; Sharma et al., 2020). As our understanding of these genetic quirks deepens, the mix between innovative editing techniques and traditional genetics is expected to steer genetic medicine toward some pretty revolutionary therapies - a future that, if one thinks about it, might rewrite the rules of healthcare (Figure 12.4).

12.1.3. Chromosomal Mutations

Chromosomal mutations significantly alter the way our bodies develop and respond to illness. They come in various forms—such as deletions, duplications, inversions, and translocations—and can affect multiple genes simultaneously, resulting in a range of outcomes.

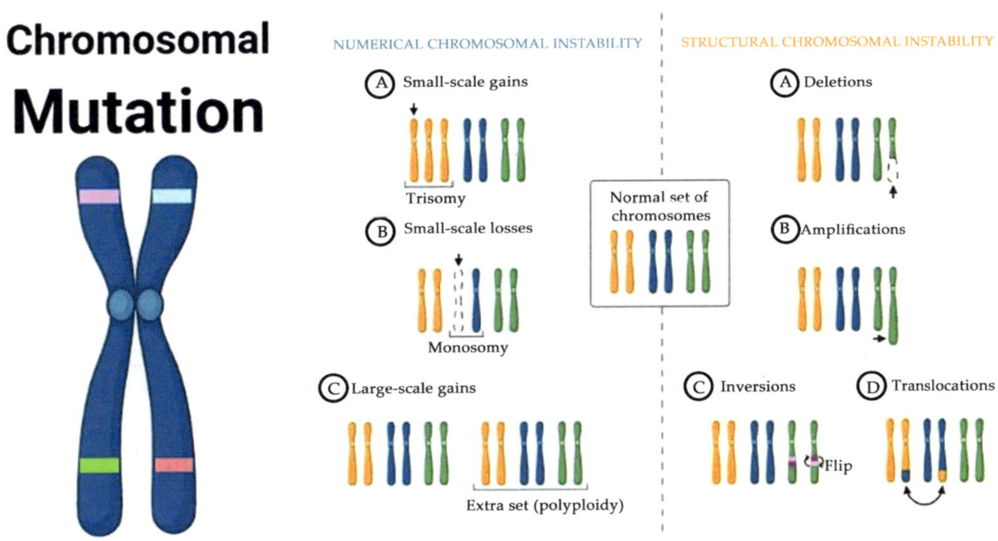

Figure 12.5. Chromosomal mutations.

Source: https://microbenotes.com/wp-content/uploads/2021/03/Chromosomal-Mutations.jpeg.

In cases like neurodevelopmental disorders, the roots are usually a complex interplay of factors; there may be changes in processes like synaptic plasticity or cell signaling emerging because these mutations disrupt these pathways. Research generally suggests that alterations to the architecture of chromosomes often lead to a connection with neurodevelopmental disorders, making it challenging to match exact genetic changes with the observed symptoms (Parenti et al., 2020). It's essential to understand how these mutations function if we're to advance diagnostic methods and treatments. NGS, for example, has significantly changed the landscape by enhancing our ability to detect these problematic mutations—making it much more sensitive at identifying abnormalities. Tools like chromosomal microarray analysis are vital for identifying copy number variations, especially in cases where children face unexplained neurodevelopmental challenges. And when scientists notice that different issues follow the same molecular pathways, it sometimes opens the door to treatments that target those specific routes. As an example, certain chromosomal missteps are tied to autism spectrum disorder, which affects about 2% of children in the United States. This highlights the importance of accurately pinpointing chromosomal mutations (Rose et al., 2018). Beyond nailing down a diagnosis, the effects of chromosomal mutations run deep, influencing how patients are managed over time. Children with these mutations often face additional conditions that further complicate their treatment plans. One model, commonly known as the two-hit hypothesis, suggests that an inherited mutation might later be wedded with a somatic one, and together they shape the overall disease picture. In most cases, disorders—including many neurodevelopmental ones—are the result of multiple mutations mixed with environmental factors, highlighting why thorough genetic counseling is so crucial. As more research delves into these relationships, we can hope for more effective interventions that ultimately lead to improved outcomes for patients and their families (Parenti et al., 2020) (Figure 12.5).

12.2. Causes of Genetic Mutations

Genetic mutations come about from a mash-up of reasons—some stir up from inside the body while others come from outside influences. DNA copying isn't perfect; the enzyme responsible for the job can occasionally slip and add the wrong component. Then there are spontaneous changes caused by the natural chemical wobble in the DNA strand, which, frankly, can scramble the usual sequence. Outside factors, such as ionizing radiation or certain chemicals, can also disrupt the DNA's structure. Take reactive oxygen species (ROS), for example—they can trigger oxidative damage that further muddles the accurate makeup of our genetic material. All these little mishaps and influences combine to help us understand why genetic changes can lead to disorders, disrupting normal gene function and overall health in unpredictable ways. Looking at conditions like neurodegenerative disorders, it quickly becomes clear that a mix of genetic predispositions and environmental conditions are at play. Studies generally show that tiny organisms—bacteria, fungi, and even viruses—may interfere with our immune system, sometimes tipping the balance and worsening symptoms. It isn't just about a faulty gene; the broader environment also plays a significant role. For example, an individual with a natural tendency toward brain-wrecking issues might suffer more when specific pathogens come into the picture, as seen in research exploring links between microbial infections and neurological problems (Dehhaghi et al., 2018). This complex interplay suggests that it is essential to consider all the contributing factors—both what's within us and what surrounds us—to understand how these conditions develop. Spinal muscular atrophy (SMA) is one clear example of how gene alterations can have serious health impacts. Essentially, when both copies of the SMN1 gene go awry, nerve cells and muscles don't function the way they should. Some people show severe signs early on, while others experience a milder form—it's all a bit unpredictable. Although SMA isn't super standard, its many facets underline how diverse genetic disorders can be, making diagnosis and tracking affected populations a real challenge. Interestingly, the number of people carrying the SMN1 mutation can vary between groups, adding another layer to the story (Verhaart et al., 2017). All of this gently reminds us that delving into genetic research is key—it can help us pinpoint the causes and eventually craft more targeted therapies that improve outcomes for patients (Figure 12.6).

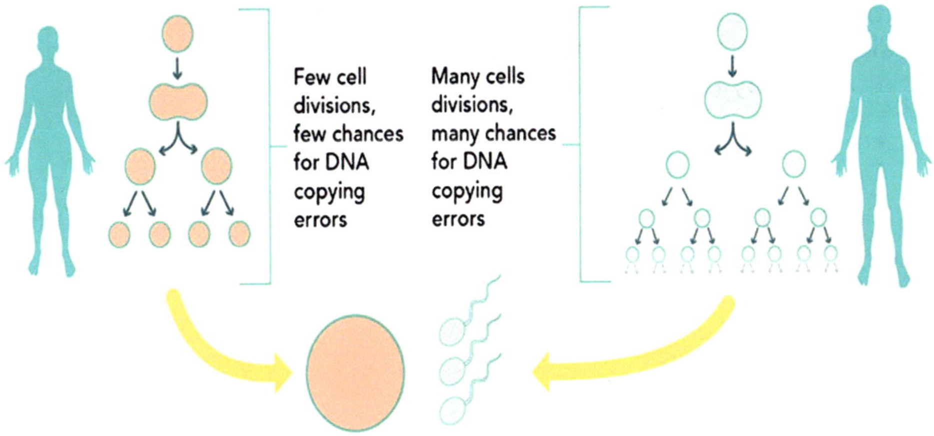

Figure 12.6. The causes of mutations.

Source: https://evolution.berkeley.edu/wp-content/uploads/2021/09/cell-divisions.jpg.

12.2.1. Spontaneous Mutations

Genetic mutations have their puzzling way of just showing up—spontaneously, without any obvious outside trigger. Often, these changes occur when DNA is copied (and the process isn't perfect) or when the cell's repair system slips up. In most cases, these unprompted mutations are key to understanding why genetic traits vary and how heritable diseases can emerge. Lately, research has shed light on de novo mutations—those that don't come from the parents—which seem to be front and center in medical genetics. For instance, the Human Gene Mutation Database (HGMD) has compiled a comprehensive list of these new, disease-associated mutations, highlighting their increasing role in both diagnosis and ongoing genetic studies. Overall, many reviews suggest that a significant number of these spontaneous changes are associated with complex disorders, indicating that they may play a substantial role in the underlying causes of developmental and psychiatric conditions (Lopes-Marques et al., 2024). Examining these spontaneous mutations provides insight into their role in congenital disorders as well. Think about it: when important genes that guide development get hit by a random mutation, the outcomes can be pretty severe. A clear example is the Microphthalmia-associated transcription factor (MITF) gene—mutations in this gene have been linked to issues in pigmentation and hearing, sometimes in unexpected ways. Animal studies, such as those on porcupines, reveal that these changes can lead to irregular pigmentation and even hearing loss; these kinds of phenotypic abnormalities naturally push scientists to dive deeper into conditions like Waardenburg Syndrome. Techniques such as Bulk Segregant Analysis (BSA) and RNA sequencing have been employed, enabling researchers to pinpoint candidate mutations and thereby gain new insights into how these spontaneous genetic glitches contribute to the overall picture (Li et al., 2024). Also, there's a fascinating evolutionary twist to consider. Generally speaking, spontaneous mutations tend to be more harmful than those passed down from one generation to the next, since inherited mutations usually get trimmed by natural selection over the years. Without the usual pressure, these random errors can persist, sometimes leading to a higher frequency of disease-linked variants in specific populations. By mapping how these spontaneous mutations occur in various genetic settings, researchers can begin to estimate their actual impact—especially on developmental and psychiatric disorders. This deeper understanding informs therapeutic strategies aimed at mitigating the effects of such mutations, and it highlights the importance of monitoring these genetic shifts in both clinical practice and future research (Lopes-Marques et al., 2024) (Figure 12.7).

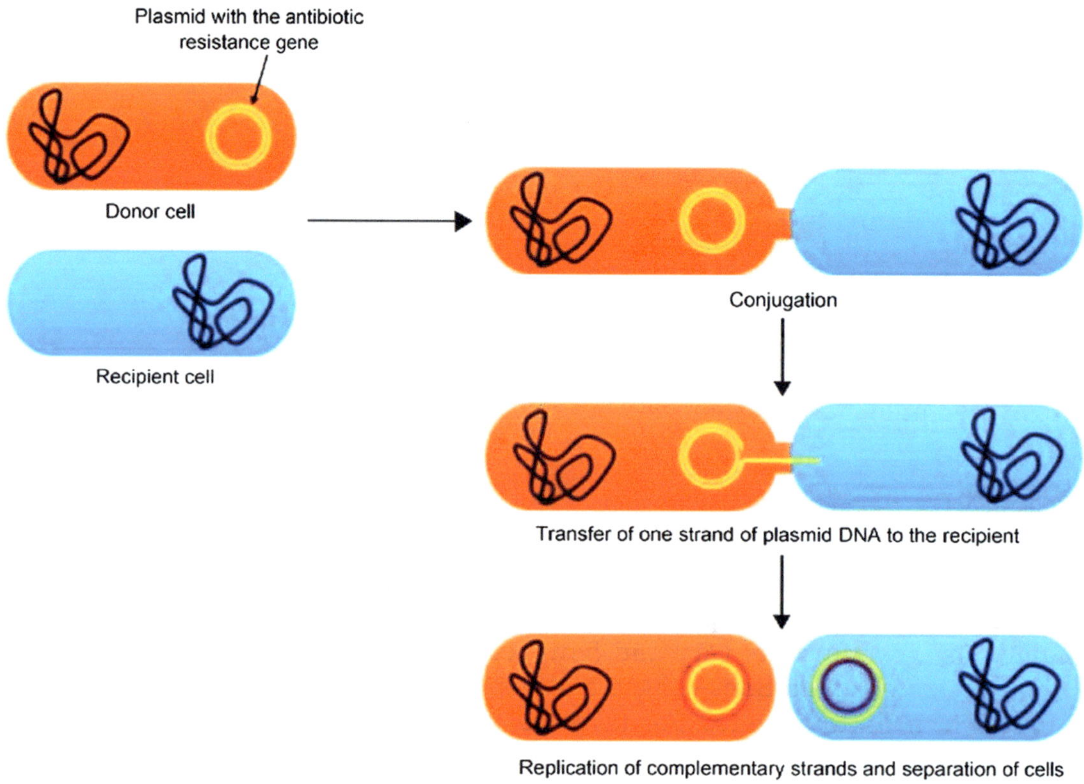

Figure 12.7. Spontaneous mutations.

Source: https://www.researchgate.net/profile/Kamila-Szudera-Konczal/publication/344722156/figure/fig2/AS:947759108608000@1602974788361/Resistance-arising-as-a-result-of-spontaneous-mutation-in-chromosomal-DNA.png.

12.2.2. Environmental Factors

Environmental factors can significantly exacerbate genetic issues, sometimes triggering problems that lie dormant within our DNA. Exposure to chemicals, poor diet, and constant stress can accelerate the onset and impact of diseases on our overall well-being. For instance, liver problems like non-alcoholic fatty liver disease—our genes and everyday choices, such as what we chow down on or simply sitting around, blend in ways that shape how the disease unfolds. These days, the increasing prevalence of metabolic issues makes it clear that we need smarter public health measures to reduce harmful exposures. This could help us decode how these diseases work and guide better treatments for individuals who may be at risk due to their genetic makeup (Mary et al., 2023). Look a bit closer and the dance between our genes and the world around us gets even messier, especially when it comes to mental health concerns like schizophrenia. Things like infections before birth or rough childhood experiences might mix with our genetic predispositions—yes, even gene quirks—to worsen symptoms or even spark these conditions. Studies suggest that early life disappointments can disrupt essential steps in brain development, affecting the systems that keep our thinking and feelings balanced. In most cases, observing how genetic cues and environmental factors interact provides us with additional insights into these complex disorders. This awareness enables us to tailor prevention and intervention plans to each person's specific risks, while also guiding future research in new directions (Guerrin et al., 2021). It's not just the mind that feels the impact—our bodies get caught in this web too. Every day elements like pollution, what we eat, and how we choose to live all play a part in long-lasting problems like obesity, diabetes, and even heart disease. For example, consuming excessive amounts of saturated fats and sugars can trigger genetic predispositions to metabolic disorders, potentially leading to serious health issues in the future. This complex interplay of genes and the environment underscores the need for a broader approach to health—one that addresses lifestyle modifications and environmental changes in conjunction with our genetic profiles. As we continue to delve deeper, there's hope that a better understanding of these interactions will spark advances in personalized medicine and more tailored public health plans aimed at alleviating the burden on those most at risk (Mary et al., 2023).

12.2.3. Inherited Mutations

Research shows that the mutations one inherits can have a surprisingly significant impact on genetic disorders, and this work pulls back the curtain on just how messy Mendelian genetics can be. In many cases, point mutations seem to be the main troublemaker—often responsible for almost half of the recessive diseases we see today. They crop up in all sorts of ways, whether as a base swap, a deletion, an insertion, or even a duplication, all of which remind us that the underlying molecular processes are pretty mixed up. It's essential to understand how these mutations work, especially when considering factors like ionizing radiation, which generally carries significant mutagenic risks. Researchers are still testing whether such radiation impacts our germ cells and how well it triggers specific DNA changes; in most cases, these studies feed into a bigger picture for public health and genetic counseling (Alexandrov et al., 2022). In communities where families are closely interrelated, the case of inherited mutations gets even more eye-catching. For example, when relatives have children, the risk of both copies of a gene being affected goes up, which naturally leads to a higher chance of recessive disorders. Detailed genetic tests in these family groups can unexpectedly reveal how these mutations travel and spread. Recent work, using exome sequencing focused on consanguineous groups, has even brought to light new mutations linked to retinal dystrophies. In one study involving 10 such families, researchers identified several harmful mutations, including some unusual variants in genes already known to be associated with these disorders. This focused approach not only showcases the power of modern genetic tools in solving these puzzles but also highlights the importance of customized genetic counseling in such cases (Shen et al., 2021). Inherited mutations don't just affect one disorder; they ripple out to shape broader public health concerns and the study of genetic trends. Understanding the patterns of these changes helps form effective strategies for prevention, early diagnosis, and intervention—measures that can make a significant difference for individuals and families alike. With our increasing exposure to environmental mutagens (ionizing radiation being a prime example), paying attention to these mutations is becoming increasingly essential. Looking ahead, future research needs to continue exploring how our genetic predispositions interact with external influences while driving advancements in genetic testing. All in all, these steps are key to uncovering meaningful insights and developing treatments that tackle the challenges of inherited genetic disorders across diverse communities (Alexandrov et al., 2022) (Figure 12.8).

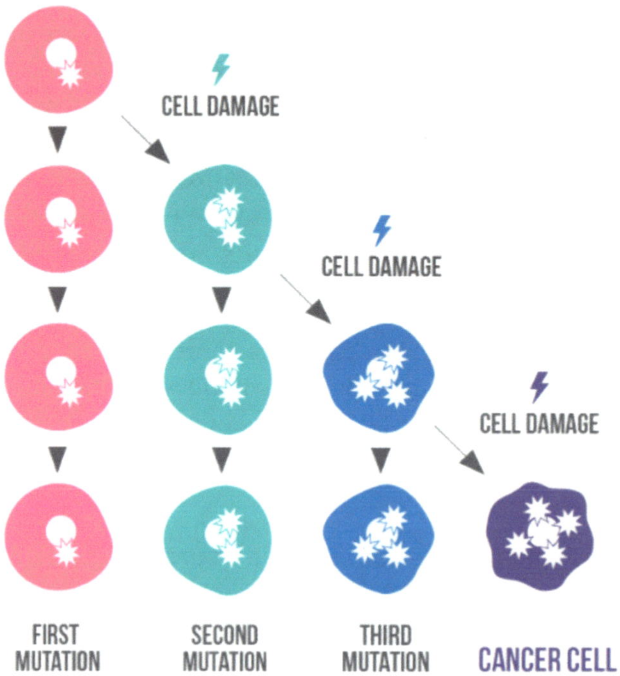

Figure 12.8. Inherited mutations and cancer.

Source: https://www.facingourrisk.org/uploads/FORCE-cell%20mutations_241220_1.png.

12.3. Mechanisms of Mutation Repair

Genetic material staying intact is key for an organism to function right. Cells run into all kinds of stress and damage on a daily basis, and over time, they've developed a mix of fixes to keep the DNA working as it should. One popular fix is NER, which essentially sweeps out those chunky DNA lesions that appear due to factors such as UV rays. Then there's BER, handling the more minor bumps that don't warp the helix—keeping replication and transcription from going off-track. If these repair systems slip up, the outcome can be messy, sometimes nudging folks toward inherited diseases or even increasing cancer risks. Looking a bit closer at how mutation fixes work, the mix of biochemical routes directs how a cell ends up. HR, for example, is impressively meticulous—it borrows a matching DNA copy to ensure accuracy. In contrast, NHEJ acts quicker but, well, it might toss in extra bits or drop some, making it less precise. The balance between these methods is razor-thin; if that gets muddled, the genome's stability can start to crumble, opening the door to the emergence of various issues. This tug-of-war not only explains why some mutations persist but also provides clues for refining treatment options for individuals with genetic abnormalities or cancers. Further consideration of DNA repair reveals some promising avenues in therapy. With tools like CRISPR now in the mix, scientists aren't just peering at the fallout of mutations—they're stepping in to fix them in cells taken straight from patients. By creating isogenic cell lines that differ by just one tiny genetic tweak, researchers can pinpoint which molecular pathways are disrupted. This fresh approach not only deepens our grasp of disease mechanisms but also builds a foundation for targeted treatments. Recent breakthroughs demonstrate that combining gene editing with cell models provides a new perspective on genetic disorders—optimizing these repair processes may one day lead to cures or more effective treatments (Bassett, 2017). Additionally, understanding how the immune system responds to errors in the DNA repair process is crucial for advancing cancer immunotherapy strategies (Ribas et al., 2018) (Figure 12.9).

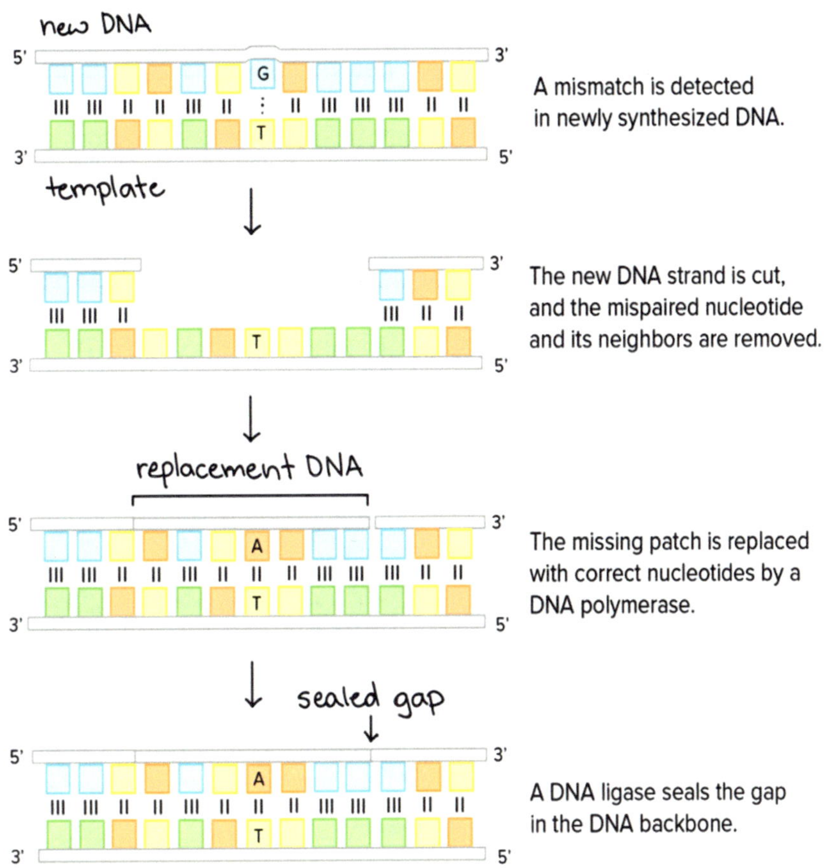

Figure 12.9. Mechanisms of mutation repair.

Source: https://i1.wp.com/cdn.kastatic.org/ka-perseus-images/0d0c2d4819f456c4e0d164e00780fd17cf84945b.png?resize=1025%2C692&ssl=1.

12.3.1. DNA Repair Pathways

DNA repair is fundamental to maintaining the integrity of our genetic material, and new studies continue to highlight the crucial role these pathways play in preventing genetic disorders. Kids with certain brain cancers, like pediatric high-grade gliomas, sometimes have odd mutations—take H3.3-

G34R/V, for example—that mess up the cell's cleanup crew. These changes lower the cell's usual repair work, making it more prone to damage and leading to a kind of messy genetic instability. Extra bits of DNA can even trigger our immune system unexpectedly, revealing a direct link between faulty DNA repair and tumor growth. This suggests not only that healthy repair processes are crucial for cell well-being, but they may also be promising targets for new treatments that combine strategies to enhance how cells respond to DNA damage (Haase et al., 2022). Problems with DNA repair aren't limited to cancer—it can also affect reproductive cells, with effects that might carry over to future generations. Researchers have found that when the repair systems are lagging, cells often accumulate more mutations. For example, deficiencies in nucleotide excision repair are linked to more base substitution errors, while glitches in specific translesion synthesis polymerases result in noticeable deletions. These recurring issues remind us that maintaining low mutation rates is a multifaceted, ongoing challenge, with repair pathways playing a crucial role in preserving genetic fidelity beyond immediate health concerns (Meier et al., 2021). Different ways in which DNA repair can falter lead to a wide range of outcomes, each pathway leaving its distinct mark on the genome. Defects in homologous recombination, for instance, can produce various types of mutations that affect not only an individual's health but also influence broader evolutionary trends. Occasionally, when checkpoint proteins don't perform their job correctly, one sees clusters of mutations forming in regions like the subtelomeric areas — a detail that adds even more complexity to the situation. All these messy interactions underscore the urgent need to develop targeted interventions aimed at strengthening these repair processes to help prevent or lessen the onset of genetic diseases (Meier et al., 2021) (Figure 12.10).

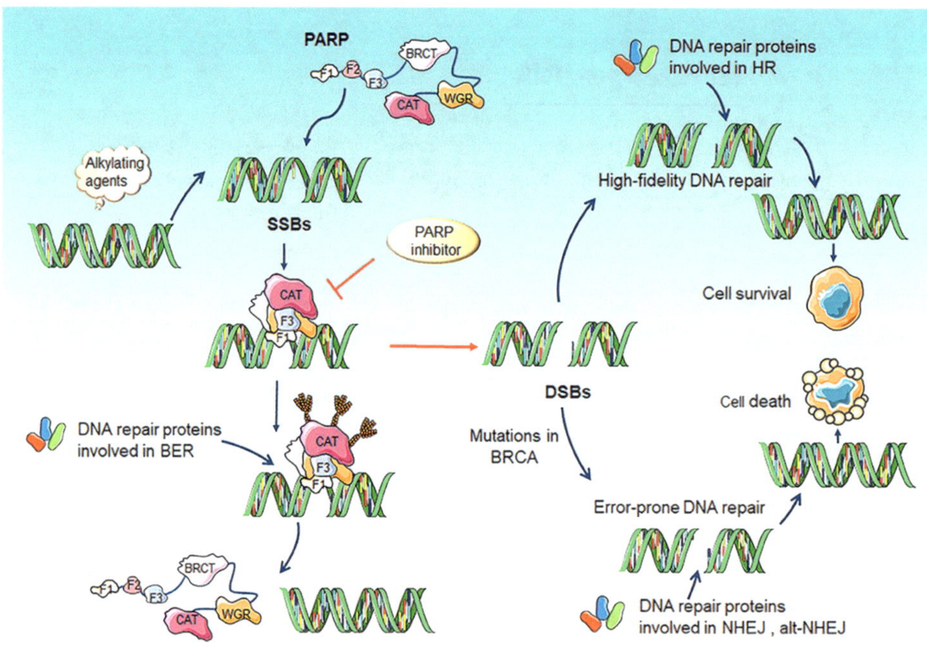

Figure 12.10. DNA repair pathways.

Source: https://external-content.duckduckgo.com/iu/?u=https%3A%2F%2Fwww.frontiersin.org%2Ffiles%2FArticles%2F629266%2Ffphar-11-629266-HTML%2Fimage_m%2Ffphar-11-629266-g002.jpg&f=1&nofb=1&ipt=01920f68608a1794752c28fa8d22e1fda001e0a4cdff67a0769c09e48fda5f56.

12.3.2. Role of Enzymes in Repair

DNA repair is crucial for maintaining the integrity of our genetic code and preventing mutations that could lead to problems. A jumble of enzymes works behind the scenes, often in unexpected ways. Take polymerase θ (POLQ) for instance – it's a core part of what's called polymerase theta-mediated end joining (TMEJ). This repair route uses tiny matching sequences, or microhomology, to help join broken DNA strands when they're split apart. Sure, the process is error-prone, but in cells where the more accurate homologous recombination isn't an option, POLQ ends up being a real lifesaver. Its increased activity, generally speaking, has been linked with poor outcomes in several cancers (Schrempf et al., 2020). Examining the broader picture of DNA repair reveals a host of enzyme families as key actors. Base excision repair (BER) is one such pathway – glycosylases first hunt down and remove damaged bases, and then DNA polymerase β steps in to extend the strand after removal. It's almost like a relay race where each runner (or enzyme) does its part; if any leg of the race stumbles, disorders like neurodegeneration or various cancers can arise. In simpler terms, when these repair systems fail to function as they should, mutations tend to accumulate, making one more susceptible to disease (Petr et al., 2020).

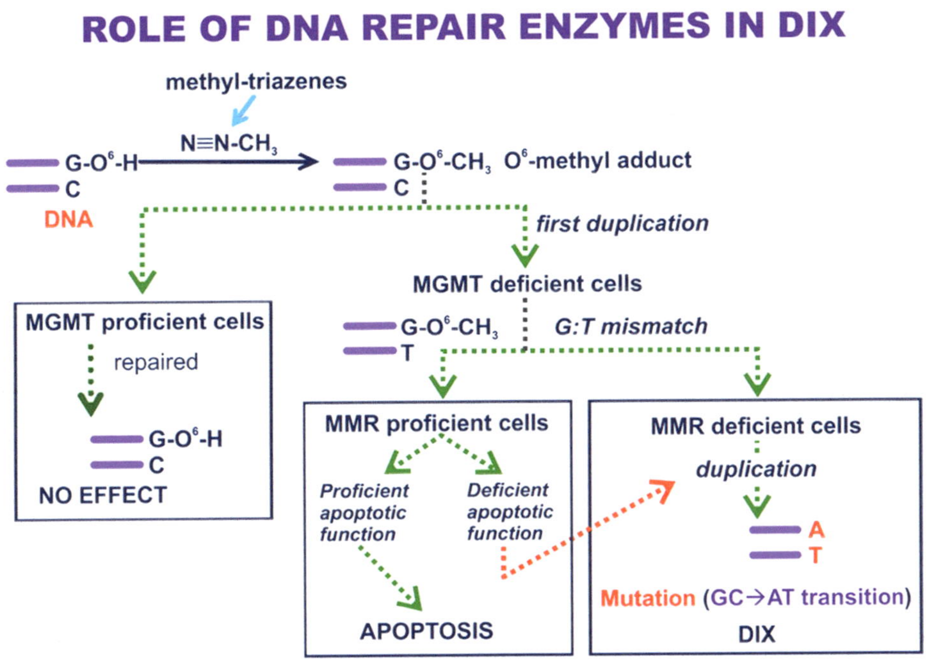

Figure 12.11. The role of DNA repair enzymes in DIX.

Source: https://www.researchgate.net/profile/Maria-Pia-Fuggetta/publication/315344156/figure/fig3/AS:728061234409472@1550594733772/The-role-of-DNA-repair-enzymes-in-DIX-The-end-metabolic-product-of-triazene-compounds-of.ppm.

Sometimes, a failure in one enzyme has a ripple effect that muddles the overall genetic stability. Then there are helicases, another crucial component that helps unravel DNA. Their role is to unwind the double helix so other repair enzymes can access and fix the strands. For instance, during double-strand break (DSB) repair, helicases get the DNA ready by opening it up in a way that's both critical and, admittedly, a bit unpredictable. The precision and hustle of these helicases aren't just about neat repair; they're also key in keeping mutations at bay. In this tangled web of repair processes, each enzyme—whether it's POLQ stitching breaks together, glycosylases spotting damage, or helicases unzipping the strand—plays a part in a dynamic network that guards our genome. Understanding how these molecules interact not only sheds light on genetic disorders but also hints at future ways we might treat them (Schrempf et al., 2020) (Figure 12.11).

12.3.3. Consequences of Repair Failure

Genetic material in good condition is essential for cells to function normally and prevent a range of issues. When the systems that repair DNA malfunction, the consequences can be varied and severe—generally speaking, mutations accumulate and disrupt essential genes. Studies have shown time and again that these mistakes in our genetic code tie in closely with problems in how cells operate, playing a part in things like cancer and even neurodegenerative conditions. As repair pathways weaken, harmful mutations accumulate, which not only jeopardize individual health but may also have ripple effects for families across generations. When cells stumble in mending their DNA, it often sets off a chain reaction inside the cell. Under stress, cells tend to crank out extra ROS – those troublesome molecules that end up damaging DNA, proteins, and lipids—sometimes even more than needed. The delicate balance between making ROS and neutralizing them with antioxidants is crucial; when things tip, oxidative stress kicks in and has been linked to a host of long-term health issues. This failure to repair DNA properly can lead to a domino effect, where initial damage ripples out into overall cellular dysfunction and eventual tissue breakdown. The impact of sloppy DNA repair isn't confined to just one cell—it can throw the whole organism off track. Genetic disorders born from faulty repair processes often sneak into families as inheritable conditions, reminding us that the stakes are high for future generations. Take, for example, mutations in repair genes that lead to syndromes like hereditary breast and ovarian cancer; such cases underscore why understanding these mechanisms matters so much. Additionally, when repair routines go awry, cells can begin multiplying unchecked, thereby opening the door to various cancers. All in all, figuring out how to boost these repair systems isn't just an academic pursuit—it's a critical step toward better, more resilient health outcomes across the board.

12.4. Genetic Disorders Caused by Mutations

Genetic mutations significantly impact health, and many of these rare ones still remain a mystery. Skeletal disorders show how troublesome things can get. In multiple epiphyseal dysplasia (MED), changes in key genes affect cartilage development by tampering with the proteins that build its matrix. People with MED often end up with a mix of features like oddly short stature, joint aches, and early arthritis—proof that mutations can show up in wildly different ways. Researchers have been experimenting with both cell cultures and mouse models to piece together these puzzles, and they continue to spot signs of endoplasmic reticulum (ER) stress. In most cases, these clues prompt further study and suggest that curbing ER stress may be a promising treatment route (Ella et al., 2020). Mutations aren't just about bones, though. Alterations in the genes for nuclear envelope proteins also appear to affect muscles and the aging process significantly. Hutchinson-Gilford Progeria Syndrome is one stark example—it speeds up aging and wrecks muscle function because of a genetic slip-up. These mutations upset essential cell structures, which can kickstart early aging in unexpected ways. Studying these proteins gives clues not only about specific disorders but also about the broader picture of how we age. This link between faulty genes and muscle weakness highlights how profoundly genetics can influence our daily strength and independence as we age. By looking closely at how these errors work, researchers hope to uncover new targets for treatments that might slow age-related muscle decline (Battey et al., 2020). The overall tangle between genetic mutations and the disorders they spawn lays out some enormous challenges for treatment and care. Some conditions are well understood, yet many remain shrouded in mystery due to their rarity and our incomplete understanding of how they work. This gap in our knowledge often means treatments fall short, leaving people with a lower quality of life. Think about it: the struggle to find effective therapies for skeletal diseases nails home the need for more dedicated research in medical genetics. As scientists slowly unravel these rare genetic quirks, the door opens wider for personalized medicine—a significant shift in how we approach these disorders. All this points to the need for deeper dives into the genetics of rare illnesses, a step that could eventually lead to better treatment methods and improved outcomes for patients (Ella et al., 2020) (Figure 12.12).

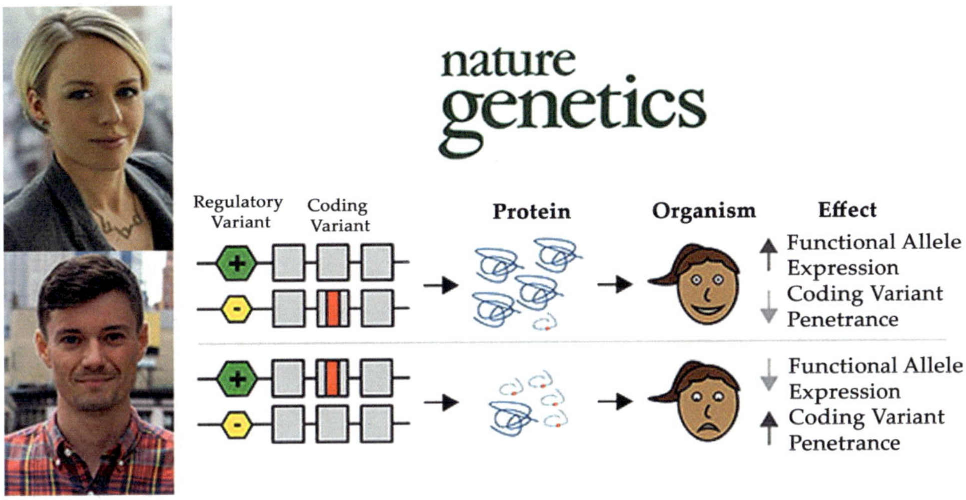

Figure 12.12. Genetic disorders caused by mutations.

Source: https://systemsbiology.columbia.edu/sites/default/files/Revised_Image_for_web_posting.jpg.

12.4.1. Single-Gene Disorders

Genetic disorders are a real maze. Sometimes, a single tiny glitch in a gene can have surprising effects on our overall health. In many cases, these issues arise when changes occur in a specific gene, resulting in a range of symptoms—some relatively mild, others severe enough to be life-threatening. These genetic shifts are tied to our core biological processes, so it's pretty essential to understand what's going on underneath. Take neurodevelopmental disorders, for example; usually grouped with single-gene problems, they tend to mess up critical brain development stages. Generally speaking, research suggests that shared molecular pathways underlie the varied manifestations of these conditions. However, pinpointing the exact genotype–phenotype relationships remains a significant challenge due to the numerous influencing factors (Parenti et al., 2020). When single-gene disorders are examined more closely, understanding how mutations affect the body becomes essential for accurate diagnosis and effective care. These issues are often sorted by inheritance patterns—like autosomal dominant, autosomal recessive, or X-linked—which each bring their traits regarding how the disease shows up and the risks it poses for families. For instance, sometimes, one encounters haploinsufficiency, where losing function in just one allele is enough to trigger symptoms; other times, even one altered copy can set things off. The genetic background of an individual can further tweak how these disorders present, suggesting that spotting common disease triggers might help pave the way for better treatments and smoother clinical management (Chalasani et al., 2017). Overall, understanding single-gene disorders calls for a mix of approaches. Advances in genomic tech, such as whole-exome sequencing, have changed the game by making it easier to pinpoint the genetic variants behind these conditions. The switch from traditional methods to NGS has opened up a broader understanding of genetic contributions, significantly enhancing diagnostic success. Yet, many patients still end up without a precise molecular diagnosis—proof of how complex our genetic landscape is. Researchers, in most cases, continue to map the disrupted pathways and investigate how environmental factors may influence outcomes, all while holding out hope for more personalized treatments and ultimately, better care for individuals with single-gene disorders (Parenti et al., 2020) (Figure 12.13).

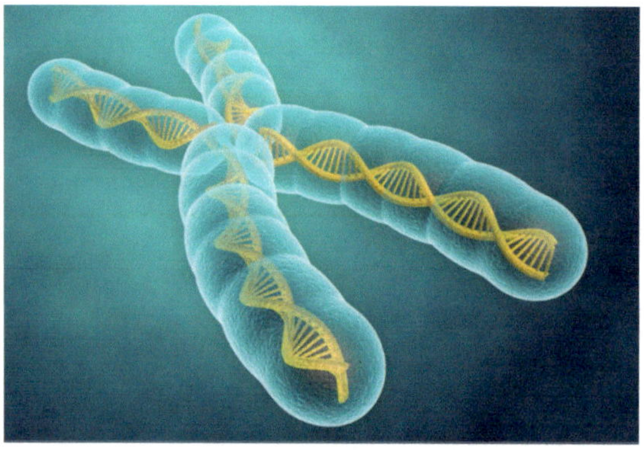

Figure 12.13. Single-gene disorders.

Source: https://fertijin.com.tr/wp-content/uploads/2024/01/what-is-single-gene-disease-1024x694.png.

12.4.2. Chromosomal Disorders

Chromosomal abnormalities often manifest in unexpected ways during human development. Sometimes a missing or extra bit in our DNA ends up giving rise to a whole set of physical traits that aren't always what one would expect. Take Turner Syndrome as an example: a 45,X karyotype typically results in shorter stature, along with a few other distinctive developmental features. Studies on the X and Y chromosomes have, generally speaking, shed light on how specific genes tucked away in the pseudo-autosomal regions might be playing a part in determining height. The SHOX gene, for instance, has clearly been mapped to these areas and has significantly shifted our approach to diagnosing issues like short stature, underscoring the importance of a thorough genetic check in linking gene changes to physical observations. All in all, these chromosomal quirks highlight the profound impact of genetic mutations on human health and development (Giordano et al., 2022). New genetic testing techniques—most notably Whole Exome Sequencing (WES)—have significantly transformed our understanding of these disorders. By examining the complex interplay of gene mutations, researchers can now illuminate the landscape of inherited conditions, including several retinal dystrophies and other conditions that sometimes fall into the syndromic category. WES identifies both the rearrangements we are already aware of and those that have remained unnoticed until now, thereby broadening the range of genetic variants associated with these disorders. For example, families with inherited retinal dystrophies have often shown us the weight of pathogenic mutations, nudging clinicians toward a more refined understanding of what constitutes syndromic versus non-syndromic conditions. In most cases, such advancements prompt a fresh look at clinical practices, boosting genetic counseling and paving the way for targeted interventions (Marta et al., 2016). Then there's the constant, messy exploration of how subtle genetic changes align with clinical realities. Finding harmful variants—such as those in the NPR2 gene—illustrates how even tiny genetic tweaks can lead to wildly different levels of disorder severity. There's a kind of not-always-straightforward link between a person's unique genetic makeup and the way a disorder shows up clinically, which makes diagnosis and management a bit of a challenge. Researchers continue to unearth more Mendelian syndromes that are linked to chromosomal differences, and with each discovery, the prospect for customized genetic therapies becomes a bit brighter. In this context, spotting alternative gene modifiers is proving crucial, as the ongoing interplay between chromosomal changes and physical outcomes remains a rich field for research—one that holds promise for improved therapies and better patient outcomes (Giordano et al., 2022) (Figure 12.14).

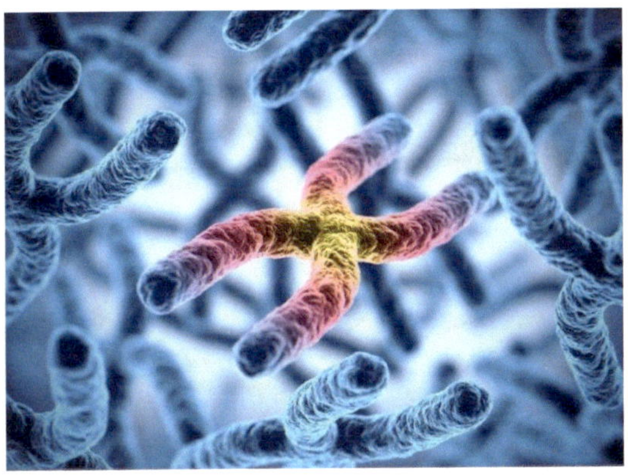

Figure 12.14. Chromosomal disorders.

Source: https://medmonks.com/home/img/blog/chromosomal-disorders.jpg.

12.4.3. Multifactorial Disorders

Genetic makeup and everyday surroundings mix in ways that make multifactorial disorders so hard to pin down. Lots of genes plus different external cues create a messy picture—look at autism spectrum disorders. Generally speaking, research suggests that issues with synapses and developmental timing may play a role. Sometimes, a genetic mutation can trigger lasting shifts in brain wiring, especially during critical growth phases. Even minor tweaks in vital developmental programs can disrupt the normal course of brain regions like the cortex and cerebellum, highlighting how genes and the world around us interact during delicate times (Guerra et al., 2024).

In most cases, this means that any treatment should move beyond a one-sided genetic view and consider everyday experiences as well. Alzheimer's disease shows a similar kind of tangled interplay. Although specific key mutations boost the risk, they don't necessarily guarantee the onset of AD. Many individuals diagnosed with it may not have a clear family history; instead, factors like age, geographical setting, and even gender quietly add up. Research suggests that, in many cases, lifestyle factors and environmental stress can significantly influence the course of the disease. The combination of these influences makes the disease's trajectory unpredictable, underscoring the need for early checkups and interventions that monitor both gene-related and everyday factors (Saragea et al., 2024).

Focusing solely on genetic mutations overlooks a good chunk of the story. By recognizing that both inherited traits and personal experiences shape health outcomes, we gain a richer, more flexible understanding of disorders. As more studies tease apart these tangled pathways in ASD and AD, it becomes clear that a one-track genetic explanation won't do. Instead, approaches that acknowledge the full range of influences not only improve how we treat patients but also inspire broader public health initiatives aimed at reducing environmental risks. In doing so, we take a more well-rounded approach that might finally bridge the gap between lab research and real-world patient care.

12.5. Diagnosis of Genetic Disorders

Genetic disorders are tricky, and figuring them out means looking not just at what can be seen but also digging deep into the genes. Symptoms can shift so much that it sometimes becomes a guessing game—one mutation might make an individual bleed, while another might cause clots, and yet another person might not show any signs at all. Take congenital fibrinogen disorders, for example; patients with different gene changes can come down with bleeding issues, clotting, or even nothing noticeable. Genomic tests, in many cases, help clarify the confusion by pinpointing the exact mutation and providing a clearer understanding of how genes relate to symptoms. By incorporating this additional information into regular diagnostic routines (Simurda et al., 2021), doctors can more accurately diagnose patients and intervene sooner, ultimately improving patient care.

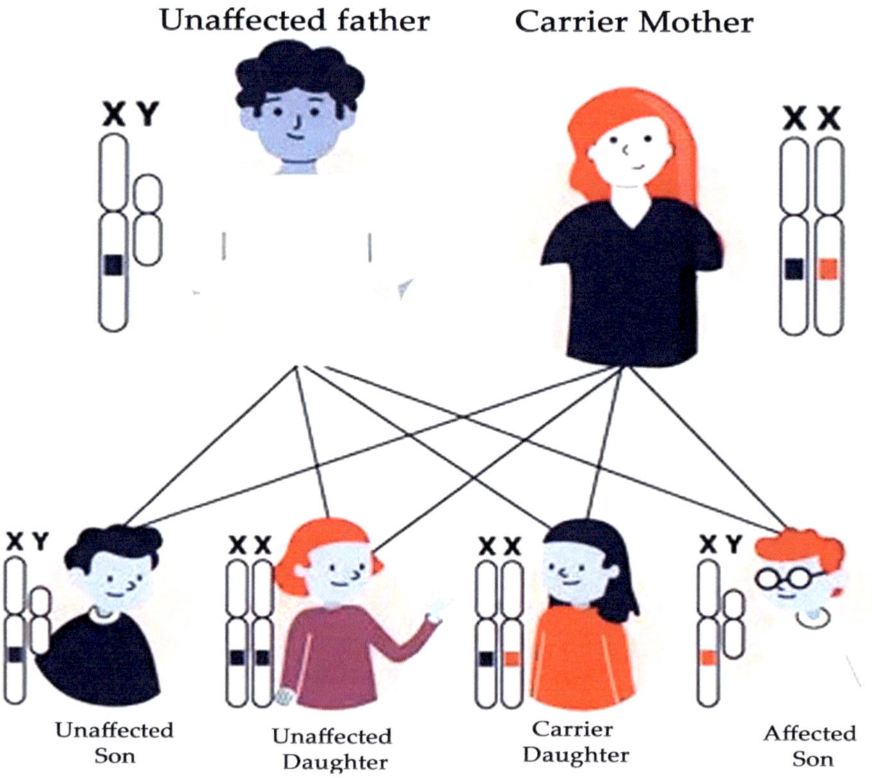

Figure 12.15. Identifying a genetic disease.

Source: https://www.asgct.org/getmedia/025513d5-2060-4979-876b-2fd7b743cbe7/GT-1-Illustrations-02.aspx?width=475&height=446.

New developments in genetic testing have provided new methods to approach these conditions, significantly changing how we approach them. NGS, lets labs scan a bunch of genes at once, turning a once slow process into a pretty speedy investigation. Consider inherited manganese transporter problems—conditions like hypermagnesemia with dystonia result from specific pairs of mutations in transporter proteins, and identifying these early is crucial. Using broad genetic panels that encompass all significant biomarkers provides clinicians with the opportunity to identify the underlying cause without wasting time, allowing treatment to commence more quickly (Anagianni et al., 2019). This method not only uncovers the condition but also paves the way for earlier, more tailored care. Pinning down the correct genetic diagnosis goes beyond just immediate medical fixes; it touches families and even raises some ethical questions. Genetic testing provides valuable insights for family members who may be at risk, enabling them to make informed choices about their futures and manage their health more effectively. In cases like congenital hypofibrinogenemia, knowing that a mutation runs in the family can mean closer check-ups and proactive steps. However, it sometimes leaves everyone a bit on edge about the findings. Deciding who gets tested and sorting out how to break the news isn't always clear-cut, as the benefits of knowing must be balanced against the possible emotional fallout. In the end, the whole deal of diagnosing genetic disorders is steeped in clinical, familial, and ethical layers, calling for a sensitive and sometimes flexible approach (Figure 12.15).

12.5.1. Genetic Testing Methods

Genetic testing now plays a crucial role in handling our many inherited quirks and health issues. NGS is one of those standout tools—it can sift through vast amounts of DNA in a flash and spot even the most minor differences that other tests might miss. It's not unusual for researchers and clinicians to uncover hidden mutations that lead to early clues about a disorder.

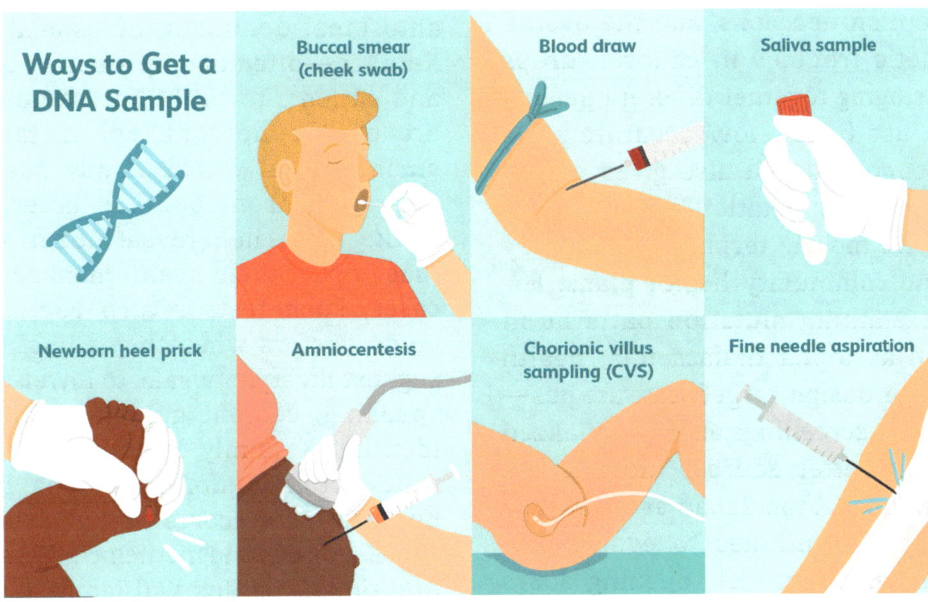

Figure 12.16. Genetic carrier testing methods.

Source: https://external-content.duckduckgo.com/iu/?u=https%3A%2F%2Fwww.verywellhealth.com%2Fthmb%2FZekL3n2fRk3S5JU_swJHKdw5vSo%3D%2F1500x0%2Ffilters%3Ano_upscale()%3Amax_bytes(150000)%3Astrip_icc()%2F2860730_color-5babc8d9c9e77c002ccae708.png&f=1&nofb=1&ipt=eef05a9dac926c4de7626b1af52ee397a62e93ae56f5f6ecb1942cd94b223dab.

For example, in Rasht City, there has been a notable rise in alpha thalassemia mutations (Ahmadabad et al., 2023), hinting that focused screening might pay off. Knowing all the ins and outs of these changes enables doctors to offer better advice about family planning and potential risks, which, generally speaking, makes genetic testing a cornerstone of modern healthcare. Another critical approach is preimplantation genetic testing for monogenic disorders (PGT-M). This method essentially checks embryos for specific genetic abnormalities to help prevent passing on risky traits to the next generation. In situations where, say, a father shows sperm DNA mosaicism, PGT-M has been quite promising in sidestepping serious, sporadic diseases in kids. One study even reported that a couple went through *in vitro* fertilization (IVF) using PGT-M, ultimately welcoming a healthy, unaffected baby (Pan et al., 2022). By using this technique, families get more information for their conception decisions, and the overall chance of genetic troubles in children drops significantly. Bringing together different genetic tests doesn't just boost how accurately we can diagnose conditions—it also gives people a better grip on their health. Tools like NGS and PGT-M aren't merely technical feats; they also help shape community health plans. For instance, by examining mutation patterns in disorders such as alpha thalassemia, health professionals can design targeted strategies—such as premarital screenings and personalized counseling—that better address these issues in local populations (Ahmadabad et al., 2023). As genetic testing continues to evolve, our knowledge base grows as well, opening doors to new treatment ideas and preventive methods. In many ways, this blend of state-of-the-art tech and everyday healthcare marks a turning point in addressing genetic mutations and disorders (Figure 12.16).

12.5.2. Role of Family History

Genetic disorders aren't just about one-off mutations; they also mix in family background clues that help us figure out risk. Family history often plays a significant role in identifying hereditary issues—it even helps in discussing possible genetic risks with others. For example, suppose an individual sees that blood clots (thrombosis) crop up often in their family. In that case, they might start worrying and end up asking for a genetic consultation to check for passed-down mutations. This early, proactive look can prompt action, allowing doctors to shape personalized prevention or treatment plans. Digging deep into a family's past sometimes reveals complex inheritance patterns that illustrate how genes and the environment interact to trigger these disorders (Deepa et al., 2022). Examining the family background in terms of genetic changes can provide valuable insights into how traits and risks are passed down. Inheritance patterns—whether they're autosomal dominant, autosomal recessive, or X-linked—often end up steering both clinicians and patients toward understanding what risks are on the horizon. For instance, consider an individual whose family has a history of heritable thrombophilia; undergoing genetic testing might help reveal hidden vulnerabilities that impact their health management. In most cases, such tests return useful details that guide doctors when they adjust treatments or suggest lifestyle tweaks to lower risk. Generally speaking, current guidelines emphasize that identifying family members with inheritable traits not only informs personal health choices but also underscores the importance of family health in genomic medicine (Wilde et al., 2022). Additionally, a detailed family history lays the groundwork for what's known as cascade screening. Essentially, suppose one relative is found to carry a gene mutation. In that case, this approach helps identify other family members who, even if they don't exhibit any symptoms, may still be at risk. This not only gives families a bit of reassurance but also identifies individuals who might otherwise go unnoticed. With recent advancements in gene technology, such screenings have become far more practical and effective in addressing a variety of genetic issues. So, keeping a well-rounded record of family history isn't just about ticking boxes—it actively influences how doctors plan treatments and even shapes public health strategies. All in all, these practices underscore the importance of understanding our family's genetic ties in today's ongoing discussion about mutations and the disorders they trigger (Deepa et al., 2022) (Figure 12.17).

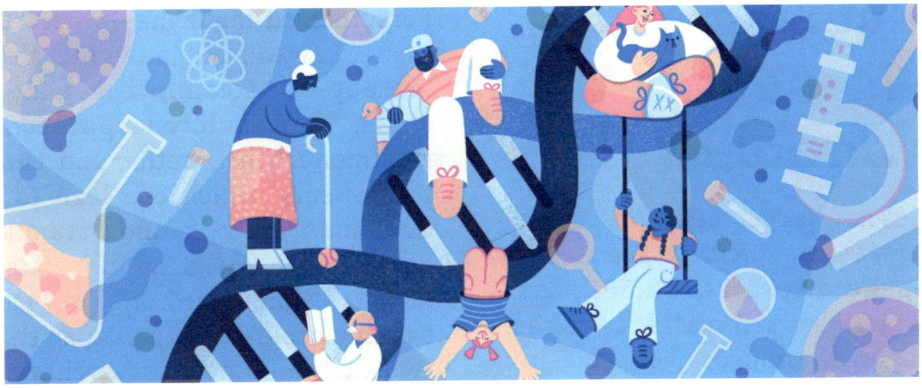

Figure 12.17. Family History of Genetic disorders.

Source: https://external-content.duckduckgo.com/iu/?u= https%3A%2F%2 Fwww. chicagobooth.edu% -%2Fmedia%2Fproject% 2Fchicago-booth%2Fchicago-booth-review%2F2021%2Fmarch%2Fchicago-booth-dna-family-cbr.jpg%3Fcx%3D0. 48%26cy%3D0.55% 26cw%3D1880%26ch%3D783%26hash% 3DD3D6B68C97A3EBAF8C38C68703BCD127&f=1&nofb =1&ipt=e2381b4dea5f375eab4224180d148af37a4fda872b8525d2230d6baa3250b2af.

12.5.3. Ethical Considerations in Testing

Genetic testing's become a real maze of moral twists, especially when it comes to choosing embryos during IVF. More couples are turning to preimplantation genetic testing for single-gene issues (PGT-M) and suddenly find themselves wrestling with which embryo to pick. Many genetic counselors, in most cases—lean toward transferring embryos known to have a monogenic condition. This choice sparks serious debate about a child's future quality of life and how society views disability. The tension hits hardest with conditions like Huntington's disease, suggesting that we need more straightforward guidelines to balance patient wishes with a doctor's duty (Gunderson et al., 2024). Looking at testing for things like Alzheimer's, the role of genetic counseling becomes even more apparent. Counselors must navigate family histories and the emotional impact of risk details while breaking down complex data into everyday language. They tailor risk assessments to fit each patient's background and emotional state, even if that means repeating some key points in slightly different ways to make the ideas stick. It's easy to misinterpret genetic signals, so patients need a clear, honest picture of their odds—helping them feel in control instead of overwhelmed (Saragea, 2024). Then there's the bigger picture of fairness and access. As genetic screening becomes more widespread and refined, the gap between those who have access and those who don't may widen further. In many cases, healthcare providers and policymakers must step up to ensure everyone—especially marginalized groups—gets a fair shot at testing. Without such balance, some communities might be left out, which could slow down progress in understanding genetic disorders. Ultimately, the challenges of genetic testing aren't just about individual choices but also raise broader questions about social justice in our healthcare system (Gunderson et al., 2024).

12.6. Treatment and Management of Genetic Disorders

Genetic therapies now target mutations directly at their source, opening up new avenues for addressing genetic disorders. CRISPR/Cas9, for example, enables scientists to tweak DNA sequences with impressive precision; however, these methods still face hurdles, such as ensuring the treatment is delivered correctly and avoiding unintended changes in other parts of the genome. AZD7648—a blocker of DNA-dependent protein kinase—has recently shown some promise by boosting the cell's natural repair process and cutting down unwanted mutations. This type of dual benefit may not only aid in addressing genetic disorders but could also serve as a model for enhancing gene therapies in numerous other cases (Wimberger et al., 2022). Understanding how genetic disorders actually work is key to crafting effective treatment plans. Take chronic lymphocytic leukemia (CLL) as an example; it demonstrates the messy relationship between genetic mistakes and what ends up happening in patients. Research tracking CLL's progression shows that when it shifts into a more aggressive lymphoma, significant changes in the genome often accompany the transformation, making treatment all the more challenging. In most cases, the molecular details behind this change—especially after earlier treatments have already been tried—suggest that a single approach won't cover it all. Additionally, the early appearance of distinct subclones indicates that identifying and targeting these critical mutations sooner may have a significant impact (Nadeu et al., 2022). Combining different fields now seems essential when it comes to treating genetic disorders. Merging insights from genomic science, personalized care that focuses on each person, and modern computational tools gives us a broader view of how diseases operate. Personalized medicine—where treatments are crafted to suit an individual's unique genetic makeup—is steadily becoming the norm in clinics. This tailored approach often means treatments work better and come with fewer side effects, which can lead to better overall outcomes. As our understanding of genetic mutations deepens, the opportunity to explore new therapies continues to grow, promising exciting progress in managing these conditions. Working together, researchers, doctors, and patients alike seem poised to make the most of these breakthroughs (Figure 12.18).

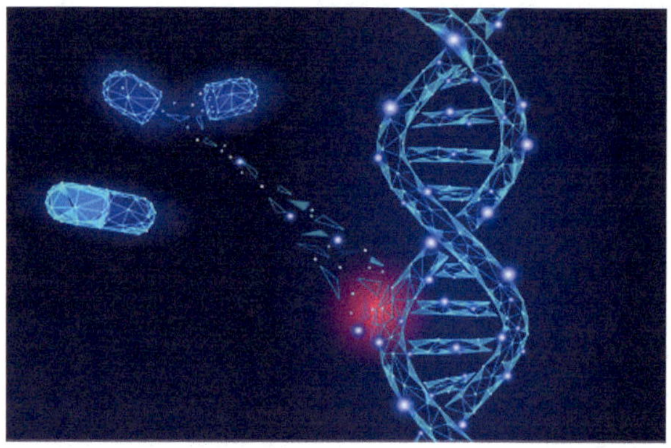

Figure 12.18. Treatment and Management of Genetic Disorders.

Source: https://geneticsinindia.com/blog/wp-content/uploads/2020/08/genetic-disorders.jpg.

12.6.1. Gene Therapy

Gene therapy is getting a lot of buzz these days as a fresh way to tackle genetic problems. Breakthroughs like CRISPR-Cas9 have turned things upside-down for scientists and doctors—

they can now target even small bits of DNA and modify them. This isn't just about masking symptoms; it's about going right to the source, like tweaking the DNA behind issues such as hypertrophic cardiomyopathy or muscular dystrophy. With these precise edits, patients may transition from merely managing symptoms to actually addressing the underlying genetic problems.

Research is moving at a breakneck pace, and in most cases, every discovery makes the idea of curing these inherited disorders look even more promising. It isn't only about heart or muscle troubles either—gene therapy reaches into a whole bunch of genetic conditions that regular treatments have mostly overlooked. Sometimes, swapping out a problematic gene for a functional one can significantly change the course of the condition, easing symptoms and, in some instances, even curing it entirely. Think about those rare inherited disorders where the usual treatments just don't cut it; here, gene therapy shows an encouraging sign of delivering results where nothing else has. This shift, from wild theory to actual clinical practice, means that what once seemed like science fiction is now starting to reshape how we approach healthcare. Still, it isn't all smooth sailing. Even if gene therapy's promise is enormous, there are plenty of hurdles to clear. Getting the gene exactly where it needs to be remains tricky, and off-target effects can sometimes cause unexpected, unwanted changes. Then we have the long-term issues—alterations that might pass on to future generations bring up serious ethical questions, with consent often remaining unresolved. Although the idea of erasing genetic disorders is highly appealing, these challenges mean that researchers still have a significant amount of work ahead. As new techniques are invented and our understanding deepens, the dream of making gene therapy a routine part of personalized medicine is inching closer, opening doors to innovative healthcare solutions (Moradi et al., 2025; Rehman, 2025) (Figure 12.19).

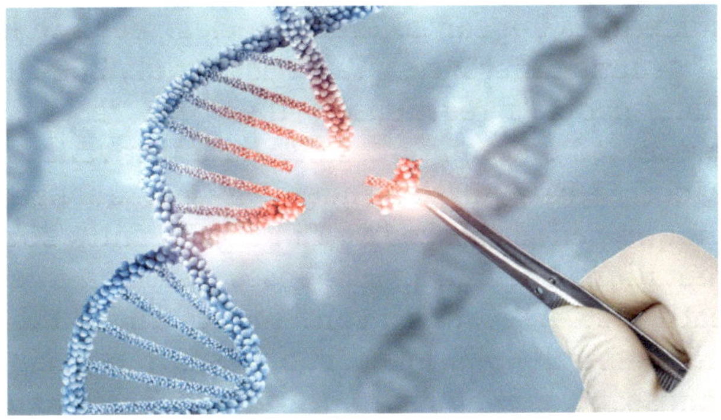

Figure 12.19. Gene therapy.

Source: https://cdn.mos.cms.futurecdn.net/97QX5fRoqwVAQD5cZ6nPoa.jpg.

12.6.2. Pharmacological Interventions

Drugs help manage problems linked to genetic mutations and often make life a bit better for many people. For instance, children with autism—usually characterized by difficulties with speaking, socializing, and a few repetitive behaviors—as one example. In a lot of cases, anxiety and thinking issues tag along with autism, so extra-focused drug plans become necessary. No current treatment effectively addresses the main challenges, but several approaches aim to alleviate these secondary issues, which in turn improve overall well-being. Studies using mouse models have given us clues about what's going on with autism's genetics, and they've spurred drug research that might calm these extra symptoms, even if a complete fix remains a work in progress (Bonetti et al., 2024). The link between gene mutations and drug treatments isn't limited to one field—it also appears in cancer care. Odd changes in gene activity, usually because of tweaks in how genes behave (not changes in the DNA itself), are a big deal when it comes to cancers that won't respond to routine methods. For example, valemetostat works by blocking the EZH1–EZH2 pair, demonstrating what epigenetic drugs might achieve. Clinical studies, as they say, indicate that the drug can shrink tumors in patients with refractory lymphomas, highlighting the promise of these approaches against diseases complicated by genetic complexity. Of course, resistant clones sometimes appear, so there's a clear need to keep creating new strategies for folks with all kinds of genetic differences (Yamagishi et al., 2024). Besides the issue of drugs losing their impact over time, people's reactions to them can vary a whole lot. Mutations can change how a drug gets processed or even how safe and effective it is, which makes handling conditions like autism and cancer a real puzzle. That's why personalized medicine—tailoring treatments to each patient's unique genetic makeup—can significantly boost outcomes. When doctors understand how these mutations affect drug responses, they can fine-tune treatment plans and choose what fits best for each case. As research continues to unveil the complex interplay between genes and medications, incorporating pharmacogenomics into regular practice appears poised to transform the treatment landscape, aiming for improved outcomes and reduced side effects (Figure 12.20).

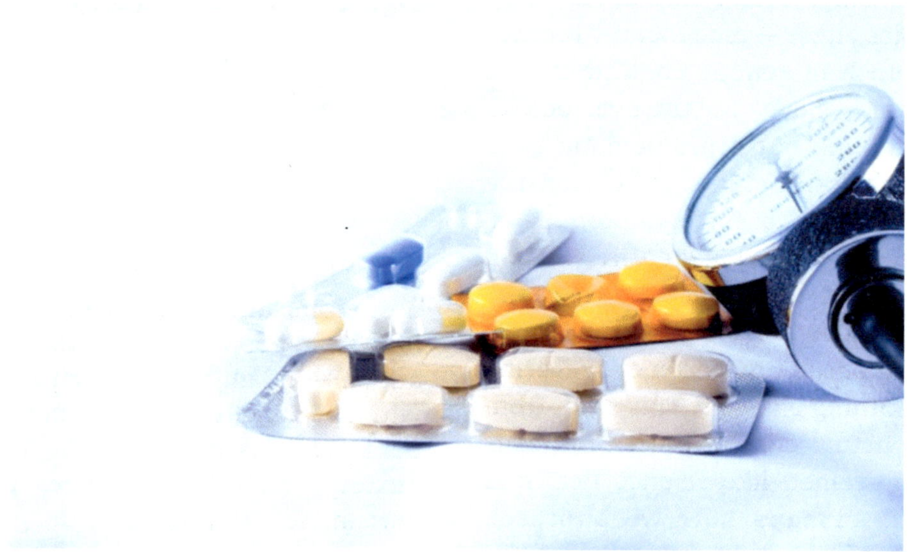

Figure 12.20. Pharmacological Interventions.

Source: https://external-content.duckduckgo.com/iu/?u=https%3A%2F%2Fd2jx2rerrg6sh3.cloudfront.net%2Fimages%2FArticle_Images%2FImageForArticle_22815_16575488716685074.jpg&f=1&nofb=1&ipt=2da05e1affbd54986866e41f7696ca7cb6ac36990a3558f8045d3e3ff10adfec.

12.6.3. Supportive Care and Lifestyle Changes

Supportive care plays a significant role in managing genetic disorders—it provides an additional form of support alongside standard medical treatments. Counseling, physical therapy, and even nutritional guidance all play their roles, each contributing in their way to ease the physical strain and mental stress that patients often face. Genetic mutations, which generally lead to additional health risks, make these supportive measures even more critical and, in most cases, can help mitigate those risks. For example, caregivers keep getting recognized for their crucial work with folks suffering from conditions like Alzheimer's disease—a situation where challenges seem to be growing fast. Simple lifestyle tweaks, such as regular exercise and stress-relief practices, can also give patients a bit more control over their health. Lifestyle improvements — such as eating balanced meals, engaging in regular physical activity, and maintaining mental wellness routines — are another essential piece of the puzzle. Studies tend to show that a healthier lifestyle may significantly reduce the impact of one's genetic predispositions. For patients with inherited heart conditions, some have seen benefits from making small adjustments to their diet, paired with specific exercise regimens aimed at boosting heart function and overall resilience (Eric et al., 2022). These lifestyle changes not only improve physical well-being but also seem to lift one's spirits, giving a renewed sense of control. In many cases, educational programs that explain these beneficial alterations are very helpful in encouraging patients to commit and feel more hopeful truly. Mixing supportive care with these lifestyle shifts can build a more rounded approach to cracking the challenges posed by genetic disorders. There's value in having different experts—such as genetic counselors, nutritionists, and physical therapists—work together to tailor solutions to each unique case. Given that genetic conditions are becoming more common, such a collaborative, sometimes even slightly improvised, approach is pretty timely. The blend of direct support and practical lifestyle changes paves the way for better health outcomes, ensuring that patients receive not only standard treatments but also the knowledge they need to manage their care. In the end, fostering a fully supportive environment is key to helping people face their genetic challenges with real resilience and a bit of confidence, even if sometimes the path isn't perfectly straight.

SUMMARY

Genetic mutations and disorders shake up healthcare in unexpected ways—they push us to improve our research and technology continually. Even tiny changes in our genes can trigger a range of problems, providing clues for prevention and possible cures. AI, for instance, is stepping in to sift through massive datasets and spot hidden patterns, which many say helps doctors fine-tune diagnoses and treatment plans. This blend of deep learning with genetic studies can lead to more precise results and even tailor treatments to individual needs, ultimately aiming for better patient outcomes. Still, one can't ignore issues like data privacy and bias; these ethical bumps remind us that responsibility is key when harnessing such innovations for personal medicine (Shuroug et al., 2023). The ripple effects of genetic disorders go well beyond the patients—they ripple through entire families and our healthcare systems. Consider Alzheimer's disease as a case in point; its rising numbers place heavy demands not just on those suffering, but also on caregivers and overall health resources. Research often shows that when family members are drawn into the caregiver role, they might end up battling their emotional strain and health declines, which only muddles the already complex care landscape. Rising costs in Alzheimer's care signal that our medical infrastructure has to shift gears soon, especially with global events worsening workforce shortages in dementia care—a gap that needs better training and recruitment efforts. In short, untangling the challenges of genetic mutations and disorders requires a multifaceted approach—a blend of scientific breakthroughs, ethical reflection, and robust support for patients and their families. It seems clear that when research labs, healthcare teams, and policymakers collaborate, they can develop interventions that alleviate the burden of these conditions. At the same time, raising public awareness about genetic illnesses may break down stigma and encourage people to get the help they need. As this field moves forward, a regular check on the ethical and social sides of emerging genetic and AI advances is, in most cases, crucial for ensuring these tools truly benefit society, paving the way for a healthier future for everyone Shuroug et al., 2023).

Exploring genetic mutations reveals surprising insights into how various disorders may develop. Mutations come in several flavors – think point changes, insertions, deletions, or even extra copies – and each one can mess with the way genes build proteins. Low-frequency variants, which appear rare but are actually common in certain groups, also play a significant role. The FinnGen project, for example, illustrates how these uncommon changes can persist through challenging population pressures, gradually increasing certain alleles that, in most cases, may influence disease risk. By analyzing data from 224,737 individuals, the study identified connections between these rare variants and various illnesses, underscoring the importance of large-scale, population-based studies in understanding the mechanisms of genetic disorders (Kurki et al., 2023). Looking beyond simply identifying these gene changes, it's also important to understand their implications for patient care. Guidelines from organizations like ESC/EAS act more like flexible road maps for handling conditions tied to genetics. They combine scientific facts with hands-on clinical evidence to help healthcare professionals make informed decisions about prevention, diagnosis, and treatment strategies – all while emphasizing that every patient is unique. Even though these recommendations offer solid insights, they still nudge us towards personalized care and encourage the integration of the latest public health advice. This sort of balanced approach between broad protocols and tailored treatment enables doctors to better cope with the complex intricacies of genetic mutations and the disorders they cause (François Mach et al., 2019). Sometimes, though, the story of genetic research isn't just about lab work; it's truly a team effort between big genomic studies and everyday medical practice. New connections between genes, identified in large-scale studies, often illuminate the way for targeted treatments and innovative ways to prevent diseases before they start. Identifying specific coding changes associated with health challenges often opens doors to innovative treatment ideas. Blending research insights into clinical guidelines builds a stronger bridge toward effective patient care, creating a healthcare environment that's both informed and adaptable. When geneticists and clinicians join forces—even if their methods don't always match perfectly—the outcome is a deeper understanding of mutations and better results for patients, proving that real progress comes from linking research with day-to-day medical work (Kurki et al., 2023).

CLOSER LOOK

HYPOFIBRINOGENEMIA

Hypofibrinogenemia is a rare hematological disorder characterized by abnormally low levels of fibrinogen, a critical glycoprotein involved in the coagulation cascade. Fibrinogen, also known as factor I, is synthesized in the liver and plays a pivotal role in hemostasis by being converted into fibrin by thrombin during the final steps of blood clot formation. In hypofibrinogenemia, the plasma concentration of fibrinogen is lower than usual—typically between 50 and 150 mg/dL, compared to the reference range of 200 to 400 mg/dL—leading to an increased risk of bleeding. This condition can be either congenital or acquired. Congenital hypofibrinogenemia is inherited in an autosomal recessive or, less commonly, autosomal dominant manner, and results from mutations in one of the three genes (FGA, FGB, or FGG) that encode the fibrinogen chains. It often presents in infancy or childhood with symptoms such as easy bruising, nosebleeds, gum bleeding, excessive menstrual bleeding, prolonged bleeding after trauma or surgery, and, in severe cases, spontaneous internal bleeding. Acquired hypofibrinogenemia, on the other hand, is more common and usually occurs as a result of underlying medical conditions such as liver disease, disseminated intravascular coagulation (DIC), massive transfusions, or severe trauma, all of which can lead to increased consumption or decreased production of fibrinogen.

Diagnosis of hypofibrinogenemia involves both clinical assessment and laboratory testing. Standard laboratory tests include measuring plasma fibrinogen concentration using methods such as the Clauss assay or immunoassays, along with coagulation screening tests like prothrombin time (PT), activated partial thromboplastin time (aPTT), and thrombin time (TT), which may all be prolonged in affected individuals. Further genetic testing may be employed to confirm congenital forms and to identify specific mutations. It is essential to distinguish hypofibrinogenemia from related fibrinogen disorders such as afibrinogenemia, in which fibrinogen is completely absent, and dysfibrinogenemia, in which fibrinogen levels may be normal but the protein is functionally defective.

Management of hypofibrinogenemia focuses on preventing and treating episodes of bleeding. In mild cases, regular monitoring and avoidance of trauma may suffice. For more severe cases or before surgical procedures, fibrinogen replacement therapy is necessary. This can be achieved using fibrinogen concentrate, cryoprecipitate, or fresh frozen plasma (FFP), with fibrinogen concentrate being the preferred option due to its standardized dose, viral inactivation, and lower risk of volume overload or allergic reactions. Prophylactic therapy may be considered in patients with a history of severe bleeding or recurrent hemorrhagic episodes. During pregnancy, women with hypofibrinogenemia require close monitoring, as the condition can increase the risk of miscarriage, placental abruption, and postpartum hemorrhage.

Although congenital hypofibrinogenemia is a lifelong condition, appropriate management and timely intervention can significantly reduce the risk of complications and improve quality of life. Research into gene therapy and newer fibrinogen replacement products offers potential for future therapeutic advancements. Overall, heightened awareness and early diagnosis are crucial for minimizing bleeding risks and ensuring optimal patient outcomes in those affected by this rare but clinically significant coagulopathy.

REFERENCES

1. Ahmadabad, M. A., Pourreza, N., Ramezanpour, S., Baghersalimi, A., Enshaei, M., Askari, M., Alizadeh, A., Izadi, E., & Darbandi, B. (2023). An analysis of the distribution and spectrum of alpha thalassemia mutations in Rasht City, North of Iran. *Frontiers in Pediatrics, 11*. https://doi.org/10.3389/fped.2023.1039148Alexandrov, I., Alexandrova, M., & Afanasyeva, K. (2022). The nature of radiation-induced inherited recessive gene mutations in *Drosophila melanogaster*. *Archives of Molecular Biology and Genetics*. https://www.semanticscholar.org/paper/7dd824d5d5ee22a68b773bf14bec3b4e33b4cfb2 (accessed on 26 May 2025).
2. Alowais, S. A., Alghamdi, S. S., Alsuhebany, N., Alqahtani, T., Alshaya, A., Almohareb, S. N., Aldairem, A., et al. (2023). Revolutionizing healthcare: The role of artificial intelligence in clinical practice. *BMC Medical Education, 23*. https://doi.org/10.1186/s12909-023-04698-z.
3. Alzheimer's Association. (2023). 2023 Alzheimer's disease facts and figures. *Alzheimer's & Dementia, 19*, 1598–1695. https://doi.org/10.1002/alz.13016.
4. An, J.-Y., Lin, K., Zhu, L., Werling, D. M., Dong, S., Brand, H., Wang, H. Z., et al. (2018). Genome-wide de novo risk score implicates promoter variation in autism spectrum disorder. *Science, 362*. https://doi.org/10.1126/science.aat6576.
5. Anagianni, S., & Tuschl, K. (2019). Genetic disorders of manganese metabolism. *Current Neurology and Neuroscience Reports, 19*. https://www.semanticscholar.org/paper/315cf3da65ee0c1d7eccd727691c9b967649ce0f (accessed on 26 May 2025).
6. Andrés, C., Pérez de la Lastra, J. M., Plou, F. J., & Pérez-Lebeña, E. (2021). The chemistry of reactive oxygen species (ROS) revisited: Outlining their role in biological macromolecules (DNA, lipids and proteins) and induced pathologies. *International Journal of Molecular Sciences, 22*, 4642. https://doi.org/10.3390/ijms22094642.
7. Arachchillage, D. J., Mackillop, L., Chandratheva, A., Motawani, J., MacCallum, P., & Laffan, M. (2022). Thrombophilia testing: A British Society for Haematology guideline. *British Journal of Haematology, 198*, 443–458. https://doi.org/10.1111/bjh.18239.
8. Bassett, A. (2017). Editing the genome of hiPSC with CRISPR/Cas9: Disease models. *Mammalian Genome, 28*, 348–364. https://doi.org/10.1007/s00335-017-9684-9.
9. Battey, E., Stroud, M., & Ochala, J. (2020). Using nuclear envelope mutations to explore age-related skeletal muscle weakness. *Clinical Science (London), 134*, 2177–2187. https://www.semanticscholar.org/paper/92cc8b638ef896259a86fe0b2a8fea259f6f92f5 (accessed on 26 May 2025).
10. Bonetti, M., Borsani, E., & Bonomini, F. (2024). The use of nutraceutical and pharmacological strategies in murine models of autism spectrum disorder. *Cells, 13*. https://www.semanticscholar.org/paper/914c2d00ae3d1c5b49c19301313d366ab6ecd362 (accessed on 26 May 2025).
11. Chalasani, N., Younossi, Z. M., Lavine, J. E., Charlton, M., Cusi, K., Rinella, M. E., Harrison, S. A., et al. (2017). The diagnosis and management of non-alcoholic fatty liver disease: Practice guidance from the American Association for the Study of Liver Diseases. *Hepatology, 67*, 328–357. https://doi.org/10.1002/hep.29367.
12. de Castro-Miró, M., Tonda, R., Escudero-Ferruz, P., Andrés, R., Mayor-Lorenzo, A., Castro, J.,

Ciccioli, M., et al. (2016). Novel candidate genes and a wide spectrum of structural and point mutations responsible for inherited retinal dystrophies revealed by exome sequencing. *PLoS ONE, 11*. https://www.semanticscholar.org/paper/451eff47e1067c078e6b0cc834e8952a6140c27c (accessed on 26 May 2025).

13. Dehhaghi, M., Kazemi Shariat Panahi, H., & Guillemin, G. J. (2018). Microorganisms' footprint in neurodegenerative diseases. *Frontiers in Cellular Neuroscience, 12*, 466. https://doi.org/10.3389/fncel.2018.00466.
14. Dennis, E. P., Greenhalgh-Maychell, P. L., & Briggs, M. (2020). Multiple epiphyseal dysplasia and related disorders: Molecular genetics, disease mechanisms, and therapeutic avenues. *Developmental Dynamics, 250*, 345–359. https://www.semanticscholar.org/paper/a9be94d6f40e19547fb65c1ce011541d3f3c2926 (accessed on 26 May 2025).
15. Giordano, M., & Stuppia, L. (2022). Editorial: Novel insights into the genetics of growth disorders. *Frontiers in Genetics, 13*. https://www.semanticscholar.org/paper/72617581f3180adfdbec2c9b1215c37f51143cdd (accessed on 26 May 2025).
16. Guerra, M., Medici, V., La Sala, G., & Farini, D. (2024). Unravelling the cerebellar involvement in autism spectrum disorders: Insights into genetic mechanisms and developmental pathways. *Cells, 13*. https://www.semanticscholar.org/paper/2a7abe7eefbfa29108b6a304b881d677ba2d2cd5 (accessed on 26 May 2025).
17. Guerrin, C. G. J., Doorduin, J., Sommer, I. E., & de Vries, E. F. J. (2021). The dual hit hypothesis of schizophrenia: Evidence from animal models. *Neuroscience & Biobehavioral Reviews, 131*, 1150–1168. https://doi.org/10.1016/j.neubiorev.2021.10.025.
18. Gunderson, S., & Gabriel, J. (2024). Transfer of embryos with positive PGT-M results: Genetic counselors' perspectives and ethical considerations. *Journal of Genetic Counseling*. https://www.semanticscholar.org/paper/b3ea9a0599b26c75752cee71507ab60b99fac64c (accessed on 26 May 2025).
19. Haase, S., Banerjee, K., Mujeeb, A. A., Hartlage, C. S., Nunez, F., Núñez, F. J., Alghamri, M. S., et al. (2022). H3.3-G34 mutations impair DNA repair and promote cGAS/STING-mediated immune responses in pediatric high-grade glioma models. *The Journal of Clinical Investigation, 132*. https://www.semanticscholar.org/paper/c247c3002c6ef23e60fdc79dd7f12d8057af9a7e (accessed on 26 May 2025).
20. Hu, B., Guo, H., Zhou, P., & Shi, Z. L. (2020). Characteristics of SARS-CoV-2 and COVID-19. *Nature Reviews Microbiology, 19*, 141–154. https://doi.org/10.1038/s41579-020-00459-7.
21. Isselbacher, E. M., Preventza, O., Black, J. H., Augoustides, J., Beck, A. W., Bolen, M. A., Braverman, A. C., et al. (2022). 2022 ACC/AHA guideline for the diagnosis and management of aortic disease: A report of the American Heart Association/American College of Cardiology Joint Committee on Clinical Practice Guidelines. *Circulation, 146*. https://doi.org/10.1161/cir.0000000000001106.
22. Kurki, M., Karjalainen, J., Palta, P., Sipilä, T. P., Kristiansson, K., Donner, K., Reeve, M. P., et al. (2023). FinnGen provides genetic insights from a well-phenotyped isolated population. *Nature, 613*, 508–518. https://doi.org/10.1038/s41586-022-05473-8.
23. Lek, M., Karczewski, K. J., Minikel, E. V., Samocha, K. E., Banks, E., Fennell, T. R., O'Donnell-Luria, A., et al. (2016). Analysis of protein-coding genetic variation in 60,706 humans. *Nature, 536*, 285–291. https://doi.org/10.1038/nature19057.

24. Li, K., Huo, C., Long, H., Tang, K., & Zhang, S. (2024). Identification of the *Mitf* gene mutation causing congenital deafness and pigmentation disorders in porcupines using BSA-Seq. *Scientific Reports, 14*. https://www.semanticscholar.org/paper/ad8d9fd951ef3916996824242e60b19d6bbfdfb1 (accessed on 26 May 2025).

25. Lilley, E., Stanford, S. C., Kendall, D., Alexander, S. P. H., Cirino, G., Docherty, J. R., George, C. H., et al. (2020). ARRIVE 2.0 and the British Journal of Pharmacology: Updated guidance for 2020. *British Journal of Pharmacology, 177*, 3611–3616. https://doi.org/10.1111/bph.15178.

26. Lipinski, K. A., Barber, L. J., Davies, M. N., Ashenden, M., Sottoriva, A., & Gerlinger, M. (2016). Cancer evolution and the limits of predictability in precision cancer medicine. *Trends in Cancer, 2*, 49–63. https://doi.org/10.1016/j.trecan.2015.11.003.

27. Lopes-Marques, M., Mort, M., Carneiro, J., Azevedo, A., Amaro, A. P., Cooper, D. N., & Azevedo, L. (2024). Meta-analysis of 46,000 germline de novo mutations linked to human inherited disease. *Human Genomics, 18*. https://www.semanticscholar.org/paper/abd4944030b9c8454d3a21f435ea4d5445eb4c0f (accessed on 26 May 2025).

28. Mach, F., Baigent, C., Catapano, A. L., Koskinas, K. C., Casula, M., Badimón, L., Chapman, M. J., et al. (2019). 2019 ESC/EAS Guidelines for the management of dyslipidemia's: Lipid modification to reduce cardiovascular risk. *European Heart Journal, 41*, 111–188. https://doi.org/10.1093/eurheartj/ehz455.

29. Meier, B., Volkova, N. V., Hong, Y., Bertolini, S., González-Huici, V., Petrova, T., Boulton, S., et al. (2021). Protection of the *C. elegans* germ cell genome depends on diverse DNA repair pathways during normal proliferation. *PLOS ONE, 16*. https://www.semanticscholar.org/paper/007a41a4eb4a59a9b4b36841c2d6560c886676ff (accessed on 26 May 2025).

30. Moradi, A., Khoshniyat, S., Nzeako, T., Khazeei Tabari, M. A., Olanisa, O. O., Tabbaa, K., Alkowati, H., et al. (2025). The future of clustered regularly interspaced short palindromic repeats (CRISPR)-Cas9 gene therapy in cardiomyopathies: A review of its therapeutic potential and emerging applications. *Cureus, 17*. https://www.semanticscholar.org/paper/3ef19a3485939fa849dcb291156769ae330f9562 (accessed on 26 May 2025).

31. Nadeu, F., Royo, R., Massoni-Badosa, R., García-Torre, B., Duran-Ferrer, M., Dawson, K., Kulis, M., et al. (2022). Abstract 3795: Early seeding of Richter transformation in chronic lymphocytic leukemia. *Cancer Research*. https://www.semanticscholar.org/paper/f7ac6d909f1ac8b379f527eaf7f5fb11d5aa19f0 (accessed on 26 May 2025).

32. Pan, J., Li, J., Chen, S., Xu, C., Huang, H., & Jin, L. (2022). Living birth following preimplantation genetic testing for monogenic disorders to prevent low-level germline mosaicism related Nicolaides–Baraitser syndrome. *Frontiers in Genetics, 13*. https://www.semanticscholar.org/paper/a29420d9ff0ca3f49c8765c2d792e5c3212f57df (accessed on 26 May 2025).

33. Parenti, I., Rabaneda, L. G., Schoen, H., & Novarino, G. (2020). Neurodevelopmental disorders: From genetics to functional pathways. *Trends in Neurosciences, 43*, 608–621. https://doi.org/10.1016/j.tins.2020.05.004.

34. Petr, M., Tulika, T., Carmona-Marin, L. M., & Scheibye-Knudsen, M. (2020). Protecting the aging genome. *Trends in Cell Biology, 30*, 117–132. https://doi.org/10.1016/j.tcb.2019.12.001.

35. Ponikowski, P., Voors, A. A., Anker, S. D., Bueno, H., Cleland, J. G. F., Coats, A. J. S., Falk, V., et al. (2016). 2016 ESC Guidelines for the diagnosis and treatment of acute and chronic heart failure. *European Heart Journal, 37*, 2129–2200. https://doi.org/10.1093/eurheartj/ehw128.

36. Rehman, S. U. (2025). Advancement in gene therapy: Current and future of gene therapy. *Kashmir Journal of Science*. https://www.semanticscholar.org/paper/b52a192a46bd071e41e3a160b10b231a04116a32 (accessed on 26 May 2025).

37. Ribas, A., & Wolchok, J. D. (2018). Cancer immunotherapy using checkpoint blockade. *Science, 359*, 1350–1355. https://doi.org/10.1126/science.aar4060.

38. Rinella, M. E., Neuschwander-Tetri, B. A., Siddiqui, M. S., Abdelmalek, M. F., Caldwell, S. H., Barb, D., Kleiner, D. E., et al. (2023). AASLD practice guidance on the clinical assessment and management of nonalcoholic fatty liver disease. *Hepatology, 77*, 1797–1835. https://doi.org/10.1097/hep.0000000000000323.

39. Rose, S., Niyazov, D., Rossignol, D. A., Goldenthal, M. J., Kahler, S. G., & Frye, R. E. (2018). Clinical and molecular characteristics of mitochondrial dysfunction in autism spectrum disorder. *Molecular Diagnosis & Therapy, 22*, 571–593. https://doi.org/10.1007/s40291-018-0352-x.

40. Saragea, P. D. (2024). Diagnosis, genetic counseling and risk assessment in Alzheimer's disease: Methodologies, implications, and ethical considerations. *International Journal for Multidisciplinary Research*. https://www.semanticscholar.org/paper/57eea0bad8c4b0d2482f0b20b3ac348bd939cf37 (accessed on 26 May 2025).

41. Saragea, P. D., & Tudose, C. (2024). Alzheimer (AD)–A multifactorial neurodegenerative disease–A cohort study. *Journal of Experimental and Molecular Biology*. https://www.semanticscholar.org/paper/49edf3ddff7e3a97027fcfa638611d5747583600 (accessed on 26 May 2025).

42. Schlieben, L. D., & Prokisch, H. (2020). The dimensions of primary mitochondrial disorders. *Frontiers in Cell and Developmental Biology, 8*. https://doi.org/10.3389/fcell.2020.600079.

43. Schrempf, A., Slyšková, J., & Loizou, J. I. (2020). Targeting the DNA repair enzyme polymerase θ in cancer therapy. *Trends in Cancer, 7*, 98–111. https://doi.org/10.1016/j.trecan.2020.09.007.

44. Sharma, G., Sharma, A. R., Bhattacharya, M., Lee, S. S., & Chakraborty, C. (2020). CRISPR-Cas9: A preclinical and clinical perspective for the treatment of human diseases. *Molecular Therapy, 29*, 571–586. https://doi.org/10.1016/j.ymthe.2020.09.028.

45. Shen, R. J., Wang, J. G., Li, Y., & Jin, Z. B. (2021). Consanguinity-based analysis of exome sequencing yields likely genetic causes in patients with inherited retinal dystrophy. *Orphanet Journal of Rare Diseases, 16*. https://www.semanticscholar.org/paper/f2a7aaed9607fe620bdab5b49f371350a14cb16c (accessed on 26 May 2025).

46. Simurda, T., Asselta, R., Žolková, J., Brunclíková, M., Dobrotová, M., Kolková, Z., Loderer, D., et al. (2021). Congenital afibrinogenemia and hypofibrinogenemia: Laboratory and genetic testing in rare bleeding disorders with life-threatening clinical manifestations and challenging management. *Diagnostics, 11*. https://www.semanticscholar.org/paper/2923255326fdee8351c3e20bd22a226d898578e9 (accessed on 26 May 2025).

47. Verhaart, I. E. C., Robertson, A., Wilson, I., Aartsma-Rus, A., Cameron, S., Jones, C. C., Cook, S. F., et al. (2017). Prevalence, incidence and carrier frequency of 5q–linked spinal muscular atrophy–A literature review. *Orphanet Journal of Rare Diseases, 12*. https://doi.org/10.1186/s13023-017-0671-8.

48. Wilde, A. A. M., Semsarian, C., Márquez, M. F., Sepehri Shamloo, A., Ackerman, M. J., Ashley, E. A., Sternick, E. B., et al. (2022). EHRA/HRS/APHRS/LAHRS expert consensus statement

on the state of genetic testing for cardiac diseases. *Heart Rhythm, 19*, e1–e60. https://doi.org/10.1016/j.hrthm.2022.03.1225.

49. Wimberger, S., Akrap, N., Firth, M., Brengdahl, J., Engberg, S., Schwinn, M. K., Slater, M., et al. (2022). Simultaneous inhibition of DNA-PK and Polθ improves integration efficiency and precision of genome editing. *bioRxiv*. https://www.semanticscholar.org/paper/cb95b5d767794819f2292c9fc2198a4281a1f8af (accessed on 26 May 2025).

50. Yamagishi, M., Kuze, Y., Kobayashi, S., Nakashima, M., Morishima, S., Kawamata, T., Makiyama, J., et al. (2024). Mechanisms of action and resistance in histone methylation-targeted therapy. *Nature, 627*, 221–228. https://www.semanticscholar.org/paper/d5275c43727fc034249589ff7bfcc499342fb372 (accessed on 26 May 2025).

INDEX

D

E

P

R

S